Drug Management of Prostate Cancer

William D. Figg · Cindy H. Chau · Eric J. Small
Editors

Drug Management of Prostate Cancer

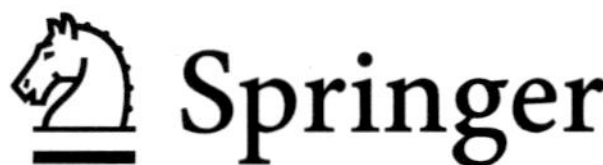

Springer

Editors
William D. Figg
National Cancer Institute
Bethesda, MD
USA

Cindy H. Chau
National Cancer Institute
Bethesda, MD
USA

Eric J. Small
University of California, San Francisco
San Francisco, CA
USA

ISBN 978-1-60327-831-7   e-ISBN 978-1-60327-829-4
DOI 10.1007/978-1-60327-829-4
Springer New York Dordrecht Heidelberg London

Library of Congress Control Number: 2010936435

Springer is part of Springer Science+Business Media (www.springer.com)

Preface

Prostate cancer is the most common noncutaneous malignancy and the second leading cause of cancer deaths among men in the United States. It is a critical public health problem and remains incurable in the metastatic setting with mortality that usually occurs as a result of castration-resistant disease.

Since Huggins and Hodges' report of the dramatic clinical effects of suppressing serum testosterone levels in men with advanced prostate cancer in 1941, hormone therapy (also called androgen deprivation therapy [ADT]) has become widely accepted as the mainstay of therapy for the treatment of advanced prostate cancer. ADT combined with radiation therapy is a standard of care in the treatment of men with locally advanced prostate cancer on the basis of evidence that shows improved survival. The role of ADT in the management of prostate cancer is controversial in that it is also used for other prostate cancer states (such as in men with biochemical recurrence after radical prostatectomy or lymph node metastases) even though the clinical effects of hormone therapy in these other settings have not been definitively proven to be beneficial. Hence the first part of this volume will focus on the role of hormone therapy in the management of advanced prostate cancer and address the controversies relevant to the role of ADT, including the time to initiate ADT, optimum duration of ADT, the benefits of combined androgen blockade, the role of intermittent ADT, and the benefits of secondary hormonal therapies.

In men whose cancer is no longer responding to hormone therapy, the treatment paradigm is shifted toward chemotherapy and other investigational options. In 2004, two landmark trials using docetaxel-based chemotherapy demonstrated for the first time a survival benefit in metastatic, castration-resistant prostate cancer. Research has revealed several distinct mechanisms of castration-resistant disease that may converge in patients with disease progression on ADT. Many approaches are currently being evaluated to improve the treatment of this condition and these findings have identified several potential targets for therapeutic intervention. These include drugs that are more active or less toxic chemotherapy agents; drugs that induce androgen deprivation; drugs that target the androgen receptor and/or androgen synthesis; drugs that target specific pathways, including angiogenesis and tyrosine kinase inhibitors, endothelin antagonists and matrix metalloproteinase inhibitors; and immunologic approaches. Many of these agents seem promising and the rationale and efficacy of these emerging therapies remain to be validated in future clinical trials.

In light of a growing array of existing and novel treatment options, this book was undertaken to capture the multidisciplinary care approach to the drug management of prostate cancer in order to optimize survival and quality of life for the patients. At this unique juncture in the treatment of prostate cancer, current standard and investigational treatment options for this disease are discussed, including hormone therapy and chemotherapy as well as rapidly evolving therapies in phase II/III trials involving antiangiogenic therapies, immunomodulatory agents, and nuclear receptor targets. It is divided into seven sections, preceded by an introduction that discusses the cell biology and molecular targets of prostate cancer. Part I describes the role of androgens and androgen deprivation therapy in prostate cancer and the several types of hormone therapy used to treat advanced prostate cancer, including luteinizing hormone-releasing hormone agonists and antagonists, and anti-androgens. Androgen receptor biology and the pharmacogenetics of the androgen metabolic pathway are also presented. Part II discusses the role of chemotherapy in prostate cancer including standard and investigational approaches as well as the clinical pharmacology and pharmacogenetics of these agents. Part III introduces the concept of angiogenesis in prostate cancer by discussing the principles of anti-angiogenic therapy, investigational angiogenesis inhibitors, and the pharmacogenetics of angiogenesis. Part IV focuses on the pathophysiology of prostate cancer bone metastasis and the agents used at this stage of the disease process. Part V continues on to describe the role of immunotherapy for advanced prostate cancer including immunotherapeutics and vaccine approaches. In Part VI, chemoprevention strategies for prostate cancer are discussed. The last section of the book, Part VII, looks at the overall drug and technological development efforts and challenges in prostate cancer.

As such, this book is a comprehensive, concisesummary of the pharmacological treatments of prostate cancer detailing knowledge of both conventional and emerging drug therapies. The chapters describe state-of-the-art information that will be appropriate for medical students, physicians in training, physicians, scientists, and members of the pharmaceutical industry. As advances in understanding the biology of prostate cancer and the mechanisms of castration-resistant disease continue over the next decade, novel drug discovery and development efforts will translate into emerging treatment paradigms in the therapeutic management of prostate cancer.

Lastly, we would like to thank our colleagues for providing their timely and important chapters. Our task of compiling this book was made easy by their high-quality contributions.

William D. Figg
Cindy H. Chau
Eric J. Small

Contents

Part IV. Bone Metastasis

Part V. Immunotherapy

Part VI. Prevention

Contributors

David E. Adelberg
Medical Oncology Branch, National Cancer Institute, Bethesda MD, USA

David B. Agus
USC, Westside Prostate Cancer Center, Keck School of Medicine of USC,
Beverly Hills, CA, USA

Ajjai S. Alva
Doctor, Hematology/Oncology Department, University of Michigan,
Ann Arbor MI, USA

Jeanny B. Aragon-Ching
Department of Medicine, George Washington University, Washington, DC, USA

Philip M. Arlen
Attending Physician Medical Oncology Branch, National Cancer Institute,
National Institutes of Health, Bethesda MD, USA

Steven P. Balk
Department of Medicine, Beth Israel Deaconess Medical Center,
Harvard Medical School, Boston MA 02215, USA

Tomasz M. Beer
Associate Professor of Medicine, Grover C. Bagby Endowed Chair for Prostate
Cancer Research Medicine/Hematology and Medical Oncology, Oregon Health &
Science University, Portland OR, USA

Norman L. Block
Clinical Director of the Endocrine, Polypeptide, and Cancer Institute, Pathology,
Urology, Oncology Miami Veterans Affairs Medical Center, Jackson Memorial
Hospital, University of Miami Hospital, University of Miami, Miami FL, USA

Guido Bocci
Assistant Professor Division of Pharmacology and Chemotherapy,
Department of Internal Medicine, University of Pisa, Pisa, Italy

Deborah A. Bradley
Assistant Professor of Medicine Department of Internal Medicine,
University of Michigan, Ann Arbor MI, USA

Ashley Brick
Clinical Research Coordinator Genitourinary Oncology,
Dana-Farber Cancer Institute, Boston, MA USA

Jackie Celestin
Internal Medicine, University of Connecticut, Farmington, CT USA

June M. Chan
Epidemiology and Biostatistics, Urology, University of California,
San Francisco, CA, USA

Cindy H. Chau
Medical Oncology Branch, Center for Cancer Research,
National Cancer Institute/NIH, Bethesda, MD, USA

Michael E. Cox
Associate Professor UBC Department of Urologic Sciences, The Vancouver
Prostate Centre, Vancouver General Hospital, University of British Columbia,
Vancouver BC, Canada

Francesco Crea
Student Division of Pharmacology and Chemotherapy,
Department of Internal Medicine, University of Pisa, Pisa, Italy

Zoran Culig
Department of Urology, Innsbruck Medical University, Innsbruck, Austria

Ramzi N. Dagher
VP Worldwide Regulatory Strategy, Global Research and Development,
Pfizer, Inc., New London CT, USA

William Dahut
Chief Genitourinary Research Section Medical Oncology Branch, CCR, NCI, NIH
Clinical Center, National Cancer Institute, Bethesda MD, USA

Romano Danesi
Division of Pharmacology and Chemotherapy, Department of Internal Medicine,
University of Pisa, Pisa, Italy

Angelo M. De Marzo
Department of Pathology, Bunting Blaustein Cancer Research,
The Johns Hopkins University School of Medicine, Baltimore MD, USA

Mario Del Tacca
Full Professor Division of Pharmacology and Chemotherapy,
Department of Internal Medicine, University of Pisa, Pisa, Italy

Giuseppe Di Lorenzo
Medical Oncology, AOU Federico II, Napoli, Italy

Antonello Di Paolo
Division of Pharmacology and Chemotherapy, Department of Internal Medicine,
University of Pisa, Pisa, Italy

Aymen A. Elfiky
Lank Center for Genitourinary Oncology, Dana-Farber Cancer Institute,
Brigham and Women's Hospital, Harvard Medical School, Boston MA, USA

Alireza Farabishahadel
Department of Internal Medicine, University of Nevada School of Las Vegas,
Las Vegas NV, USA

William D. Figg
Medical Oncology Branch, Center for Cancer Research,
National Cancer Institute, National Institute of Health, Bethesda, MD, USA

Antonio Tito Fojo
Experimental Therapeutics Section, Medical Oncology Branch,
Center for Cancer Research, National Cancer Institute, Bethesda, MD, USA

Lawrence Fong
Associate Professor Department of Medicine, Division of Hematology/Oncology,
University of California San Francisco, San Francisco CA, USA

Terence W. Friedlander
Department of Medicine, Division of Hematology/Oncology,
University of California San Francisco Medical Center, San Francisco CA, USA

Mark W. Frohlich
Sr. Vice President, Clinical Affairs and Chief Medical Officer
Dendreon Corporation, Seattle WA, USA

Erin R. Gardner
SAIC-Frederick, Inc., Clinical Pharmacology Program, National Cancer Institute,
Frederick MD, USA

Edward P. Gelmann
Division of Hematology/Oncology, Herbert Irving Comprehensive Cancer Center,
Columbia University, New York, NY, USA

Martin E. Gleave
UBC Department of Urologic Sciences, The Vancouver Prostate Center,
Vancouver General Hospital,
University of British Columbia, Vancouver, BC, Canada

Oscar B. Goodman
Jr., Assistant Professor Clinical Oncology, Nevada Cancer Institute,
Las Vegas NV, USA

Mitchell Gross
Director of Experimental Therapeutics Louis Warschaw Prostate Cancer Center,
Cedars-Sinai Medical Center, Los Angeles CA, USA

James L. Gulley
Laboratory of Tumor Immunology and Biology, Medical Oncology Branch,
National Cancer Institute, Bethesda, MD, USA

Christopher L. Hall
Research Investigator Department of Urology, University of Michigan,
Ann Arbor MI, USA

Patricia Halterman
Clinical Pharmacy, Nevada Cancer Institute, Las Vegas, NV, USA

Andrea L. Harzstark
Department of Medicine, Division of Hematology/Oncology,
University of California San Francisco, San Francisco, CA, USA

Hannelore V. Heemers
Department of Urology, Rosewell Park Cancer Institute, Buffalo, NY 14263, USA

Celestia S. Higano
University of Washington, Seattle Cancer Care Alliance, Seattle, WA, USA

Margaret G. House
Nurse Consultant Division of Cancer Prevention, Department of Health and
Human Services, National Cancer Institute, Rockville MD, USA

Ann W. Hsing
Senior Investigator Division of Cancer Epidemiology and Genetics,
National Cancer Institute, National Institutes of Health, Bethesda MD, USA

Jiaoti Huang
Professor Pathology Department, UCLA David Geffen School of Medicine,
Los Angeles CA, USA

Maha Hussain
Comprehensive Cancer Center, University of Michigan, Ann Arbor, MI, USA

Ana R. Jensen
Sections of Hematology/Oncology, Department of Medicine,
University of Chicago, Chicago IL, USA

Evan T. Keller
Department of Urology, University of Michigan, Ann Arbor, MI, USA

William Kevin Kelly
Solid Tumor Oncology, Department of Medical Oncology, Associate Director of
Translation Research, Jefferson Kimmel Cancel Center, Thomas Jefferson
University, Suite 314, Philadelphia, PA 19107, USA

James R. Lambert
Assistant Professor Pathology Department,
University of Colorado Denver, Aurora CO, USA

Marshall Scott Lucia
Department of Pathology, University of Colorado, Denver, Aurora, CO, USA

Ravi A. Madan
Assistant Clinical Investigator Laboratory of Tumor Immunology and Biology,
Medical Oncology Branch, National Cancer Institute, Bethesda MD, USA

Francine Zanchetta Coelho Marques
Plunkett Chair of Molecular Biology (Medicine) Anatomy Department, The
University of Sydney, Sydney NSW, Australia

Joel B. Nelson
Department of Urology, University of Pittsburgh, Pittsburgh, PA, USA

Edward Macrohon Nepomuceno
Fellow in Medical Oncology and Hematology Olive View,
Department of Medicine, UCLA Medical Center, Sylmar CA, USA

Yang-Min Ning
Office of Oncology Drug Products, The U.S. Food and Drug Administration,
Silver Spring MD, USA

Junyang Niu
Professor Pathology Department, Anhui Provincial Hospital,
Hefei, Anhui Province, China

William K. Oh
Division of Hematology and Medical Oncology,
Dana-Farber Cancer Institute, New York, 10029 NY, USA

Howard L. Parnes
Prostate and Urologic Cancer Research Group, NCI-Division of Cancer Prevention,
Center for Cancer Research, National Cancer Institute, Bethesda, MD, USA

Guiseppe Pasqualetti
Post-doctoral Fellow Division of Pharmacology and Chemotherapy,
Department of Internal Medicine, University of Pisa, Pisa, Italy

Lalit R. Patel
Research Coordinator Prostate Cancer Foundation, Santa Monica CA, USA

Richard Pazdur
Director Office of Oncology Drug Products, The U.S. Food and Drug
Administration, Silver Spring MD, USA

Daniel P. Petrylak
Columbia University Medical Center, New York, NY

Courtney K. Phillips
Assistant Professor of Urology Urology Department, Mount Sinai School of
Medicine, New York NY, USA

Elizabeth A. Platz
Department of Epidemiology, Johns Hopkins Bloomberg School of Public Health,
Baltimore MD, USA

Edwin M. Posadas
Section of Hematology/Oncology, Department of Medicine,
University of Chicago, Chicago, IL 60637, USA

Douglas K. Price
Medical Oncology Branch, National Cancer Institute, National Institutes of Health,
Bethesda, MD, USA

Juergen K.V. Reichardt
Plunkett Chair of Molecular Biology (Medicine),
The University of Sydney, Sydney, NSW, Australia

Erin L. Richman
Nutrition Department, Harvard School of Public Health, Boston MA, USA

Jonathan Rosenberg
Lank Center for Genitourinary Oncology, Dana-Farber Cancer Institute,
Boston, MA, USA

Charles J. Ryan
Department of Medicine, University of California San Francisco,
San Francisco CA, USA

Oliver Sartor
Departments of Medicine and Urology, Tulane Medical School,
New Orleans, LA, USA

Philip J. Saylor
Department of Medicine, Division of Hematology/Oncology,
Massachusetts General Hospital Cancer Center, Boston, MA, USA

Andrew V. Schally
Department of Veterans Affairs, VA Research Services, Veterans Affairs Medical
Center, Miami FL, USA, and Division of Hematology/Oncology and Division of
Endocrinology,
Departments of Pathology and Medicine, Miller School of Medicine,
University of Miami, Miami, FL, USA

Jeffrey Schlom
Chief Laboratory of Tumor Immunology and Biology,
Center for Cancer Research, National Cancer Institute,
National Institutes of Health, Bethesda MD, USA

Nima Sharifi
Division of Hematology/Oncology, University of Texas Southwestern Medical
Center, Dallas, TX, USA

Howard C. Shen
Research Fellow Department of Medicine, Bth Israel Deaconess Medical Center,
Harvard Medical School, Boston MA, USA

Jonathan W. Simons
Prostate Cancer Foundation, Santa Monica, CA, USA

Tristan M. Sissung
Medical Oncology Branch, Center for Cancer Research, National Cancer Institutes,
National Institute of Health, Bethesda MD, USA

Matthew R. Smith
Associate Professor Division of Hematology/Oncology, Department of Medicine,
Massachusetts General Hospital Cancer Center, Harvard Medical School,
Boston MA, USA

Russell Z. Szmulewitz
Instructor Sections of Hematology/Oncology, Department of Medicine,
University of Chicago, Chicago IL, USA

Joseph A. Tangrea
Program Director Department of Health and Human Services,
National Cancer Institute, Rockville MD, USA

Mary-Ellen Taplin
Associate Professor of Medicine Lank Center for Genitourinary,
Oncology, Harvard Medical School, Dana-Farber Cancer Institute,
Boston MA, USA

Donald J. Tindall
Professor Department of Urology Research,
Mayo Clinic, Rochester MN, USA

Damerla R. Venugopal
Section of Hematology-Oncology, Department of Medical Oncology,
Tulane Medical School, New Orleans LA, USA

Nicholas J. Vogelzang
Professor, Director Medical Oncology, Nevada Cancer Institute,
University of Nevada School of Medicine, Las Vegas NV, USA

Yuzhuo Wang
Senior Scientist The Vancouver Prostate Centre, Vancouver General Hospital,
University of British Columbia, Vancouver BC, Canada

Chapter 1
Cell Biology of Prostate Cancer and Molecular Targets

Martin E. Gleave, Michael E. Cox, and Yuzhuo Wang

Abstract While not appreciated at the time, the Nobel Prize-winning work of Huggins and Hodges in the 1940s illustrated the androgen dependence of prostate cancer and credentialized the first "targeted" (in this case, the androgen receptor) anticancer therapy. Androgen deprivation therapy induces long-term remission in most patients, but development of castration-resistant prostate cancer (CRPC) is inevitable. Most treatments for CRPC have been approved for symptomatic benefit, with only docetaxel shown to improve overall survival. Mechanisms underlying shift to castrate resistance have been attributed to a complex interplay of clonal selection, reactivation of AR axis despite castrate levels of serum T, adaptive upregulation of antiapoptotic and survival gene networks, stress-induced cytoprotective chaperones, and alternative growth factor pathways. CRPC tumors develop compensatory mechanisms during androgen deprivation, tailored to the synthesis of intratumoral androgens, which along with ligand-independent mechanisms involving cofactors or growth factor pathways, cooperatively trigger AR activation and thus disease progression. Over the last few years, numerous gene targets involved with CRPC that regulate apoptosis, proliferation, angiogenesis, cell signaling, and tumor-bone stromal interactions have been identified, and many novel compounds have entered clinical trials either as single agents or in combination with cytotoxic chemotherapy. In this review, several genes and pathways involved in CRPC progression will be reviewed, with particular emphasis on preclinically credentialized genes and pathways that are currently the targets of novel inhibitors in later stages of clinical development. These include the AR axis, molecular chaperones, tumor vasculature, bone stroma, and signal transduction pathways such as those triggered by IGF-1 and IL-6.

Keywords Castration-resistant prostate cancer • Androgen receptor • Clusterin • Hsp27 • IGF-1

Introduction

Prostate cancer (CaP) cell proliferation and survival are regulated through complex interactions between cell surface receptor-mediated cell signaling and transcription factor regulation of gene expression. Androgens are principal factors in CaP carcinogenesis and progression, regulating gene and signaling networks that promote cell survival through binding with the androgen receptor (AR), a ligand-responsive transcription factor. Testicular synthesis of testosterone (T) accounts for 90% of the dihydrotestosterone (DHT) formed in the prostate, with the remainder derived from less potent adrenal androgens. Once intracellular, T is converted to DHT by 5α-reductase, binding to and activating the AR that subsequently dimerizes, translocates to the nucleus, and interacts with promoter regions of specific genes to regulate transcription and hence protein synthesis, cell proliferation, survival, and differentiation.

Though not appreciated at the time, the Nobel Prize-winning work of Huggins and Hodges [1] in the 1940s credentialized the first "targeted" (in this case, the AR) anticancer therapy by confirming the androgen

M.E. Gleave (✉)
UBC Department of Urologic Sciences,
The Vancouver Prostate Center, Vancouver General Hospital,
University of British Columbia, Vancouver, BC, Canada,
and
The Vancouver Prostate Center, Vancouver General Hospital,
Vancouver, BC, Canada
e-mail: m.gleave@ubc.ca

W.D. Figg et al. (eds.), *Drug Management of Prostate Cancer*,
DOI 10.1007/978-1-60327-829-4_1, © Springer Science+Business Media, LLC 2010

dependence of CaP. Following androgen deprivation therapy (ADT), benign and malignant prostate epithelial cells undergo apoptotic regression leading to >80% objective response and prolonging median overall survival from ~18 to ~36 months in men with metastatic disease [2]. Serum PSA, an AR-regulated gene, remains the most useful marker of response and prognosis to ADT; PSA nadir levels above 4 µg/L after 6 months of ADT are associated with a median survival of 18 months compared with 40 months when nadirs below 4 µg/L are seen [3]. Despite high initial response rates, remissions are temporary because surviving tumor cells usually recur with castration-resistant prostate cancer (CRPC) phenotype. The earliest signal of CRPC is a rising PSA while on ADT, predating clinical progression by 6–12 months and death by 18-24 months [2, 4]. Thus, one of the main obstacles to the cure of advanced CaP by androgen ablation is progression to CRPC, a complex process involving variable combinations of clonal selection [5, 6], adaptive upregulation of antiapoptotic survival genes [6–11], AR transactivation from low levels of androgen, mutations or increased levels of coactivators [12–14], and alternative growth factor pathways [15–20] (Fig. 1.1). If we are to have a significant impact on survival, new therapeutic strategies designed to inhibit the emergence of this acquire treatment-resistant phenotype must be developed.

Improved understanding of the molecular basis underlying bone-specific metastases and resistance to ADT or chemotherapy will facilitate the rational design of targeted therapeutics. In addition to castrate-resistant disease, a second unique characteristic of CaP progression is bone-predominant metastatic progression. Bone provides a rich microenvironment for establishment of CaP metastasis, at least in part, because of its dense reservoir of growth regulatory factors, extracellular matrix proteins, and hydroxyapatite scaffolds to support tumor growth. Over the last few years, numerous gene targets that regulate apoptosis, proliferation, angiogenesis, cell signaling, and tumorbone stromal interactions have been identified, and many novel compounds have entered clinical trials either as single agents or in combination with cytotoxic chemotherapy. Because of rapid progress of this field, it is beyond the scope of this chapter to review all compounds under investigation. This review will focus on molecular and cellular mechanisms involved in CaP progression, metastases, and treatment resistance, with particular emphasis on preclinically credentialized genes and pathways that are currently the targets of novel inhibitors. These include the AR axis, molecular chaperones, tumor vasculature, bone stroma, and signal transduction pathways such as IGF-1 and IL-6.

AR Axis

The AR is a ligand-dependent transcription factor and member of the class I subgroup of the nuclear receptor superfamily that plays a key role in prostate carcinogenesis and progression [21, 22]. The classical model of androgen-regulated AR transcriptional activity has not fully defined the many diverse effects of androgens on CaP cell survival and growth. In response to androgen, cytoplasmic AR rapidly translocates to the nucleus and interacts with sequence-specific androgen response elements (ARE) in the transcriptional regulatory regions of target genes [22, 23]. In addition to this transcriptional genomic action, androgens and other steroid hormones such as progesterone and estrogen can exert rapid nongenomic effects that are not mediated through nuclear receptors but rather initiated at the plasma membrane, presumably through surface receptors [24–26].

Androgens and AR are essential for CaP progression, and in many cases CRPC maintains many aspects of AR function by increased AR expression and/or mutagenesis resulting in increased sensitivity to androgens, permissive activation by nonandrogenic steroids, de novo steroid synthesis, and/or ligand-independent activation [6, 12–15]. Moreover, AR activation controls CaP proliferation and survival by upregulating responsiveness to autocrine and paracrine growth factor and cognate receptor loops [20, 27–30] discussed further below.

Almost uniformly, CRPC involves the reactivation of the AR, as illustrated by sentinel upregulation of PSA, a discretely androgen-regulated gene. Experimental models and molecular profiles of human CaP indicate that the AR becomes reactivated in most CRPC [31–35]. Several groups [12–14, 31, 32] reported that androgen-regulated genes become constitutively reexpressed in the absence of testicular androgens during "AI" progression. Moreover, downregulation of AR using siRNA can suppress "AI" tumor growth [14, 36], and many enzymes and gene networks implicated in

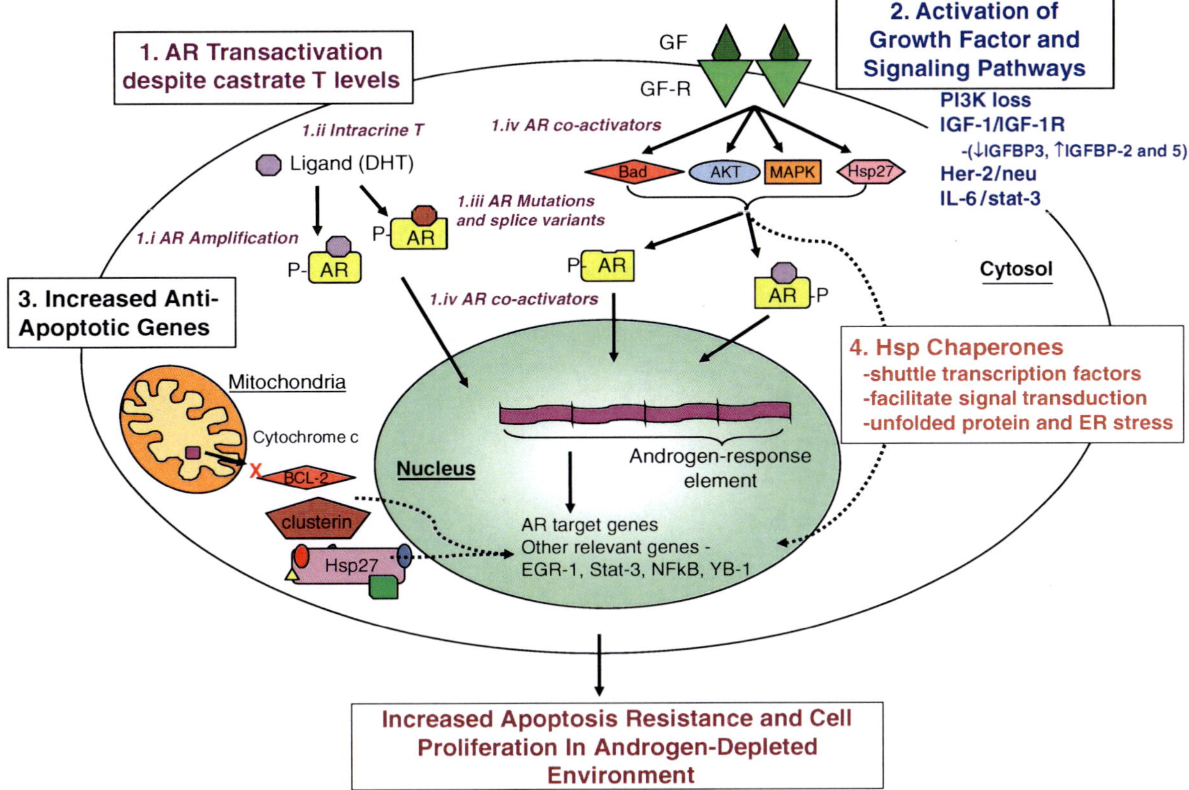

Fig. 1.1 Schematic of molecular mechanisms contributing to castration-resistant disease. (1) Increased androgen receptor (AR) transcriptional activity in the presence of castrate levels of serum testosterone via (a) overamplification and increased hypersensitivity of AR; (b) de novo intracrine synthesis of DHT and other androgens via the backdoor pathways; (c) mutations in ligand-binding domain of AR leading to promiscuous activation by other ligands or splice variants lacking ligand-binding domain leading to ligand-independent AR transactivation; (d) increased coactivators (e.g., SRC, TIF-2, Ack1) that enhance AR activity. (2) Activation of proliferative growth factor and signaling pathways, notably insulin-like growth factor-1 (IGF-1) and interleukin-6 (IL-6). (3) Upregulation of cell survival genes that inhibit apoptotic pathway activation, including Bcl-2, clusterin, Hsp27, YB-1, and NF-kB. (4) Molecular chaperones (e.g., clusterin, Hsp27, Hsp90) facilitate protein interactions to shuttle transcriptional factors (e.g., AR), phosphorylation of signaling events, and suppress stress-induced cytochrome c release through interactions with proapoptotic Bcl family genes. Another mechanism includes selective outgrowth of subpopulations of preexisting androgen-independent CaP cells (clonal selection)

steroidogenesis are upregulated, leading to reactivation of AR [12, 37]. These data suggest that CRPC progression may not be entirely independent of androgen-driven activity of the AR, but in fact other sources of androgens are being capitalized upon for AR activation. Recent data suggests that at least two hypotheses may account for these observations: that the AR is activated independent of ligand (by mutations, over-amplification, signaling pathways, or increased AR coactivators) or that androgen-regulated pathways within CaP cells are activated by alternative sources of androgenic steroids. These mechanisms are not mutually exclusive and expose the clinical problem of developing therapies that can account for the complex adaptive capacity of CRPC.

(1) Persistent or reactivated AR signaling under ligand-deprived (or- independent) conditions may result from (a) amplified or elevated AR expression [38, 39]; (b) AR mutations in the ligand-binding domain that enhance AR promiscuity [40–43]; (c) expression of AR splice variants that lack a ligand-binding domain and are constitutively active in a ligand-independent manner [44, 45] (d) altered expression or activity of AR coactivator [46, 47] or chaperone [48] proteins, and (e) AR activation by certain kinases or signal transduction pathways that enhance AR activation in response

to low levels of androgen [49–54]. Previous studies established that the AR is phosphorylated at multiple serine/threonine sites [52, 55–57] and at several tyrosine residues. Tyrosine phosphorylation is mediated by at least two tyrosine kinases, Src and Ack1, and enhances AR responses to low androgen levels [58–60].

(2) An important factor contributing to CRPC via the AR axis also includes suboptimal reduction of natural AR ligands by traditional ADT. Early studies by Geller and colleagues [61] indicated that concentrations of androgens sufficient to activate the AR remained in the prostate gland despite surgical or medical castration, and more recently, these were confirmed and extended using LC-MS by Mohler et al. [33, 34] and others [13, 31, 35]. Adrenal androgens were initially believed to be the sole source of androgens utilized by CaP tumors [33, 34, 37]. An alternative hypothesis is that cholesterol and its derivatives can be converted to androgens in prostate tumor cells through a series of well-characterized stepwise enzymatic events. Androgen synthesis is often described in terms of the classical steroidogenic pathway through DHEA and testosterone (T) (Fig. 1.2). A recently described "backdoor pathway" may serve as an alternative synthesis pathway, which utilizes progesterone as the primary steroidal precursor of DHT, thereby bypassing T as an intermediate [63]. Using the

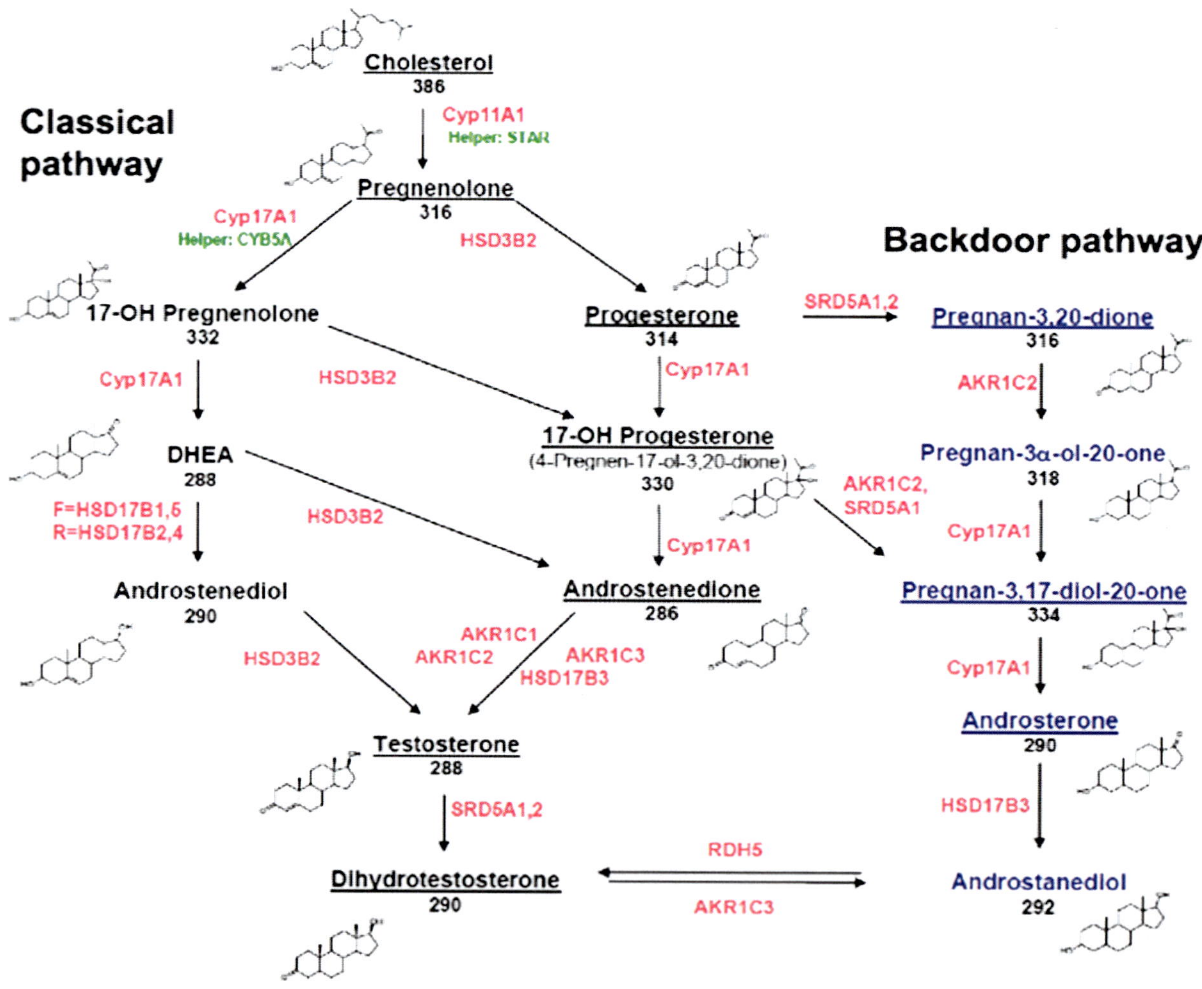

Fig. 1.2 Intracrine de novo synthesis of testosterone. Steroidogenesis pathway converts cholesterol to DHT via the pathways involving the steroidal intermediates and interlinked enzymatic reactions. Steroids are portrayed in black (classical steroidogenesis pathway) and blue (backdoor steroidogenesis pathway), and enzymes are portrayed in pink and green. Some of the pathways are reversible while others are irreversible as indicated by the direction of the arrows

LNCaP xenograft model, Locke et al. [13] reported that tumor androgens, like PSA, increase during castrate-resistant progression. As mice do not synthesize adrenal androgens, LNCaP tumors themselves were investigated as the source of increased androgens. All enzymes necessary for androgen synthesis were expressed in castrate-resistant tumors, which were capable of de novo conversion of [^{14}C]-acetic acid to DHT and [^{3}H]-progesterone to six other steroids upstream of DHT. This evidence suggests that de novo androgen synthesis may be one of the mechanisms leading to CaP progression following castration.

Collectively, these studies suggest that CRPC tumors develop compensatory mechanisms during androgen starvation, tailored to the synthesis of intratumoral androgens, which along with ligand-independent or AR-sensitizing mechanisms outlined above, cooperatively trigger AR activation to facilitate disease progression. Hence, despite the failure of maximal androgen blockage trials using nonsteroid antiandrogens such as flutamide or bicalutamide, CRPC tumors are not uniformly hormone refractory and may remain sensitive to therapies directed against the AR axis. Several new classes of AR-targeting agents are now in clinical development, including more potent AR antagonists (e.g., MDV3100), inhibitors of steroidogenesis (abiraterone), and AR-disrupting agents that target AR chaperones such as Hsp90 (17-AAG analogs) or Hsp27 (OGX-427).

AR Antagonists

First generation nonsteroidal antiandrogens (flutamide and bicalutamide) compete with T and DHT in binding to AR's steroid binding domain. However, these antiandrogens do not sufficiently inhibit AR transactivation in CRPC. Second generation antagonists have been identified that more potently block AR activity in CRPC. For example, MDV3100 is a novel AR antagonist [14, 64] that demonstrates antitumor activity in models with *AR* amplification and resistance to bicalutamide. Clinical activity has been observed in a phase 1 trial of MDV3100 in patients with both castration-resistant and docetaxel-refractory disease. This drug is currently in Phase II trials with PSA response rates exceeding 40% in CRPC and will move into Phase III registration trials in 2010 [64].

Inhibitors of Androgen Synthesis

Historical attempts to suppress adrenal (as well as intracrine) androgen production have met with limited success. Ketoconazole inhibits several adrenal enzymes involved with adrenal androgen synthesis, but only modest therapeutic activities in CRPC were observed [65]. Abiraterone acetate is a potent steroidal irreversible inhibitor of CYP17 [17α hydroxylase/C17,20-lyase], blocking two important enzymatic activities in the synthesis of testosterone [66–68]. Pharmacodynamic studies demonstrated that its effects on adrenal steroid synthesis were consistent with its mechanism of action. In Phase II studies of chemotherapy-naïve men with CRPC, declines in PSA ≥ 30%, ≥50%, and ≥90% were observed in 80, 70, and 24% of patients, respectively, reflecting decreases in ligand-dependent AR transactivation. Consistent with abiraterone's mechanism of action, hypertension (HTN), hypokalemia, and lower extremity edema were the most commonly observed drug-related adverse events. Phase III trials of abiraterone in CRPC began in 2008 and data should be available by early 2011.

AR Chaperone Inhibitors

Molecular chaperones are involved in processes of folding, activation, trafficking, and transcriptional activity of most steroid receptors, including AR. In the absence of ligand, AR is predominately cytoplasmic, maintained in an inactive, but highly responsive state by a large dynamic heterocomplex composed of heat-shock proteins (Hsp), cochaperones, and tetratricopeptide repeat (TPR)-containing proteins. Ligand binding leads to a conformational change in the AR and dissociation from the large Hsp complex [69–74]. Subsequently, the AR translocates to the nucleus, interacts with coactivators, dimerizes, and binds to ARE to transactivate target gene expression. Dissociation of the AR–chaperone complex after ligand binding is viewed as a general regulatory mechanism of AR signaling.

Several agents targeting AR-associated chaperones are in development. For example, Hsp90 inhibitors such as geldanamycin induce steroid receptor degradation by directly binding to the ATP-binding pocket of Hsp90 to inhibit its function [70, 71]. Several Hsp90 inhibitors are in Phase I-II trials in CRPC. Hsp27 is a cytoprotective chaperone expressed in response to many stress signals to regulate key effectors of the apoptotic machinery including the apoptosome, the caspase activation complex [75, 76], and proteasome-mediated degradation of apoptosis-regulatory proteins [77, 78]. Recently, a feed-forward loop was reported whereby androgen-bound AR induces rapid Hsp27 phosphorylation that in turn cooperatively facilitates genomic activity of the AR, thereby enhancing CaP cell survival. Antisense knockdown of Hsp27 (OGX-427) delays CRPC xenograft progression [10, 11], in part, by destabilizing the AR through ubiquitin-proteasome-mediated AR degradation [48] (Fig. 1.3). Interestingly, OGX-427 induces degradation of Hsp27, AR, and Hsp90, while geldanamycin inhibition of Hsp90 induces degradation of client proteins [71], but is accompanied by stress-activated increases in Hsp70 and Hsp27 [79]. A dose escalation Phase I trial of single agent OGX-427 in Hsp27-positive cancers was completed in 2008 and showed that OGX-427 was well tolerated. Decreases in PSA and CA-125, as well as CTC counts, suggest single-agent activity in CRPC and ovarian cancer, respectively. OGX-427 will move into Phase II trials in CRPC in 2010 [80].

Regulation of Apoptosis

In mammals, programmed cell death can be initiated by extrinsic or intrinsic death pathways. The extrinsic pathway is triggered by extracellular ligands that induce oligomerization of death receptors such as Fas or other members of the TNF receptor superfamily, resulting in activation of a caspase cascade leading to apoptosis. The instrinsic pathway is triggered in response to a variety of apoptotic stimuli that induce damage within the cell including anticancer agents, oxidative damage, UV irradiation, and growth factor withdrawal and is mediated through the mitochondria. These stimuli induce the loss of mitochondrial membrane integrity and result in the release of proapoptotic molecules, including cytochrome c (cyt c), which associates with Apaf-1 and caspase-9 to promote caspase activation, and SMAC/Diablo and Omi/HtrA2 that promote caspase activation by eliminating inhibition by IAPs (inhibitors of apoptosis proteins) [81–85].

Fas-induced death is the best understood extrinsic apoptotic pathway both in terms of mechanism and its physiological importance in vivo [86]. Multivalent cross-linking of the Fas receptor as a result of FasL binding to preassociated Fas receptor trimers triggers the recruitment of a set of effector proteins to the receptor, resulting in the formation of the death-inducing signaling complex (DISC). The DISC is composed of intracellular signaling proteins including FADD/MORT1, a death domain-containing adaptor protein, and Caspase-8 (also known as FLICE/MACH). Upon recruitment to the DISC, caspase-8 is autoproteolytically cleaved and activated, which then directly activates caspase-3 leading to execution of apoptosis. Caspase-8 also leads to activation of the mitochondrial amplification loop by proteolytic cleavage of the proapoptotic Bcl-2 member, Bid. The truncated Bid then translocates to the mitochondria and promotes cytochrome c release into the cytosol. In association with APAF-1 and pro-caspase-9, cytochrome c forms the apoptosome complex leading to the activation of caspase-9 that subsequently cleaves and activates effector caspases.

The propensity of tumor cells to undergo stress-induced apoptosis determines their susceptibility to biologic and cytotoxic therapies [85]. Adaptations achieved by progressively accumulating genetic mutations increase tumor heterogeneity and decrease susceptibility to treatment. Many of these adaptations involve changes in intrinsic and extrinsic apoptotic machinery, including Bcl family members, inhibitors of apoptosis, cytoprotective molecular chaperones, and/or activation of growth factor-mediated and convergent downstream prosurvival signaling cascades.

Bcl-2

The *bcl-2* gene, initially identified in follicular B-cell lymphoma due to a characteristic t14;18 translocation [87], is a mitochondrial membrane protein that heterodimerizes with Bax and other proapoptotic regulators to prevent cytochrome c release from the mitochondria and subsequent activation of the intrinsic apoptotic cascade [88]. Competitive dimerization between pairs of pro and antiapoptotic *bcl-2* family members (and other chaperones such as clusterin) determines how a cell responds to an apoptotic signal.

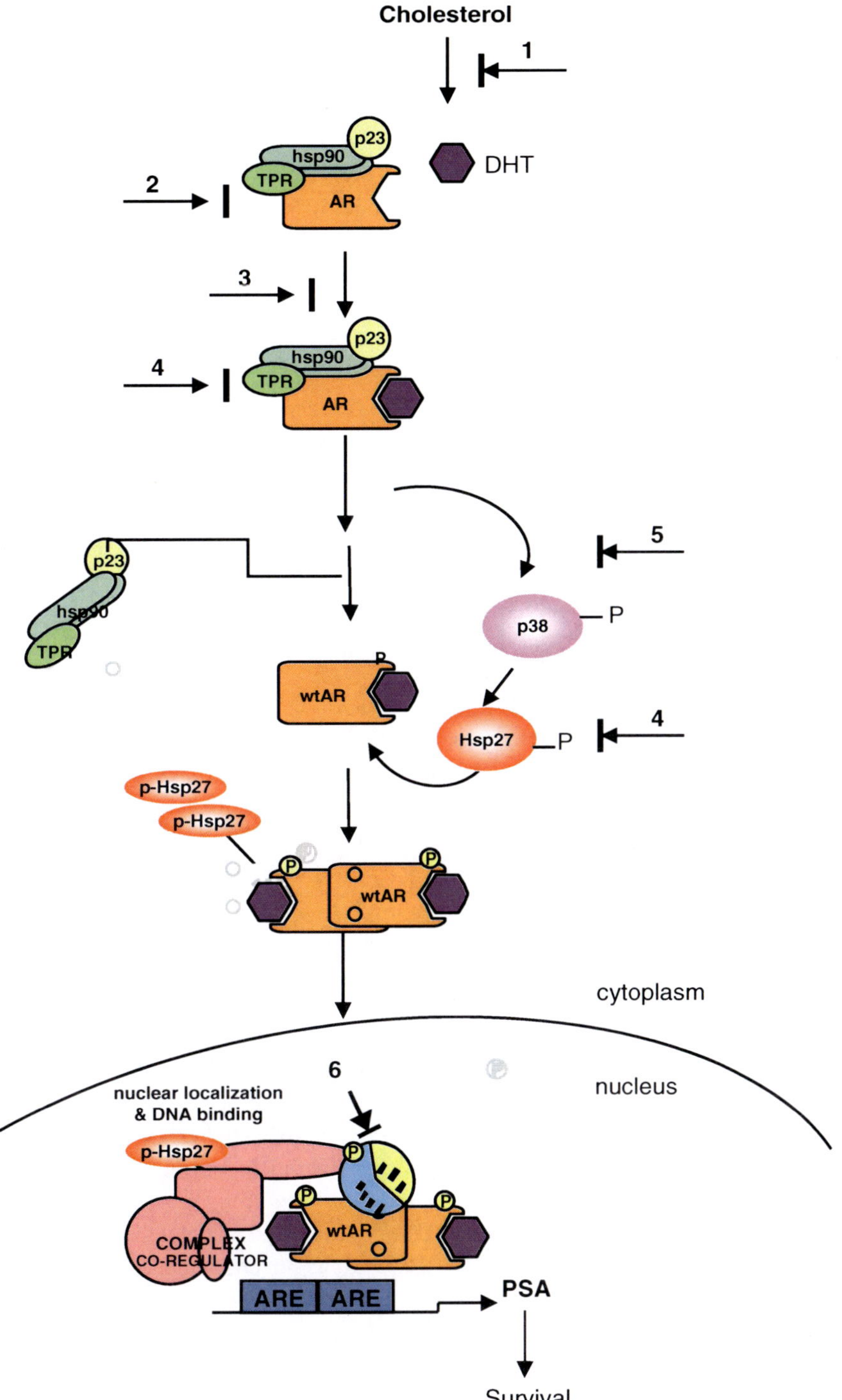

Fig. 1.3 AR transactivation in castration-resistant prostate cancer and potential points of therapeutic intervention. Ligand-binding to the steroid-binding domain of the AR leads to dissociation of heat-shock proteins, p38 kinase-mediated phosphorylation of Hsp27 that replaces Hsp90 as the predominant AR chaperone to shuttle the dimerized and phosphorylated AR into the nucleus. Several mechanisms converge to support AR signaling in a castrate environment and are potential targets of therapeutic intervention. (1) Inhibitors of de novo androgen synthesis using abiraterone or 5 alpha reductase inhibitors to block enzymes involved in the synthesis and metabolism of androgens. (2) Target AR synthesis (antisense oligonucleotides or siRNA) or maturation [histone deacetylase (HDAC) inhibitors, e.g., SAHA]. (3) Potent second generation AR antagonists that block ligand-binding domain and prevent dimerization and nuclear translocation (e.g., MDV3100). (4) Target AR chaperones to destabilize and increase AR ubiquitination and degradation rates using inhibitors against Hsp90 (e.g., 17-allylaminogeldanamycin) or Hsp27 (OGX-427). (5) Inhibitors of nonnuclear AR signaling (e.g., SRC). (6) Coactivator inhibition

Many studies link overexpression of bcl-2 with treatment resistance [88–92], highlighting bcl-2 as the target to enhance chemotherapy-induced apoptosis. Targeted inhibition of bcl-2 was initially accomplished using antisense oligonucleotides (ASOs) with many reporting good hormone or chemosensitization activity in preclinical models [8, 93–96]. G3139, also referred to as oblimersen sodium or Genasense (Genta Inc.), is a first generation 18-mer phosphorothioate ASO evaluated in many clinical trials based on promising activity in preclinical models of many cancers [97–101]. Unfortunately, randomized Phase II or III trials in CRPC [101] and melanoma [102] or myeloma [103] did not show clear evidence of anticancer efficacy. These negative results have put future trials with this agent on hold. Issues persist about the dosing and regimen of this first generation ASO, and whether 6 days of 7 mg/kg/day treatment are enough to suppress target sufficiently.

Bcl-xL is another antiapoptotic bcl-2 family member. In tumors where bcl-2 and Bcl-xL are coexpressed, it is difficult to predict which of the two proteins is more critical for survival, and some tumor cells have been reported to switch expression from Bcl-2 to Bcl-xL [104]. Bcl-xL ASOs have been reported to sensitize various tumor cells, including prostate, to chemotherapy [105–109].

BH3 mimetics are a novel class of anticancer agents moving forward in clinical development that induce apoptosis in tumor cells, regardless of their p53 or Bcl-2 status by enhancing the proapoptotic potential of BH3-only proteins or bypassing the need for BH3-only proteins by directly blocking interactions of Bcl-2-like prosurvival molecules with Bax and/or Bak [110, 111].

CLU

Human clusterin gene is located in chromosome 8p21-p12, where it is organized into nine exons [3] and encodes for two transcriptional isoforms in humans (Isoform 1, NM_001831 [GenBank]; Isoform 2, NM_203339 [GenBank]). These isoforms result from different transcriptional initiation sites and are produced only in humans and primates. In humans, clusterin exists as both an intracellular truncated 55-kDa nuclear splice variant (nCLU) and a 80-kDa secreted heterodimer disulfide-linked glycoprotein, making

clusterin the only known secreted chaperone [112–114]. Clusterin isoform 2 (sCLU-2) is the predominant isoform and is highly conserved across species, while sCLU-1 is expressed only in primate species. sCLU is a multifunctional stress-activated molecular chaperone possessing chaperone-like properties similar to small heat-shock proteins that stabilize and/or scaffold multimeric protein conformations during times of cell stress. A low abundant proapoptotic nuclear (nCLU) splice variant with properties that can regulate DNA repair has also been described [115–117]. Hsp and CLU facilitate degradation of terminally misfolded proteins by the ubiquitin-proteasomal degradation or aggresome-autophagy systems [118]. The 60 kD cytoplasmic CLU interacts with and inhibits conformationally altered Bax in response to cytotoxic stress, impeding Bax oligomerization and intrinsic pathway activation [119, 120]. Cytoplasmic CLU also regulates NF-κB activation, a stress-regulated transcription factor that controls inflammatory and innate immune responses, as well as many aspects of oncogenesis. NF-κB is activated in cancer cells by chemo- and radiation therapy and associated with acquired anticancer treatment resistance, including CRPC [121–123]. In its inactive form, NF-κB is sequestered in the cytoplasm by members of the IκB family. In the canonical pathway, IKK complex phosphorylates IκB, which is then ubiquitinated and degraded in the 26S proteosome, exposing nuclear localization signals on NF-κB subunits with subsequent NF-κB dimer translocation to the nucleus and transactivation of NF-κB-regulated genes. CLU functions as a ubiquitin binding protein that enhances COMMD1 and I-κB proteasomal degradation through its interaction with members of the SCF-bTrCP E3 ligase family, which leads to increased NF-κB nuclear translocation and transcriptional activity.

Many mechanisms in heterogeneous cancers contribute to acquired resistance including stress-activated prosurvival genes transcriptionally activated by heat-shock factor 1 (HSF1). HSF1 is the key regulator of the heat-shock response, a highly conserved protective mechanism for eukaryotic cells under stress, and has been associated with oncogenic transformation, proliferation, and survival [124]. Targeting HSF1 [125] or multifunctional genes regulated by HSF1 that are associated with cancer progression and treatment resistance is a rational therapeutic strategy. CLU is transcriptionally activated by HSF1 [126, 127], IGF-1 signaling [128], and androgen [129] and is antiapoptotic in response to hormone-, radiation-, and chemotherapy [9, 130–132]. Knockdown of CLU in CaP cells increases activated Bax levels with increased cytochrome c release from the mitochondria and subsequent activation of the intrinsic apoptotic cascade, as well as stabilization of I-κB with cytoplasmic NF-κB sequestration and decreased NF-κB activity. These data link stress-induced CLU expression with several antiapoptotic pathways relevant to acquired anticancer treatment resistance and mark CLU as an anticancer target.

Clusterin is overexpressed in a variety of human cancers, including those of the breast, lung, bladder, kidney, colon/rectum, and prostate [133–138]. Antisense- or siRNA-induced CLU knockdown enhances treatment-induced apoptosis and delays progression in many cancer models [9, 130, 139–141]. OGX-011 is a second-generation ASO that incorporates the 2′ MOE modification with four 2′ MOE-modified nucleosides at the 3′ and 5′ ends of the oligomer [141, 142] that decrease CLU levels >90% [143]. A randomized phase II study in chemo-naïve CRPC reported that OGX-011+docetaxel prolonged overall survival by 7 months (16.9–23.8 months) and reduced death rates by 39%, compared with docetaxel alone [144]. Phase III trials are set to begin in 2010.

Hsp27

Heat-shock protein 27 (Hsp27) is a 27-kDa molecular chaperone induced and phosphoactivated in response to a variety of biological, chemical, and physical stressors including heat-shock, oxidative stress, cytokines, and hormone- or chemotherapy [145]. Increased expression of Hsp27 during stress suppresses apoptosis, in part, from its role as a molecular chaperone to prevent protein aggregation or facilitate elimination of misfolded proteins. In addition, Hsp27 can act as a scaffolding protein to facilitate protein interactions and phosphorylation of signaling events [146]. Hsp27 is a multifunctional suppressor of apoptosis through interactions with Bid [75], procaspase-3 [147], cytochrome c [75], Smac/Diablo [148], and Daxx [149]. In addition, Hsp27 modulates the actin cytoskeleton [150] and intracellular levels of reactive oxygen species [151], interacts with several key client proteins involved in cell survival signals including IκBα [152], IKKβ [153], STAT-3 [11], AR [48], and Akt [154–156]. Akt

is a key serine–threonine kinase that enhances the survival and proliferation of cells by regulating the function of proapoptotic proteins such as BAD and caspase-9, cell cycle regulators such as p27kip1, and mediators that control apoptosis and/or proliferation, such as MDM2, FOXO, GSK3, TSC2, and PRAS40 [156].

Hsp27 is frequently overexpressed in numerous malignancies, including prostate, [10, 157] and associated with poor clinical prognosis and therapeutic resistance [10, 158, 159]. Not only is Hsp-27 a powerful biomarker of aggressive CaP, but it is also a potential target for novel therapeutic intervention. Knockdown of Hsp27 suppresses tumor growth and sensitizes cancer cells to hormone-, chemo-, and radiotherapy [10, 11, 159]. The biphenyl isoxasole KRIBB3 inhibits protein kinase C-dependent phosphorylation of Hsp27 to induce mitotic arrest and enhances apoptosis [160]. Recently, pyrrolo-pyrimidones, a novel class of p38 MAPK/MAPK-activated protein kinase 2 (MK2) inhibitors, have been shown to inhibit phosphorylation of Hsp-27 at Ser78 and Ser82 by the MAPKAP kinase MK5 [161, 162]. Not only is the MAPKAPK2/Hsp-27 pathway a promising potential target for therapeutic intervention but the isoflavone genistein, an estrogen analog and candidate chemotherapeutic agent, inhibits cell migration by blocking activation of this pathway [163]. Recently, OGX-427, a selective, second-generation ASO inhibitor of Hsp27 has recently advanced into phase I/II clinical trials for treatment of a variety of cancers [80]. OGX-427 was well tolerated as a monotherapy and demonstrated declines in circulating tumor cells as well as reduction in PSA levels in three patients with CRPC. Reductions in both circulating tumor cells and tumor markers suggest single-agent activity warranting further clinical investigation.

Signal Transduction Pathways

IGF and IGF-1R in CaP Progression

The IGF axis is an important regulator of growth, survival, and metastatic potential in a variety of malignancies and is strongly implicated in CaP etiology [164–167]. This endocrine system consists of the ligands IGF-I and IGF-II, the receptor tyrosine kinase (IGF-1R) and the mannose-6-phosphate receptor (IGF-IIR), and a family of high-affinity IGF-binding proteins

(IGFBPs) and IGFBP-related proteins, which modulate IGF/IGF receptor biological activities, any of which change in many disease states [168–170]. IGF-1R overexpression has been found in a range of tumor types and is a predictor of poor prognosis in many cancers. IGF-1R signaling plays critical roles in the development and progression of cancer by allowing cells to overcome the propensity to die via apoptosis, necrosis, or autophagy in response to uncontrolled replication, loss of substrate adhesion, hypoxia, and therapeutic stress (Fig. 1.4).

Ligand activation of IGF-1R results in phosphorylation and membrane recruitment of insulin receptor substrate proteins (IRSs) and activation of intracellular signaling pathways including Ras/mitogen-activated protein kinase (MAPK) and phosphatidylinositol-3 kinase (PI3K)/AKT/mTOR that in turn control the various IGF-mediated biological effects [171]. IGFs are potent mitogens and antiapoptotic factors for many normal and malignant tissues [172]. Both receptor activation and these downstream signaling cascades are therapeutic target candidates.

Perturbations in intrinsic expression of IGF axis components are implicated in susceptibility and progression of CaP [173–181]. IGF-1R expression is elevated in metastatic [177] and CRPC [17, 20]. Furthermore, maintaining IGF-I responsiveness facilitates CaP survival and growth and is achieved

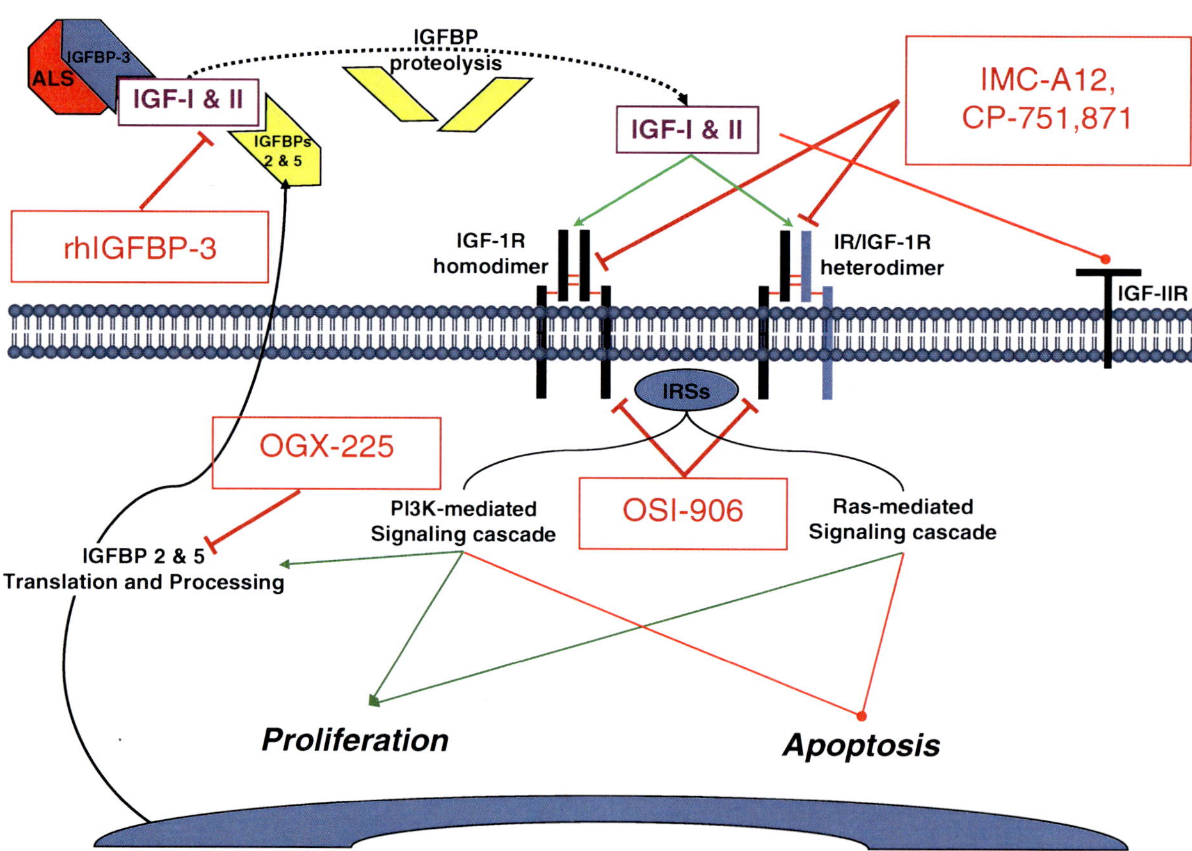

Fig. 1.4 Rational Therapeutic Targeting of Insulin-like Growth Factor Axis. Insulin-like growth factors I and II (IGF-I & II) are sequestered in circulation by IGF-binding protein (IGFBP)-3/acid-labile subunit (ALS). IGFBPs -2 and -5 produced by tumor cells extract IGFs from IGFBP-3/ALS complex and release IGFs into the pericellular space upon proteolysis to facilitate IGF receptor binding and activation of proliferative and survival signaling via PI3K and Ras cascades. Retention of IGFs in the pericellular space can be competitively suppressed by administration of recombinant human IGFBP-3 (rhIGFBP-3) and by suppression of IGFBP-2 & -5 expression by OGX-225 antisense oligonucleotide. IGF-1R activation can be blocked by small molecule tyrosine kinase inhibitors such as OSI-906 and by induction of internalization and degradation by humanized anti-IGF-1R antibodies such as IMC-A12 and CP-751,871

through androgen-modulated IGF-1R expression [20, 182, 183]. While CaP cells can adapt to enhance IGF responsiveness, accumulating evidence indicates that paracrine sources of IGF-I and IGFBPs are also important mediators of CaP progression [184–187]. Such observations directly implicate the IGF axis as a mediator of CRPC progression and mark IGF-related signaling an attractive therapeutic target [188–192]. The clinical potential of a number of immunologic, antisense, and small molecules is now being investigated. As previously reviewed, these approaches convincingly demonstrate that perturbing IGF-1R availability significantly impacts growth and survival of in vitro and xenograft model systems.

The long list of TKIs and antibodies targeting IGF-1R highlights the high level of enthusiasm for this target in prostate and many other cancers. Many humanized antibodies targeting the IGF-1R are in early clinical development in CRPC and include IMC-A12 and CP-751,871 [193, 194]. IGF1R is highly homologous to insulin receptors (IRs) with 100% homology in the ATP-binding cleft commonly targeted for small molecule inhibitors. Because of their structural similarities, TKIs and Abs directed at IGF-1R often also affect signaling of IR. Small molecule IGF-1R kinase inhibitors, such as NVP-AEW541 [195, 196], initially showed great promise in preferentially targeting IGF-1R from its close homologue, the IR; however, the clinical use of such agents is hampered by off-target toxicity. Preclinical data of newly emerging agents, such as OSI-906 that showed strong antitumor activity and reduced incidence of IR-mediated side effects, and this TKI that is in Phase 1 trials are forthcoming [197].

IGFBPs and CRPC

IGFBPs are a family of six circulating proteins that bind IGF-I and -II with equal or greater affinity than that of the IGF receptors and regulate IGF distribution, function, and activity [198, 199]. IGFBPs-2, 3, 4, 5, and 6 are expressed in prostatic tissues and cell lines [200–204]. IGFBP-2, 4, and 5 levels are correlated, while IGFBP-3 levels are inversely associated, with poor prognosis [200, 204]. The correlation between changes in IGFBP levels and concomitant changes in IGF-1R and IGF levels, disease state, and androgen ablation therapy implicates these adaptive responses in influencing disease progression.

Although it is clear that increased IGFBP-3 and 4 levels antagonize IGF signaling and increase sensitivity to apoptotic stress [205–207], other IGFBPs have been suggested to both inhibit and enhance IGF-1R-mediated signaling [208–211]. IGFBP-2 is one such factor whose expression is elevated in patients undergoing androgen ablation therapy [19]. Inhibiting IGFBP-2 expression in LNCaP cells increased androgen withdrawal-induced apoptosis and suppressed xenograft growth in castrated hosts [19]. Additionally, overexpressing IGFBP-5 accelerated AI progression of LNCaP tumors [18], while inhibiting IGFBP-5 expression decreased AI progression and IGF-I-dependent growth [212]. However, while elevated IGFBP-2 and 5 levels appear to contribute to disease progression at least in part by enhancing IGF responsiveness, IGFBPs have also been attributed with IGF-1R-independent activities that may contribute to prostatic oncogenesis [18, 208, 213–215] suggesting that binding and modulation of integrin signaling may also be critical to both IGF-1R-dependent and -independent IGFBP activities.

The primary IGF-binding protein, IGFBP-3, has also been attributed with IGF-dependent and -independent antiproliferative and proapoptotic activities on human cancer cells. In preclinical cancer models, recombinant human IGFBP-3 (rhIGFBP-3) is able to suppress growth of Herceptin-resistant breast, as well as lung and colon cancer xenografts as a single agent and on the latter xenograft model, augmented antitumor activity of irinotecan in combination [216, 217]. Consistent with the role of IGFBPs in modulating IGF signaling, these antitumor activities are correlated with suppression of AKT signaling in these models. In the CaP xenograft model, LAPC-4, rhIGFBP-3 synergized with the retinoid X receptor-alpha ligand VTP194204, to dramatically inhibit tumor growth by induction of apoptosis [218].

Also targeting IGFBPs is OGX-225, an ASO that effectively suppresses expression of IGFs -2, -3, and -5. Since IGFBP-2 and -5 are reproducibly upregulated in breast and CaPs, targeting their expression can selectively disrupt IGF signaling in tumor cells. Preclinical studies in human prostate, bladder, glioma, and breast cancer models indicate that reducing IGFBP-2 and IGFBP-5 production with OGX-225 promotes apoptosis and sensitize all of these tumor types to chemotherapy [219]. OGX-225 has completed preclinical pharmacology and is being evaluated for clinical trials.

Phosphatidylinositol 3-Kinase-Mediated Survival Signaling in CaP

A key oncogenic feature of IGF signaling is protection against cytotoxic stress mediated by PI3K/AKT/PTEN signal transduction-triggered intracellular signaling cascades [190, 220]. The serine/threonine kinase, AKT, is a prominent node in the convergence of various growth and survival-promoting intracellular signaling cascades. Its activation is triggered by PI3K and generation of phosphatidylinositol 3-, 4-, 5-triphosphate (PIP-3), which serves to recruit pleckstrin homology (PH) domain-containing proteins to the plasma membrane, including the S/T kinases, PDK-1 and -2, or ILK and AKT [221, 222].

A signature event impacting PI3K signaling in ~50% of advanced CaP is homozygous loss of the tumor-suppressor gene, *PTEN* [223] and among those patients who are not *PTEN* null, many exhibit loss of one *PTEN* allele [224]. Recently, hemizygous *PTEN* loss combined with the presence of TMPRSS2:ERG gene rearrangements were reported to increase the risk of biochemical progression [225]. PTEN is a tumor suppressor that functions as a 3′ phosphatase of PIP3. It acts as a negative regulator of cell migration, cell survival, and cell cycle progression [226] and is associated with increased resistance to chemotherapy and increased angiogenesis [227, 228]. Its loss results in aberrant accumulation of PIP3 and subsequent survival signals [224, 229, 230]. Demonstration that prostate-specific PTEN knock-out mice develop metastatic CaP [231] and that ectopic expression of PTEN reduces CaP cell growth and induces apoptosis [232–234] underscores the importance of PTEN in PCa establishment and progression. However, while loss of PTEN expression appears to be a prominent means by which CaP cells promote AI growth, which and how selection for hyperactivated PI3K signaling is invoked remains to be elucidated.

PI3K-induced recruitment and activation of AKT is a central antiapoptotic pathway triggered by growth factors [reviewed in235]. AKT directly phosphorylates and inactivates several proapoptotic factors, including Bad [236], procaspase-9 [237], GSK3β, and Forkhead transcription factors [238, 239] and activates c-FLIP, MDM2, mTOR, and the antiapoptotic transcription factor, NFκB [240]. In turn, mTOR complexed with rictor can regulate activation of AKT [241]. Association of constitutive AKT activation with resistance to chemo- and radiotherapeutics in diverse cancers, particularly CaP, has promoted research into the role(s) of subsequent downstream signaling in regulation of these phenomena [242, 243].

The mammalian target of rapamycin (mTOR) is an S/T kinase that regulates cell growth and division by integrating information regarding nutrient sufficiency, energy levels, and mitogenic signaling [244, 245]. mTOR relays proliferative signals from the PI3K pathway and information on amino acid sufficiency to critical mediators of protein translation. Inhibition of mTOR can reverse AKT-dependent malignant transformation of murine prostate [246] and doxorubicin resistance in CaP cell lines [227]. These downstream mediators, the 40S ribosomal subunit protein kinase (S6K1) and the eukaryotic initiation factor 4E binding protein-1 (4EBP1), are required for ribosomal biosynthesis and the production of proteins required for G_1/S transition [247, 248]. Monitoring the activation state of terminal kinase targets such as S6 and 4EBP1 can therefore be used as pharmacodynamic endpoints for activation of upstream signaling cascades due to loss of PTEN function, and in response to therapeutics that target proximal PI3K activation.

Angiogenesis

Angiogenesis is critically important for the growth and metastatic development of tumors. It involves migration and proliferation of endothelial cells from the microvasculature, controlled expression of proteolytic enzymes, breakdown and reassembly of extracellular matrix, and endothelial tube formation. Stimuli such as hypoxia can drive tumor, inflammatory, and connective tissue cells to generate a variety of angiogenic factors, including growth factors, cytokines, proteases, and cell adhesion molecules. Regulation of angiogenesis is thought to be largely dependent on a balance between pro- and antiangiogenic factors during the vascular network formation [249]. Angiogenesis plays an essential role in CaP development and metastasis. Therapy targeting tumor neovasculature therefore represents a promising area of research aimed at developing anticancer and antimetastasis therapeutics with many anti-angiogenic agents being evaluated in various phases of clinical trials [250].

Among the various proangiogenic factors, vascular endothelial growth factor (VEGF) is a major angiogenesis promoting factor, primarily acting on endothelial cells to induce their migration and proliferation via activation of tyrosine kinase receptors, VEGFR1 and VEGFR2. Increased expression of VEGF by tumors, resulting from e.g., hypoxia, can lead to tumor angiogenesis. As such, VEGF and its receptors represent key targets for new antiangiogenic drugs for treatment of cancer and have evoked a lot of interest [251, 252]. The VEGF level in plasma can serve as an independent prognostic factor in men with metastatic CRPC [253]. Antiangiogenic agents utilizing specific anti-VEGF monoclonal antibodies, such as bevacizumab (Avastin®), have been evaluated in CRPC. Interestingly, most antiangiogenic drugs failed to demonstrate significant activity as single agents in CRPC, but when bevacizumab was combined with docetaxel a 65% PSA response was achieved [254]. Unfortunately, a phase III study with accrual of 1,050 patients (CALGB 90401) recently reported that the addition of bevacizumab to docetaxel did not prolong OS.

In addition to VEGF, platelet-derived growth factor (PDGF) has been implicated in the progression of CaP and bone metastasis and is expressed in 80% of CRPC lesions [255]. Preclinical studies indicated that imatinib mesylate (Gleevec®), a PDGF inhibitor, is active in CaP cell lines, and a phase I trial of 21 patients with metastatic CRPC reported a 38% PSA response rate [256]. However, a randomized Phase II trial of imatinib and docetaxel in patients with CRPC showed increased toxicity without delaying progression. Sunitinib (Sutent®) and sorafenib (Nexavar®) are oral multitargeted tyrosine kinase inhibitors that inhibit RAF kinase, VEGF receptor tyrosine kinase, and the PDGF receptor; both are currently approved for the treatment of metastatic renal cell carcinoma [257]. Several phase II studies evaluated the activity of sorafenib in CRPC [258–260], demonstrating single agent decreases in PSA. Phase III trials of sunitinib and sorafenib are either planned or underway as second line therapy in docetaxel recurrent CRPC. Despite negative results with bevacizumab, the use of angiogenesis inhibitors continues to be evaluated as a promising treatment strategy for a variety of solid tumors, including CRPC.

Inflammation

Increasing evidence suggests that cancer-associated inflammation should be viewed as a seventh hallmark of cancer [261]. Most recently, such inflammation has been functionally linked to metastasis [262]. In fact, a number of inflammation-associated proteins, including tumor necrosis factor (TNF)-α, interleukin-1 (IL-1), interleukin-6 (IL-6), interleukin-11 (IL-11), TGFβ, cyclooxygenase 2 (COX-2), NFκB, Stat3, stromal-derived factor-1 (SDF1) and hedgehog, have been shown to facilitate CaP growth, tissue invasion and importantly, metastasis. Furthermore, inhibition of, for example, the COX-2 enzyme, which catalyzes the conversion of arachidonic acid to prostaglandins, i.e., important inflammatory mediators, has led to inhibition of tumor growth and suppression of metastasis in multiple cancers, including CaP [263]. Accordingly, inhibition of cancer-associated inflammation has emerged as a most promising new approach for treatment of metastatic CaP.

The nuclear transcription factor, NFκB, is a key regulator of immune, inflammatory and acute phase responses and has also been implicated in the control of cell proliferation and apoptosis [264]. It is overexpressed in many human cancers, including metastatic CaP [265, 266]. Stat3, which is both a cytoplasmic signaling molecule and a nuclear transcription factor, belongs to the seven-member Stat gene family of transcription factors. Recently, it has been reported that Stat3 is activated in clinical CaP metastasis and in recurrent CaP and may have a major effect on metastatic dissemination of the disease [267]. In view of this, NFkB and Stat3 could act as potential targets for inhibition of metastatic progression of CaP. RTA 402, an NFκB and Stat3 inhibitor, has demonstrated anticancer activity in preclinical studies and a recent clinical Phase I pancreatic cancer trial [268]. This inhibitor is now moving into Phase II trials. Moreover, several small molecule inhibitors for such targets are under preclinical development [269].

The chemokine stroma-derived factor, SDF-1/CXCL12, plays multiple roles in tumor pathogenesis. It has been demonstrated that CXCL12 promotes CaP growth, enhances tumor angiogenesis, contributes to immunosuppressive networks within the tumor microenvironment, and participates in tumor metastasis [270, 271]. The interaction of CXCL12 and its receptor CXCR4 leads to mitogen-activated protein kinase and phosphoinositide 3-kinase/Akt–mediated MMP-9 expression, migration, and tissue invasion of CaP cells [272]. Therefore, it stands to reason that the CXCL12/CXCR4 pathway is an important target for development of novel antimetastasis therapies. A wide variety of strategies, based on peptides (e.g., T22) [273], small molecules (e.g., AMD3100) [274], antibodies [275], and small interfering RNAs [276], have been used to target this pathway. Treatments in combination with current therapies seem to be especially promising in preclinical studies, and compounds are advancing into early stages of clinical development [277].

The hedgehog pathway has also been implicated in CaP development and metastasis [278]. The multi transmembrane protein, Patched (PTCH), is the receptor for various hedgehog ligands (Sonic, Indian, and Desert). In the absence of hedgehog, PTCH inhibits Smoothened (SMO), a G protein-coupled receptor protein encoded by the SMO gene of the hedgehog pathway [279]. When hedgehog binds to PTCH, SMO is disinhibited and initiates a signaling cascade that results in activation of GLI transcription factors and increased expression of target genes (including PTCH and GLI1). Inhibition of the hedgehog pathway induces apoptosis and decreases tumor invasiveness of CaP cells. For example, IPI-926 (Infinity Pharmaceuticals, Inc.), a small molecule inhibitor of the hedgehog signaling pathway, has shown potent efficacy and specific inhibition of the hedgehog pathway in multiple preclinical animal cancer models. Currently, IPI-926 is in a clinical Phase 1 trial for patients with advanced and/or metastatic solid tumors. GLI2 knockdown in preclinical models induces apoptosis, inhibits cancer growth, and chemosensitizes cells to chemotherapy in vitro and in vivo, providing preclinical proof-of-principle for CRPC [280]. The approach of regulating cancer-associated inflammation will be one of the most promising treatment strategies for a variety of tumors, including CaP.

Bone Metastases

Bone is the most frequent site for metastases of CaP. While the precise mechanism by which cancer cells home to bone is still unclear, it is generally accepted that bone can express certain chemo-attractants (e.g., SDF-1) or growth factors [e.g., TGFβ, IGF] that selectively retain/promote circulating CaP cells. As well, the cancer cells secrete many factors (e.g., uPA, TGFβ, FGFs, BMPs, PDGF, IGF, PTHrP, ET1) that activate bone stromal components, thus establishing a complex interplay between tumor and bone tissue.

Advances in the understanding of the biology of CaP, bone and interactions between tumor and bone stroma have led to the development of drugs directed against specific molecular sites in the CaP and host cells in the bone environment. Bone remodeling is a tightly regulated process of osteoclast-mediated bone resorption, counterbalanced by osteoblast-mediated bone formation. Disruption of this balance can lead to excessive bone loss or extra bone formation. Recently, a triad of key regulators of bone remodeling in bone oncology was discovered. It consists of the receptor activator of NF-κB (RANK), an essential receptor for osteoclast formation, its ligand RANKL, and the decoy receptor osteoprotegerin (OPG). OPG, a member of the tumor necrosis factor (TNF) receptor superfamily, can bind to RANKL and thus prevents activation of osteoclastic bone resorption. RANK, RANKL, and OPG are critical determinants of osteoclastogenesis, and increased RANK signaling is involved in metastasis of various cancers, including CaP [281–283]. These findings highlight the potential of RANKL inhibition as a novel treatment for patients with bone diseases and metastatic CaP [283–287]. Denosumab, a human monoclonal antibody, inhibits osteoclastic bone destruction by binding and neutralizing RANKL and has been evaluated in a randomized Phase 2 trial of CaP patients with bone metastases [288]. Denosumab suppressed bone turnover markers (BTMs) in CaP patients with bone metastases and elevated BTMs. Phase 3 trials of denosumab in patients with bone metastases of CaP are in progress (e.g., ClinicalTrials. gov Identifier: NCT00286091).

Endothelins (ETs) and their receptors (i.e., ET-B and ET-A) have emerged as potential targets for therapeutic intervention of CaP bone metastasis [289, 290]. Several clinical trial studies have shown that use of ET-A receptor antagonists (e.g., atrasentan, ZD4054) led to a significant increase in the time to disease progression [291]. While atrasentan failed to achieve its primary endpoints in two Phase III trials, indicators of anticancer activity were seen. Currently, the SWOG-S0421 trial is testing this further in patients with metastatic CRPC in a randomized phase III trial to compare the efficacy of docetaxel and prednisone with or without atrasentan. Several phase III trials of ZD4054 monotherapy or in combination with docetaxel are underway in CRPC.

c-Met is a receptor tyrosine kinase involved in multiple pathways linked to cancer, such as cell migration, tissue invasion, and metastasis and is upregulated in a large number of human cancers, including metastatic

CaP [292, 293]. Multiple agents to target c-Met or its ligand hepatocyte growth factor (HGF, scatter factor) are under development [294]. Like c-Met, the nonreceptor tyrosine kinase, Src, is considered part of the metastatic process [295]. Consequently, a number of Src inhibitors are under development. PSCA [296, 297], MEK5 [298], CDK5 [299], ASAP1 [300], and ID1 [301] have also been proposed as potential therapeutic targets for metastatic CRPC.

References

1. Huggins C, Hodges CV. Studies on prostatic cancer: I. The effect of castration, of estrogen and of androgen injection on serum phosphatases in metastatic carcinoma of the prostate. Cancer Res 1941;1:293–7.

2. Eisenberger MA, Blumenstein BA, Crawford ED, Miller G, McLeod DG, Loehrer PJ, Wilding G, Sears K, Culkin DJ, Thompson IM Jr, Bueschen AJ, Lowe BA. Bilateral orchiectomy with or without flutamide for metastatic prostate cancer. N Engl J Med. 1998;339(15):1036–42.

3. Hussain M, Tangen CM, Higano C, Schelhammer PF, Faulkner J, Crawford ED, Wilding G, Akdas A, Small EJ, Donnelly B, MacVicar G, Raghavan D; Southwest Oncology Group Trial 9346 (INT-0162). Absolute prostate-specific antigen value after androgen deprivation is a strong independent predictor of survival in new metastatic prostate cancer: data from Southwest Oncology Group Trial 9346 (INT-0162). J Clin Oncol. 2006;24(24):3984–90.

4. Berthold DR, Pond GR, Soban F, de Wit R, Eisenberger M, Tannock IF. Docetaxel plus prednisone or mitoxantrone plus prednisone for advanced prostate cancer: updated survival in the TAX 327 study. J Clin Oncol. 2008;26(2):242–5.

5. Isaacs, J.T., Wake, N., Coffey, D.S. and Sandberg, A.A. Genetic instability coupled to clonal selection as a mechanism for progression in prostatic cancer. Cancer Res. 1982; 42: 2353–71.

6. Feldman BJ and Feldman D. The development of androgen-independent prostate cancer. Nature Rev 2001;1:34–45.

7. Bruchovsky, N., Rennie, P.S., Coldman, A.J., Goldenberg, S.L., and Lawson, D.: Effects of androgen withdrawal on the stem cell composition of the Shionogi carcinoma. Cancer Res. 1990;50:2275–82.

8. Miyake H, Tolcher A, Gleave ME. Antisense Bcl-2 oligodeoxynucleotides delay progression to androgen-independence after castration in the androgen dependent Shionogi tumor model. Cancer Res 1999;59:4030–4.

9. Miyake H, Rennie P, Nelson C, Gleave ME. Testosterone-Repressed Prostate Message-2 (TRPM-2) is an Antiapoptotic Gene that confers resistance to androgen ablation in Prostate Cancer Xenograft Models. Cancer Res 2000;60:170–6.

10. Rocchi P, So A, Kojima S, Signaevsky M, Beraldi E, Fazli L, Hurtado-Coll A, Yamanka K and Gleave ME. heat shock protein 27 increases after androgen ablation and plays a cytoprotective role in hormone refractory prostate cancer. Cancer Res 2004;64(18):6595–602 IF 7.672.

11. Rocchi P, Beraldi E, Ettinger S, Fazli L, Vessella RL, Nelson C, M Gleave. Increased Hsp27 after androgen ablation facilitates androgen independent progression in prostate cancer via stat3-mediated suppression of apoptosis. Cancer Res 2005;65(23):11083–93.

12. Ettinger SL, Sobel R, Whitmore T, Akbari M, Bradley DR, Gleave ME and Nelson CC. Dysregulation of sterol response element binding proteins and downstream effectors in prostate cancer during progression to androgen-independence. Cancer Res 2004;64(6):2212–21. IF 7.672.

13. Locke JA, Guns ES, Lubik AA, Adomat HH, Hendy SC, Wood CA, Ettinger SL, Gleave ME, Nelson CC. Androgen levels increase by intratumoral de novo steroidogenesis during progression of castration-resistant prostate cancer. Cancer Res 2008;68(15):6407–15. IF 7.672.

14. Chen CD, Welsbie DS, Tran C, Baek SH, Chen R, Vessella R, Rosenfeld MG, Sawyers CL. Molecular determinants of resistance to antiandrogen therapy. Nat Med. 2004;10(1):33–9.

15. Craft N, Shostak Y, Carey M, and Sawyers C. A mechanism for hormone-independent prostate cancer through modulation of androgen receptor signaling by the HER-2/neu tyrosine kinase. Nat Med 1999;5:280–5.

16. Nickerson T, Miyake H, Gleave M, Pollak M. Castration-Induced Apoptosis of Androgen-Dependent Shionogi Carcinoma is Associated With Increased Expression of Genes Encoding Insulin-Like Growth Factor Binding Proteins Cancer Res 1999;59:3392–5.

17. Nickerson T, Chang F, Lorimer D, Smeekens SP, Sawyers CL, Pollak M. In vivo progression of LAPC-9 and LNCaP prostate cancer models to androgen independence is associated with increased expression of insulin-like growth factor I (IGF-I) and IGF-I receptor (IGF-IR). Cancer Res. 2001;61(16):6276–80.

18. Miyake H, Nelson C, Rennie P, Gleave ME. Overexpression of insulin-like growth factor binding protein-5 helps accelerate progression to androgen-independence in the human prostate LNCaP tumor model through activation of phosphatidylinositol 3'-kinase pathway. Endocrinology 2000;141:2257–65.

19. Kiyama S, Morrison K, Zellweger T, et al. Castration-induced increases in insulin-like growth factor-binding protein 2 promotes proliferation of androgen-independent human prostate LNCaP tumors. Cancer Res 2003;63:3575–84.

20. Krueckl SL, Sikes RA, Edlund NM, Bell RH, Hurtado-Coll A, Fazli L, Gleave ME, Cox ME. Increased insulin-like growth factor I receptor expression and signaling are components of androgen-independent progression in a lineage-derived prostate cancer progression model. Cancer Res. 2004;64(23):8620–9.

21. Simental JA, Sar M, Lane MV, French FS, Wilson EM. Transcriptional activation and nuclear targeting signals of the human androgen receptor. J Biol Chem 1991;266: 510–8.

22. Tsai MJ, O'Malley BW. Molecular mechanisms of action of steroid/thyroid receptor superfamily members. Ann Rev Biochem 1994;63:451–86.

23. Rennie PS, Bruchovsky N, Leco KJ, Sheppard PC, McQueen SA, Cheng H, Snoek R, Hamel, A, Bock, ME, MacDonald, BS, Nickel, BE, Chang, C, Liao, S, Cattini, PA & Matusik, RJ Characterization of two cis-acting DNA

elements involved in the androgen regulation of the proba-sin gene. Mol Endocrinol 1993;7:23–36.

24. Sun M, Yang L, Feldman RI, et al. Activation of phosphatidylinositol 3-kinase/Akt pathway by androgen through interaction of p85a, androgen receptor, and Src. J Biol Chem 2003;278:42992–3000.

25. Heinlein CA, Chang C. The roles of androgen receptors and androgen-binding proteins in nongenomic androgen actions. Mol Endocrinol 2002;16:2181–7.

26. Kousteni S, Bellido T, Plotkin LI, et al. Nongenotropic, sex-nonspecific signaling through the estrogen or androgen receptors: dissociation from transcriptional activity. Cell 2001;104:719–30.

27. Zhu ML and Kyprianou N. Androgen receptor and growth factor signaling cross-talk in prostate cancer cells. Endocr Relat Cancer 2008;15:841–49.

28. Fan W, Yanase T, Morinaga H, Okabe T, Nomura M, Daitoku H, Fukamizu A, Kato S, Takayanagi R and Nawata H. Insulin-like growth factor 1/insulin signaling activates androgen signaling through direct interactions of Foxo1 with androgen receptor. J Biol Chem 2007;282:7329–38.

29. Hobisch A, Eder IE, Putz T, Horninger W, Bartsch G, Klocker H and Culig Z. Interleukin-6 regulates prostate-specific protein expression in prostate carcinoma cells by activation of the androgen receptor. Cancer Res 1998;58:4640–5.

30. Culig Z, Hobisch A, Cronauer MV, Radmayr C, Trapman J, Hittmair A, Bartsch G and Klocker H. Androgen receptor activation in prostatic tumor cell lines by insulin-like growth factor-I, keratinocyte growth factor, and epidermal growth factor. Cancer Res 1994;54:5474–8.

31. Mostaghel EA, Page ST, Lin DW, Fazli L, Coleman IM, True LD, Knudsen B, Hess DL, Nelson CC, Matsumoto AM, Bremner WJ, Gleave ME and Nelson PS. Intraprostatic androgens and androgen-regulated gene expression persist after testosterone suppression: therapeutic implications for castration-resistant prostate cancer. Cancer Res. 2007;67:5033–41.

32. Gregory CW, Johnson RT,Jr, Mohler JL, French FS and Wilson EM. Androgen receptor stabilization in recurrent prostate cancer is associated with hypersensitivity to low androgen. Cancer Res. 2001;61:2892–8.

33. Mohler JL, Gregory CW, Ford OH III, Kim D, Weaver CM, Petrusz P, Wilson EM and French FS. The androgen axis in recurrent prostate cancer. Clin Cancer Res 2004;10:440–8.

34. Titus MA, Schell MJ, Lih FB, Tomer KB and Mohler JL. Testosterone and dihydrotestosterone tissue levels in recurrent prostate cancer. Clin Cancer Res 2005;11:4653–7.

35. Labrie F. Adrenal androgens and intracrinology. Semin Reprod Med 2004;22:299–309.

36. Snoek R, Cheng H, Margiotti K, Wafa LA, Wong CA, Wong EC, Fazli L, Nelson CC, Gleave ME, Rennie PS. In vivo knockdown of the androgen receptor results in growth inhibition and regression of well-established, castration-resistant prostate tumors. Clin Cancer Res 2009;15(1):39–47.

37. Stanbrough M, Bubley GJ, Ross K, Golub TR, Rubin MA, Penning TM, Febbo PG and Balk SP. Increased expression of genes converting adrenal androgens to testosterone in androgen-independent prostate cancer. Cancer Res 2006;66:2815–25.

38. Visakorpi T, Hyytinen E, Koivisto P, Tanner M, Keinanen R, Palmberg C, Palotie A, Tammela T, Isola J and Kallioniemi O. In vivo amplification of the androgen receptor gene and progression of human prostate cancer. Nat Genet 1995;9:401–6.

39. Koivisto P, Kononen J, Palmberg C, Tammela T, Hyytinen E, Isola J, Trapman J, Cleutjens K, Noordzij A, Visakorpi T, Kallioniemi OP. Androgen receptor gene amplification: a possible molecular mechanism for androgen deprivation therapy failure in prostate cancer. Cancer Res 1997;57:314–9.

40. Culig Z, Hobisch A, Cronauer MV, Cato AC, Hittmair A, Radmayr C, Eberle J, Bartsch G, Klocker H. Mutant androgen receptor detected in an advanced-stage prostatic carcinoma is activated by adrenal androgens and progesterone. Mol Endocrinol 1993;7:1541–50.

41. Taplin ME, Bubley GJ, Shuster TD, Frantz ME, Spooner AE, Ogata GK, Keer HN, Balk SP. Mutation of the androgen-receptor gene in metastatic androgen- independent prostate cancer. N Engl J Med 1995;332:1393–8.

42. Taplin ME, Bubley GJ, Ko YJ, Small EJ, Upton M, Rajeshkumar B, Balk SP. Selection for androgen receptor mutations in prostate cancers treated with androgen antagonist. Cancer Res 1999;59:2511–5.

43. Zhao XY, Malloy PJ, Krishnan AV, Swami S, Navone NM, Peehl DM, Feldman D. Glucocorticoids can promote androgen-independent growth of prostate cancer cells through a mutated androgen receptor. Nat Med 2000;6:703–6.

44. Hu R, Dunn TA, Wei S, Isharwal S, Veltri RW, Humphreys E, Han M, Partin AW, Vessella RL, Isaacs WB, Bova GS, Luo J. Ligand-independent androgen receptor variants derived from splicing of cryptic exons signify hormone-refractory prostate cancer. Cancer Res 2009;69(1):16–22.

45. Steinkamp MP, O'Mahony OA, Brogley M, Rehman H, Lapensee EW, Dhanasekaran S, Hofer MD, Kuefer R, Chinnaiyan A, Rubin MA, Pienta KJ, Robins DM. Treatment-dependent androgen receptor mutations in prostate cancer exploit multiple mechanisms to evade therapy. Cancer Res 2009;69(10):4434–42.

46. Gregory CW, He B, Johnson RT, Ford OH, Mohler JL, French FS, Wilson EM. A mechanism for androgen receptor-mediated prostate cancer recurrence after androgen deprivation therapy. Cancer Res 2001;61:4315–9.

47. Tillman JE, Yuan J, Gu G, Fazli L, Ghosh R, Flynt AS, Gleave M, Rennie PS, Kasper S. DJ-1 binds androgen receptor directly and mediates its activity in hormonally treated prostate cancer cells. Cancer Res 2007;67(10): 4630–7.

48. Zoubeidi A, Zardan A, Beraldi E, Fazli L, Sowery R, Rennie P, Nelson C, Gleave M: Cooperative interactions between androgen receptor (AR) and heat-shock protein 27 facilitate AR transcriptional activity. Cancer Res 2007; 67(21):10455–65.

49. Nazareth LV, Weigel NL. Activation of the human androgen receptor through a protein kinase A signaling pathway. J Biol Chem 1996;271:19900–7.

50. Sadar MD. Androgen-independent induction of prostate-specific antigen gene expression via cross-talk between the androgen receptor and protein kinase A signal transduction pathways. J Biol Chem 1999;274:7777–83.

51. Yeh S, Lin HK, Kang HY, Thin TH, Lin MF, Chang C. From HER2/Neu signal cascade to androgen receptor and its coactivators: a novel pathway by induction of androgen target genes through MAP kinase in prostate cancer cells. Proc Natl Acad Sci USA 1999;96:5458–63.

52. Chen S, Xu Y, Yuan X, Bubley GJ, Balk SP. Androgen receptor phosphorylation and stabilization in prostate cancer by cyclin-dependent kinase 1. Proc Natl Acad Sci USA 2006;103:15969–74.

53. Mellinghoff IK, Vivanco I, Kwon A, Tran C, Wongvipat J, Sawyers CL. HER2/neu kinase-dependent modulation of androgen receptor function through effects on DNA binding and stability. Cancer Cell 2004;6:517–27.

54. Signoretti S, Montironi R, Manola J, Altimari A, Tam C, Bubley G, Balk S, Thomas G, Kaplan I, Hlatky L, Hahnfeldt P, Kantoff P, Loda M. Her-2-neu expression and progression toward androgen independence in human prostate cancer. J Natl Cancer Inst 2000;92:1918–25.

55. Kuiper GG, Brinkmann AO. Phosphotryptic peptide analysis of the human androgen receptor: detection of a hormone-induced phosphopeptide. Biochemistry 1995;34:1851–7.

56. Zhou ZX, Kemppainen JA, Wilson EM. Identification of three proline-directed phosphorylation sites in the human androgen receptor. Mol Endocrinol 1995;9:605–15.

57. Gioeli D, Ficarro SB, Kwiek JJ, Aaronson D, Hancock M, Catling AD, White FM, Christian RE, Settlage RE, Shabanowitz J, Hunt DF, Weber MJ. Androgen receptor phosphorylation. Regulation and identification of the phosphorylation sites. J Biol Chem 2002;277:29304–14.

58. Guo Z, Dai B, Jiang T, Xu K, Xie Y, Kim O, Nesheiwat I, Kong X, Melamed J, Handratta VD, Njar VC, Brodie AM, Yu LR, Veenstra TD, Chen H, Qiu Y. Regulation of androgen receptor activity by tyrosine phosphorylation. Cancer Cell 2006;10:309–19.

59. Kraus S, Gioeli D, Vomastek T, Gordon V, Weber MJ. Receptor for activated C kinase 1 (RACK1) and Src regulate the tyrosine phosphorylation and function of the androgen receptor. Cancer Res 2006;66:11047–54.

60. Mahajan NP, Liu Y, Majumder S, Warren MR, Parker CE, Mohler JL, Earp HS, Whang YE. Activated Cdc42- associated kinase Ack1 promotes prostate cancer progression via androgen receptor tyrosine phosphorylation. Proc Natl Acad Sci USA 2007;104:8438–43.

61. Geller J, Albert JD, Nachtsheim DA, Loza D. Comparison of prostatic cancer tissue dihydrotestosterone levels at the time of relapse following orchiectomy or estrogen therapy. J Urol 1984;132:693–6.

62. Page ST, Lin DW, Mostaghel EA, Hess DL, True LD, Amory JK, Nelson PS, Matsumoto AM, Bremner WJ. Persistent intraprostatic androgen concentrations after medical castration in healthy men. J Clin Endocrinol Metab 2006;91:3850–6.

63. Auchus RJ. The backdoor pathway to dihydrotestosterone. Trends Endocrinol Metab 2004;15(9):432–8.

64. Tran C, Ouk S, Clegg NJ, Chen Y, Watson PA, Arora V, Wongvipat J, Smith-Jones PM, Yoo D, Kwon A, Wasielewska T, Welsbie D, Chen CD, Higano CS, Beer TM, Hung DT, Scher HI, Jung ME, Sawyers CL. Development of a second-generation antiandrogen for treatment of advanced prostate cancer. Science. 2009;324(5928):787–90.

65. Small EJ, Ryan CJ. The case for secondary hormonal therapies in the chemotherapy age. J Urol 2006;176(6 Pt 2):S66–71.

66. Attard G, Reid AH, Yap TA, Raynaud F, Dowsett M, Settatree S, Barrett M, Parker C, Martins V, Folkerd E, Clark J, Cooper CS, Kaye SB, Dearnaley D, Lee G, de Bono JS. Phase I clinical trial of a selective inhibitor of CYP17, abiraterone acetate, confirms that castration-resistant prostate cancer commonly remains hormone driven. J Clin Oncol 2008;26(28):4563–71.

67. Attard G, Reid AH, A'hern R, Parker C, Oommen NB, Folkerd E, Messiou C, Molife LR, Maier G, Thompson E, Olmos D, Sinha R, Lee G, Dowsett M, Kaye SB, Dearnaley D, Kheoh T, Molina A, de Bono JS. Selective Inhibition of CYP17 With Abiraterone Acetate Is Highly Active in the Treatment of Castration-Resistant Prostate. Cancer J Clin Oncol 2009;27(23);3742–8.

68. Attard G, Reid AH, Olmos D, de Bono JS. Antitumor activity with CYP17 blockade indicates that castration-resistant prostate cancer frequently remains hormone driven. Cancer Res 2009;69(12):4937–40.

69. Georget V, Térouanne B, Nicolas JC, Sultan C. Mechanism of antiandrogen action: key role of hsp90 in conformational change and transcriptional activity of the androgen receptor.Biochemistry. 2002;41(39):11824–31.

70. Buchanan G, Ricciardelli C, Harris JM, Prescott J, Yu ZC, Jia L, Butler LM, Marshall VR, Scher HI, Gerald WL, Coetzee GA, Tilley WD. Control of androgen receptor signaling in prostate cancer by the cochaperone small glutamine rich tetratricopeptide repeat containing protein alpha. Cancer Res 2007;67(20):10087–9.

71. Solit DB, Zheng FF, Drobnjak M, Münster PN, Higgins B, Verbel D, Heller G, Tong W, Cordon-Cardo C, Agus DB, Scher HI, Rosen N. 17-Allylamino-17-demethoxygeldanamycin induces the degradation of androgen receptor and HER-2/neu and inhibits the growth of prostate cancer xenografts. Clin Cancer Res. 2002;8(5):986–93.

72. Shatkina L, Mink S, Rogatsch H, et al. The cochaperone Bag-1 L enhances androgen receptor action via interaction with the NH2-terminal region of the receptor. Mol Cell Biol 2003;23:7189–97.

73. Cheung-Flynn J, Prapapanich V, Cox MB, Riggs DL Suarez-Quian C, Smith DF. Physiological role for the cochaperone FKBP52 in androgen receptor signaling. Mol Endocrinol 2005;19:1654–66.

74. Yang Z, Wolf IM, Chen H, et al. FK506-binding protein 52 is essential to uterine reproductive physiology controlled by the progesterone receptor A isoform. Mol Endocrinol 2006;20:2682–94.

75. Paul C, Manero F, Gonin S, Kretz-Remy C, Virot S, Arrigo AP. Hsp27 as a negative regulator of cytochrome C release. Mol Cell Biol 2002;22:816–34.

76. Concannon CG, Orrenius S, Samali A. Hsp27 inhibits cytochrome c-mediated caspase activation by sequestering both pro-caspase-3 and cytochrome c. Gene Expr 2001; 9:195–201.

77. Parcellier A, Schmitt E, Gurbuxani S, et al. HSP27 is a ubiquitin-binding protein involved in I-nBa proteasomal degradation. Mol Cell Biol 2003;23:5790–802.

78. Chauhan D, Li G, Podar K, et al. The bortezomib/ proteasome inhibitor PS-341 and triterpenoid CDDO-Im induce

synergistic anti-multiple myeloma (MM) activity and overcome bortezomib resistance. Blood 2004;103:3158–66.

79. McCollum AK, Teneyck CJ, Sauer BM, Toft DO, Erlichman C. Up-regulation of heat shock protein 27 induces resistance to 17-allylamino-demethoxygeldanamycin through a glutathione-mediated mechanism. Cancer Res 2006;66(22):10967–75.

80. Hotte SJ, Yu EY, Hirte HW, Higano CS, Gleave M, Chi KN. OGX-427, a 2'methoxyethyl antisense oligonucleotide (ASO), against HSP27: Results of a first-in-human trial. J Clin Oncol 2009;27:15s, (suppl. abstr 3506).

81. Jin Z, El-Deiry WS.Overview of cell death signaling pathways. Cancer Biol Ther 2005;4(2):139–63.

82. Russo A, Terrasi M, Agnese V, Santini D, Bazan V. Apoptosis: a relevant tool for anticancer therapy. Ann Oncol 2006; Suppl. 7:vii115–23. Review.

83. Letai AG. Diagnosing and exploiting cancer's addiction to blocks in apoptosis. Nat Rev Cancer 2008;8(2):121–32.

84. Danson S, Dean E, Dive C, Ranson M. IAPs as a target for anticancer therapy. Curr Cancer Drug Targets 2007;7(8):785–94.

85. Lowe SW, Lin AW. Apoptosis in cancer. Carcinogenesis. 2000;21(3):485–95.

86. Wajant H. The Fas signaling pathway: more than a paradigm. Science 2002;296(5573):1635–6.

87. Tsujimoto Y & Croce CM. Analysis of the structure, transcripts, and protein products of bcl-2, the gene involved in human follicular lymphoma. Proc Natl Acad Sci USA 1986;83:5214–8.

88. Reed JC. Bcl-2 and the regulation of programmed cell death. J Cell Biol 124, 1-6 (1994).

89. Miyashita T & Reed JC. Bcl-2 oncoprotein blocks chemotherapy-induced apoptosis in a human leukemia cell line. Blood 1993;81:151–7.

90. McDonnell TJ et al. Expression of the protooncogene bcl-2 in the prostate and its association with emergence of androgen-independent prostate cancer. Cancer Res 1992;52:6940–4.

91. Kyprianou N, King ED, Bradbury D & Rhee JG. bcl-2 over-expression delays radiation-induced apoptosis without affecting the clonogenic survival of human prostate cancer cells. Int J Cancer 1997;70:341–8.

92. Raffo AJ et al. Overexpression of bcl-2 protects prostate cancer cells from apoptosis in vitro and confers resistance to androgen depletion in vivo. Cancer Res 1995;55:4438–45.

93. Gleave M et al. Progression to androgen independence is delayed by adjuvant treatment with antisense Bcl-2 oligodeoxynucleotides after castration in the LNCaP prostate tumor model. Clin Cancer Res 1999;5:2891–8.

94. Zangemeister-Wittke U et al. A novel bispecific antisense oligonucleotide inhibiting both bcl-2 and bcl-xL expression efficiently induces apoptosis in tumor cells. Clin Cancer Res 2000;6:2547–55.

95. Jansen B et al. bcl-2 antisense therapy chemosensitizes human melanoma in SCID mice. Nat Med 1998;4:232–4.

96. Jansen B et al. Chemosensitisation of malignant melanoma by BCL2 antisense therapy. Lancet 2000;356:1728–33.

97. Rai KR & Moore JO. Phase 3 randomized trial of fludarabine/cyclophosphamide chemotherapy with or without oblimersen sodium (Bcl-2 antisense; genasense; G3139) for patients with relapsed or refractory chronic lymphocytic leukemia (CLL). Blood 2004;104:100a.

98. Chanan-Khan A et al. Randomized Multicenter Phase 3 Trial of High-Dose Dexamethasone (dex) with or without Oblimersen Sodium (G3139; Bcl-2 antisense; Genasense) for Patients with Advanced Multiple Myeloma (MM). Blood 2004;104:413a.

99. Chi KN et al. A phase I dose-finding study of combined treatment with an antisense Bcl-2 oligonucleotide (Genasense) and mitoxantrone in patients with metastatic hormone-refractory prostate cancer. Clin Cancer Res 2001;7:3920–7.

100. Tolcher AW, Chi K, Kuhn J, Gleave M, Patnaik A, Takimoto C, Schwartz G, Thompson I, Berg K, D'Aloisio S, Murray N, Frankel SR, Izbicka E, Rowinsky E. A phase II, pharmacokinetic, and biological correlative study of oblimersen sodium and docetaxel in patients with hormone-refractory prostate cancer. Clin Cancer Res 2005;11(10):3854–61.

101. Sternberg CN, Dumez H, Van Poppel H, Skoneczna I, Sella A, Daugaard G, Gil T, Graham J, Carpentier P, Calabro F, Collette L, Lacombe D; for the EORTC Genitourinary Tract Cancer Group. Docetaxel plus oblimersen sodium (Bcl-2 antisense oligonucleotide): an EORTC multicenter, randomized phase II study in patients with castration-resistant prostate cancer. Ann Oncol. 2009 Mar 17.

102. Bedikian AY, Millward M, Pehamberger H, Conry R, Gore M, Trefzer U, Pavlick AC, DeConti R, Hersh EM, Hersey P, Kirkwood JM, Haluska FG; Oblimersen Melanoma Study Group. Bcl-2 antisense (oblimersen sodium) plus dacarbazine in patients with advanced melanoma: the Oblimersen Melanoma Study Group. J Clin Oncol 2006;24(29):4738–45.

103. Chanan-Khan AA, Niesvizky R, Hohl RJ, Zimmerman TM, Christiansen NP, Schiller GJ, Callander N, Lister J, Oken M, Jagannath S. Phase III randomised study of dexamethasone with or without oblimersen sodium for patients with advanced multiple myeloma. Leuk Lymphoma 2009;50(4):559–65.

104. Han Z et al. Isolation and characterization of an apoptosis-resistant variant of human leukemia HL-60 cells that has switched expression from Bcl-2 to Bcl-xL. Cancer Res 1996;56:1621–8.

105. Leech, S.H. et al. Induction of apoptosis in lung-cancer cells following bcl-xL anti-sense treatment. Int J Cancer 2000;86:570–6.

106. Simoes-Wust, AP et al. Bcl-xl antisense treatment induces apoptosis in breast carcinoma cells. Int J Cancer 2000;87:582–90.

107. Lebedeva I, Rando R, Ojwang J, Cossum P & Stein CA. Bcl-xL in prostate cancer cells: effects of overexpression and down-regulation on chemosensitivity. Cancer Res 2000;60:6052–60.

108. Leung S, Miyake H, Zellweger T, Tolcher A & Gleave ME. Synergistic chemosensitization and inhibition of progression to androgen independence by antisense Bcl-2 oligodeoxynucleotide and paclitaxel in the LNCaP prostate tumor model. Int J Cancer 2001;91:846–50.

109. Miyake H, Monia BP & Gleave ME. Inhibition of progression to androgen-independence by combined adjuvant treatment with antisense BCL-XL and antisense Bcl-2 oligonucleotides plus taxol after castration in the Shionogi tumor model. Int J Cancer 2000;86:855–62.

110. Cragg MS, Harris C, Strasser A, Scott CL. Unleashing the power of inhibitors of oncogenic kinases through BH3 mimetics. Nat Rev Cancer 2009;9(5):321–6.

111. Labi V, Grespi F, Baumgartner F, Villunger A.Targeting the Bcl-2-regulated apoptosis pathway by BH3 mimetics: a breakthrough in anticancer therapy? Cell Death Differ 2008;15(6):977–87.

112. Jones SE, Jomary C. Clusterin. Int J Biochem Cell Biol 2002;34:427–31.

113. Trougakos IP, Gonos ES. Clusterin/apolipoprotein J in human aging and cancer. Int J Biochem Cell Biol 2002;34:1430–48.

114. Shannan B, Seifert M, Leskov K, Willis J, Boothman D, Tilgen W, Reichrath J. Challenge and promise: roles for clusterin in pathogenesis, progression and therapy of cancer. Cell Death Differ 2006;13(1):12–9.

115. Yang CR, Leskov K, Hosley-Eberlein K, Criswell T, Pink JJ, Kinsella TJ, Boothman DA. Nuclear clusterin/XIP8, an x-ray-induced Ku70-binding protein that signals cell death. Proc Natl Acad Sci USA 2000;97:5907–12.

116. Zhang Q, Zhou W, Kundu S, et al. The leader sequence triggers and enhances several functions of clusterin and is instrumental in the progression of human prostate cancer in vivo and in vitro. BJU Int 2006;98:452–60.

117. Leskov KS, Klokov DY, Li J, et al. Synthesis and functional analyses of nuclear clusterin, a cell death protein. J Biol Chem 2003;278:11590–600.

118. Carver JA, Rekas A, Thorn DC, Wilson MR. Small heat-shock proteins and clusterin: intra- and extracellular molecular chaperones with a common mechanism of action and function? IUBMB Life 2003;55:661–8.

119. Zhang H, Kim JK, Edwards CA, et al. Clusterin inhibits apoptosis by interacting with activated Bax. Nat Cell Biol 2005;7:909–15.

120. Trougakos IP, Lourda M, Antonelou MH, Kletsas D, Gorgoulis VG, Papassideri IS, Zou Y, Margaritis LH, Boothman DA, Gonos ES. Intracellular clusterin inhibits mitochondrial apoptosis by suppressing p53-activating stress signals and stabilizing the cytosolic Ku70-Bax protein complex. Clin Cancer Res 2009;15(1):48–59.

121. Nakanishi C, Toi M. Nuclear factor-kappaB inhibitors as sensitizers to anticancer drugs. Nat Rev Cancer 2005;5:297–309.

122. Beg AA, Baltimore D. An essential role for NF-kappaB in preventing TNF-alpha-induced cell death. Science 1996;274:782–4.

123. Jin RJ, Lho Y, Connelly L, et al. The nuclear factor-kappaB pathway controls the progression of prostate cancer to androgen-independent growth. Cancer Res 2008;68:6762–9.

124. Dai C, Whitesell L, Rogers AB, Lindquist S. Heat shock factor 1 is a powerful multifaceted modifier of carcinogenesis. Cell 2007;130(6):1005–1.

125. Whitesell L, Lindquist S. Inhibiting the transcription factor HSF1 as an anticancer strategy. Expert Opin Ther Targets 2009;13(4):469–78.

126. Bayon Y, Ortiz MA, Lopez-Hernandez FJ, Howe PH, Piedrafita FJ. The retinoid antagonist MX781 induces clusterin expression in prostate cancer cells via heat shock factor-1 and activator protein-1 transcription factors. Cancer Res 2004;64:5905–12.

127. Loison F, Debure L, Nizard P, le Goff P, Michel D, le Drean Y. Up-regulation of the clusterin gene after proteotoxic stress: implication of HSF1-HSF2 heterocomplexes. Biochem J 2006;395:223–31.

128. Criswell T, Beman M, Araki S, Leskov K, Cataldo E, Mayo LD, Boothman DA. Delayed activation of insulin-like growth factor-1 receptor/Src/MAPK/Egr-1 signaling regulates clusterin expression, a pro-survival factor. J Biol Chem 2005;280(14):14212–21.

129. Cochrane DR, Wang Z, Muramaki M, Gleave ME, Nelson CC: Differential regulation of clusterin and its isoforms by androgens in prostate cells. J Biol Chem 2007;282(4):2278–87.

130. Sensibar JA, Sutkowski DM, Raffo A, et al. Prevention of cell death induced by tumor necrosis factor alpha in LNCaP cells by overexpression of sulfated glycoprotein-2 (clusterin). Cancer Res 1995;55:2431–7.

131. Zellweger T, Chi K, Miyake H, et al. Enhanced radiation sensitivity in prostate cancer by inhibition of the cell survival protein clusterin. Clin Cancer Res 2002;8:3276–84.

132. Miyake H, Chi KN, Gleave ME. Antisense TRPM-2 oligodeoxynucleotides chemosensitize human androgen-independent PC-3 prostate cancer cells both in vitro and in vivo. Clin Cancer Res 2000;6:1655–63.

133. Redondo M, Villar E, Torres-Munoz J, et al. Overexpression of clusterin in human breast carcinoma. Am J Path 2000;157:393–9.

134. Miyake H, Gleave M, Kamidono S, et al. Overexpression of clusterin in transitional cell carcinoma of the bladder is related to disease progression and recurrence. Urology 2002;59:150–4.

135. July LV, Beraldi E, So A, et al. Nucleotide-based therapies targeting clusterin chemosensitize human lung adenocarcinoma cells both in vitro and in vivo. Mol Cancer Ther 2004;3:223–32.

136. Miyake H, Hara S, Arakawa S, et al. Over expression of clusterin is an independent prognostic factor for nonpapillary renal cell carcinoma. J Urol 2002;167:703–6.

137. Chen X, Halberg RB, Ehrhardt WM, et al. Clusterin as a biomarker in murine and human intestinal neoplasia. Proc Natl Acad Sci USA 2003;100:9530–5.

138. Steinberg J, Oyasu R, Lang S, et al. Intracellular levels of SGP-2 (Clusterin) correlate with tumor grade in prostate cancer. Clin Cancer Res 1997;3:1707–11.

139. Cao C, Shinohara ET, Li H, et al. Clusterin as a therapeutic target for radiation sensitization in a lung cancer model. Int J Radiat Oncol Biol Phys 2005;63:1228–36.

140. Gleave M, Jansen B. Clusterin and IGFBPs as antisense targets in prostate cancer. Ann N Y Acad Sci 2003;1002:95–104.

141. Chi KN, Zoubeidi A, Gleave ME. Custirsen (OGX-011): a second-generation antisense inhibitor of clusterin for the treatment of cancer. Expert Opin Investig Drugs. 2008;17(12):1955–62.

142. Zellweger T, Miyake H, Cooper S, et al. Antitumor activity of antisense clusterin oligonucleotides is improved in vitro and in vivo by incorporation of 2'-O-(2-methoxy)ethyl chemistry. J Pharmacol Exp Ther 2001;298:934–40.

143. Chi KN, Eisenhauer E, Fazli L, Jones EC, Goldenberg SL, Powers J, Tu D, Gleave ME. A phase I pharmacokinetic and pharmacodynamic study of OGX-011, a 2'-methoxy-ethyl antisense oligonucleotide to clusterin, in patients with localized prostate cancer. J Natl Cancer Inst. 2005;97(17):1287–96.

144. Chi KN, Hotte SJ, Yu E, Tu D, Eigl B, Tannock I, Saad F, North S, Powers J, Eisenhauer E. Mature results of a

randomized phase II study of OGX-011 in combination with docetaxel/prednisone versus docetaxel/prednisone in patients with metastatic castration-resistant prostate cancer. J Clin Oncol 2009;27:15s (Suppl; abstr 5012).

145. Garrido C, Brunet M, Didelot C, Zermati Y, Schmitt E, and Kroemer G. Heat shock proteins 27 and 70: anti-apoptotic proteins with tumorigenic properties. Cell Cycle 2006;5:2592–601.

146. Wu R, Kausar H, Johnson P, Montoya-Durango DE, Merchant M, and Rane MJ. Hsp27 regulates Akt activation and polymorphonuclear leukocyte apoptosis by scaffolding MK2 to Akt signal complex. J Biol Chem 2007;282:21598–608.

147. Pandey P, Farber R, Nakazawa A, Kumar S, Bharti A, Nalin C, Weichselbaum R, Kufe D, and Kharbanda S. Hsp27 functions as a negative regulator of cytochrome c-dependent activation of procaspase-3. Oncogene 2000;19:1975–81.

148. Chauhan D, Li G, Hideshima T, Podar K, Mitsiades C, Mitsiades N, Catley L, Tai YT, Hayashi T, Shringarpure R, Burger R, Munshi N, Ohtake Y, Saxena S, and Anderson KC. Hsp27 inhibits release of mitochondrial protein Smac in multiple myeloma cells and confers dexamethasone resistance. Blood 2003;102:3379–86.

149. Charette SJ, Lavoie JN, Lambert H, and Landry J. Inhibition of Daxx-mediated apoptosis by heat shock protein 27. Mol Cell Biol. 2000;20:7602–12.

150. Guay J, Lambert H, Gingras-Breton G, Lavoie JN, Huot J, and Landry J. 1997. Regulation of actin filament dynamics by p38 map kinase-mediated phosphorylation of heat shock protein 27. J Cell Sci 1997;110 (Pt 3):357–68.

151. Arrigo, AP, Virot S, Chaufour S, Firdaus W, Kretz-Remy C, and Diaz-Latoud C. Hsp27 consolidates intracellular redox homeostasis by upholding glutathione in its reduced form and by decreasing iron intracellular levels. Antioxid Redox Signal. 2005;7:414–22.

152. Parcellier A, Schmitt E, Gurbuxani S, Seigneurin-Berny D, Pance A, Chantome A, Plenchette S, Khochbin S, Solary E, and Garrido C. HSP27 is a ubiquitin-binding protein involved in I-kappaBalpha proteasomal degradation. Mol Cell Biol 2003;23:5790–802.

153. Park KJ, Gaynor RB, and Kwak YT. Heat shock protein 27 association with the I kappa B kinase complex regulates tumor necrosis factor alpha-induced NF-kappa B activation. J Biol Chem 2003;278:35272–8.

154. Konishi H, Matsuzaki H, Tanaka M, Takemura Y, Kuroda S, Ono Y, and Kikkawa U. Activation of protein kinase B (Akt/RAC-protein kinase) by cellular stress and its association with heat shock protein Hsp27. FEBS Lett 1997;410:493–8.

155. Rane, MJ, Pan Y, Singh S, Powell DW, Wu R, Cummins T, Chen Q, McLeish KR, and Klein JB. Heat shock protein 27 controls apoptosis by regulating Akt activation. J Biol Chem 2003;278:27828–35.

156. Manning BD, and Cantley LC. AKT/PKB signaling: navigating downstream. Cell 2007;129:1261–74.

157. Ciocca DR, and Calderwood SK. Heat shock proteins in cancer: diagnostic, prognostic, predictive, and treatment implications. Cell Stress Chaperones. 2005;10:86–103.

158. Garrido C, Fromentin A, Bonnotte B, Favre N, Moutet M, Arrigo AP, Mehlen P, and Solary E. 1998. Heat shock protein 27 enhances the tumorigenicity of immunogenic rat colon carcinoma cell clones. Cancer Res 1998;58:5495–9.

159. Kamada M, So A, Muramaki M, Rocchi P, Beraldi E, Gleave M. Hsp27 knockdown using nucleotide-based therapies inhibit tumor growth and enhance chemotherapy in human bladder cancer cells. Mol Cancer Ther 2007;1:299–308.

160. Shin KD, Yoon YJ, Kang YR, Son KH, Kim HM, Kwon BM, Han DC. KRIBB3, a novel microtubule inhibitor, induces mitotic arrest and apoptosis in human cancer cells. Biochem Pharmacol 2008;75(2):383–94.

161. Kostenko S, Johannessen M, Moens U.PKA-induced F-actin rearrangement requires phosphorylation of Hsp27 by the MAPKAP kinase MK5. Cell Signal 2009;21(5):712–8.

162. Schlapbach A, Feifel R, Hawtin S, Heng R, Koch G, Moebitz H, Revesz L, Scheufler C, Velcicky J, Waelchli R, Huppertz C. Pyrrolo-pyrimidones: a novel class of MK2 inhibitors with potent cellular activity. Bioorg Med Chem Lett 2008;18(23):6142–6.

163. Xu L, Bergan RC. Genistein inhibits matrix metalloproteinase type 2 activation and prostate cancer cell invasion by blocking the transforming growth factor beta-mediated activation of mitogen-activated protein kinase-activated protein kinase 2-27-kDa heat shock protein pathway. Mol Pharmacol 2006;70(3):869–77.

164. LeRoith D, Roberts CT, Jr. The insulin-like growth factor system and cancer. Cancer Lett 2003;195:127–37.

165. Baserga R, Peruzzi F, Reiss K. The IGF-1 receptor in cancer biology. Int J Cancer 2003;107:873–7.

166. Papatsoris AG, Karamouzis MV, Papavassiliou AG. Novel insights into the implication of the IGF-1 network in prostate cancer. Trends Mol Med 2005;11:52–5.

167. Ryan CJ, Haqq CM, Simko J, et al. Expression of insulin-like growth factor-1 receptor in local and metastatic prostate cancer. Urol Oncol 2007;25:134–40.

168. Baserga R. The IGF-I receptor in cancer research. Exp Cell Res 1999;253:1–6.

169. Lopez-Bermejo A, Buckway CK, Devi GR, et al. Characterization of insulin-like growth factor-binding protein-related proteins (IGFBP-rPs) 1, 2, and 3 in human prostate epithelial cells: potential roles for IGFBP-rP1 and 2 in senescence of the prostatic epithelium. Endocrinology 2000;141:4072–80.

170. Rosenzweig SA. What's new in the IGF-binding proteins? Growth Horm IGF Res 2004;14:329–36.

171. Butler AA, Yakar S, Gewolb IH, Karas M, Okubo Y, LeRoith D. Insulin-like growth factor-I receptor signal transduction: at the interface between physiology and cell biology. Comp Biochem Physiol B Biochem Mol Biol 1998;121:19–26.

172. Scott CD, Martin JL, Baxter RC. Rat hepatocyte insulin-like growth factor I and binding protein: effect of growth hormone in vitro and in vivo. Endocrinology 1985;116:1102–7.

173. Pollak M. Insulin-like growth factor physiology and cancer risk. Eur J Cancer 2000;36:1224–8.

174. DiGiovanni J, Kiguchi K, Frijhoff A, et al. Deregulated expression of insulin-like growth factor 1 in prostate epithelium leads to neoplasia in transgenic mice. Proc Natl Acad Sci USA 2000;97:3455–60.

175. Chan JM, Stampfer MJ, Ma J, et al. Insulin-like growth factor-I (IGF-I) and IGF binding protein-3 as predictors of advanced-stage prostate cancer. J Natl Cancer Inst 2002;94:1099–106.

176. Grimberg A. Mechanisms by which IGF-I may promote cancer. Cancer Biol Ther 2003;2:630–5.

177. Hellawell GO, Turner GD, Davies DR, Poulsom R, Brewster SF, Macaulay VM. Expression of the type 1 insulin-like growth factor receptor is up-regulated in primary prostate cancer and commonly persists in metastatic disease. Cancer Res 2002;62:2942–50.

178. Scorilas A, Plebani M, Mazza S, et al. Serum human glandular kallikrein (hK2) and insulin-like growth factor 1 (IGF-1) improve the discrimination between prostate cancer and benign prostatic hyperplasia in combination with total and %free PSA. Prostate 2003;54:220–9.

179. Oliver SE, Barrass B, Gunnell DJ, et al. Serum insulin-like growth factor-I is positively associated with serum prostate-specific antigen in middle-aged men without evidence of prostate cancer. Cancer Epidemiol Biomarkers Prev 2004;13:163–5.

180. Frasca F, Pandini G, Sciacca L, et al. The role of insulin receptors and IGF-I receptors in cancer and other diseases. Arch Physiol Biochem 2008;114:23–37.

181. Hellawell GO, Ferguson DJ, Brewster SF, Macaulay VM. Chemosensitization of human prostate cancer using antisense agents targeting the type 1 insulin-like growth factor receptor. BJU Int 2003;91:271–7.

182. Huynh H, Seyam RM, Brock GB. Reduction of ventral prostate weight by finasteride is associated with suppression of insulin-like growth factor I (IGF-I) and IGF-I receptor genes and with an increase in IGF binding protein 3. Cancer Res 1998;58:215–8.

183. Pandini G, Mineo R, Frasca F, et al. Androgens up-regulate the insulin-like growth factor-I receptor in prostate cancer cells. Cancer Res 2005;65:1849–57.

184. Yonou H, Aoyagi Y, Kanomata N, et al. Prostate-specific antigen induces osteoplastic changes by an autonomous mechanism. Biochem Biophys Res Commun 2001;289:1082–7.

185. Goya M, Miyamoto S, Nagai K, et al. Growth inhibition of human prostate cancer cells in human adult bone implanted into nonobese diabetic/severe combined immunodeficient mice by a ligand-specific antibody to human insulin-like growth factors. Cancer Res 2004;64:6252–8.

186. Kawada M, Inoue H, Masuda T, Ikeda D. Insulin-like growth factor I secreted from prostate stromal cells mediates tumor-stromal cell interactions of prostate cancer. Cancer Res 2006;66:4419–25.

187. Xu C, Graf LF, Fazli L, et al. Regulation of global gene expression in the bone marrow microenvironment by androgen: androgen ablation increases insulin-like growth factor binding protein-5 expression. Prostate 2007;67:1621–9.

188. Burfeind P, Chernicky CL, Rininsland F, Ilan J. Antisense RNA to the type I insulin-like growth factor receptor suppresses tumor growth and prevents invasion by rat prostate cancer cells in vivo. Proc Natl Acad Sci USA 1996;93:7263–8.

189. Denley A, Cosgrove LJ, Booker GW, Wallace JC, Forbes BE. Molecular interactions of the IGF system. Cytokine Growth Factor Rev 2005;16:421–39.

190. Baserga R. The insulin-like growth factor-I receptor as a target for cancer therapy. Expert Opin Ther Targets 2005;9:753–68.

191. Plymate SR, Haugk K, Coleman I, et al. An antibody targeting the type I insulin-like growth factor receptor enhances the castration-induced response in androgen-dependent prostate cancer. Clin Cancer Res 2007;13:6429–39.

192. LeRoith D, Helman L. The new kid on the block(ade) of the IGF-1 receptor. Cancer Cell 2004;5:201–2.

193. Cohen BD, Baker DA, Soderstrom C, et al. Combination therapy enhances the inhibition of tumor growth with the fully human anti-type 1 insulin-like growth factor receptor monoclonal antibody CP-751,871. Clin Cancer Res 2005;11:2063–73.

194. Sachdev D, Yee D. Disrupting insulin-like growth factor signaling as a potential cancer therapy. Mol Cancer Ther 2007;6:1–12.

195. Mitsiades CS, Mitsiades NS, McMullan CJ, et al. Inhibition of the insulin-like growth factor receptor-1 tyrosine kinase activity as a therapeutic strategy for multiple myeloma, other hematologic malignancies, and solid tumors. Cancer Cell 2004;5:221–30.

196. Garcia-Echeverria C, Pearson MA, Marti A, et al. In vivo antitumor activity of NVP-AEW541-A novel, potent, and selective inhibitor of the IGF-IR kinase. Cancer Cell 2004;5:231–9.

197. Wu J, Li W, Craddock BP, et al. Small-molecule inhibition and activation-loop trans-phosphorylation of the IGF1 receptor. EMBO J 2008;27:1985–94.

198. Baxter RC. Changes in the IGF-IGFBP axis in critical illness. Best Pract Res Clin Endocrinol Metab 2001;15:421–34.

199. Clemmons DR. Use of mutagenesis to probe IGF-binding protein structure/function relationships. Endocr Rev 2001;22:800–17.

200. Figueroa JA, De Raad S, Tadlock L, Speights VO, Rinehart JJ. Differential expression of insulin-like growth factor binding proteins in high versus low Gleason score prostate cancer. J Urol 1998;159:1379–83.

201. Thomas LN, Cohen P, Douglas RC, Lazier C, Rittmaster RS. Insulin-like growth factor binding protein 5 is associated with involution of the ventral prostate in castrated and finasteride-treated rats. Prostate 1998;35:273–8.

202. Goossens K, Esquenet M, Swinnen JV, Manin M, Rombauts W, Verhoeven G. Androgens decrease and retinoids increase the expression of insulin-like growth factor-binding protein-3 in LNcaP prostatic adenocarcinoma cells. Mol Cell Endocrinol 1999;155:9–18.

203. Kimura G, Kasuya J, Giannini S, et al. Insulin-like growth factor (IGF) system components in human prostatic cancer cell-lines: LNCaP, DU145, and PC-3 cells. Int J Urol 1996;3:39–46.

204. Kanety H, Madjar Y, Dagan Y, et al. Serum insulin-like growth factor-binding protein-2 (IGFBP-2) is increased and IGFBP-3 is decreased in patients with prostate cancer: correlation with serum prostate-specific antigen. J Clin Endocrinol Metab 1993;77:229–33.

205. Angelloz-Nicoud P, Binoux M. Autocrine regulation of cell proliferation by the insulin-like growth factor (IGF) and IGF binding protein-3 protease system in a human prostate carcinoma cell line (PC-3). Endocrinology 1995;136:5485–92.

206. Damon SE, Maddison L, Ware JL, Plymate SR. Overexpression of an inhibitory insulin-like growth factor binding protein (IGFBP), IGFBP-4, delays onset of prostate tumor formation. Endocrinology 1998;139:3456–64.

207. Rajah R, Valentinis B, Cohen P. Insulin-like growth factor (IGF)-binding protein-3 induces apoptosis and mediates the effects of transforming growth factor-beta1 on programmed cell death through a p53- and IGF-independent mechanism. J Biol Chem 1997;272:12181–8.

208. Jones JI, Clemmons DR. Insulin-like growth factors and their binding proteins: biological actions. Endocr Rev 1995;16:3–34.

209. Perks CM, Holly JM. The insulin-like growth factor (IGF) family and breast cancer. Breast Dis 2003;18:45–60.

210. Schneider MR, Zhou R, Hoeflich A, et al. Insulin-like growth factor-binding protein-5 inhibits growth and induces differentiation of mouse osteosarcoma cells. Biochem Biophys Res Commun 2001;288:435–42.

211. Hoeflich A, Wu M, Mohan S, et al. Overexpression of insulin-like growth factor-binding protein-2 in transgenic mice reduces postnatal body weight gain. Endocrinology 1999;140:5488–96.

212. Miyake H, Pollak M, Gleave ME. Castration-induced upregulation of insulin-like growth factor binding protein-5 potentiates insulin-like growth factor-I activity and accelerates progression to androgen independence in prostate cancer models. Cancer Res 2000;60:3058–64.

213. Nam T, Moralez A, Clemmons D. Vitronectin binding to IGF binding protein-5 (IGFBP-5) alters IGFBP-5 modulation of IGF-I actions. Endocrinology 2002;143:30–6.

214. Schutt BS, Langkamp M, Rauschnabel U, Ranke MB, Elmlinger MW. Integrin-mediated action of insulin-like growth factor binding protein-2 in tumor cells. J Mol Endocrinol 2004;32:859–68.

215. Clemmons DR, Maile LA. Interaction between insulin-like growth factor-I receptor and alphaVbeta3 integrin linked signaling pathways: cellular responses to changes in multiple signaling inputs. Mol Endocrinol 2005;19:1–11.

216. Jerome L, Alami N, Belanger S, et al. Recombinant human insulin-like growth factor binding protein 3 inhibits growth of human epidermal growth factor receptor-2-overexpressing breast tumors and potentiates herceptin activity in vivo. Cancer Res 2006;66:7245–52.

217. Alami N, Page V, Yu Q, et al. Recombinant human insulin-like growth factor-binding protein 3 inhibits tumor growth and targets the Akt pathway in lung and colon cancer models. Growth Horm IGF Res 2008;18:487–96.

218. Liu B, Lee KW, Li H, et al. Combination therapy of insulin-like growth factor binding protein-3 and retinoid X receptor ligands synergize on prostate cancer cell apoptosis in vitro and in vivo. Clin Cancer Res 2005;11:4851–6.

219. So AI, Levitt RJ, Eigl B, Fazli L, Muramaki M, Leung S, Cheang MC, Nielsen TO, Gleave M, Pollak M. Insulin-like growth factor binding protein-2 is a novel therapeutic target associated with breast cancer. Clin Cancer Res 2008;14(21):6944–54.

220. Sansal I, Sellers WR. The biology and clinical relevance of the PTEN tumor suppressor pathway. J Clin Oncol 2004;22:2954–63.

221. Shepherd PR, Withers DJ, Siddle K. Phosphoinositide 3-kinase: the key switch mechanism in insulin signalling. Biochem J 1998;333 (Pt 3):471–90.

222. Persad S, Attwell S, Gray V, et al. Inhibition of integrin-linked kinase (ILK) suppresses activation of protein kinase B/Akt and induces cell cycle arrest and apoptosis of PTEN-mutant prostate cancer cells. Proc Natl Acad Sci USA 2000;97:3207–12.

223. Muller M, Rink K, Krause H, Miller K. PTEN/MMAC1 mutations in prostate cancer. Prostate Cancer Prostatic Dis 2000;3:S32.

224. Trotman LC, Niki M, Dotan ZA, et al. Pten dose dictates cancer progression in the prostate. PLoS Biol 2003;1:E59.

225. Yoshimoto M, Joshua AM, Cunha IW, et al. Absence of TMPRSS2:ERG fusions and PTEN losses in prostate cancer is associated with a favorable outcome. Mod Pathol 2008.

226. McMenamin ME, Soung P, Perera S, Kaplan I, Loda M, Sellers WR. Loss of PTEN expression in paraffin-embedded primary prostate cancer correlates with high Gleason score and advanced stage. Cancer Res 1999;59:4291–6.

227. Grunwald V, DeGraffenried L, Russel D, Friedrichs WE, Ray RB, Hidalgo M. Inhibitors of mTOR reverse doxorubicin resistance conferred by PTEN status in prostate cancer cells. Cancer Res 2002;62:6141–5.

228. Giri D, Ittmann M. Inactivation of the PTEN tumor suppressor gene is associated with increased angiogenesis in clinically localized prostate carcinoma. Hum Pathol 1999;30:419–24.

229. Vivanco I, Sawyers CL. The phosphatidylinositol 3-Kinase AKT pathway in human cancer. Nat Rev Cancer 2002;2:489–501.

230. Culig Z, Klocker H, Bartsch G, Hobisch A. Androgen receptor mutations in carcinoma of the prostate: significance for endocrine therapy. Am J Pharmacogenomics 2001;1:241–9.

231. Wang S, Gao J, Lei Q, et al. Prostate-specific deletion of the murine Pten tumor suppressor gene leads to metastatic prostate cancer. Cancer Cell 2003;4:209–21.

232. Zhao H, Dupont J, Yakar S, Karas M, LeRoith D. PTEN inhibits cell proliferation and induces apoptosis by downregulating cell surface IGF-IR expression in prostate cancer cells. Oncogene 2004;23:786–94.

233. Davies MA, Kim SJ, Parikh NU, Dong Z, Bucana CD, Gallick GE. Adenoviral-mediated expression of MMAC/PTEN inhibits proliferation and metastasis of human prostate cancer cells. Clin Cancer Res 2002;8:1904–14.

234. Bertram J, Peacock JW, Tan C, et al. Inhibition of the phosphatidylinositol 3'-kinase pathway promotes autocrine Fas-induced death of phosphatase and tensin homologue-deficient prostate cancer cells. Cancer Res 2006;66:4781–8.

235. Song G, Ouyang G, Bao S. The activation of Akt/PKB signaling pathway and cell survival. J Cell Mol Med 2005;9:59–71.

236. Datta SR, Dudek H, Tao X, et al. Akt phosphorylation of BAD couples survival signals to the cell-intrinsic death machinery. Cell 1997;91:231–41.

237. Cardone MH, Roy N, Stennicke HR, et al. Regulation of cell death protease caspase-9 by phosphorylation. Science 1998;282:1318–21.

238. Brunet A, Bonni A, Zigmond MJ, et al. Akt promotes cell survival by phosphorylating and inhibiting a Forkhead transcription factor. Cell 1999;96:857–68.

239. Kops GJ, Burgering BM. Forkhead transcription factors are targets of signalling by the proto-oncogene PKB (C-AKT). J Anat 2000;197 Pt 4:571–4.

240. Mitsiades CS, Mitsiades N, Poulaki V, et al. Activation of NF-kappaB and upregulation of intracellular anti-apoptotic proteins via the IGF-1/Akt signaling in human multiple myeloma cells: therapeutic implications. Oncogene 2002;21:5673–83.

241. Sarbassov DD, Guertin DA, Ali SM, Sabatini DM. Phosphorylation and regulation of Akt/PKB by the rictor-mTOR complex. Science 2005;307:1098–101.

242. Lee JT, Steelman LS, Chappell WH, McCubrey JA. Akt inactivates ERK causing decreased response to chemotherapeutic drugs in advanced CaP cells. Cell Cycle 2008;7:631–6.

243. Priulla M, Calastretti A, Bruno P, et al. Preferential chemosensitization of PTEN-mutated prostate cells by silencing the Akt kinase. Prostate 2007;67:782–9.

244. Fingar DC, Blenis J. Target of rapamycin (TOR): an integrator of nutrient and growth factor signals and coordinator of cell growth and cell cycle progression. Oncogene 2004;23:3151–71.

245. Martin KA, Blenis J. Coordinate regulation of translation by the PI 3-kinase and mTOR pathways. Adv Cancer Res 2002;86:1–39.

246. Majumder PK, Febbo PG, Bikoff R, et al. mTOR inhibition reverses Akt-dependent prostate intraepithelial neoplasia through regulation of apoptotic and HIF-1-dependent pathways. Nat Med 2004;10:594–601.

247. Hara K, Yonezawa K, Weng QP, Kozlowski MT, Belham C, Avruch J. Amino acid sufficiency and mTOR regulate p70 S6 kinase and eIF-4E BP1 through a common effector mechanism. J Biol Chem 1998;273:14484–94.

248. Mita MM, Mita A, Rowinsky EK. Mammalian target of rapamycin: a new molecular target for breast cancer. Clin Breast Cancer 2003;4:126–37.

249. Battegay EJ. Angiogenesis: mechanistic insights, neovascular diseases, and therapeutic prospects. J Mol Med 1995;73:333–46.

250. Aragon-Ching JB, Dahut WL. The role of angiogenesis inhibitors in prostate cancer. Cancer J 2008;14: 20–5.

251. Cao Y. Positive and negative modulation of angiogenesis by VEGFR1 ligands. Sci Signal 2009;2(59): re1.

252. Rundhaug JE. Matrix metalloproteinases and angiogenesis. J Cell Mol Med 2005;9:267–85.

253. George DJ, Halabi S, Shepard TF, Vogelzang NJ, Hayes DF, Small EJ, Kantoff PW. Prognostic significance of plasma vascular endothelial growth factor levels in patients with hormone-refractory prostate cancer treated on Cancer and Leukemia Group B 9480. Clin Cancer Res 2001;7:1932–6.

254. Di Lorenzo G, Figg WD, Fossa SD, Mirone V, Autorino R, Longo N, Imbimbo C, Perdona S, Giordano A, Giuliano M, Labianca R, De Placido S. Combination of bevacizumab and docetaxel in docetaxel-pretreated hormone-refractory prostate cancer: a phase 2 study. Eur Urol 2008;54:1089–94.

255. George D. Platelet-derived growth factor receptors: a therapeutic target in solid tumors. Semin Oncol 2001;28:27–33.

256. Mathew P, Thall PF, Jones D, Perez C, Bucana C, Troncoso P, Kim SJ, Fidler IJ, Logothetis C. Platelet-derived growth factor receptor inhibitor imatinib mesylate and docetaxel: a modular phase I trial in androgen-independent prostate cancer. J Clin Oncol 2004;22:3323–9.

257. Grandinetti CA, Goldspiel BR. Sorafenib and sunitinib: novel targeted therapies for renal cell cancer. Pharmacotherapy 2007;27:1125–44.

258. Chi KN, Ellard SL, Hotte SJ, Czaykowski P, Moore M, Ruether JD, Schell AJ, Taylor S, Hansen C, Gauthier I, Walsh W, Seymour L. A phase II study of sorafenib in patients with chemo-naive castration-resistant prostate cancer. Ann Oncol 2008;19:746–51.

259. Dahut WL, Scripture C, Posadas E, Jain L, Gulley JL, Arlen PM, Wright JJ, Yu Y, Cao L, Steinberg SM, Aragon-Ching JB, Venitz J, Jones E, Chen CC, Figg WD (2008) A phase II clinical trial of sorafenib in androgen-independent prostate cancer. Clin Cancer Res 2008;14:209–14.

260. Steinbild S, Mross K, Frost A, Morant R, Gillessen S, Dittrich C, Strumberg D, Hochhaus A, Hanauske AR, Edler L, Burkholder I, Scheulen M. A clinical phase II study with sorafenib in patients with progressive hormone-refractory prostate cancer: a study of the CESAR Central European Society for Anticancer Drug Research-EWIV. Br J Cancer 2007;97:1480–5.

261. Mantovani A. Cancer: Inflaming metastasis. Nature 2009;457:36–7.

262. Kim S, Takahashi H, Lin WW, Descargues P, Grivennikov S, Kim Y, Luo JL, Karin M. Carcinoma-produced factors activate myeloid cells through TLR2 to stimulate metastasis. Nature 2009;457:102–6.

263. Giannitsas K, Konstantinopoulos A, Perimenis P. Non-steroidal anti-inflammatory drugs in the treatment of genitourinary malignancies: focus on clinical data. Expert Opin Investig Drugs 2007;16:1841–9.

264. Rayet B, Gelinas C. Aberrant rel/nfkb genes and activity in human cancer. Oncogene 1999;18:6938–47.

265. McDonnell TJ, Chari NS, Cho-Vega JH, Troncoso P, Wang X, Bueso-Ramos CE, Coombes K, Brisbay S, Lopez R, Prendergast G, Logothetis C, Do KA. Biomarker expression patterns that correlate with high grade features in treatment naive, organ-confined prostate cancer. BMC Med Genomics 2008;1:1.

266. Savli H, Szendroi A, Romics I, Nagy B. Gene network and canonical pathway analysis in prostate cancer: a microarray study. Exp Mol Med 2008;40:176–85.

267. Abdulghani J, Gu L, Dagvadorj A, Lutz J, Leiby B, Bonuccelli G, Lisanti MP, Zellweger T, Alanen K, Mirtti T, Visakorpi T, Bubendorf L, Nevalainen MT. Stat3 promotes metastatic progression of prostate cancer. Am J Pathol 2008;172:1717–28.

268. Molckovsky A, Siu LL. First-in-class, first-in-human phase I results of targeted agents: Highlights of the 2008 American Society of Clinical Oncology meeting. J Hematol Oncol 2008;1:20.

269. Bhasin D, Cisek K, Pandharkar T, Regan N, Li C, Pandit B, Lin J, Li PK. Design, synthesis, and studies of small molecule STAT3 inhibitors. Bioorg Med Chem Lett 2008;18:391–5.

270. Chinni SR, Yamamoto H, Dong Z, Sabbota A, Bonfil RD, Cher ML. CXCL12/CXCR4 transactivates HER2 in lipid rafts of prostate cancer cells and promotes growth of metastatic deposits in bone. Mol Cancer Res 2008;6:446–57.

271. Kryczek I, Wei S, Keller E, Liu R, Zou W. Stroma-derived factor (SDF-1/CXCL12) and human tumor pathogenesis. Am J Physiol Cell Physiol 2007;292:C987–95.

272. Chinni SR, Sivalogan S, Dong Z, Filho JC, Deng X, Bonfil RD, Cher ML. CXCL12/CXCR4 signaling activates Akt-1 and MMP-9 expression in prostate cancer cells: the role of bone microenvironment-associated CXCL12. Prostate 2006;66:32–48.

273. Murakami T, Maki W, Cardones AR, Fang H, Tun Kyi A, Nestle FO, Hwang ST. Expression of CXC chemokine receptor-4 enhances the pulmonary metastatic potential of murine B16 melanoma cells. Cancer Res 2002;62:7328–34.

274. Kajiyama H, Shibata K, Terauchi M, Ino K, Nawa A, Kikkawa F. Involvement of SDF-1alpha/CXCR4 axis in the enhanced peritoneal metastasis of epithelial ovarian carcinoma. Int J Cancer 2008;122:91–9.

275. Sun YX, Schneider A, Jung Y, Wang J, Dai J, Cook K, Osman NI, Koh-Paige AJ, Shim H, Pienta KJ, Keller ET, McCauley LK, Taichman RS. Skeletal localization and neutralization of the SDF-1(CXCL12)/CXCR4 axis blocks prostate cancer metastasis and growth in osseous sites in vivo. J Bone Miner Res 2005;20:318–29.

276. Balkwill F. The significance of cancer cell expression of the chemokine receptor CXCR4. Semin Cancer Biol 2004;14:171–9.

277. Wong D, Korz W. Translating an Antagonist of Chemokine Receptor CXCR4: from bench to bedside. Clin Cancer Res 2008;14:7975–80.

278. Karhadkar SS, Bova GS, Abdallah N, Dhara S, Gardner D, Maitra A, Isaacs JT, Berman DM, Beachy PA. Hedgehog signalling in prostate regeneration, neoplasia and metastasis. Nature 2004;431:707–12.

279. Xie J, Murone M, Luoh SM, Ryan A, Gu Q, Zhang C, Bonifas JM, Lam CW, Hynes M, Goddard A, Rosenthal A, Epstein EH, Jr., de Sauvage FJ. Activating Smoothened mutations in sporadic basal-cell carcinoma. Nature 1998;391:90–2.

280. Narita S, So A, Ettinger S, Hayashi N, Muramaki M, Fazli L, Kim Y, Gleave ME. GLI2 knockdown using an antisense oligonucleotide induces apoptosis and chemosensitizes cells to paclitaxel in androgen-independent prostate cancer. Clin Cancer Res 2008;14:5769–77.

281. Brown JM, Corey E, Lee ZD, True LD, Yun TJ, Tondravi M, Vessella RL. Osteoprotegerin and rank ligand expression in prostate cancer. Urology 2001;57:611–6.

282. Chen G, Sircar K, Aprikian A, Potti A, Goltzman D, Rabbani SA. Expression of RANKL/RANK/OPG in primary and metastatic human prostate cancer as markers of disease stage and functional regulation. Cancer 2006;107:289–98.

283. Fili S, Karalaki M, Schaller B. Mechanism of bone metastasis: The role of osteoprotegerin and of the host-tissue microenvironment-related survival factors. Cancer Lett 2009;283(1):10–19.

284. Ando K, Mori K, Redini F, Heymann D. RANKL/RANK/OPG: key therapeutic target in bone oncology. Curr Drug Discov Technol 2008;5:263–8.

285. Armstrong AP, Miller RE, Jones JC, Zhang J, Keller ET, Dougall WC. RANKL acts directly on RANK-expressing prostate tumor cells and mediates migration and expression of tumor metastasis genes. Prostate 2008;68:92–104.

286. Miller RE, Roudier M, Jones J, Armstrong A, Canon J, Dougall WC. RANK ligand inhibition plus docetaxel improves survival and reduces tumor burden in a murine model of prostate cancer bone metastasis. Mol Cancer Ther 2008;7: 2160–9.

287. Saad F, Markus R, Goessl C. Targeting the receptor activator of nuclear factor-kappaB (RANK) ligand in prostate cancer bone metastases. BJU Int 2008;101:1071–5.

288. Fizazi K, Lipton A, Mariette X, Body JJ, Rahim Y, Gralow JR, Gao G, Wu L, Sohn W, Jun S. Randomized phase II trial of denosumab in patients with bone metastases from prostate cancer, breast cancer, or other neoplasms after intravenous bisphosphonates. J Clin Oncol 2009;27(10):1564–1571.

289. Carducci MA, Jimeno A. Targeting bone metastasis in prostate cancer with endothelin receptor antagonists. Clin Cancer Res 2006;12:6296s–6300s.

290. Nelson JB, Hedican SP, George DJ, Reddi AH, Piantadosi S, Eisenberger MA, Simons JW. Identification of endothelin-1 in the pathophysiology of metastatic adenocarcinoma of the prostate. Nat Med 1995;1:944–9.

291. Warren R, Liu G. ZD4054: a specific endothelin A receptor antagonist with promising activity in metastatic castration-resistant prostate cancer. Expert Opin Investig Drugs 2008;17:1237–45.

292. Knudsen BS, Gmyrek GA, Inra J, Scherr DS, Vaughan ED, Nanus DM, Kattan MW, Gerald WL, Vande Woude GF. High expression of the Met receptor in prostate cancer metastasis to bone. Urology 2002;60:1113–7.

293. Pisters LL, Troncoso P, Zhau HE, Li W, von Eschenbach AC, Chung LW. c-met proto-oncogene expression in benign and malignant human prostate tissues. J Urol 1995;154:293–8.

294. Toschi L, Janne PA. Single-agent and combination therapeutic strategies to inhibit hepatocyte growth factor/MET signaling in cancer. Clin Cancer Res 2008;14: 5941–6.

295. Park SI, Zhang J, Phillips KA, Araujo JC, Najjar AM, Volgin AY, Gelovani JG, Kim SJ, Wang Z, Gallick GE. Targeting SRC family kinases inhibits growth and lymph node metastases of prostate cancer in an orthotopic nude mouse model. Cancer Res 2008;68:3323–33.

296. Raff AB, Gray A, Kast WM. Prostate stem cell antigen: A prospective therapeutic and diagnostic target. Cancer Lett 2008;277(2):123–32.

297. Saffran DC, Raitano AB, Hubert RS, Witte ON, Reiter RE, Jakobovits A Anti-PSCA mAbs inhibit tumor growth and metastasis formation and prolong the survival of mice bearing human prostate cancer xenografts. Proc Natl Acad Sci USA 2001;98:2658–63.

298. Mehta PB, Jenkins BL, McCarthy L, Thilak L, Robson CN, Neal DE, Leung HY. MEK5 overexpression is associated with metastatic prostate cancer, and stimulates proliferation, MMP-9 expression and invasion. Oncogene 2003;22:1381–9.

299. Strock CJ, Park JI, Nakakura EK, Bova GS, Isaacs JT, Ball DW, Nelkin BD. Cyclin-dependent kinase 5 activity controls cell motility and metastatic potential of prostate cancer cells. Cancer Res 2006;66:7509–15.

300. Lin D, Watahiki A, Bayani J, Zhang F, Liu L, Ling V, Sadar MD, English J, Fazli L, So A, Gout PW, Gleave M, Squire JA, Wang YZ. ASAP1, a gene at 8q24, is associated with prostate cancer metastasis. Cancer Res 2008;68: 4352–9.

301. Forootan SS, Wong YC, Dodson A, Wang X, Lin K, Smith PH, Foster CS, Ke Y. Increased Id-1 expression is significantly associated with poor survival of patients with prostate cancer. Hum Pathol 2007;38:1321–9.

Part I
Hormone Therapy

Chapter 2
Luteinizing Hormone-Releasing Hormone and Its Agonistic, Antagonistic, and Targeted Cytotoxic Analogs in Prostate Cancer

Andrew V. Schally and Norman L. Block

Abstract Chronic administration of luteinizing hormone-releasing hormone I (LHRH-I) or its agonistic analogs leads to downregulation of pituitary receptors for LHRH, and a gradual suppression of circulating levels of gonadotropins and sex steroids. The creation of a state of sex-hormone deprivation produced by periodic administration of sustained delivery system of LHRH agonists forms the basis of therapy for advanced prostate cancer and other malignant neoplasms. LHRH antagonists developed in recent decades bind competitively to LHRH receptors and cause an immediate inhibition of the release of gonadotropins and sex steroids. This rapid induction of sex-hormone deprivation by LHRH antagonists makes them useful for the treatment of prostate cancer and other sex steroid-dependent cancers. Potent LHRH-I antagonists are finding important clinical applications in urology, oncology, and gynecology. In addition to their suppressive effects on sex-hormone secretion induced by the downregulation of pituitary LHRH receptors, LHRH agonists and antagonists also exert direct inhibitory actions on tumors, which are mediated by tumoral LHRH receptors. These direct actions contribute to the therapeutic effects of LHRH analogs on cancers and in the case LHRH-I antagonists are also utilized for the treatment of benign prostatic hyperplasia (BPH). In this chapter, we review some selected endocrine and antitumoral effects of LHRH agonists and antagonists and clinical trials on prostate cancer and BPH. Experimental studies and early clinical trials with targeted cytotoxic LHRH analogs developed recently for targeted chemotherapy of tumors expressing LHRH receptors are also described.

Keywords LH secretion • FSH secretion • Sex steroid • Gonadotropin • Chemical castration • Anticancer effects • Tumor growth • Cell proliferation • LHRH-receptor

Introduction

Luteinizing hormone-releasing hormone I (LHRH-I) also called gonadotropin-releasing hormone (GnRH) plays a key role in the regulation of reproduction by controlling the secretion of luteinizing hormone (LH) and follicle stimulating hormone (FSH) from the anterior pituitary gland [1, 2]. Thus, LHRH regulates gametogenesis and sex steroid hormone secretion from the gonads [1–7].

The isolation, determination of structure (Fig. 2.1), and synthesis of decapeptide (LHRH I) in the laboratory of one of us (AVS) in 1971 has had a major impact on endocrinology, gynecology, and oncology [1, 2, 6, 7]. Various agonistic analogs of LHRH were rapidly developed in view of their expected medical applications [2, 6, 7]. The effects of LHRH are mediated by high-affinity G protein-coupled receptors found on pituitary gonadotrophs and various extrapituitary sites [3–5]. Responses to LHRH vary under different conditions and depend on administration and doses delivered to the gonadotroph cells. Continuous administration

$$pGlu\text{-}His\text{-}Trp\text{-}Ser\text{-}Tyr\text{-}Gly\text{-}Leu\text{-}Arg\text{-}Pro\text{-}Gly\text{-}NH_2$$

Fig. 2.1. The amino acid sequence of LHRH-I

A.V. Schally (✉)
Department of Veterans Affairs, VA Research Services, Veterans Affairs Medical Center, Miami, FL, USA,
and
Division of Hematology/Oncology and Division of Endocrinology, Departments of Pathology and Medicine, Miller School of Medicine, University of Miami, Miami, FL, USA
e-mail: andrew.schally@va.gov

W.D. Figg et al. (eds.), *Drug Management of Prostate Cancer*,
DOI 10.1007/978-1-60327-829-4_2, © Springer Science+Business Media, LLC 2010

of LHRH or its potent agonistic analogs, such as Decapeptyl, Leuprolide, Goserelin, and Buserelin, leads to downregulation of pituitary receptors for LHRH and suppression of circulating levels of LH, FSH, and sex steroids [5–7]. Treatment of central precocious puberty, polycystic ovarian disease, and in vitro fertilization and embryo-transfer programs (IVF-ET) are based on the suppression of gonadotropin secretion (selective medical hypophysectomy) [6, 7]. The deprivation of sex hormones induced by chronic administration of LHRH analogs can be used for therapy of hormone-dependent tumors as well as conditions such as leiomyomas and endometriosis. Thus, therapy of breast cancer and prostate cancers is based on reversible medical castration [6, 7]. Several LHRH agonists have found important clinical applications in gynecology and oncology. Potent antagonists of LHRH have also been developed [6–8]. Single administration of these competitive LHRH receptor antagonists causes an immediate inhibition of sex steroid secretion [8, 9]. The elimination of the potentially dangerous transient increase in circulating sex steroid levels (flare effect) caused by LHRH agonists makes the LHRH antagonists possibly more effective for the treatment of hormone-sensitive cancers [6–13]. LHRH agonists and antagonists can also exert a direct inhibitory effect on various cancer cells and some benign genitourinary tissues through local LHRH receptors. Thus, LHRH antagonists can be used for therapy of benign prostatic hyperplasia (BPH), endometriosis, and leiomyomas. This direct inhibitory effect may contribute to the composite therapeutic effects of LHRH analogs in the treatment of cancer and other conditions [6–9, 13, 14].

In addition to agonists and antagonists, a new class of cytotoxic LHRH analogs has been developed for targeted therapy of cancers expressing LHRH receptors [15–18]. Elevated levels of receptors for LHRH, and other peptides, found on tumor cells, can serve as targets for LHRH analogs linked to cytotoxic agents such as doxorubicin [6, 7, 15–18]. These analogs thereby can be used as carriers to deliver cytotoxic agents directly to tumors. This direct delivery augments levels of the chemotherapeutic agents in the tumor cells while sparing normal tissues from the toxicity of these drugs. One such carrier hormone used for targeted tumor therapy is the decapeptide [(D-Lys^6)] LHRH [6, 7, 16–18].

We will review some selected endocrine and antitumoral effects of agonists and antagonists of LHRH-I with special reference to treatment of prostate cancer. Anticancer effects of the cytotoxic LHRH analogs will also be discussed. However, a second form of LHRH (LHRH-II), also known as chicken LHRH, that is expressed in the brain and other tissue [5], and its agonists and antagonists will not be discussed because of space limitations as well as because they are not in clinical use, the receptors for LHRH-II being absent in man.

Agonists of LHRH

In the course of the isolation and synthesis of LHRH-I, in 1971, the work in the laboratory of one of us (AVS) showed that both the natural LHRH-I and synthetic LHRH-I possessed high LH- and FSH-releasing properties [19–21]. The concept that LHRH regulates the secretion of both pituitary gonadotropins, LH and FSH, [21] was confirmed by much experimental and clinical evidence [1, 2, 6, 7, 22]. The name gonadotropin-releasing hormone and the abbreviation GnRH likewise proposed by us [21] are used now by many scientists and clinicians [5, 14]. However, the abbreviation GnRH leads to confusion with the abbreviation GHRH (growth hormone-releasing hormone) so the use of the original name, LHRH, is favored.

The half-life of LHRH-I is short; thus, more potent and longer-acting analogs were immediately considered to be essential for clinical applications. The studies on the relationship between structure and biologic activity showed that histidine in position 2 and tryptophan in position 3 play a functional role, and simple substitutions or deletions in this active center decrease or abolish LHRH activity [13, 23, 24]. However, the tripeptide pyroGlu-His-Trp, or its amide, is inactive. High LHRH activity can be generated by the substitution of these amino acids by structures with similar acid–base and hydrogen-bonding capacity. Amino acids in positions 1 and 4–10 are essential for binding to the receptors and exerting conformational effects [13,23,24]. Substitutions in positions 6 and 10 can produce superactive peptides. Thus, several LHRH analogs substituted in positions 6, 10, or both are much more active than LHRH and also possess protracted activity [6, 13, 23, 24]. Of these, the most important are: [D-Trp^6]LHRH (Decapeptyl, triptorelin), [D-Leu^6,Pro^9-NHET]LHRH (Leuprolide, Lupron), [D-Ser(But)^6,Pro^9-NHET]LHRH (Buserelin), and [D-Ser(But^6),Aza-Gly^{10}]LHRH (Zoladex, Goserelin).

These agonists are 50–100 times more potent than native LHRH [6, 13, 23–27]. This greater biological activity of the analogs is due to increased resistance to enzymatic degradation as well as an enhancement in receptor affinity. The substitution of Gly^6 by D-amino acids renders the analog more resistant to degradation by endopeptidases, which split LHRH at this position [23].

Principles of Oncological and Gynecological Use of LHRH-1 Agonists

An acute injection of superactive agonists of LHRH-I induces a marked release of LH and FSH, but paradoxically, chronic administration produces inhibitory effects [2, 4–7, 13, 23–27]. This can be explained by the facts that LHRH secretion is pulsatile and physiologic stimulation of secretion of gonadotropins requires intermittent LHRH release [6]. Continuous stimulation of the pituitary with LHRH-1 or its superactive agonists produces inhibition of hypophyseal–gonadal axis through the process of downregulation (a reduction in the number) of pituitary receptors for LHRH, decrease in expression of LHRH receptor gene, desensitization of the pituitary gonadotrophs, and a suppression of circulating levels of LH, FSH, and sex steroids [2, 4–7, 13, 23, 27]. The molecular and cellular basis of the LHRH action on the pituitary and signal transduction pathways of LHRH receptors have been reviewed expertly [3–5]. The cloning of DNA for mouse, rat, and human LHRH type I receptor and the organization of LHRH receptor gene have been reported [5, 28, 29].

Sustained Delivery Systems for LHRH Analogs

Initially, agonists of LHRH were administered to patients daily by the subcutaneous (s.c.) route or intranasally [6, 7, 13]. However, daily administration is inconvenient. Subsequently, long-acting delivery systems for [D-Trp^6] LHRH (Decapeptyl) and other agonists in microcapsules of poly(dl-lactide-co-glycolide) or different polymers were developed [6, 7, 13, 27]. These microcapsules were designed to release a controlled dose of the peptide (usually 100 μg) over a 30-day period.

These spherical microcapsules contain 2–6% analog dispersed in biodegradable polymer. Other forms of sustained delivery system consist of microgranules or cylindrical rods containing the peptide analogs.

For administration, the microcapsules or microgranules are suspended in an injection vehicle containing 2% carboxymethyl cellulose or d-Mannitol and 1% Tween 20 or 80 in water and injected i.m. through an18–22 gauge needle [6, 13]. Preparations of Decapeptyl and Lupron depot microspheres containing 3.75 mg of peptide injectable i.m., or of Zoladex (Goserelin, 3.6 mg) in cylindrical rods of the polymer poly(dl-lactide-co-glycolide) [13, 27] injectable s.c. through a 16-gauge needle, and polyhydroxybutyrate tablets containing 3.6–5 mg of Buserelin, which are implantable s.c., have been developed [6]. Improved depot preparations, which release the analogs for 60–180 days have been developed more recently. Six-month depot formulation of leuprolide acetate 22.5 mg (Eligard) and Triptorelin Pamoate (Trelstar LA) containing 11.25 mg of the active drug to be administered every 12 weeks are now available. These formulations release the drugs for several months at the same daily dose as the monthly preparations. There are also implantable devices (Viadur containing 65 mg Leuprolide) for year-long release. Zoladex 3-month implant contains 10.8 mg of Goserelin and is designed for subcutaneous implantation with continuous release over a 12-week period. It is supplied as a 1.5-mm-diameter cylinder, preloaded in a single-use syringe with a 14-gauge needle. Microcapsules and other sustained delivery systems permit the delivery of peptides into the blood stream at a controlled rate over an extended period of time. The agonist Histrelin (Vantas®) has been formulated to deliver the analog for 1 year by using Hydron® technology [30]. The delivery systems developed for administration of LHRH analogs are practical and convenient and ensure patient compliance [6, 13].

Antagonistic Analogs of LHRH

The concept of modified structures, which exhibit little intrinsic activity, but which can compete with a biologically active ligand for the same receptor sites, has been used to design a number of drugs. The use of LHRH antagonists, instead of agonists, would be indicated in clinical conditions where a prompt and significant inhibition of gonadotropin and/or sex steroid hormones is desired. The development of antagonistic LHRH analogs with required safety and pharmacodynamic characteristics has taken several decades. Since 1972, hundreds of LHRH antagonists have been synthesized and tested [6, 8, 13, 23, 24]. Early first-generation LHRH antagonists were hydrophilic and contained replacements or deletions for His in position 2 and Trp in position 3 but had a low potency [23, 24]. Later, it was found that the incorporation of a d-amino acid in position 6 increased the inhibitory activity of the second-generation antagonists. [D-Phe^2,D-Trp^3,D-Phe^6] LHRH was the first antagonist clinically [13, 23, 24] active. Insertion of d-arginine or related basic residues in position 6 of LHRH antagonists increased the inhibitory activity, but the antagonists of this type induced histamine liberation resulting in transient edema and other anaphylactoid reactions [13, 23, 24].

In the third generation of LHRH antagonists, further replacements at positions 1, 10, and other positions were introduced.

To eliminate the undesirable edematogenic effect, new analogs with neutral d-ureidoalkyl amino acids, such as D-Cit at position 6, were synthesized in our laboratory [31]. Among these antagonists devoid of any significant edematogenic effects, [Ac-D-Nal(2)^1, D-Phe(4CI)^2, D-Pal(3)^3, D-Cit^6, D-Ala^{10}]-LHRH (Cetrorelix) had the highest inhibitory activity and receptor binding affinity [6, 13, 31, 32].

Other groups have also reported different structural modifications that preserve high activity and diminish anaphylactoid activity. Antagonists such as antide [N-Ac-D-Nal(2)^1, D-Phe(4CI)^2, D-Pal(3)^3, Lys(Nic)^5, D-Lys(Nic)^6, Lys(iPr)^8, D-Ala^{10}]-LHRH (103) and Nal-Glu antagonist [Ac-D-Nal(2)^1, D-Phe(4C1)^2, D-Pal(3)^3, Arg^5, D-Glu^6(AA), D-Ala^{10}]-LHRH were also potent, although antide had low solubility and Nal-Glu antagonist caused some clinical side effects [13]. Other LHRH antagonists that were developed included Azaline B [Ac-D-Nal(2)^1, D-Phe(4C1)^2, D-Pal(3)l^3, Aph^5(Atz), Aph^6(Atz), Ilys^8, D-Ala^{10}]-LHRH, Ganirelix [N-Ac-D-Nal(2)^1, D-p-C1-Phe^2, D-Pal(3)^3, D-hArg(Et$_2$)^6, L-hArg(Et$_2$)^8, D-A1a^{10}]-LHRH [33], and Abarelix [N-Ac-D-Nal(2)-D-(p-C1-Phe)-D-Pal(3)-Ser-NMeTyr-Asn-Leu-Ilys-Pro-Gly-NH$_2$] [34]. These compounds inhibited ovulation in rats at low doses (1–5 µg), were devoid of edematogenic side effects, and on chronic administration to rats induced a

reversible suppression in the circulating level of sex steroids [31, 35].

Recently, a new powerful LHRH antagonist, Degarelix, with a high therapeutic index, and its various analogs were synthesized [36] and evaluated experimentally in vivo and in vitro as well as clinically [37]. Its chemical structure is: *N*-acetyl-3(naphtalen-2-yl)-D-alanyl-4-chloro-D-phenylalanyl-3-(pyridin-3-yl)-D-alanyl-L-seryl-4((((4S)-2,6-dioxohexahydropyrimidin-4-yl) carbonyl)amino)-L-phenylalanyl-4-(carbamoylamino)-D-phenylalanyl-L-leucyl-N6-(1-methylethyl)-L-lysyl-L-prolyl-D-alaninamide [36, 37].

The antagonist cetrorelix first made in our laboratory [6, 7, 13, 31, 32] and later developed for clinical use by Asta-Medica, then Zentaris, Frankfurt, Germany, and Ganirelix [33] (Syntex Research), and Abarelix (Praecis Pharmaceuticals), USA [34] were shown to be safe and effective in patients and have already been useful in clinical practice [38]. Because parenteral administration of peptide LHRH antagonists may be inconvenient for some patients, nonpeptide antagonists that can be given orally were also recently developed [39].

Principles of Gynecological and Oncological Use of LHRH Antagonists

Effects on the Pituitary LHRH Receptors

Because native LHRH stimulates the secretion of both gonadotropins, LHRH antagonists were expected to inhibit the release of both LH and FSH. While the inhibitory effect of LHRH antagonists on LH is immediate in onset, however, that on the FSH is not as instantaneous [10–12, 40]. A single injection of an LHRH antagonist at a high dose causes an immediate and long-lasting suppression of serum LH and a smaller and delayed decrease in the FSH levels [10–12, 40]. Thus, in rats, LHRH antagonists are not able to completely block the release of FSH in vivo, and other mechanisms may contribute to the regulation of FSH secretion. However, extensive clinical findings indicate that chronic treatment with LHRH antagonists at high doses results in a profound decrease in both LH and FSH as well as a reduction in sex steroid hormone levels [6–9, 32].

The receptor mechanisms through which the LHRH antagonists suppress LH and FSH release were elucidated in the laboratory of one of us [35, 41–44]. In our initial study [41], male rats were implanted subcutaneously with osmotic minipumps releasing Cetrorelix. The treatment with Cetrorelix reduced serum LH and testosterone levels, but 90 days after cessation of treatment, LH and testosterone returned to control levels [41]. Immediately after the discontinuation of Cetrorelix, a significant downregulation of the pituitary LHRH receptors was found, but 90 days later, this phenomenon was reversed [41]. These findings indicate that the recovery of hormonal levels parallels the return of pituitary LHRH receptor numbers to normal values [41].

In another investigation, a single subcutaneous administration of a large dose of Cetrorelix to male rats suppressed serum testosterone and LH levels and produced a significant downregulation of binding sites for LHRH 7 days after administration, but a complete recovery in LHRH receptor levels occurred within 60 days [42].

To determine if the treatment with Cetrorelix affects the concentration of measurable LHRH binding sites, we used an in vitro method for desaturation of receptors based on chaotropic agents such as NH_4SCN [43]. Six hours after the administration of Cetrorelix, occupied LHRH receptors represented only 10% of total receptors, but later, no occupied receptors could be detected. Receptor assays carried out after desaturation of LHRH binding sites demonstrated that pituitary LHRH receptors in rats were significantly downregulated for at least 72 h after the administration of Cetrorelix [43]. The downregulation of LHRH binding sites induced by Cetrorelix was accompanied by suppression of serum LH and testosterone. These results demonstrate that the LHRH antagonist Cetrorelix produces a clear downregulation of pituitary receptors for LHRH and not merely an occupancy of binding sites [43].

In another study [44], we treated one group of male rats daily for 4 weeks with Cetrorelix. Another group of rats received a single intramuscular injection of 4.5 mg of depot Cetrorelix pamoate. An intravenous stimulation test with LHRH was performed after 4 weeks of treatment [44]. LHRH-stimulated LH secretion at 30 min was completely suppressed in rats treated with either regimen of Cetrorelix. The concentration

of pituitary receptors for LHRH was reduced in both Cetrorelix treated groups by 77–82%. Depot Cetrorelix pamoate also led to a 75–80% decrease in the levels of mRNA for pituitary LHRH receptors [44]. These results demonstrate that administration of the LHRH antagonist Cetrorelix causes a marked decrease in the levels of LHRH receptors and in the expression of the LHRH receptor gene [44].

Using Cetrorelix at high doses in vivo in ovariectomized rats as well as in vitro in the superfused pituitary cell system, we demonstrated that LHRH antagonists, in addition to the blockade of the pituitary LHRH receptors downregulate the mRNA expression for the LHRH receptors indirectly, by counteracting the stimulatory effect of endogenous LHRH [10–12]. Thus, in the rat pituitary cell system in vitro, which is devoid of LHRH, Cetrorelix caused no change in the gene expression of the pituitary LHRH receptors [10, 11]. However, when Cetrorelix was used in vivo at low doses, it suppressed the pituitary–gonadal axis only by a competitive receptor blockade but no downregulation of the LHRH receptors occurred [12].

Clinical Findings

Extensive clinical data indicate that a downregulation of pituitary receptors occurs in a clinical setting under a variety of conditions after the administration of agonistic analogs of LHRH [6, 13]. Some clinical results suggest that LHRH antagonists may also lead to pituitary downregulation. Behre and coworkers [45] injected men with a loading dose of 10 mg of Cetrorelix for 5 days followed by administration of 1–2 mg of Cetrorelix once or twice daily for 3 weeks. Initial administration of Cetrorelix suppressed serum levels of LH, FSH, and testosterone, and this reduction was maintained during the low-dose maintenance therapy in all groups [45]. In comparison with the first week, lower levels of LH, FSH, and testosterone were detected during the second and third weeks [45]. Observation that low doses of LHRH antagonist, which are ineffective initially can suppress gonadotropins effectively during subsequent treatment suggest that LHRH antagonists produce receptor downregulation in addition to competitive receptor occupancy [45].

Receptors for LHRH Type I on Tumors

Besides their actions on the pituitary, LHRH agonists and antagonists exert direct effects on tumor cells [6, 13]. The evidence for direct action of LHRH analogs on tumors is based on the detection of high-affinity binding sites for LHRH in various cancers, the inhibitory effects of analogs on tumor cell lines in cultures [6, 13], and clinical findings. Receptors for LHRH have been found in various rodent and human cancers [6, 13]. Binding sites for LHRH and the expression of mRNA for LHRH receptors have been detected in specimens of human prostate cancer [46–48] and prostate cancer lines [46, 49, 50]. Various investigators have reported the presence of LHRH receptors in human mammary carcinoma cell lines [51, 52]. We found high-affinity LHRH binding sites in 52% of human breast cancer specimen [53]. LHRH receptors were similarly detected in about 80% of human ovarian epithelial cancer samples, in ovarian cancer lines [54, 55], in nearly 80% of human endometrial carcinomas [56], and in endometrial cancer lines [54, 57]. The expression of LHRH receptor gene in human breast, endometrial, ovarian tumors, and the respective cancer cell lines was also demonstrated by reverse transcription-polymerase chain reaction (RT-PCR) [58–61]. In addition, LHRH receptors were also demonstrated in surgical specimens of human renal cell carcinomas, lymphomas, and melanomas by immunohistochemistry and/or RT-PCR [32, 57]. LHRH receptors on human cancers appear to be similar to pituitary LHRH receptors [28]. These results provide a rationale for the use of targeted cytotoxic LHRH analogs in malignancies in which receptors for LHRH are expressed [15, 16, 18]. In addition, the presence of receptors for LHRH on tumors may expound the effect of LHRH analogs seen in vitro and occasional responses to LHRH agonists in postmenopausal women with breast cancer [6].

Direct Effects of LHRH Analogs on Tumors

LHRH analogs can exert direct effects on prostate, breast, ovarian, endometrial and other cancers mediated through specific LHRH receptors on tumor cells [5–7, 13, 14, 46, 49, 51, 52, 58, 61, 62]. Inhibition of growth of cultured tumor cells by LHRH analogs supports the view of their direct effects. Suppression of human mammary, ovarian, endometrial, and prostatic cancer cell lines by LHRH agonists and LHRH antagonists, such as Cetrorelix in vitro, is now well documented [6, 7, 13, 51, 52, 58, 61, 63]. These results suggest a regulatory role for LHRH in tumor growth. The production of an LHRH-like peptide or expression of mRNA for LHRH was demonstrated in human prostatic, mammary, endometrial, and ovarian cancer lines, suggesting that local LHRH may be involved in the growth of these tumors [6, 7, 49, 50, 64]. The existence of functional regulatory LHRH loops in prostate cancer and ovarian cancer has also been postulated [49, 50, 64].

Mechanism of Action of LHRH-I and Its Analogs

The actions of LHRH-I are mediated by type I LHRH receptors localized on the plasma membranes of the pituitary gonadotrophs [3–5, 13, 58]. The initial step in the action of LHRH is the binding to its receptors [3, 4, 65]. The binding causes a microaggregation of receptors and complex formation. The complex formed is then internalized and degraded [3, 4, 65]. In the pituitary, the LHRH receptors are coupled to G proteins (αq) that activate phospholipase C, which leads to the production of inositol phosphates and diacylglycerol [3, 4]. This process induces Ca++ mobilization and activation of protein kinase C, resulting in the release of LH and FSH. However in cancers, after binding of the ligand, the LHRH receptors couple to G protein αi and activate a phosphotyrosine phosphatase [58, 61, 66–69], which dephosphorylates epidermal growth factor (EGF) receptors. Thus, mitogenic signaling induced by binding of EGF to its receptor is abolished leading to an inhibition of mitogen-activated protein kinase (MAPK) [58, 61] and EGF-induced proliferation [58, 61]. The signaling mechanism of type I LHRH receptor has been reviewed extensively [3–5, 58, 61, 65, 68].

Clinical Applications of LHRH Antagonists

LHRH antagonists can be used in clinical conditions when suppression of endogenous gonadotropin/sex steroid levels is indicated. The applications of LHRH antagonists include the treatment of nonmalignant tumorous conditions such as endometriosis, and leiomyomas [70], central precocious puberty [71], as well as of BPH, and breast, ovarian, and prostatic cancers [6, 7, 13, 32, 57, 70, 72–76]. Another important application is the prevention of premature LH surge in protocols for controlled ovarian stimulation (COS) for assisted reproductive technology (ART) used for IVF-ET [8, 9, 38]. At this time, LHRH antagonists are approved for the use in COS-ART and are in phase III trials for BPH. The applications for endometriosis and myomas have approval pending.

Use of LHRH Antagonists in BPH

LHRH antagonists should be beneficial for patients with BPH since the decrease in testosterone levels by LHRH agonists and antagonists leads to reduction in prostate size. However, the effects of LHRH agonists on BPH are only transient [32, 57, 71–76].

Several studies and clinical trials [74–76] have documented that therapy with LHRH antagonist Cetrorelix causes a marked and long-lasting improvement in lower urinary tract symptoms (LUTS) in men with symptomatic BPH without impairment of gonadal function [74–76]. This improvement, including the lowering of international prostate symptom score (IPSS), reduction in prostate volume, and increase in urinary peak flow rate, appears to be superior to that achieved with alpha-blockers or 5-alpha-reductase inhibitors. Low doses of Cetrorelix used in current clinical trials cause only a temporary downregulation of pituitary receptors for LHRH and a partial suppression of pituitary–gonadal axis and testosterone levels [32, 57, 77]. The improvement in LUTS could be due to direct inhibitory effects of Cetrorelix on the prostate exerted through prostatic LHRH receptors and possible alterations in levels of growth factors. Thus, Cetrorelix appears to reduce various growth factors in the prostate, and in doses which, do not induce castration levels of testosterone, can lower prostate weights. Experimental and clinical studies with LHRH agonists, antagonist, and cytotoxic analogs in prostate cancer will be described separately.

Targeted Cytotoxic LHRH Analogs

Targeted chemotherapy represents a modern oncological approach designed to improve the effectiveness of cytotoxic drugs and decrease peripheral toxicity. The first concept of targeted therapy, so-called *Magic Bullets*, was proposed by Paul Ehrich more than 100 years ago (for review see [15]). However, this approach remained unexplored for many decades. In the early 1990s, we put forward the hypothesis that the receptors for peptide hormones on tumor cells could serve as targets for peptide ligands linked to various cytotoxic agents [15]. On the basis of the presence of specific receptors for LHRH on tumor cells, we developed a new class of targeted antitumor agents by linking cytotoxic radicals to analogs of LHRH and other peptides [15–18].

Therapy with targeted cytotoxic analog therapy can produce an accumulation of the cytotoxic agent in the cancer cells, thus producing a localized cytocidal effect and reducing peripheral toxicity [7, 13, 15–18, 50, 78–80]. Our early conjugates contained cisplatin, methotrexate, or melphalan [15]. Later, we developed much more potent LHRH analogs containing doxorubicin or its derivatives [80]. In the targeted cytotoxic LHRH analog, AN-152, doxorubicin hemiglutarate was coupled to the agonist [D-Lys^6] LHRH. Another targeted cytotoxic LHRH analog, AN-207, contained (2-pyrrolino)-doxorubicin (AN-201) coupled to the same [D-Lys^6] LHRH carrier. Both cytotoxic analogs preserved high binding affinity of the [D-Lys^6] LHRH to LHRH receptors and the powerful cytocidal activity of the cytotoxic agent [13, 79] and exhibited a high antitumor activity in various experimental cancer models [15–18, 32, 57]. Other groups developed different types of cytotoxic LHRH analogs by designing LHRH-containing chimeric toxic protein complexes, which were effective against various cancers [81].

Cytotoxic LHRH analogs are internalized by rat pituitary cells as well as by human ovarian, endometrial, and breast cancer cells [17, 18]. The binding of AN-152 to the LHRH receptors, its entry into the cells, and its localization in the cytoplasm, followed by appearance in the nucleus were demonstrated by confocal laser scanning microscopy and by coupling a two-photon-emitting fluorophore to the compound [17, 18, 82, 83]. The internalization process depends on the presence of LHRH receptors on cells since it does not occur in cancer cells, which do not express LHRH receptors [18].

LHRH Agonists in Therapy of Prostate Cancer

LHRH agonists have had a great therapeutic impact on treatment of prostate cancer [6, 7]. Carcinoma of the prostate is the most common noncutaneous malignancy in the American male and is the second leading cause of cancer-related deaths among men [6, 72]. About 70% of human prostate cancers are androgen dependent [6, 72]. The therapy of advanced prostate cancer is based on the androgen dependence of the tumor. Previous therapies included orchiectomy and administration of estrogens [6, 72, 84]. However, surgical castration is associated with a psychological impact, and diethylstilbestrol has serious cardiovascular, hepatic, and mammotropic side effects. About 27 years ago, we introduced a new endocrine therapy for advanced prostate cancer based on the use of agonistic analogs of LHRH [85, 86]. Medical castration produced by chronic administration of LHRH analogs accounts for most therapeutic benefits derived from this therapy [6, 72, 84–86], but LHRH agonists and antagonists also exert direct effects on prostate tumor cells [6, 72].

First, in our experimental studies, we demonstrated that chronic administration of the agonist [D-Trp^6] LHRH reduced serum levels of LH, FSH, and testosterone and suppressed tumor growth in rats with Dunning R-3327-H prostate cancers [85]. This demonstration led to clinical trials. The efficacy of palliative therapy with the agonistic analog of LHRH in men with advanced prostate cancer was first shown in 1980–1981 in collaboration with Tolis et al. [86] in a clinical trial in Montreal. Our study revealed a fall in testosterone levels and marked subjective and objective improvement in patients with advanced prostate carcinoma after therapy with agonistic LHRH analogs, Decapeptyl and Buserelin [86]. These results were confirmed and extended by further clinical trials with LHRH agonists in patients with prostate cancer [6, 72, 87]. The LHRH analogs used clinically for therapy of advanced prostate cancer include Decapeptyl, Buserelin, Leuprolide, and Zoladex [6, 72, 87]. Initially, agonists of LHRH were given daily by the s.c. or even intranasal route. Subsequently, we developed a long-acting delivery system for Decapeptyl based on microcapsules designed to release 100 µg/day of the peptide over a 30-day period [6, 72] after the i.m. injection of 3.7 mg of the analog in these microcapsules. The efficacy of the slow-release formulation of microcapsules of LHRH agonists in the treatment of advanced prostatic carcinoma was documented in clinical trials [6, 72] Development of microcapsules and other sustained-release formulations, such as implants that can be administered periodically, made the treatment of patients with prostate cancer more convenient, and efficacious [6].

Treatment with agonists of LHRH is now also recommended in men with a rising prostate-specific antigen (PSA) level after surgery or radiotherapy. LHRH agonists can be also used in combination with an antiandrogen prior to radical prostatectomy or at the beginning of external-beam radiotherapy. Intermittent therapy with LHRH agonists may improve the quality of life in patients with prostate cancer. The therapy with agonists of LHRH is presently the preferred method of treatment for men with advanced prostate cancer, and in ≈70% of cases, LHRH agonists are selected for primary treatment [6].

Side effects caused by chronic administration of LHRH agonists include impotence, loss of libido, and hot flushes and are due to androgen deprivation. An occasional "flare" in the disease with an increase in bone pain in the first few days after administration of LHRH agonists has been reported in ≈10–20% of patients [6, 72, 87]. This flare can be prevented by pretreatment with antiandrogens. Long-term androgen deprivation therapy may also be associated with osteoporosis and an increased incidence of cardiovascular disease and diabetes.

Total androgen blockade is based on the use of a combination of LHRH agonist with antiandrogen for the treatment of prostate cancer. Combinations of LHRH agonists with antiandrogens, such as nilutamide, bicalutamide, or flutamide, are used clinically [88]. The benefits of this combination are still controversial as antiandrogens are expensive and may be toxic to the liver. Moreover, the combination of LHRH agonists and antiandrogen cannot prevent an eventual relapse.

Use of LHRH Antagonists in Prostate Cancer

The use of LHRH antagonists would avoid the temporary clinical "flare" of the disease that can occur in ≈10–20% of prostate cancer patients when the LHRH agonists are given as single agents [6, 88]. We first investigated inhibitory effects of the antagonist Cetrorelix on the growth of experimental prostate cancers in rats bearing Dunning R-3327-H prostate carcinoma. Cetrorelix caused a greater inhibition of prostate cancer growth than [D-Trp[6]]LHRH [72]. We also treated male nude mice bearing xenografts of human androgen-dependent prostate adenocarcinoma PC-82 with microcapsules of the agonist [D-Trp[6]]LHRH or microgranules of Cetrorelix. Cetrorelix, again caused a greater decrease in tumor weight and volume [72], induced more enhanced apoptosis in prostate tumors, and lowered serum levels of testosterone and PSA better than the LHRH agonist. These studies demonstrated the efficacy of Cetrorelix in inhibiting growth of androgen-dependent prostate cancers [72].

Clinical trials demonstrated that an inhibition of testosterone and PSA levels and a decrease in prostate size are achieved in patients with advanced prostatic cancer treated with the antagonist Cetrorelix [74]. In the first study, the responses to 500 µg of Cetrorelix given b.i.d. were evaluated in patients with advanced prostatic cancer [74]. Therapy with Cetrorelix produced a decrease in bone pain, relief in urinary outflow obstruction, reduction in serum testosterone, and a decrease in PSA levels. The second study involved 36 patients with advanced prostate cancer with elevated PSA and bone pain [89]. Group I consisted of 16 patients, who received 500 µg of Cetrorelix b.i.d. for up to 37 months. Thirteen patients responded but later five patients relapsed [89]. Group II included 20 patients who received a loading dose of Cetrorelix, 5 mg b.i.d. for the first 2 days and thereafter 800 µg b.i.d. for up to 20 months. Nineteen patients showed a clinical remission but later three relapsed. Five of six patients who were paraplegic due to metastatic invasion of spinal cord showed neurologic improvement during therapy with Cetrorelix [90]. Cetrorelix may be indicated for patients with prostate cancer and metastases to the spinal cord, bone marrow, and other sites in whom the LHRH agonists cannot be used as single drugs because of the possibility of flare-up [6, 72, 73, 90].

Other studies have demonstrated that administration of a depot formulation of the LHRH antagonist abarelix produces a faster reduction in testosterone levels than is achieved with Leuprolide, with or without concomitant antiandrogens [91, 92]. Leuprolide and abarelix were equally effective in maintaining serum testosterone at castration levels and in decreasing PSA levels [91, 92]. However, some patients treated with abarelix experience allergic reactions. Treatment of patients with androgen-independent prostate cancer with abarelix does not fully suppress serum FSH or lower PSA levels [93]. Thus, LHRH antagonists are of

no therapeutic benefits in patients with relapsed prostate cancer [6, 72].

Clinical phase II trials with a new LHRH antagonist, degarelix, in men with prostate cancer indicate that the LHRH receptor blocker administered at initial doses of 200–240 mg and subsequently at monthly maintenance doses of 80–160 mg suppresses serum testosterone levels to ≤0.5 ng/ml [37a]. A 90% reduction in PSA was achieved in 8 weeks and after 1 year PSA levels were decreased by 97–98%. Degarelix shows a similar efficacy to Leuprolide but it acts much more rapidly. Degarelix's effectiveness in attaining and maintaining serum testosterone suppression to medical castration levels and with no evidence of testosterone surge during 12 months of treatment in a phase III trial led to its US FDA approval at the end of 2008 for the treatment of patients with advanced prostate cancer [37b]. Phase I or II studies in men with prostate cancer with other LHRH receptor antagonists, teverelix, acycline, and ozarelix have been also completed. Orally active LHRH antagonists are also being developed [39]. Because of their prompt action LHRH antagonists would be even better suited for intermittent therapy than the agonists; however, in men with prostate cancer, LHRH antagonists have to be given at larger doses than LHRH agonists and thus would entail greater costs.

In conclusion, it has been documented in thousands of patients with advanced prostate cancer that LHRH agonists provide an effective palliative therapy. LHRH antagonists may also find an application for treatment of prostate cancer. However, all hormonal therapies aimed at androgen deprivation, including castration and LHRH agonists or antagonists, provide only a palliation and disease remission with a limited duration, and most patients with advanced prostatic carcinoma eventually relapse [6, 72, 73].

The treatment of relapsed castration-resistant prostate cancer remains a major oncological challenge. One of the approaches for improving the therapeutic response and its duration could be based on combining LHRH agonists or antagonist with other peptides such as GHRH antagonists [94, 95] or the use of cytotoxic LHRH analogs [18, 96, 97].

Use of Cytotoxic LHRH Analogs in Prostate Cancer

Because most of human prostate cancers exhibited receptors for LHRH [47], targeted cytotoxic analogs were extensively studied in various models of prostate cancer. In rats bearing Dunning R-3327-H or androgen-independent R-3327-AT-1 prostate cancers, significant growth inhibition was observed after administration of AN-207 [18]. In PC-82 human prostate cancers xenografted into nude mice, AN-207 induced a major reduction in tumor volume and a fall in serum PSA levels [18]. Radical AN-201 had only a minor effect and was toxic. Cytotoxic analog AN-207 also inhibited growth of MDA-PCa-2b human prostate cancers [97]. Cytotoxic analog AN-152 also strongly suppressed the growth of androgen-sensitive LNCaP and MDA-PCa-2b prostate cancers and was more effective than doxorubicin [96]. In nude mice with androgen-independent intraosseous C4-2 prostate cancers, AN-152 decreased serum PSA levels but doxorubicin had no effect [96]. Thus, targeted chemotherapy with cytotoxic LHRH analogs should be more efficacious than systemic chemotherapy in patients with relapsed prostate cancers, and clinical trials are pending. Cytotoxic analogs of LHRH might also be indicated for primary therapy of patients with advanced prostate cancer [6, 72].

Side Effects

Cytotoxic LHRH analogs have fewer side effects than do the respective cytotoxic radicals doxorubicin and AN-201. Side effects caused by cytotoxic analogs and the cytotoxic moiety that dissociated from the peptide carrier in the circulation may affect normal cells expressing LHRH receptor. Pituitary cells secreting LH and FSH are the principal nontumoral targets of cytotoxic LHRH analogs. However, the damage to these cells may not be detrimental since patients with hormone-dependent cancers have tolerated treatment by hypophysectomy in the past years [6, 15, 16, 18, 50]. Furthermore, our investigations showed that treatment with AN-207 causes only a transient decrease in levels of LHRH receptors or gonadotrophs, and pituitary function recovers after cessation of treatment [50, 78, 98, 99]. These results indicate that the therapy with cytotoxic LHRH analogs will not inflict permanent damage on pituitary functions. The main side effect of cytotoxic LHRH analogs is myelotoxicity [6, 16, 18]. In clinical phase I studies, women with gynecologic cancers expressing receptors for LHRH were given AN-152 by intravenous infusion in escalating doses up

to 267 mg/m^2. Leukocytopenia was observed but it was rapidly reversible [100]. Cytotoxic LHRH analog AN-152 is now in clinical phase II trials in women with ovarian and endometrial cancers. Clinical trials with AN-152 in men with relapsed prostate cancers are in a planning stage. A new drug, abiraterone, which can be used orally and which might better control advanced prostatic disease is now in clinical trials in UK.

Acknowledgment Experimental studies cited in this review were supported by the Medical Research Service of the Veterans Affairs Department.

References

1. Schally AV, Arimura A, Kastin AJ. Hypothalamic FSH and LH-regulating hormone: Structure, physiology and clinical studies. Fertil Steril 1971;22:703–721.
2. Schally AV. Aspects of hypothalamic regulation of the pituitary gland. Science 1978;202:18–28.
3. Clayton RN, Catt KJ. GnRH receptors: Characterization, physiologic regulation and relationship to reproductive functions. Endocr Rev 1981;2(2):186–209.
4. Conn PM, Huckle WR, Anders WV, McArdle CA. The molecular mechanism of action of gonadotropin releasing hormone (GnRH) in the pituitary. Recent Prog Horm Res 1987;43:29–68.
5. Millar RP, Lu ZL, Pawson AJ, Flanagan CA, Morgan K, Maudsley SR. Gonadotropin-releasing hormone receptors. Endocr Rev 2004;25;235–275.
6. Schally AV, Comaru-Schally AM. Hypothalamic and other peptide hormones. In: Holland JF, Frei E, Bast RC, Kufe DE, Pollock RE, Weichselbaum RR, Hait WN, Hong WK, eds. Cancer medicine. 7th ed. Hamilton, ON: BC Dekker, 2006:802–816.
7. Schally AV, Comaru-Schally AV, Nagy A, et al. Hypothalamic hormones and cancer. Front Neuroendocrinol 2001;22:248–291.
8. Reissmann T, Schally AV, Bouchard P, Riethmuller H, Engel J. The LHRH antagonist cetrorelix: A review. Hum Reprod Update 2000;6:322–331.
9. Griesinger G, Felberbaum R, Diedrich K. GnRH-antagonists in reproductive medicine. Arch Gynecol Obstet 2005;273:71–78.
10. Kovács M, Schally AV. Comparison of mechanism of action of LHRH antagonist cetrorelix and LHRH agonist triptorelin on the gne expression of pituitary LHRH receptors in rats. Proc Natl Acad Sci USA 2001;987:12197–12202.
11. Kovács M, Schally AV, Csernus B, Rekasi Z. LHRH antagonist cetrorelix downregulates the mRNA expression of pituitary receptors for LHRH by counteracting the stimulatory effect of endogenous LHRH. Proc Natl Aca Sci USA 2001;98:1829–1834.
12. Horvath JE, Bajo AM, Schally AV, Kovács M, Herbert F, Groot K. Effects of long-term treatment with the luteinizing hormone-releasing hormone (LHRH) agonist Decapeptyl

and the LHRH antagonist Cetrorelix on the level of pituitary LHRH receptors and their mRNA expression in rats. Proc Natl Acad Sci U S A 2002;99:15048–15053.

13. Schally AV. Luteinizing hormone releasing-hormone analogues: Their impact on the control of tumorigenesis. Peptides 1999;20:1247–1262.

14. Maudsley S, Davidson L, Pawson AJ, Chan R, Lopez de Maturana R, Millar RP. Gonadotropin-releasing hormone (GnRH) antagonists promote proapoptotic signaling in peripheral reproductive tumor cells by activating a Galphai-coupling state of the type I GnRH receptor. Cancer Res 2004;64:7533–7544.

15. Schally AV, Nagy A. Cancer chemotherapy based on targeting of cytotoxic peptide conjugates to their receptors on tumors. Eur J Endocrinol 1999;141:1–14.

16. Schally AV, Nagy A. New approaches to treatment of various cancers based on cytotoxic analogs of LHRH, somatostatin and bombesin. Life Sci 2003;72:2305–2320.

17. Krebs JL, Wang X, Pudavar HE, et al. Regulation of targeted chemotherapy with cytotoxic LHRH analog by epidermal growth factor. Cancer Res 2000;60:4194–4199.

18. Schally AV, Nagy A. Chemotherapy targeted to cancers through tumoral hormone receptors. Trends Endocrinol Metab 2004;15:300–310.

19. Schally AV, Arimura A, Baba Y, et al. Isolation and properties of the FSH- and LH-releasing hormone. Biochem Biophys Res Commun 1971;43:393–399.

20. Matsuo H, Baba Y, Nair RMG, Arimura A, Schally AV. Structure of the porcine LH- and FSH-releasing hormone. I. The proposed amino acid sequence. Biochem Biophys Res Commun 1971;43:1334–1339.

21. Schally AV, Arimura A, Kastin A, et al. The gonadotropin-releasing hormone: One polypeptide regulates secretion of luteinizing and follicle-stimulating hormones. Science 1971;173:1036–1038.

22. Kastin AJ, Schally AV, Gual C, Midgley AR Jr, Bowers CY, Gomez-Perez E. Administration of LH-releasing hormone to selected human subjects. Am J Obstet Gynecol 1970;108: 177–182.

23. Karten MJ, Rivier JE. Gonadotropin-releasing hormone analog design. Structure-function studies toward the development of agonists and antagonists: Rationale and perspective. Endocr Rev 1986;7:44–66.

24. Schally AV, Kastin AJ, Coy DH, Edward T. Tyler Prize Oration. LH-releasing hormone and its analogs: recent basic and clinical investigations. Int J Fertil 1976;21:1–30.

25. Coy DH, Vilchez-Martinez JA, Coy EJ, Schally AV. Analogs of luteinizing hormone-releasing hormone with increased biological activity produced by D-amino acid substitutions in position 6. J Med Chem 1976;19: 423–425.

26. Fujino M, Fukuda T, Shinagawa S, et al. Synthetic analogs of luteinizing hormone-releasing hormone (LHRH) substituted in positions 6 and 10. Biochem Biophys Res Commun 1974;57:1248–1256.

27. Dutta AN. Luteinizing hormone-releasing hormone (LHRH) agonists. Drugs Future 1988;13:43–57.

28. Kakar SS, Grizzle WE, Neill JD. The nucleotide sequences of human GnRH receptors in breast and ovarian tumors are identical in that found in pituitary. Mol Cell Endocrinol 1994;106:145–149.

29. Neill JD. GnRH and GnRH receptor genes in the human genome. Endocrinology 2002;143:737–743.

30. Schlegel PN. Efficacy and safety of histrelin subdermal implant in patients with advanced prostate cancer. J Urol 2006;175:1353–1358.

31. Bajusz S, Kovács M, Gazdag M, eta al. Highly potent antagonists of luteinizing hormone-releasing hormone free of edematogenic effects. Proc Natl Acad Sci USA 1988;85:1637–1641.

32. Schally AV, Engel J. Analogs of luteinizing hormone-releasing hormone (LHRH) in cancer. In: Handbook of biologically active peptides. Kastin AJ, ed. Academic Press: New York, 2006:421–427.

33. Nelson LR, Fujimoto VY, Jaffe RB, Monroe SE. Suppression of follicular phase pituitary gonadal function by a potent new gonadotropin-releasing hormone antagonist with reduced histamine-releasing properties (ganirelix). Fertil Steril 1995;63:963–969.

34. Molineaux CJ, Sluss PM, Bree MP, Geefter ML, Sullivan LM, Garnick BM. Suppression of plasma gonadotropins by Abarelix: A potent new LHRH antagonist. Mol Urol 1998;2:265–268.

35. Pinski J, Yano T, Szepesházi K, Groot K, Schally AV. Recovery of pituitary-gonadal function in male rats after long-term suppression induced by a single injection of microcapsules of LH-RH antagonist cetrorelix SB-75. J Androl 1993;14:164–169.

36. Samant MP, Hong DJ, Croston G, Rivier C, Rivier J. Novel analogues of degarelix incorporating hydroxyl-, methoxy- and pegylated-urea moieties at positions 3,5,6 and the N-Terminus. J Med Chem 2006;49:3536–3543.

37. Van Poppel H, Tombal B, de la Rosette JJ, Persson BE, Jensen JK, Kold OT. Degarelix: a novel gonadotropin-releasing hormone (GNRH) receptor blocker-results from a 1-yr, multicentre, randomized, phase 2 dosage-finding study in the treatment of prostate cancer. Eur Urol 2008;54:805–813.

37a. Gittelman M, Pommerville PJ, Persson BE, et al. A 1-year, open label, randomized phase II dose finding study of degarelix for the treatment of prostate cancer in North America. J Urol 2008;180(5):1986–1992.

37b. Klotz L, Boccon-Gibod L, Shore ND, et al. The efficacy and safety of degarelix: a 12-month, comparative, randomized, open-label, parallel-group phase III study in patients with prostate cancer. BJU Int 2008;102(11):1531–1538.

38. Tarlatzis BC, Fauser BC, Kolibianakis EM, Diedrich K, Rombauts L, Devroey P. GnRH antagonists in ovarian stimulation for IVF. Hum Reprod Update 2006;12:333–340.

39. Armer RE, Smelt KH. Non-peptidic GnRH receptor antagonists. Curr Med Chem 2004;11:3017–3026.

40. Kovács M, Koppán M, Mező I, Teplán I. Diverse effects of a potent LHRH antagonist on the LH and FSH release. Acta Biol Hung 1994;45:285–296.

41. Bokser L, Srkalovic G, Szepeshazi K, et al. Recovery of pituitary-gonadal function in male and female rats after prolonged administration of a potent antagonist of luteinizing hormone-releasing hormone (SB-75). Neuroendocrinology 1991;54:136–145.

42. Pinski J, Yano T, Groot K, et al. Comparison of biological effects of a sustained delivery system and nonecapsulated LH-RH antagonist SB-75 in rats. Peptides 1992;13:905–911.

43. Halmos G, Schally AV, Pinski J, et al. Down-regulation of pituitary receptors for luteinizing hormone-releasing hormone (LH-RH) in rats by LH-RH antagonist Cetrorelix. Proc Natl Acad Sci USA 1996;93:2398–2402.

44. Pinski J, Lamharzi N, Halmos G, et al. Chronic administration of luteinizing hormone-releasing hormone (LHRH) antagonist Cetrorelix decreases gonadotrope responsiveness and pituitary LHRH receptor messenger ribonucleic acid levels in rats. Endocrinology 1996;137:3430–3436.

45. Behre HM, Kliesch S, Pühse G, et al. High loading and low maintenance doses of a gonadotropin-releasing hormone antagonist effectively suppress serum luteininzing hormone, follicle-stimulating hormone, and testosterone in normal men. J Clin Endocrinol Metab 1997;82:1403–1408.

46. Qayum A, Gullick W, Clayton RC, Sikora K, Waxman J. The effects of gonadotropin-releasing hormone analogues in prostate cancer are mediated through specific tumour receptors. Br J Cancer 1990;62:96–99.

47. Halmos G, Arenciba JM, Schally AV, Davis R, Bostwick DG. High incidence of receptors for luteinizing hormone-releasing hormone (LH-RH) and LH-RH receptor gene expression in human prostate cancers. J Urology 2000;163:623–629.

48. Straub B, Müller M, Krause H, et al. Increased incidence of LHRH receptor gene messenger RNA expression in hormone-refractory human prostate cancers. Clin Cancer Res 2001;7:2340–2343.

49. Limonta P, Dondi D, Roberta M, et al. Expression of luteinizing hormone-releasing hormone mRNA in the human prostatic cancer cell line LNCaP. J Clin Endocrinol Metab 1993;76:797–800.

50. Schally AV, Halmos G, Rekasi Z, Arencibia-Jimenez JM. The actions of luteinizing hormone-releasing hormone agonists, antagonists, and cytotoxic analogues on the luteinizing hormone-releasing hormone receptors on the pituitary and tumors. Infert Reprod Med Clin North Amer 2001;12:17–44.

51. Eidne KA, Flanagan CA, Millar RP. Gonadotropin-releasing hormone binding sites in human breast carcinoma. Science 1985;229:989–991.

52. Miller WR, Scott WN, Morris R, Fraser HM, Sharpe RM. Growth of human breast cancer cells inhibited by a luteinizing hormone-releasing hormone agonist. Nature 1985;313:231–233.

53. Fekete M, Wittliff JL, Schally AV. Characteristics and distribution of receptors for [D-Trp^6]-luteinizing hormone-releasing hormone, somatostatin, epidermal growth factor and sex steroids in 500 biopsy samples of human breast cancer. J Clin Lab Anal 1989;3:137–147.

54. Emons G, Schally AV. The use of luteinizing hormone releaseing hormone agonists and antagonists in gynaecological cancers. Reproduction 1994;9:1364–1379.

55. Srkalovic G, Schally AV, Wittliff JL, Day G, Jenison EL. Presence and characteristics of receptors for [D-Trp^6]-luteinizing hormone-releasing hormone and epidermal growth factor in human ovarian cancer. Int J Oncol 1998;12:489–498.

56. Srkalovic G, Wittliff JL, Schally AV. Detection and partial characterization of receptors for [D-Trp6]luteinizing hormone-releasing hormone in human endometrial carcinoma. Cancer Res 1990;50:1841–1846.

57. Engel J B, Schally AV. Drug insight: clinical use of agonists and antagonists of luteinizing hormone-releasing hormone. Nat Clin Pract Endocrinol Metab 2007;3:157–167.

58. Emons G, Ortmann O, Schulz KD, et al. Growth-inhibitory actions of analogues of luteinizing hormone releasing hormone on tumor cells. Trends Endocrinol Metab 1997;8:355–362.

59. Irmer G, Burger C, Ortmann O, Schulz KD, Emmons G. Expression of luteinizing hormone-releasing hormone and its mRNA in human endometrial cancer cell lines. J Clin Endocrinol Metab 1994;79:916–919.

60. Harris NS, Dutlow C, Eidne K, et al. Gonadotropin-releasing hormone gene expression in MDA-MB-231 and ZR-75-1 breast carcinoma cell lines. Cancer Res 1991;51:2577–2581.

61. Emons G, Müller V, Ortmann O, Schultz KD. Effects of LHRH analogues on mitogenic signal transduction in cancer cells. J Steroid Biochem Mol Biol 1998;65:199–205.

62. Tang X, Yano T, Osuga Y, et al. Cellular mechanisms of growth inhibition of human epithelial ovarian cancer cell line by LH-releasing hormone antagonist Cetrorelix. J Clin Endocrinol Metab 2002;87:3721–3727.

63. Sharoni Y, Bosin E, Minster A, et al. Inhibition of growth of human mammary tumor cells by potent antagonists of luteinizing hormone-releasing hormone. Proc Natl Acad Sci USA 1989;86:1648–1651.

64. Dondi D, Limonta P, Moretti RM, Marelli MM, Garattini E, Motta M. Antiproliferative effects of LHRH agonists on the human androgen-independent prostate cancer cell line DU 145: Evidence for an autocrine inhibitory LHRH loop. Cancer Res 1994;54:4091–4095.

65. Hawes BE, Conn PM. Assessment of the role of G proteins and inositol phosphate production in the action of gonadotropin-releasing hormone. Clin Chem 1993;39:325–332.

66. Völker P, Gründker C, Schmidt O, Schultz K-D, Emons G. Expression of receptors for luteinizing hormone-releasing hormone in human ovarian and endometrial cancers: Frequency, autoregulation, and correlation with direct antirproliferative activity of luteinizing hormone-releasing hormone analogs. Am J Obstet Gynecol 2002;186:171–179.

67. Shedgley KR, Finch AR, Caunt CJ, McArdle CA. Intracellular gonadotropin-releasing hormone receptors in breast and gonadotrope lineage cells. J Endocrinol 2006;191:625–636.

68. Cheng CK, Leung PCK. Molecular biology of gonadotropin-releasing hormone (GnRH)-I, GnRH-II, and their receptors in humans. Endocr Rev 2005;26:283–306.

69. Gründker C, Gunthert AR, Westphalen S, Emons G. Biology of the gonadotropin-releasing hormone system in gynecological cancers. Eur J Endocrinol 2002;146:1–14.

70. Emons G, Grundker C, Gunthert AR, Westphalen S, Kavanagh J, Verschraegen C. GnRH antagonists in the treatment of gynecological and breast cancers. Endocr Relat Cancer 2003;10:291–299.

71. Schally AV. LH-RH analogues. I. Their impact on reproductive medicine. Gynecol Endocrinol 1999;13:401–409.

72. Schally AV, Comaru-Schally AM, Plonowski A, Nagy A, Halmos G, Rekasi Z. Peptide analogs in the therapy of prostate cancer. Prostate 2000;45:158–166.

73. Schally AV. Luteinizing hormone-releasing hormone analogues and hormone ablation for prostate cancer: state of the art. Br J Urol 2007;100(S2):2–4.

74. Gonzalez-Barcena D, Vadillo-Buenfil M, Gomez-Orta F. Responses to the antagonistic analog of LHRH (Cetrorelix) in patients with benign prostatic hyperplasia and prostatic cancer. Prostate 1994;24:84–92.

75. Comaru-Schally AM, Brannan W, Schally AV, Colcolough M, Monga M. Efficacy and safety of luteinizing hormone-releasing hormone antagonist Cetrorelix in the treatment of symptomatic benign prostatic hyperplasia. J Clin Endocrinol Metab1998;83:3826–3831.

76. Debruyne F, Gress AA, Arustamov DL. Placebo-controlled dose-ranging phase 2 study of subcutaneously administered LHRH antagonist cetrorelix in patients with symptomatic benign prostatic hyperplasia. Eur Urol 2008;54:170–177.

77. Horvath JE, Toller GL, Schally AV, Bajo AM, Groot K. Effect of long-term treatment with low doses of the LHRH antagonist Cetrorelix on pituitary receptors for LHRH and gonadal axis in male and female rats. PNAS 2004;101:4996–5001.

78. Nagy A, Schally AV. Targeting of cytotoxic LHRH analogs to breast, ovarian, endometrial and prostate cancers. Biol Reprod 2005;73:851–859.

79. Nagy A, Schally AV. Targeting cytotoxic conjugates of somatostatin, luteinizing hormone-releasing hormone and bombesin to cancers expressing their receptors: A "smarter" chemotherapy. Curr Pharm Des 2004;14:1167–1180.

80. Nagy A, Schally AV, Armatis P, et al. Cytotoxic analogs of luteinizing hormone-releasing hormone containing doxorubicin or 2-pyrrolinodoxorubicin, a derivative 500-1000 times more potent. Proc Natl Acad Sci USA 1996;93:7269–7273.

81. Eaveri R, Ben-Yehudah A, Lorberboum-Galski H. Surface antigens/receptors for targeted cancer treatment: the GnRH receptor/binding site for targeted adenocarcinoma therapy. Curr Cancer Drug Targets 2004;4:673–687.

82. Wang X, Krebs LJ, Al-Nuri M, et al. A chemically labeled cytotoxic agent: Two-photon fluorophore for optical tracking of cellular pathway in chemotherapy. Proc Natl Acad Sci USA 1999;96:11081–11084.

83. Gunthert AR, Grundker C, Bongertz T, Schlott T, Nagy A, Schally AV. Internalization of cytotoxic luteinizing hormone-releasing hormone analog AN-152 induces multi drug resistance 1 (MDR-1) independent apoptosis in human endometrial and ovarian cancer cell lines. Am J Obstet Gynecol 2004;191:1164–1172.

84. Peeling WB. Phase III studies to compare goserelin (Zoladex) with orchiectomy and with diethylstilbestrol in treatment of prostatic carcinoma. Urology 1989;33(S):45–52.

85. Redding TW, Schally AV. Inhibition of prostate tumour growth in two rat models by chronic administration of D-Trp⁶-LH-RH. Proc Natl Acad Sci USA 1981;78:6509–6512.

86. Tolis G, Ackman D, Stellos A, et al. Tumor growth inhibition in patients with prostatic carcinoma treated with luteinizing hormone-releasing agonists. Proc Natl Acad Sci USA 1982;79:1658–1662.

87. Sogani PC, Fair WR. Treatment of advanced prostate cancer. Urol Clin North Am 1987;14:253–271.

88. Crawford ED, Eisenberger MA, McLeod DG, et al. A controlled trial of leuprolide with and without flutamide in prostatic carcinoma. N Engl J Med 1989;321:419–424.

89. Gonzalez-Barcena D, Schally AV, Comaru-Schally AM, Cortez-Morales A, Vadillo-Buenfil M, Molina-Ayala MA. Treatment of patients with advanced prostate cancer with LH-RH antagonist Cetrorelix. In: Filicori M, Flamigni C, eds. Treatment with GnRH analogs: Controversies & perspectives, London/New York: Parthenon, 1996;139–144.

90. Gonzalez-Barcena D, Vadillo-Buenfil M, Cortez-Morales A, et al. Luteinizing hormone-releasing hormone antagonist SB-75 (Cetrorelix) as primary single therapy in patients with advanced prostatic cancer and paraplegia due to metastatic invasion of spinal cord. Urology 1995;45:275–281.

91. Trachtenberg J, et al. A phase 3, multicenter, open label, randomized study of abarelix versus leuprolide plus daily antiandrogen in men with prostate cancer. J Urol 2002;167:1670–1674.

92. Garnick MB, Campion M. Abarelix Depot, a GnRH antagonist, v LHRH superagonists in prostate cancer: differential effects on follicle-stimulating hormone. Abarelix study group. Mol Urol 2000;4:275–277.

93. Beer TM, Ryan C, Bhat G, Garnick M, Abarelix Study Group. Dose-escalated abarelix in androgen-independent prostate cancer: A phase I study. Anti-Cancer Drugs 2006;17:1075–1079.

94. Schally AV, Varga JL, Engel JB. Drug Insight: Antagonistic growth hormone-releasing hormone: An emerging new therapy for cancer. Nat Clin Pract Endocrinol Metab 2008;4:33–43.

95. Stangelberger A, Schally AV, Zarandi M, et al. The combination of antagonists of LHRH with antagonists of GHRH improves inhibition of androgen sensitive MDA-Pca-2b and LuCaP-35 prostate cancers. Prostate 2007;67:1339–1353.

96. Letsch M, Schally AV, Szepeshazi K, Halmos G, Nagy A. Preclinical evaluation of targeted cytotoxic luteinizing hormone-releasing hormone analogue AN-152 in androgen-sensitive and insensitive prostate cancers. Clin Cancer Res 2003;9:4505–4513.

97. Plonowski A, Schally AV, Nagy A, et al. Inhibition of in vivo proliferation of MDA-Pca-2b human prostate cancer by targeted cytotoxic analog of luteinizing hormone-releasing hormone AN-207. Cancer Lett 2002;176:57–63.

98. Kovács M, Schally AV, Nagy A, Koppán M, Groot K. Recovery of pituitary function after treatment with a targeted cytotoxic analog of luteinizing hormone-releasing hormone. Proc Natl Acad Sci USA 1997;94:1420–1425.

99. Kovács M, Schally AV, Csernus B, Busto R, Rékási Z, Nagy A. Targeted cytotoxic analogue of luteinizing hormone-releasing hormone (LH-RH) only transiently decreases the gene expression of pituitary receptors for LH-RH. J Neuroendocrinol 2002;14:5–13.

100. Emons G, Kauffmann M, Gunthert AR, et al. Phase I study of Zen-008 (AN-152), a targeted cytotoxic LHRH analog in female patients with cancers expressing LHRH receptors. J Clin Oncol, ASCO Annual Meeting Proceedings 2007;25(18S):3571.

Chapter 3
Nuclear Receptor Coregulators: Promising Therapeutic Targets for the Treatment of Prostate Cancer

Hannelore V. Heemers and Donald J. Tindall

Abstract The concept that androgens exert control over the prostate and prostate disease dates back to the eighteenth century, when the first observations of seasonal variations in the size of the prostate gland were observed in animals. Since then, a direct link between testis-derived androgens and prostate growth was established, leading to the seminal study of Charles Huggins who demonstrated that surgical or medical castration is able to inhibit the growth of metastatic and advanced prostate cancer (CaP). Today, more than six decades after Huggins' original groundbreaking report, so-called androgen deprivation therapies are still the preferred treatment option for CaP patients who do not benefit from surgery or radiation therapy. While such treatment regimes initially result in a clinical favorable response and an overall decrease in tumor burden in a majority of patients, disease regression is not complete, and androgen deprivation is therefore not curative. Recent findings of physiologically relevant tissue levels of androgens in castration-recurrent prostate cancer (CRPC) have led to a paradigm shift that CaP, which recurs following androgen deprivation therapy, is not androgen-independent and has rekindled research into alternative means of blocking androgen action as a therapeutic option during prostate cancer progression. Here, we explore the possibility of targeting coregulator proteins, which are critical determinants for androgenic responses, as an indirect means of blocking androgen action in CaP cells.

Keywords Androgen receptor • Androgen • Coactivator • Corepressor • Cell proliferation

H.V. Heemers (✉)
Department of Urology, Roswell Park Cancer Institute,
Buffalo, NY 14263, USA
e-mail: hannelore.heemers@roswellpark.org

Introduction

The concept that androgens exert control over the prostate and prostate disease dates back to the eighteenth century, when observations of seasonal variations in the size of the prostate gland were made in animals. Since then, several reports established a direct link between testis-derived androgens and prostate growth. Investigators proposed and implemented androgen ablation strategies as a means to manage the prostate (reviewed in [1]). These efforts, combined with increased knowledge regarding endocrine physiology, and the functional relationships within the hypothalamus–pituitary–testes hormonal axis in particular, culminated in the seminal study of Charles Huggins who demonstrated that surgical or medical castration inhibits the growth of metastatic and advanced prostate cancer (CaP) [1]. Today, more than six decades after Huggins' original groundbreaking report, androgen deprivation therapies are still the preferred treatment option for CaP patients who do not benefit from surgery or radiation therapy [2] (as addressed in more detail in Chap. 9). While such treatment regimes initially result in a clinically favorable response and an overall decrease in tumor burden in the majority of patients, disease regression is not complete. Thus, androgen deprivation is not curative, a fact that was recognized by Dr. Huggins [1]. Recent findings of physiologically relevant tissue levels of androgens in castration-recurrent prostate cancer (CRPC) [3] led to a paradigm shift that recurrent CaP following androgen deprivation therapy is not androgen-independent [4] and rekindled research into alternative means of blocking androgen action throughout prostate cancer progression. Here, we explore the possibility of targeting coregulator proteins, which are

W.D. Figg et al. (eds.), *Drug Management of Prostate Cancer*,
DOI 10.1007/978-1-60327-829-4_3, © Springer Science+Business Media, LLC 2010

critical determinants for androgenic responses, as an indirect means of interfering with androgen action in CaP cells.

Androgens, the Androgen Receptor, and Prostate Cancer

The discovery of the androgen receptor (AR), a nuclear receptor that mediates the cellular effects of androgens, and the subsequent identification and characterization of critical components of the AR transcriptional complex has considerably increased our understanding of the mechanism by which androgens affect target cells. Along with the continuously evolving insights into the synthesis and metabolism of androgens in CaP cells, this knowledge may provide a template needed for novel therapeutic strategies in the fight against CaP.

Androgens: Synthesis and Metabolites

Testosterone is synthesized by the testes and is the principal androgen in the male circulation (~95% of circulating androgen). The remaining androgens in the bloodstream [principally dehydroepiandrosterone (DHEA), androstenediol, and androstenedione] are either produced by the adrenal cortex and converted into testosterone in peripheral tissues or [as is the case for dihydrotestosterone (DHT)] are derived from peripheral conversion from testosterone [5, 6]. Synthesis of androgens is tightly regulated by the hypothalamic–pituitary–gonadal axis. Pulsatile secretion of luteinizing hormone (LH)-releasing hormone (LHRH) by the hypothalamus stimulates secretion of LH by the anterior pituitary, which in turn induces testicular Leydig cells to produce testosterone. Testosterone acts through a negative feedback loop to prevent LHRH release by the hypothalamus and to decrease the sensitivity of the pituitary to LHRH. Only 1–2% of circulating testosterone exists in an unbound, free form as the majority of testosterone in the bloodstream is bound to carrier proteins such as sex hormone-binding globulin (SHBG) and albumin [5–8].

Basic Mechanism of Androgen Action

Unbound, lipophilic testosterone diffuses into its target cell where it is rapidly and irreversibly converted into its more potent metabolite DHT by 5α-reductase (either type I or II, depending on the target tissue) [9]. Both testosterone and DHT exert their activities by binding to the AR, a 110-kDa member of the nuclear receptor superfamily of ligand-activated transcription factors. Since DHT binds the AR with higher affinity, its biological activity exceeds that of testosterone by up to ten times [10]. In addition, DHT dissociates from the AR more slowly than testosterone, and AR bound to DHT is more stable [11]. Apart from their local conversion into more active androgens, adrenal androgens can stimulate the AR by direct binding, albeit with low affinity [12]. In its basal, unliganded state, the AR is found primarily in the cytoplasmic compartment in a complex with heat shock proteins (Hsps) and immunophilin chaperones. Upon ligand binding, the composition of this Hsp complex is altered, and the AR undergoes a conformational change, which allows nuclear translocation of the AR [13]. Inside the nucleus, the activated AR binds to specific recognition sequences known as androgen response elements (AREs) in the promoter and enhancer regions of target genes. Two AR monomers in head-to-head conformations bind as homodimers to AREs [14], which are direct or indirect repeats of the core 5′-TGTTCT-3′, or more complex response elements harboring diverse arrangements of AREs [15, 16]. Activated ARE-bound AR dimers can either interact directly with components of the transcription preinitiation complex or recruit other components that promote such functional interactions (Fig. 3.1) (reviewed in [17]). Coregulators are among those critical recruits engaged by the AR to facilitate transcription of target genes. As a general definition, coregulators are proteins that are recruited by a transcription factor, which either enhance (i.e., coactivators) or reduce (i.e., corepressors) its transactivation but do not significantly alter the basal transcription rate and do not typically possess DNA-binding ability. Instead, coregulators such as those associated with the AR influence transcription by facilitating DNA occupancy, chromatin remodeling, and/or recruitment of general transcription factors associated with RNA polymerase II at the regulatory sites of target genes. Alternatively, coregulatory proteins govern transcription by assuring the competency of the AR to directly

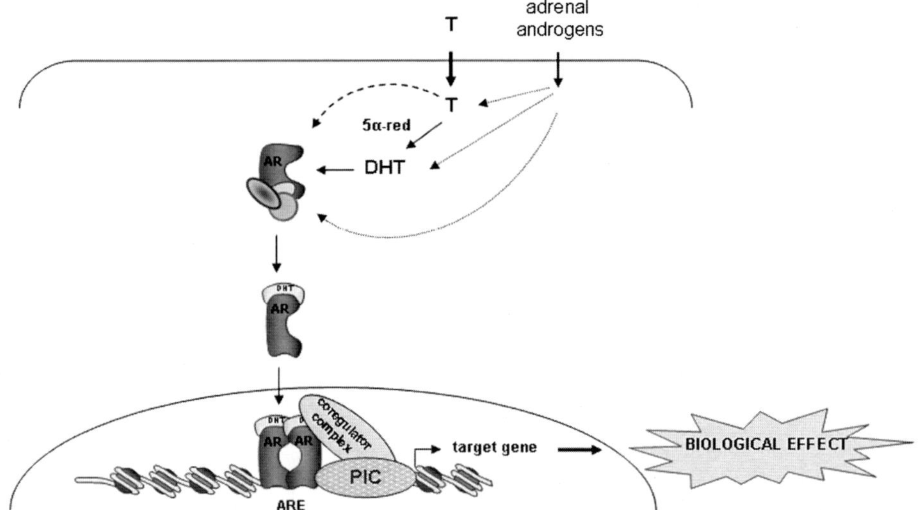

Fig. 3.1 Mechanism by which androgens regulate the expression of target genes. Upon transportation by the blood to its target tissues, unbound, lipophilic T diffuses into its target cell where it can be rapidly and irreversibly converted into a more potent metabolite DHT by 5α-reductase (5α-red). Both T and DHT bind to their cognate receptor, the androgen receptor (AR), which is stabilized by a heat shock (Hsp) complex. Androgen precursors of adrenal origin can be converted into more active androgens or weakly interact with the AR themselves. Upon ligand binding, the AR undergoes a conformational change, which allows it to dissociate from components of the Hsp complex and translocates to the cell nucleus. Inside the nucleus, the activated AR forms homodimers and binds to specific recognition sequences known as androgen response elements (AREs) in the promoter and enhancer regions of target genes. ARE-bound AR interacts with basal transcription factors and recruits coregulators to achieve AR target gene transcription, and ultimately, the appropriate biological response to the androgenic stimulus

enhance gene expression. The latter can be achieved by modulation of the proper folding of the AR, ensuring its stability or correct subcellular localization [17].

The different modes in which coregulators can affect AR-mediated transcription are reflected in the remarkable functional diversity observed in ~170 AR-associated coregulators that have been identified to date. AR-associated coregulators fulfill activities that are directly related to a role in transcription. They can alleviate the constraints imposed by the chromatin structure (by chromatin remodeling and histone modifications), affect localization, stability, and/or turnover of components of the AR transcriptional complex (by ubiquitination and sumoylation), induce maturation and processing of transcripts (by roles in the spliceosome and RNA metabolism), or remove and repair obstacles and DNA lesions. Interestingly, some AR-associated coregulators possess functions that are harder to reconcile with active transcription taking place in the cell nucleus, such as endocytosis, cytoskeletal organization, protein folding, signal transduction and integration, scaffolds, and adaptors. The remarkable functional diversity displayed by AR-associated proteins and the number of cellular pathways with which they are involved offer a glimpse of the extraordinary level of complexity of protein–protein interactions involved in generating an AR-mediated transcriptional response [17].

The Androgen Receptor: Structure and Function

Like other members of the nuclear receptor superfamily, the AR consists of four functional domains: an N-terminal domain (NTD), a DNA-binding domain (DBD), a hinge region, and a ligand-binding domain (LBD) [18, 19]. The AR NTD contains the major transactivation function (AF) of the AR, termed AF-1. AF-1 functions in a ligand-independent manner, that, when separated from the LBD, gives rise to a constitutively active AR. The AF-1 domain undergoes induced folding when contacted by basal transcription factors, resulting in a more compact and active conformation that enables coregulator recruitment and transcription [20]. In addition, the NTD harbors a variable number of homopolymeric repeats, the most important of which is a polyglutamine repeat that ranges from 8 to 31 repeats in normal individuals, with an average length of 20. Shorter polyglutamine stretches give rise to a more transcriptionally active AR and have been suggested to be associated with a predisposition for CaP [21].

The centrally located DBD is the most conserved region within the nuclear receptor family. This region forms two zinc fingers, which determine the specificity of DNA recognition and AR dimerization. A C-terminal extension of the DBD is important for the overall three-dimensional structure of the DBD and plays a role in mediating the AR selectivity of DNA interaction [15, 22].

The hinge region is involved in DNA binding as well as AR dimerization and has been suggested to attenuate transcriptional activity by the AR [23, 24]. A ligand-dependent bipartite nuclear localization signal (NLS) is located in the carboxy terminal part of the DBD and the hinge region, implicating the hinge region in AR nuclear translocation [25, 26].

Similar to the LBD of other nuclear receptors, the AR LBD consists of 12 discrete α-helices. The outermost α-helix (helix-12) of the unliganded receptor is positioned further away from the ligand-binding pocket. Insertion of an agonist into the ligand-binding pocket changes the conformation of the LBD in such a way that helix-12 folds back on top of the ligand-binding site, serving as a lid to retard dissociation of the captured ligand. This movement creates a shallow hydrophobic groove at the top of the ligand-binding pocket, generally referred to as AF-2. AF-2 is the major protein–protein interaction surface used by nuclear receptors to recruit LXXLL-motif containing coactivators [27]. The AR, however, differs from other nuclear receptors in this respect and interacts with coactivators in a unique manner [28]. The hydrophobic pocket within the AR LBD facilitates intramolecular and intermolecular interaction between the AR NTD and its C-terminus and is apparently not readily available for coactivator binding. It has been suggested that competition exists between these regulatory proteins and the NTD for binding to the AF-2. The implications of such competition and the association of NTD and LBD are not clear, but suggest that additional surfaces outside this well-defined coactivator pocket enable the AR to interact with its coactivators and that different classes of coactivators may interact with different AR surfaces. Experiments delineating the various domains within the AR with which coregulator proteins interact

support this hypothesis (reviewed in [17]). Overall, the AF-2 in the AR LBD displays relatively weak ligand-dependent transactivating properties when compared to the AF-2 of other nuclear receptors. Nonetheless, mutation or deletion of AF-2 markedly reduces transcriptional activation in response to ligand. Noteworthy, the two major therapeutic approaches used to achieve androgen deprivation in CaP patients, i.e., surgical or medical castration, which prevent the production of ligands for the AR or administration of AR antagonists, which compete with androgenic ligands for binding to the AR, are both targeted toward the AR LBD.

Clinical Relevance and Therapeutic Potential of the AR Signaling Axis in CaP

The therapeutic potential of the AR signaling pathway in hormone-naïve prostate cancer has been evident since Charles Huggins' work established castration as a systemic treatment for CaP [1, 2]. Over the last decade, several lines of investigation have led to the recognition that the AR is a critical determinant for CRPC cell proliferation and therefore is an attractive target for therapeutic intervention in CRPC, despite the castrate levels of circulating androgens in these patients [29–31]. Immunohistochemical assessment of castration recurrent specimens confirmed the presence of the AR in the nucleus of CRPC cells, where it was found to be expressed at levels similar to those in androgen-stimulated CaP and benign prostate. In addition, expression profiling of CaP from castration recurrent patients has demonstrated high expression levels of genes known to be under androgen control, indicating activation of the AR transcriptional program in CRPC cells. More importantly, several preclinical studies using cultured cell and xenograft CaP models demonstrated that CRPC cells rely on the presence of a functional AR to proliferate. The "reactivation" of the AR in CRPC cells has been attributed to mechanisms of AR hypersensitivity (AR amplification and/or mutations that render the AR more sensitive to lower levels of ligands), promiscuous activation of the AR (by adrenal androgens, nonandrogenic steroids, and even antiandrogens), and outlaw AR pathways (AR activated by growth factors and cytokines, thereby bypassing the need for androgens) [29, 30]. Moreover, measurements of physiologically relevant androgen concentrations and observations of overexpression of enzymes, which are able to catalyze the conversion of adrenal androgen precursors into active androgens in CRPC indicate a critical role for intracrine production of androgens in CRPC [4, 31]. These findings as well as the realization that routinely used continuous androgen deprivation therapies are not effective for treating castration recurrent disease, and arguably may induce a more aggressive phenotype, have led to the concept that alternative means of targeting AR-mediated signaling should be explored for the treatment of CRPC. In this respect, therapies directed against components of the AR transcriptional complex that interfere with AR signaling make sense. A growing body of literature suggests that AR-associated coregulator proteins could serve as attractive alternative targets [32].

Clinical Relevance and Therapeutic Potential of Coregulators in CaP

The appreciation of coregulators as potential therapeutic targets in the treatment of CaP stems mainly from observations of deregulated coregulator expression in CaP. Immunohistochemical analysis of CaP specimens has revealed deregulated expression of more than 50 AR-associated coregulators during disease progression (Table 3.1). In most cases, such altered coregulator expression involves increased expression of coactivators in CaP when compared to benign prostate. Using in vitro model systems for CaP, investigators have shown that increased coactivator expression contributes substantially to the mechanism of AR activation in CRPC [32]. Overexpression of most, if not all, of the coactivators in CaP is capable of inducing AR transactivation in the presence of low levels of androgens, other steroids, and even antiandrogens, irrespective of the mutational status of the AR. In addition, such overexpression has been shown to enhance the agonistic properties of antiandrogens (CBP, [33]) and to induce coregulator association with AF-2, which is not observed during normal androgen-dependent AR activation (SRC-2, [34]) resulting in increased activity through this otherwise weak activation function. These observations suggest that elevated coactivator expression in CaP could lead to a more active AR signaling pathway, and hence, a more aggressive disease. This hypothesis is consistent with data derived from clinical studies linking coregulator expression with pathological information and patient follow-up data. These studies show that deregulated coregulator expression correlates with more aggressive disease features (such as larger tumor volumes, extraprostatic disease at time of surgery, increased cell proliferation indices, etc.) and shorter disease-free survival after prostatectomy (see Table 3.1). It is tempting to speculate that decreases in corepressor expression, such as those observed for LATS2/KPM, also result in a more active AR signaling axis in CaP. Noteworthy, expression of a small number of coactivators has been reported to be decreased, rather than increased in CaP specimens. It has been suggested that these coactivator proteins are selectively involved in the transcriptional regulation of genes involved with cell proliferation and apoptosis although definite proof for this hypothesis is pending.

Alterations in coregulator expression during progression of CaP are not only limited to changes in expression levels but also can involve shifts in their subcellular distribution patterns, for example, the evolution in expression patterns of the corepressor Hey1 and the coactivator Tip60 during the progression of CaP. The immunohistochemical staining profile of Tip60 in androgen-dependent CaP varies widely, ranging from high expression in both cellular compartments to a complete lack of expression. In some specimens, solely nuclear or cytoplasmic Tip60 staining is also observed. In contrast, Tip60 is expressed almost exclusively in the nucleus in CRPC samples [35]. Hey1, on the other hand, colocalizes with AR in the epithelia of patients with benign prostatic hyperplasia, where it is found in both the cytoplasm and the nucleus. In CaP, however, a shift in Hey1 expression is observed, where Hey1 is excluded from the nucleus [36]. Thus, alterations in the subcellular localization of coregulators may affect their ability to interact with the AR and components of the AR transcriptional complex, and consequently their capacity to modulate AR-driven transcription. It should be noted that the coactivators described here not only interact exclusively with the AR but also influence transcription mediated by numerous other nuclear receptors and transcription factors. Thus, overexpression of these coregulatory proteins in CaP may also affect expression of genes by signaling mechanisms that do not necessarily involve the AR. Conversely, some level of intrinsic, nuclear receptor-independent activity by individual coactivators cannot be excluded at this time.

Table 3.1 AR-associated coregulators that are aberrantly expressed in CaP

Coregulator	coA/coR	Function	CaP expr/loc	Aggressive disease	References
α-actinin-4	coA/coR	cytoskel	–		[57]
ARA55	coA	int/transd	Stromal		[58]
ARA70	coA	Diverse	+		[46]
ART-27	coA	Diverse	–		[59]
BAF57	coA	chrom remod	+		[47]
BAF155	coA	chrom remod	+	yes	[60]
Bag-1L	coA	(co)chap	+	yes	[61, 62]
BRG1	coA	chrom remod	+	yes	[63]
β-catenin	coA	int/transd	+ (N,C)	yes	[64, 65]
CARM1/PRMT5	coA	HMT	+		[66]
Caveolin-1	coA	Endocytosis	+	yes	[67]
CBP	coA	HAT	+		[33]
cdc25B	coA	Cell cycle	+		[68]
Cdc37	coA	(co)chap	+		[69]
cyclin D1	coR	Cell cycle	+		[70]
DJ-1/PARK7	coA	Diverse		CR development	[71]
L-dopa-decarboxylase	coA	Diverse	NE		[72]
E6-AP	coA	ub/prot	–		[73]
FHL2	coA	int/transd	+ (C–N)	yes	[74]
GAK/auxillin2	coA	Endocytosis		CR development	[75]
gelsolin	coA	cytoskel	–		[76]
Hey1	coR	int/transd	N–C		[36]
HIP1	coA	Endocytosis	+	yes	[77]
Hsp90	coA	(co)chap	+		[78]
JARID1B	coA	HMT	+		[79]
LATS2/KPM	coR	Diverse	–		[80]
LSD1	coA	HMT	+	yes	[74]
MED1/TRAP220	coA	Diverse	+		[81]
p44/MEP50	coA	RNA met	+ (N–C)	yes	[82]
p300	coA	HAT	+	yes	[55, 56]
PAK6	coR	int/transd	+		[83]
par-4	coA	Apoptosis	+		[84]
PELP1/MNAR	coA	int/transd	+		[85]
PIAS3	coA/coR	Sumoylation	+		[86]
PIRH2	coA	ub/prot	+	yes	[87]
PRK1	coA	int/transd	+	yes	[88]
Rad9	coR	DNA repair	+	yes	[89]
Sam68	coA	RNA met	+		[90]
SENP1	coA	Sumoylation	+		[37]
α-SGT	coR	(co)chap	+(primary), –(met)		[91]
SIRT1	coR	HAT	+		[92]
Smad3	coA/coR	int/transd	+	yes	[93]
SRC-1	coA	HAT		yes	[34, 94]
SRC-2	coA	HAT*		yes	[34, 40]
SRC-3	coA	HAT	+	yes	[95, 96]
STAT3	coA	int/transd	+	yes	[97]
Tip30	coA	Diverse	+	yes	[98]
Tip60	coA	HAT	C–N	yes	[35]
TRIM68	coA	ub/prot	+		[99]
vav3	coA	int/transd	+		[100]

*Belongs to family of HAT proteins although significant HAT activity has not been demonstrated

coA coactivator, *coR* corepressor, *cytoskel* cytoskeleton, *int/transd* signal integrator or transducer, *chrom remod* chromatin remodeling, *(co)chap* (co)chaperone, *HMT* histone methyl transferase, *ub/prot* ubiquitination/proteasome, *RNA met* RNA metabolism, *HAT* histone acetyl transferase, – decreased expression, + overexpression, *N* nuclear, *C* cytoplasmic, *N–C* from nucleus to cytoplasm, *C–N* from cytoplasm to nucleus, *NE* neuroendocrine phenotype, *CR* castration recurrence, *met* metastatic CaP, *CaP expr/loc* coregulator expression or localization pattern in CaP, *aggressive disease* correlation of coregulator expression with aggressive disease

Potential Approaches to Target Coregulators in CaP

Targeting Coregulator Expression

Given the clinical relevance and the therapeutic potential of coregulators in CaP, a better understanding of the factors or circumstances that underlie the increase in expression of these critical cofactors in CaP disease progression and/or the signaling events that affect their activity could lead to novel approaches for treating this devastating disease. To our knowledge, no evidence of amplification of coregulator genes in CaP has been reported. Instead, a growing body of evidence suggests that circumstances such as changes in the local CaP cell milieu, even treatment-induced changes, could affect coregulator expression levels [37–42]. Insights into the signals and signaling pathways that mediate these effects could lead to valid methods for targeting coregulator gene expression. In view of the importance of androgens in the natural history of CaP and their central role in the approaches for therapeutic intervention in this disease, the impact of androgen signaling on coregulator gene expression is increasingly being investigated. Thus far, changes in androgen levels have been shown to either positively or negatively affect the expression of a few coregulators (SENP1 [37], NRIP1 [38], FHL2 [39], SRC-2 [40], p300 [41], and CBP [42], respectively). Interestingly, molecular dissection of the mechanisms by which changes in the androgenic milieu alter coregulator expression indicates that at least three coactivator genes (SRC-2, SENP1, and NRIP1) are direct targets for androgen action [37, 38, 40] as their androgen dependency is mediated through interaction of the AR with AREs within the regulatory regions of these genes. Thus, identifying mechanisms by which androgens control coregulator gene expression that involve the activity of secondary, intermediary factors might provide therapeutical potential. Recently, our laboratory identified NF-kappaB and serum response factor (SRF) as critical determinants for androgen-induced downregulation and upregulation, respectively, of the expression of the coactivator genes p300 and FHL2 [39, 41]. Importantly, NF-kappaB has been implicated in ligand-independent AR signaling in CaP cells and has been reported to bind DNA more readily in CRPC xenografts than in androgen-dependent xenografts [43–45]. In addition, we have shown that SRF activity is crucial for the proliferation of both androgen-stimulated and CRPC cells [39]. Further work is needed to fully understand the molecular machinery that coordinates androgen signaling with activity of NF-kappaB and SRF. Such studies may provide a foundation for targeting coregulator expression in treating this disease.

Targeting Coregulator Activity

Apart from strategies directed against coregulator expression, efforts to prevent the interaction of the coregulator complex with the AR could provide an effective means of targeting coregulators of AR in CaP. In this respect, an approach aimed at disrupting the molecular interaction between the AR and its coregulators or at disturbing coregulator–coregulator interaction, or a combination of both, might be appropriate. At least under in vitro experimental conditions, such strategies using fragments derived from ARA70 and BAF57 show promise. Indeed, an ARA70 fragment, harboring its AR interacting motif, has been shown to prevent AR N/C termini interaction, as well as recruitment of SRC-2 coactivator to the AR and AR transactivation [46]. Similarly, an inhibitor derived from BAF57, termed BAF57 inhibitory peptide (BIPep), which blocks AR residence on chromatin and resultant AR-dependent gene activation, was sufficient to inhibit androgen-dependent CaP cell proliferation [47]. In order to be successfully translated into the clinic, drug design using AR-coregulator interaction sites as a template for the generation of small peptides that interfere with and compete for coregulator binding would necessarily depend on a detailed understanding of the interaction of individual coactivators with the AR and with each other.

Functionally disrupting the AR-coregulator complex may not depend on a mechanical interference as discussed above. A growing body of evidence suggests that coregulators are subject to posttranslational modifications, which determine their ability to interact with the AR and fulfill their role as regulators of AR-mediated transactivation. Strikingly, several of these modifications are executed by signaling pathways and cascades that are overly active in CaP. Such modifications are under investigating for therapeutic intervention in CaP. For instance, serum levels of some growth factors such as epidermal growth factor (EGF) and cytokines such as interleukin 6 (IL-6) are elevated in patients with CRPC [48]. Stimulation of CaP cells with EGF leads to phosphorylation of the AR-associated coactivators SRC-2 [49] and MAGEA11 [50]. Moreover, EGF stimulation also results in ubiquitination of MAGEA11 [50]. In addition, IL-6 treatment induces phosphorylation of SRC-1 [51]. These modifications result in stronger AR-coregulator interaction and increased AR-mediated transcription. The effects of EGF and IL-6 stimulation on coregulator modification are mediated by the MAPK kinase signaling cascade [49, 51], the activity of which is known to be increased during CaP progression [48]. MAPK activity has also been shown to lead to phosphorylation of MED1, which in turn stimulates the intrinsic coactivation properties of MED1 [52]. Another example of the impact of cytokine-induced signaling cascades on the composition and activity of the AR transcriptional complex is illustrated by the effects of macrophage-derived cytokine IL-1beta on CaP cells. In CaP cells treated with AR antagonists, IL-1beta leads to activation of MEKK1, MEKK1-mediated removal of the coregulator TAB2 from a corepressor complex interacting with the AR NTD, and subsequent recruitment of coactivator proteins to the AR. In this case, cytokine-mediated activation of MEKK1 turns an AR antagonist into a potent agonist [53]. Apart from regulating the composition of the AR-associated coregulator complex, clinically relevant signaling pathways can affect the intrinsic enzymatic moieties of coactivators. For instance, Src and PKCδ signal transduction regulate the histone acetyl transferase (HAT) activity of p300 [54], a coactivator we have shown to be critical for CaP proliferation and to correlate with aggressive disease [55, 56]. Several coregulators possess enzymatic activities that introduce posttranslational modifications in the AR and govern its transcriptional activity. Inhibition of these signaling cascades could therefore represent an attractive therapeutic option to silence AR-mediated transcription in CaP cells.

Conclusions and Future Perspectives

The AR is currently under intense investigation as a target for novel therapeutic strategies for the treatment of CaP. Apart from strategies aimed at targeting the expression, stability, or degradation of the AR itself, the data presented in the chapter suggest that targeting AR transcriptional complex may hold promise for therapeutic strategy. A thorough understanding of the mechanisms and signaling events that control the expression, subcellular localization, and interaction of coregulators will be essential to reach the goal of novel coregulator-targeted therapies for CaP.

References

1. Denmeade SR, Isaacs JT. A history of prostate cancer treatment. Nat Rev Cancer 2002;2:389–96.
2. Miyamoto H, Messing EM, Chang C. Androgen deprivation therapy for prostate cancer: current status and future prospects. Prostate 2004;61:332–53.
3. Mohler JL, Gregory CW, Ford 3rd OH, Kim D, Weaver CM, Petrusz P, et al. The androgen axis in recurrent prostate cancer. Clin Cancer Res 2004;10:440–8.
4. Mohler JL. Castration-recurrent prostate cancer is not androgen-independent. Adv Exp Med Biol 2008;617:223–34.
5. Davison SL, Bell R. Androgen physiology. Semin Reprod Med 2006;24:71–7.
6. Rainey WE, Carr BR, Sasano H, Suzuki T, Mason JI. Dissecting human adrenal androgen production. Trends Endocrinol Metab 2002;13:234–9.
7. Vermeulen A. Reflections concerning biochemical parameters of androgenicity. Aging Male 2004;7:280–9.
8. Pardridge WM. Serum bioavailability of sex steroid hormones. Clin Endocrinol Metab 1986;15:259–78.
9. Russell DW, Wilson JD. Steroid 5 alpha-reductase: two genes/two enzymes. Annu Rev Biochem 1994;63:25–61.
10. Deslypere JP, Young M, Wilson JD, McPhaul MJ. Testosterone and 5 alpha-dihydrotestosterone interact differently with the androgen receptor to enhance transcription of the MMTV-CAT reporter gene. Mol Cell Endocrinol 1992; 88:15–22.
11. Wilson EM, French FS. Binding properties of androgen receptors. Evidence for identical receptors in rat testis, epididymis, and prostate. J Biol Chem 1976;251:5620–9.
12. Mizokami A, Koh E, Fujita H, Maeda Y, Egawa M, Koshida K, et al. The adrenal androgen androstenediol is present in prostate cancer tissue after androgen deprivation therapy and activates mutated androgen receptor. Cancer Res 2004;64: 765–71.
13. Prescott J, Coetzee GA. Molecular chaperones throughout the life cycle of the androgen receptor. Cancer Lett 2006; 231:12–9.
14. Shaffer PL, Jivan A, Dollins DE, Claessens F, Gewirth DT. Structural basis of androgen receptor binding to selective androgen response elements. Proc Natl Acad Sci U S A 2004; 101:4758–63.
15. Verrijdt G, Tanner T, Moehren U, Callewaert L, Haelens A, Claessens F. The androgen receptor DNA-binding domain determines androgen selectivity of transcriptional response. Biochem Soc Trans 2006;34:1089–94.

16. Reid KJ, Hendy SC, Saito J, Sorensen P, Nelson CC. Two classes of androgen receptor elements mediate cooperativity through allosteric interactions. J Biol Chem 2001;276: 2943–52.

17. Heemers HV, Tindall DJ. Androgen receptor (AR) coregulators: a diversity of functions converging on and regulating the AR transcriptional complex. Endocr Rev 2007;28: 778–808.

18. Tsai MJ, O'Malley BW. Molecular mechanisms of action of steroid/thyroid receptor superfamily members. Annu Rev Biochem 1994;63:451–86.

19. White R, Parker MG. Molecular mechanisms of steroid hormone action. Endocr Relat Cancer 1998;5:1–14.

20. Lavery DN, McEwan IJ. The human androgen receptor AF1 transactivation domain: interactions with transcription factor IIF and molten-globule-like structural characteristics. Biochem Soc Trans 2006;34:1054–7.

21. Giovannucci E, Stampfer MJ, Krithivas K, Brown M, Dahl D, Brufsky A, et al. The CAG repeat within the androgen receptor gene and its relationship to prostate cancer. Proc Natl Acad Sci USA 1997;94:3320–3.

22. Schoenmakers E, Verrijdt G, Peeters B, Verhoeven G, Rombauts W, Claessens F. Differences in DNA binding characteristics of the androgen and glucocorticoid receptors can determine hormone-specific responses. J Biol Chem 2000;275:12290–7.

23. Wang Q, Lu J, Yong EL. Ligand- and coactivator-mediated transactivation function (AF2) of the androgen receptor ligand-binding domain is inhibited by the cognate hinge region. J Biol Chem 2001;276:7493–9.

24. Haelens A, Tanner T, Denayer S, Callewaert L, Claessens F. The hinge region regulates DNA binding, nuclear translocation, and transactivation of the androgen receptor. Cancer Res 2007;67:4514–23.

25. Jenster G, Trapman J, Brinkmann AO. Nuclear import of the human androgen receptor. Biochem J 1993;293:761–8.

26. Zhou ZX, Sar M, Simental JA, Lane MV, Wilson EM. A ligand-dependent bipartite nuclear targeting signal in the human androgen receptor. Requirement for the DNA-binding domain and modulation by NH_2-terminal and carboxyl-terminal sequences. J Biol Chem 1994;269: 13115–23.

27. Heery DM, Kalkhoven E, Hoare S, Parker MG. A signature motif in transcriptional co-activators mediates binding to nuclear receptors. Nature 1997;387:733–6.

28. Chang CY, McDonnell DP. Androgen receptor–cofactor interactions as targets for new drug discovery. Trends Pharmacol Sci 2005;26:225–8.

29. Grossmann ME, Huang H, Tindall DJ. Androgen receptor signaling in androgen-refractory prostate cancer. J Natl Cancer Inst 2001;93:1687–97.

30. Debes JD, Tindall DJ. Mechanisms of androgen-refractory prostate cancer. N Engl J Med 2004;351:1488–90.

31. Mohler JL. A role for the androgen-receptor in clinically localized and advanced prostate cancer. Best Pract Res Clin Endocrinol Metab 2008;22:357–72.

32. Heemers HV, Tindall DJ. Androgen receptor coregulatory proteins as potential therapeutic targets in the treatment of prostate cancer. Curr Cancer Ther Rev 2005;1:175–86.

33. Comuzzi B, Lambrinidis L, Rogatsch H, Godoy-Tundidor S, Knezevic N, Krhen I, et al. The transcriptional co-activator cAMP response element-binding protein-binding protein is expressed in prostate cancer and enhances androgen and anti-androgen-induced androgen receptor function. Am J Pathol 2003;162:233–41.

34. Gregory CW, He B, Johnson RT, Ford OH, Mohler JL, French FS, et al. A mechanism for androgen receptor-mediated prostate cancer recurrence after androgen deprivation therapy. Cancer Res 2001;61:4315–9.

35. Halkidou K, Gnanapragasam VJ, Mehta PB, Logan IR, Brady ME, Cook S, et al. Expression of Tip60, an androgen receptor coactivator, and its role in prostate cancer development. Oncogene 2003;22:2466–77.

36. Belandia B, Powell SM, García-Pedrero JM, Walker MM, Bevan CL, Parker MG. Hey1, a mediator of notch signaling, is an androgen receptor corepressor. Mol Cell Biol 2005; 25:1425–36.

37. Bawa-Khalfe T, Cheng J, Wang Z, Yeh ET. Induction of the SUMO-specific protease 1 transcription by the androgen receptor in prostate cancer cells. J Biol Chem 2007;282: 37341–9.

38. Chen PH, Tsao YP, Wang CC, Chen SL. Nuclear receptor interaction protein, a coactivator of androgen receptors (AR), is regulated by AR and Sp1 to feed forward and activate its own gene expression through AR protein stability. Nucleic Acids Res 2008;36:51–66.

39. Heemers HV, Regan KM, Dehm SM, Tindall DJ. Androgen induction of the androgen receptor coactivator four and a half LIM domain protein-2: evidence for a role for serum response factor in prostate cancer. Cancer Res 2007;67: 10592–9.

40. Agoulnik IU, Vaid A, Nakka M, Alvarado M, Bingman 3rd WE, Erdem H, et al. Androgens modulate expression of transcription intermediary factor 2, an androgen receptor coactivator whose expression level correlates with early biochemical recurrence in prostate cancer. Cancer Res 2006; 66:10594–602.

41. Heemers HV, Sebo TJ, Debes JD, Regan KM, Raclaw KA, Murphy LM, et al. Androgen deprivation increases p300 expression in prostate cancer cells. Cancer Res 2007;67: 3422–30.

42. Comuzzi B, Nemes C, Schmidt S, Jasarevic Z, Lodde M, Pycha A, et al. The androgen receptor co-activator CBP is up-regulated following androgen withdrawal and is highly expressed in advanced prostate cancer. J Pathol 2004;204: 159–66.

43. Shukla S, MacLennan GT, Marengo SR, Resnick MI, Gupta S. Constitutive activation of PI3K-Akt and NF-κB during prostate cancer progression in autochtonous transgenic mouse model. Prostate 2005;64:224–39.

44. Lee SO, Lou W, Nadiminty N, Lin X, Gao AC. Requirement for NF-(kappa)B in interleukin-4-induced androgen receptor activation in prostate cancer cells. Prostate 2005;64: 160–7.

45. Chen CD, Sawyers CL. NF-kappa B activates prostate-specific antigen expression and is upregulated in androgen-independent prostate cancer. Mol Cell Biol 2002;22: 2862–70.

46. Hu YC, Yeh S, Yeh SD, Sampson ER, Huang J, Li P, et al. Functional domain and motif analyses of androgen receptor coregulator ARA70 and its differential expression in prostate cancer. J Biol Chem 2004;279:33438–46.

47. Link KA, Balasubramaniam S, Sharma A, Comstock CE, Godoy-Tundidor S, Powers N, et al. Targeting the BAF57 SWI/SNF subunit in prostate cancer: a novel platform to control androgen receptor activity. Cancer Res 2008;68: 4551–8.

48. Culig Z. Androgen receptor cross-talk with cell signalling pathways. Growth Factors 2004;22:179–84.

49. Gregory CW, Fei X, Ponguta LA, He B, Bill HM, French FS, et al. Epidermal growth factor increases coactivation of the androgen receptor in recurrent prostate cancer. J Biol Chem 2004;279:7119–30.

50. Bai S, Wilson EM. Epidermal-growth-factor-dependent phosphorylation and ubiquitinylation of MAGE-11 regulates its interaction with the androgen receptor. Mol Cell Biol 2008;28:1947–63.

51. Ueda T, Mawji NR, Bruchovsky N, Sadar MD. Ligand-independent activation of the androgen receptor by interleukin-6 and the role of steroid receptor coactivator-1 in prostate cancer cells. J Biol Chem 2002;277:38087–94.

52. Pandey PK, Udayakumar TS, Lin X, Sharma D, Shapiro PS, Fondell JD. Activation of TRAP/mediator subunit TRAP220/Med1 is regulated by mitogen-activated protein kinase-dependent phosphorylation. Mol Cell Biol 2005; 25:10695–710.

53. Zhu P, Baek SH, Bourk EM, Ohgi KA, Garcia-Bassets I, Sanjo H, et al. Macrophage/cancer cell interactions mediate hormone resistance by a nuclear receptor derepression pathway. Cell 2006;124:615–29.

54. Gong J, Zhu J, Goodman Jr OB, Pestell RG, Schlegel PN, Nanus DM, et al. Activation of p300 histone acetyltransferase activity and acetylation of the androgen receptor by bombesin in prostate cancer cells. Oncogene 2006;25: 2011–21.

55. Debes JD, Sebo TJ, Lohse CM, Murphy LM, Haugen DA, Tindall DJ. p300 in prostate cancer proliferation and progression. Cancer Res 2003;63:7638–40.

56. Debes JD, Sebo TJ, Heemers HV, Kipp BR, Haugen DL, Lohse CM, et al. p300 modulates nuclear morphology in prostate cancer. Cancer Res 2005;65:708–12.

57. Hara T, Honda K, Shitashige M, Ono M, Matsuyama H, Naito K, et al. Mass spectrometry analysis of the native protein complex containing actinin-4 in prostate cancer cells. Mol Cell Proteomics 2007;6:479–91.

58. Heitzer MD, DeFranco DB. Hic-5/ARA55, a LIM domain-containing nuclear receptor coactivator expressed in prostate stromal cells. Cancer Res 2006;66:7326–33.

59. Taneja SS, Ha S, Swenson NK, Torra IP, Rome S, Walden PD, et al. ART-27, an androgen receptor coactivator regulated in prostate development and cancer. J Biol Chem 2004;279:13944–52.

60. Heebøll S, Borre M, Ottosen PD, Andersen CL, Mansilla F, Dyrskjøt L, et al. SMARCC1 expression is upregulated in prostate cancer and positively correlated with tumour recurrence and dedifferentiation. Histol Histopathol 2008;23:1069–76.

61. Krajewska M, Turner BC, Shabaik A, Krajewski S, Reed JC. Expression of BAG-1 protein correlates with aggressive behavior of prostate cancers. Prostate 2006;66:801–10.

62. Mäki HE, Saramäki OR, Shatkina L, Martikainen PM, Tammela TL, van Weerden WM, et al. Overexpression and gene amplification of BAG-1L in hormone-refractory prostate cancer. J Pathol 2007;212:395–401.

63. Sun A, Tawfik O, Gayed B, Thrasher JB, Hoestje S, Li C, et al. Aberrant expression of SWI/SNF catalytic subunits BRG1/BRM is associated with tumor development and increased invasiveness in prostate cancers. Prostate 2007;67:203–13.

64. Chen G, Shukeir N, Potti A, Sircar K, Aprikian A, Goltzman D, et al. Up-regulation of Wnt-1 and beta-catenin production in patients with advanced metastatic prostate carcinoma: potential pathogenetic and prognostic implications. Cancer 2004;101:1345–56.

65. Whitaker HC, Girling J, Warren AY, Leung H, Mills IG, Neal DE. Alterations in beta-catenin expression and localization in prostate cancer. Prostate 2008;68:1196–205.

66. Hong H, Kao C, Jeng MH, Eble JN, Koch MO, Gardner TA, et al. Aberrant expression of CARM1, a transcriptional coactivator of androgen receptor, in the development of prostate carcinoma and androgen-independent status. Cancer 2004;101:83–9.

67. Karam JA, Lotan Y, Roehrborn CG, Ashfaq R, Karakiewicz PI, Shariat SF. Caveolin-1 overexpression is associated with aggressive prostate cancer recurrence. Prostate 2007;67: 614–22.

68. Ngan ES, Hashimoto Y, Ma ZQ, Tsai MJ, Tsai SY. Overexpression of Cdc25B, an androgen receptor coactivator, in prostate cancer. Oncogene 2003;22:734–9.

69. Stepanova L, Yang G, DeMayo F, Wheeler TM, Finegold M, Thompson TC, et al. Induction of human Cdc37 in prostate cancer correlates with the ability of targeted Cdc37 expression to promote prostatic hyperplasia. Oncogene 2000;19: 2186–93.

70. Drobnjak M, Osman I, Scher HI, Fazzari M, Cordon-Cardo C. Overexpression of cyclin D1 is associated with metastatic prostate cancer to bone. Clin Cancer Res 2000;6:1891–5.

71. Tillman JE, Yuan J, Gu G, Fazli L, Ghosh R, Flynt AS, et al. DJ-1 binds androgen receptor directly and mediates its activity in hormonally treated prostate cancer cells. Cancer Res 2007;67:4630–7.

72. Wafa LA, Palmer J, Fazli L, Hurtado-Coll A, Bell RH, Nelson CC, et al. Comprehensive expression analysis ofl-dopa decarboxylase and established neuroendocrine markers in neoadjuvant hormone-treated versus varying Gleason grade prostate tumors. Hum Pathol 2007;38:161–70.

73. Gao X, Mohsin SK, Gatalica Z, Fu G, Sharma P, Nawaz Z. Decreased expression of e6-associated protein in breast and prostate carcinomas. Endocrinology 2005;146:1707–12.

74. Kahl P, Gullotti L, Heukamp LC, Wolf S, Friedrichs N, Vorreuther R, et al. Androgen receptor coactivators lysine-specific histone demethylase 1 and four and a half LIM domain protein 2 predict risk of prostate cancer recurrence. Cancer Res 2006;66:11341–7.

75. Ray MR, Wafa LA, Cheng H, Snoek R, Fazli L, Gleave M, et al. Cyclin G-associated kinase: a novel androgen receptor-interacting transcriptional coactivator that is overexpressed in hormone refractory prostate cancer. Int J Cancer 2006; 118:1108–19.

76. Lee HK, Driscoll D, Asch H, Asch B, Zhang PJ. Downregulated gelsolin expression in hyperplastic and neoplastic lesions of the prostate. Prostate 1999;40:14–9.

77. Rao DS, Hyun TS, Kumar PD, Mizukami IF, Rubin MA, Lucas PC, et al. Huntingtin-interacting protein 1 is overexpressed in prostate and colon cancer and is critical for cellular survival. J Clin Invest 2002;110:351–60.

78. Cardillo MR, Ippoliti F. IL-6, IL-10 and HSP-90 expression in tissue microarrays from human prostate cancer assessed by computer-assisted image analysis. Anticancer Res 2006;26:3409–16.

79. Xiang Y, Zhu Z, Han G, Ye X, Xu B, Peng Z, et al. JARID1B is a histone H3 lysine 4 demethylase up-regulated in prostate cancer. Proc Natl Acad Sci U S A 2007;104:19226–31.

80. Powzaniuk M, McElwee-Witmer S, Vogel RL, Hayami T, Rutledge SJ, Chen F, et al. The LATS2/KPM tumor suppressor is a negative regulator of the androgen receptor. Mol Endocrinol 2004;18:2011–23.

81. Vijayvargia R, May MS, Fondell JD. A coregulatory role for the mediator complex in prostate cancer cell proliferation and gene expression. Cancer Res 2007;67:4034–41.

82. Peng Y, Chen F, Melamed J, Chiriboga L, Wei J, Kong X, et al. Distinct nuclear and cytoplasmic functions of androgen receptor cofactor p44 and association with androgen-independent prostate cancer. Proc Natl Acad Sci U S A 2008;105:5236–41.

83. Kaur R, Yuan X, Lu ML, Balk SP. Increased PAK6 expression in prostate cancer and identification of PAK6 associated proteins. Prostate 2008;68(14):1510–6.

84. Black PC, Mize GJ, Karlin P, Greenberg DL, Hawley SJ, True LD, et al. Overexpression of protease-activated receptors-1,-2, and-4 (PAR-1, -2, and -4) in prostate cancer. Prostate 2007;67:743–56.

85. Nair SS, Guo Z, Mueller JM, Koochekpour S, Qiu Y, Tekmal RR, et al. Proline-, glutamic acid-, and leucine-rich protein-1/modulator of nongenomic activity of estrogen receptor enhances androgen receptor functions through LIM-only coactivator, four-and-a-half LIM-only protein 2. Mol Endocrinol 2007;21:613–24.

86. Wang L, Banerjee S. Differential PIAS3 expression in human malignancy. Oncol Rep 2004;11:1319–24.

87. Logan IR, Gaughan L, McCracken SR, Sapountzi V, Leung HY, Robson CN. Human PIRH2 enhances androgen receptor signaling through inhibition of histone deacetylase 1 and is overexpressed in prostate cancer. Mol Cell Biol 2006;26:6502–10.

88. Metzger E, Yin N, Wissmann M, Kunowska N, Fischer K, Friedrichs N, et al. Phosphorylation of histone H3 at threonine 11 establishes a novel chromatin mark for transcriptional regulation. Nat Cell Biol 2008;10:53–60.

89. Zhu A, Zhang CX, Lieberman HB. Rad9 has a functional role in human prostate carcinogenesis. Cancer Res 2008;68:1267–74.

90. Rajan P, Gaughan L, Dalgliesh C, El-Sherif A, Robson CN, Leung HY, et al. The RNA-binding and adaptor protein Sam68 modulates signal-dependent splicing and transcriptional activity of the androgen receptor. J Pathol 2008;215:67–77.

91. Buchanan G, Ricciardelli C, Harris JM, Prescott J, Yu ZC, Jia L, et al. Control of androgen receptor signaling in prostate cancer by the cochaperone small glutamine rich tetratricopeptide repeat containing protein alpha. Cancer Res 2007;67:10087–96.

92. Huffman DM, Grizzle WE, Bamman MM, Kim JS, Eltoum IA, Elgavish A, et al. SIRT1 is significantly elevated in mouse and human prostate cancer. Cancer Res 2007;67:6612–8.

93. Lu S, Lee J, Revelo M, Wang X, Lu S, Dong Z. Smad3 is overexpressed in advanced human prostate cancer and necessary for progressive growth of prostate cancer cells in nude mice. Clin Cancer Res 2007;13:5692–702.

94. Agoulnik IU, Vaid A, Bingman 3rd WE, Erdeme H, Frolov A, Smith CL, et al. Role of SRC-1 in the promotion of prostate cancer cell growth and tumor progression. Cancer Res 2005;65:7959–67.

95. Zhou HJ, Yan J, Luo W, Ayala G, Lin SH, Erdem H, et al. SRC-3 is required for prostate cancer cell proliferation and survival. Cancer Res 2005;65:7976–83.

96. Gnanapragasam VJ, Leung HY, Pulimood AS, Neal DE, Robson CN. Expression of RAC 3, a steroid hormone receptor co-activator in prostate cancer. Br J Cancer 2001;85:1928–36.

97. Tam L, McGlynn LM, Traynor P, Mukherjee R, Bartlett JM, Edwards J. Expression levels of the JAK/STAT pathway in the transition from hormone-sensitive to hormone-refractory prostate cancer. Br J Cancer 2007;97:378–83.

98. Zhang H, Zhang Y, Duan HO, Kirley SD, Lin SX, McDougal WS, et al. TIP30 is associated with progression and metastasis of prostate cancer. Int J Cancer 2008;123:810–6.

99. Miyajima N, Maruyama S, Bohgaki M, Kano S, Shigemura M, Shinohara N, et al. TRIM68 regulates ligand-dependent transcription of androgen receptor in prostate cancer cells. Cancer Res 2008;68:3486–94.

100. Dong Z, Liu Y, Lu S, Wang A, Lee K, Wang LH, et al. Vav3 oncogene is overexpressed and regulates cell growth and androgen receptor activity in human prostate cancer. Mol Endocrinol 2006;20:2315–25.

Chapter 4
Androgens and Prostate Cancer

Douglas K. Price and Ann W. Hsing

Abstract Prostate cancer is the most common nonskin cancer among American men and the third leading cause of cancer deaths. Research data over many years of study support the role of androgen in driving prostate cancer growth, proliferation, and progression. Androgens are steroid hormones that induce the differentiation and maturation of the male reproductive organs. Testosterone is the principal androgen in circulation, while dihydrotestosterone (DHT) is the primary nuclear androgen, and the action of DHT in the prostate is mediated by the androgen receptor. Within the prostate, DHT binds to the androgen receptor to form an intracellular complex that binds to androgen-response elements in the DNA of prostate cells inducing proliferation. Testosterone deficiency is common among aging American males, and a number of men suffering from testosterone deficiency may be relieved of their symptoms, receiving a boost in their quality of life, but are often denied treatment due to the fear that the addition of higher testosterone from replacement therapy may cause growth of occult prostate cancer. Several small studies show that, with the right patient population, testosterone replacement after curative therapy is safe. However, a large placebo-controlled prospective trial to provide the definitive study is needed.

Keywords Prostate cancer • Androgens • Testosterone • Replacement therapy

D.K. Price (✉)
Medical Oncology Branch, National Cancer Institute,
National Institutes of Health, Bethesda, MD, USA
e-mail: dkprice@mai.nih.gov

Introduction

Prostate cancer is the most common nonskin cancer among American men and the third leading cause of cancer deaths, behind lung and colorectal cancer [1]. Despite its high morbidity and mortality, few risk factors have been established other than age, race, and family history [2]. Recently, several genome-wide association studies (GWAS) have identified a number of genomic regions, including several in 8q24, that have been consistently linked to prostate cancer risk in several populations [3–9], although the function of the variants are unclear. Both clinical and laboratory data suggest that androgens play a pivotal role in prostate growth, maintenance, and carcinogenesis [10, 11]. However, data from serum-based epidemiologic studies in human are inconclusive [12–14].

Androgen and the Prostate

Biosynthesis and Metabolism of Androgens

Androgens are steroid hormones that induce the differentiation and maturation of the male reproductive organs and the development of male secondary sex characteristics. In men, androgens are formed primarily in the testes and the adrenal gland, and to a lesser extent in peripheral tissues, such as the prostate and skin. Biosynthesis of androgens in the endocrine glands occurs by well-characterized biosynthetic pathways as shown in Fig. 4.1.

W.D. Figg et al. (eds.), *Drug Management of Prostate Cancer*,
DOI 10.1007/978-1-60327-829-4_4, © Springer Science+Business Media, LLC 2010

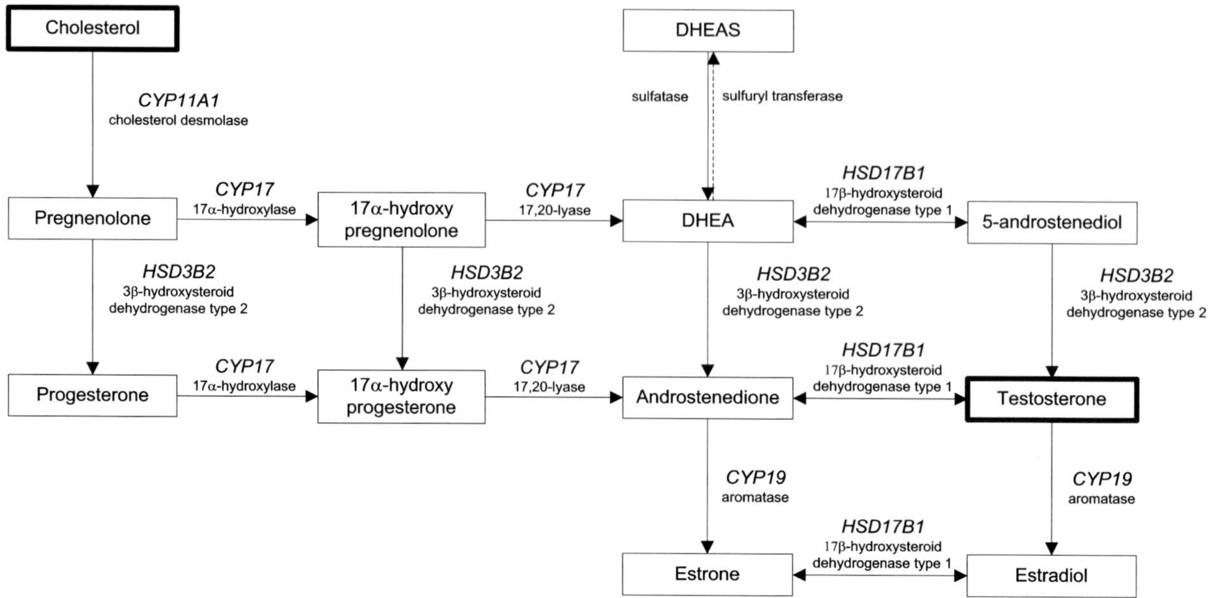

Fig. 4.1 Androgen metabolism pathways in the endocrine system. Androgen biosynthesis and metabolism within and outside the prostate gland

Testosterone (T) is the principal androgen in circulation, while dihydrotestosterone (DHT) is the primary nuclear androgen and the most potent androgen in tissue. In the circulation of adult males, roughly 44% of testosterone is bound with high affinity to sex hormone binding globulin (SHBG), 54% is bound with low affinity to albumin, and only 1–2% of testosterone exists in a free (unbound) state. About 25% of the DHT in the circulation is secreted by the testes while most (65–75%) arises from conversion of testosterone in peripheral tissue in a reaction catalyzed by the enzyme steroid 5α-reductase or from circulating inactive androgens, such as androstenedione, dehydroepiandrosterone (DHEA), and DHEA sulfate (DHEAS). In humans, two steroid 5α-reductase isoenzymes have been identified. The type 1 enzyme (encoded by the *SRD5A1* gene) is expressed mostly in skin and hair, whereas the type 2 enzyme (encoded by the *SRD5A2* gene) is localized primarily in androgen target tissue, including genital skin and the prostate [15].

In men, the prostate is a major site of nontesticular DHT production from testosterone. Free testosterone in circulation enters prostate cells by passive diffusion, whereas albumin-bound testosterone, because of its low affinity for albumin, can disassociate from albumin, allowing it to enter prostatic cells. Figure 4.2 shows the metabolic pathways of androgens within the prostate gland.

In androgen-sensitive tissue, including the prostate and skin, DHT (see Fig. 4.1), the metabolite of T, is the most potent androgen. Intracellularly, T is irreversibly metabolized to DHT. DHT is then bound by an intracellular cytosolic receptor, the androgen receptor (AR). This complex is translocated to the cell nucleus, where it activates transcription of genes with hormone-responsive elements in their promoters and initiates a cascade of androgenic action. DHT can be inactivated in the prostate by further reduction to 3α- or 3β-androstanediol. DHT homeostasis is regulated by its (1) biosynthesis and (2) degradation (see Fig. 4.1). Both processes involve multiple enzymatic steps, including the reactions catalyzed by the gene products of *CYP17A1*, *HSD17B3*, *HSD3B2*, *SRD5A2*, *CYP3A* genes, *UGT* genes, and *SULT* genes. Variation in these genes may be one endogenous source of variation in androgen action.

Androgen Action on the Prostate

The action of DHT in the prostate is mediated by the AR (see Fig. 4.2). Within the prostate, DHT binds to the AR to form an intracellular complex, which binds to androgen-response elements in the DNA of prostate

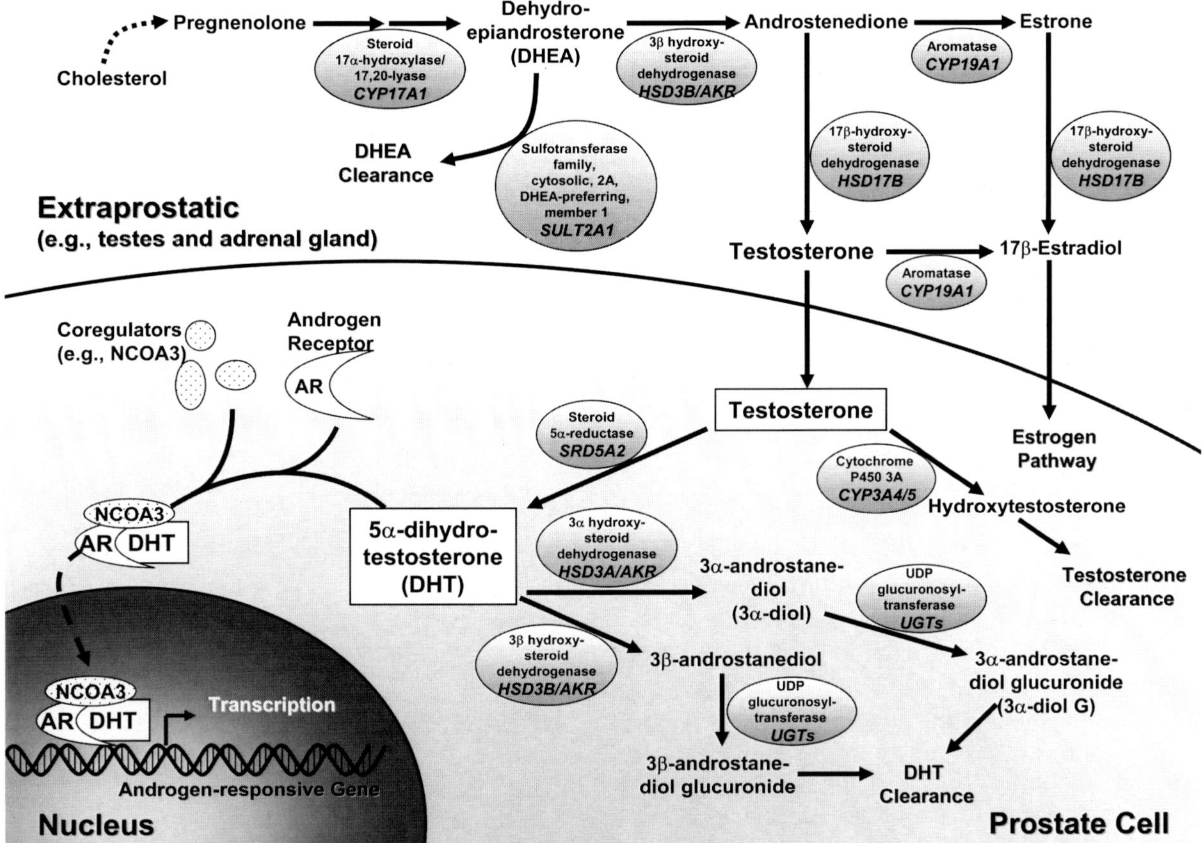

Fig. 4.2 Androgen action within the prostate cell

cells, ultimately inducing proliferation. Though the tissue concentration of DHT necessary to initiate the androgen cascade is unknown, just a minute amount is required to trigger androgenic action in prostate cancer patients who have undergone androgen ablation treatment, perhaps because such patients have hypersensitive ARs [16]. In the absence of androgen, nonandrogenic hormones including estradiol, vitamin D, and insulin-like growth factors (IGFs) can bind ARs, triggering androgenic action [17, 18]. In addition, the activity of the AR is modulated by a series of coactivator proteins, including ARA54, ARA55, ARA70, ARA160, p160, BRCA1, AIB1, and CBP, which can enhance AR transcriptional activity several-fold [9–21]. Thus, androgenic action within the prostate is determined not only by androgen concentration but also by numerous other factors, including factors yet to be identified. However, no epidemiologic studies have directly assessed tissue hormone levels or androgenic action within the prostate, due in part to the difficulty

in collecting prostate tissue from control subjects in case–control studies, or from men at baseline in cohort studies.

Androgen and Prostate Cancer

Data from animal, clinical, and prevention studies support the role of androgen in prostate cancer growth, proliferation, and progression. However, serum-based epidemiologic studies in human have been inconclusive. Part of the inconsistency in these findings stems from differences in study population, assay accuracy, intraperson variation, and limited sample size. Recently, in a pooled analysis of 18 prospective studies, Roddam and the Endogenous Hormone and Prostate Cancer Collaborative Group reported no association between blood levels of total testosterone and prostate cancer risk based on data from 3,886 men with prostate cancer and

6,438 controls [22]. It is the largest serum-based study with the most elegant and comprehensive analysis to date to test a central hypothesis in prostate cancer etiology. It is not surprising that the pooled analysis did not find a positive link between circulating levels of total testosterone and prostate cancer risk since, individually, few of the 18 studies included in the pooled analysis reported a significant positive association.

Most recently, three prospective studies have each evaluated a large number (>500) of cases in their nested case–control studies to clarify further the role of androgen in prostate cancer [16, 23, 24]. Overall, there is no convincing evidence of an association between serum androgens and total prostate cancer. However, there were suggestive associations between serum androgen and prostate cancer in certain disease subtypes. The Health Professional's Follow-up study (460 case–control pairs) reported a suggestive association between total and free testosterone with an increased risk of low-grade disease [23]. The European Prospective Investigation into Cancer and Nutrition (EPIC) study (with 643 case-control pairs) found a significant inverse association of androstenedione concentration and risk for advanced prostate cancer, and weak positive associations between free testosterone concentration and risk for total prostate cancer among young men and risk for high-grade disease [16]. The Prostate, Lung, Colorectal, and Ovarian (PLCO) Cancer Screening Trial (the largest study to date with 727 incident Caucasian prostate cancer cases and 889 matched controls) found that a higher testosterone-to-SHBG ratio (T:SHBG) was related to increased risk primarily in men 65 years of age or older [24], but there was no association with total prostate cancer. None of the subtype findings appeared in more than one of these three studies.

Several reasons contribute to the mixed results from epidemiologic studies. First, serum androgen levels are indirect indicators of intraprostatic androgen levels and may not be an accurate reflection of androgen action within the prostate [25]. In addition, relatively large assay variation, intraperson variation, differences in study population, and heterogeneity of prostate cancer in these studies may contribute to the inability of epidemiologic studies to replicate results. Furthermore, genetic susceptibility in the androgen metabolic and signaling pathways may contribute to the effects that androgens have on prostate cancer. Therefore, future studies on the enigmatic relationship between androgens and prostate cancer should take these issues into account.

Testosterone Replacement Therapy and the Risk of Prostate Cancer

Since the historic findings establishing prostate cancer's dependence on androgens put forth by Huggins and Hodges in 1941, the interaction between testosterone and prostate cancer has been at the forefront of prostate cancer treatment. This Nobel Prize-winning initial work showed that prostate cancer regressed when serum testosterone (T) was reduced to castrate levels, and that an increase in T caused growth of prostate cancer [10]. Based on this discovery, surgical or chemical androgen blockade became the mainstay of hormonal treatment of prostate cancer.

Since this landmark discovery, the idea that higher serum T levels in patients cause an increase in prostate cancer growth has been ingrained in the minds of physicians and researchers, and it seems that this entrenched idea may have clouded a more important connection between low serum T and prostate cancer. The theory of increased T causing increased prostate cancer growth appears to be based on the idea that, because a reduction of T during castration causes regression of prostate cancer growth, then an increase in T should cause prostate cancer cells to grow. If this were true, the literature would be full of reports showing that testosterone replacement therapy (TRT) is associated with prostate cancer. However, a review of the present literature has failed to provide any evidence to support this theory. This belief in the unproven serum T "dogma" has, in turn, made TRT in hypogonadal men at risk for prostate cancer a rarely used treatment option.

Testosterone deficiency, also known as androgen deficiency of the aging male (ADAM), late-onset hypogonadism (LOH) and andropause, is common among aging American males, present in up to 39% of men between the ages of 45 and 85 [26]. This condition has been characterized by low serum testosterone, depression, a decrease in libido, lack of energy, decreased muscle mass, changes in bone mineral density, anemia, and cardiovascular risk factors (reviewed by Tostain and Blanc) [27]. A large number of men suffering from T deficiency who might be relieved of their symptoms and could also receive a boost in their quality of life are often denied treatment, if they are thought to be at risk to develop prostate cancer due to the fear that the addition of higher T from TRT may cause growth of occult prostate cancer. However, several reports have shown that there is no direct correlation between levels of T in serum, and the risk of developing prostate cancer [28, 29], and that ethnicities with lower incidence of prostate cancer have higher serum T levels [30, 31]. Actually, it has been shown that low, not high, levels of T are associated with prostate cancer [26, 32–34], high Gleason grade cancer, advanced stage at initial presentation, and decreased survival [35–38]. Another argument against high levels of serum T and an association with prostate cancer can be made with the epidemiology of prostate cancer. Clinical diagnosis of carcinoma of the prostate is rare in young men (in their 20s and 30s) when serum T levels are at their highest but are much more common in aging men when serum T levels are much lower.

In the last 10 years, there have been many published reports investigating the treatment of hypogonadism in males using different formulations of testosterone, and for varying amounts of treatment and time of follow-up, and none of these studies has shown an increased risk of developing prostate cancer ([39–43], and reviewed by Rhoden and Morgentaler [44]). One example of these studies is the work done by Rhoden and Morgentaler in patients thought to be at high risk due to prostatic intraepithelial neoplasia (PIN). The authors reviewed charts of 75 men (20 with PIN and 55 without PIN), who presented with hypogonadal symptoms, and had a documented low serum T level. All 75 men reviewed had been on TRT for 1 year. Prostate cancer was diagnosed in only one man in the PIN arm, and none were diagnosed in the hypogonadal men without presence of PIN [43]. This 1% detection rate in the study group is similar to that found in screening trials [44, 45]. In addition, PSA values have not been shown to increase significantly [40, 46], nor has there been a change in concentration of DHT within the prostate following TRT [47].

Testosterone Replacement Therapy Following Treatment for Prostate Cancer

While there have not been any large studies with long-term follow-up looking at the effects of TRT after primary treatment for prostate cancer, there has been several small studies. In the first study, Kaufman and Graydon identified seven men who had undergone a radical prostatectomy and had clinical symptoms of hypogonadism [48]. In all seven men, including four who had received T supplementation prior to prostate cancer diagnosis, all men had serum T levels in the eugonadal range prior to diagnosis, and were graded with Gleason 6 or 7 scores. At the time of publication, TRT had been shown to be safe, with no reported recurrences or metastases in a follow-up period that ranged from 1 to 12 years [48].

Agarwal and Oefelein also presented their findings of ten men, with clear symptoms of hypogonadism, who were treated with TRT following a radical prostatectomy for organ confined disease [49]. These ten men had no postoperative evidence of disease or rising PSA, but suffered from symptoms that included decreased libido, erectile dysfunction, and decreased quality of life. Upon determination of baseline PSA and serum T, all were started on T supplementation. The patients were routinely followed for both clinical and quality of life measurements. While all patients had the intended rise in serum T, none of these men had a detectable PSA. The median follow-up was 19 months and there was not a single recurrence observed. The authors noted that patients responded well to the increase in serum T with an increase in sexual function and overall energy level, and a reduction in hot flashes [49].

The third study evaluated TRT after brachytherapy for early prostate cancer [50]. In this study, Sarosdy retrospectively reviewed 31 patients who had undergone TRT for hypogonadism following brachytherapy for prostate cancer. The TRT was initiated from 0.5 to 4.5 (median 2.0 years) following radioactive seed implantation. These patients received TRT for 0.5–8.5 years (median 4.5 years) and were followed for 1.5–9.0 years (median 5.0 years). None of the 31 patients stopped TRT due to cancer recurrence or progression [50].

All authors of the above-mentioned studies agreed that while controversial, a history of prostate cancer should not absolutely preclude one from TRT as long as the patient has no detectable prostate cancer, and/or has had prior curative therapy. In all cases, the patients who are to receive TRT should be carefully selected, and should be at a low risk for recurrence. Hypogonadal candidates for TRT after therapy should only include those with minimal initial disease, possess low Gleason scores, and a negligible PSA. Monitoring of these patients should be more frequent, a PSA and total T determination every 1–3 months, at least for the first year has been suggested [49].

While the above studies showing positive results after radical prostatectomy and brachytherapy have been completed, no similar study has been done on patients who were treated with radiation alone. It has been suggested that TRT following radiation may not be a viable approach due to the residual prostatic tissue that remains following radiation therapy, which could be more susceptible to T supplementation [49]. These small studies together show that, with the right patient population that TRT after curative therapy is safe, and they show the need for a large placebo-controlled prospective trial to provide the definitive study.

Conclusion

While there is a large amount of evidence regarding the role of testosterone in the growth, proliferation, and progression of prostate cancer, more information is still needed. Mixed results in clinical studies have been inconsistent due to differences in the study population, accuracy issues in serum-based assays, sample size, and sample acquisition and storage. More uniform standards would enhance epidemiological studies in the future. Also, there is a great need for a definitive study investigating testosterone replacement, both to fully understand the risk of prostate cancer associated with this treatment, and recurrence after primary therapy for prostate cancer, in order to convince clinicians that TRT is a viable option for patients in need of testosterone replacement.

Acknowledgment This work was supported by the Intramural Research Program of the NIH, National Cancer Institute.

References

1. Hsing AW, Chokkalingam AP. Prostate cancer epidemiology. Front Biosci 2006;11:1388–413.
2. Chokkalingam AP, et al. Molecular epidemiology of prostate cancer: hormone-related genetic loci. Front Biosci 2007;12: 3436–60.
3. Freedman ML, et al. Admixture mapping identifies 8q24 as a prostate cancer risk locus in African-American men. Proc Natl Acad Sci U S A 2006;103(38):14068–73.
4. Gudmundsson J, et al. Genome-wide association study identifies a second prostate cancer susceptibility variant at 8q24. Nat Genet 2007;39(5):631–7.
5. Haiman CA, et al. Multiple regions within 8q24 independently affect risk for prostate cancer. Nat Genet 2007; 39(5):638–44.
6. Suuriniemi M, et al. Confirmation of a positive association between prostate cancer risk and a locus at chromosome 8q24. Cancer Epidemiol Biomarkers Prev 2007;16(4):809–14.
7. Witte JS. Multiple prostate cancer risk variants on 8q24. Nat Genet 2007;39(5):579–80.
8. Yeager M, et al. Genome-wide association study of prostate cancer identifies a second risk locus at 8q24. Nat Genet 2007;39(5):645–9.
9. Zheng SL, et al. Association between two unlinked loci at 8q24 and prostate cancer risk among European Americans. J Natl Cancer Inst 2007;99(20):1525–33.
10. Huggins C, Hodges CV. The effects of castration, of estrogen and androgen injection on serum phosphatases in metastatic carcinoma of the prostate. Cancer Res 1941;1: 293–7.
11. Sharifi N, Gulley JL, Dahut WL. Androgen deprivation therapy for prostate cancer. JAMA 2005;294(2):238–44.
12. Chu LW, Reichardt JK, Hsing AW. Androgens and the molecular epidemiology of prostate cancer. Curr Opin Endocrinol Diabetes Obes 2008;15(3):261–70.
13. Hsing AW, Reichardt JK, Stanczyk FZ. Hormones and prostate cancer: current perspectives and future directions. Prostate 2002;52(3):213–35.
14. Platz EA, Giovannucci E. The epidemiology of sex steroid hormones and their signaling and metabolic pathways in the etiology of prostate cancer. J Steroid Biochem Mol Biol 2004;92(4):237–53.
15. Stanczyk FZ, et al. Alterations in circulating levels of androgens and PSA during treatment with Fiansteride in men at high risk for prostate cancer. In: Li JJ, et al., editors. Hormonal carcinogenesis II. New York: Springer; 1996.
16. Travis RC, et al. Serum androgens and prostate cancer among 643 cases and 643 controls in the European prospective investigation into cancer and nutrition. Int J Cancer 2007;121(6):1331–8.
17. Chamberlain NL, Driver ED, Miesfeld RL. The length and location of CAG trinucleotide repeats in the androgen receptor N-terminal domain affect transactivation function. Nucleic Acids Res 1994;22(15):3181–6.
18. Richter E, Srivastava S, Dobi A. Androgen receptor and prostate cancer. Prostate Cancer Prostatic Dis 2007;10(2): 114–8.
19. Culig Z, et al. Hyperactive androgen receptor in prostate cancer: what does it mean for new therapy concepts? Histol Histopathol 1997;12(3):781–6.
20. Hsing AW, et al. Polymorphic CAG/CAA repeat length in the AIB1/SRC-3 gene and prostate cancer risk: a population-based case-control study. Cancer Epidemiol Biomarkers Prev 2002;11(4):337–41.
21. Rahman M, Miyamoto H, Chang C. Androgen receptor coregulators in prostate cancer: mechanisms and clinical implications. Clin Cancer Res 2004;10(7):2208–19.
22. Roddam AW, et al. Endogenous sex hormones and prostate cancer: a collaborative analysis of 18 prospective studies. J Natl Cancer Inst 2008;100(3):170–83.

23. Platz EA, et al. Sex steroid hormones and the androgen receptor gene CAG repeat and subsequent risk of prostate cancer in the prostate-specific antigen era. Cancer Epidemiol Biomarkers Prev 2005;14(5):1262–9.

24. Weiss JM, et al. Endogenous sex hormones and the risk of prostate cancer: a prospective study. Int J Cancer 2008; 122(10):2345–50.

25. Hsing AW, Chu LW, Stanczyk FZ. Androgen and prostate cancer: is the hypothesis dead? Cancer Epidemiol Biomarkers Prev 2008;17(10):2525–30.

26. Mulligan T, et al. Prevalence of hypogonadism in males aged at least 45 years: the HIM study. Int J Clin Pract 2006;60(7):762–9.

27. Tostain JL, Blanc F. Testosterone deficiency: a common, unrecognized syndrome. Nat Clin Pract Urol 2008;5(7): 388–96.

28. Carter HB, et al. Longitudinal evaluation of serum androgen levels in men with and without prostate cancer. Prostate 1995;27(1):25–31.

29. Slater S, Oliver RT. Testosterone: its role in development of prostate cancer and potential risk from use as hormone replacement therapy. Drugs Aging 2000;17(6):431–9.

30. Ross RK, et al. 5-Alpha-reductase activity and risk of prostate cancer among Japanese and US white and black males. Lancet 1992;339(8798):887–9.

31. Wu AH, et al. Serum androgens and sex hormone-binding globulins in relation to lifestyle factors in older African-American, white, and Asian men in the United States and Canada. Cancer Epidemiol Biomarkers Prev 1995;4(7): 735–41.

32. Morgentaler A, Bruning 3rd CO, DeWolf WC. Occult prostate cancer in men with low serum testosterone levels. JAMA 1996;276(23):1904–6.

33. Morgentaler A, Rhoden EL. Prevalence of prostate cancer among hypogonadal men with prostate-specific antigen levels of 4.0 ng/mL or less. Urology 2006;68(6):1263–7.

34. Yamamoto S, et al. Preoperative serum testosterone level as an independent predictor of treatment failure following radical prostatectomy. Eur Urol 2007;52(3):696–701.

35. Hoffman MA, DeWolf WC, Morgentaler A. Is low serum free testosterone a marker for high grade prostate cancer? J Urol 2000;163(3):824–7.

36. Schatzl G, et al. High-grade prostate cancer is associated with low serum testosterone levels. Prostate 2001;47(1):52–8.

37. Massengill JC, et al. Pretreatment total testosterone level predicts pathological stage in patients with localized prostate cancer treated with radical prostatectomy. J Urol 2003;169(5):1670–5.

38. Ribeiro M, Ruff P, Falkson G. Low serum testosterone and a younger age predict for a poor outcome in metastatic prostate cancer. Am J Clin Oncol 1997;20(6):605–8.

39. Sih R, et al. Testosterone replacement in older hypogonadal men: a 12-month randomized controlled trial. J Clin Endocrinol Metab 1997;82(6):1661–7.

40. Svetec DA, et al. The effect of parenteral testosterone replacement on prostate specific antigen in hypogonadal men with erectile dysfunction. J Urol 1997;158(5): 1775–7.

41. Kenny AM, et al. Effects of transdermal testosterone on bone and muscle in older men with low bioavailable testosterone levels. J Gerontol A Biol Sci Med Sci 2001;56(5): M266–72.

42. Snyder PJ, et al. Effects of testosterone replacement in hypogonadal men. J Clin Endocrinol Metab 2000;85(8): 2670–7.

43. Rhoden EL, Morgentaler A. Testosterone replacement therapy in hypogonadal men at high risk for prostate cancer: results of 1 year of treatment in men with prostatic intraepithelial neoplasia. J Urol 2003;170(6 Pt 1):2348–51.

44. Rhoden EL, Morgentaler A. Risks of testosterone-replacement therapy and recommendations for monitoring. N Engl J Med 2004;350(5):482–92.

45. Makinen T, et al. Second round results of the Finnish population-based prostate cancer screening trial. Clin Cancer Res 2004;10(7):2231–6.

46. Grober ED, et al. Correlation between simultaneous PSA and serum testosterone concentrations among eugonadal, untreated hypogonadal and hypogonadal men receiving testosterone replacement therapy. Int J Impot Res 2008; 20(6):561–5.

47. Marks LS, et al. Effect of testosterone replacement therapy on prostate tissue in men with late-onset hypogonadism: a randomized controlled trial. JAMA 2006;296(19):2351–61.

48. Kaufman JM, Graydon RJ. Androgen replacement after curative radical prostatectomy for prostate cancer in hypogonadal men. J Urol 2004;172(3):920–2.

49. Agarwal PK, Oefelein MG. Testosterone replacement therapy after primary treatment for prostate cancer. J Urol 2005;173(2):533–6.

50. Sarosdy MF. Testosterone replacement for hypogonadism after treatment of early prostate cancer with brachytherapy. Cancer 2007;109(3):536–41.

Chapter 5
Androgen Receptor Biology in Prostate Cancer

Edward P. Gelmann

Abstract Androgens are essential development and survival factors for prostate epithelial cells. Prostate cancer cells retain androgen dependence and, for some period of time, are suppressed by androgen deprivation. Castration-resistant prostate cancer (CRPC) arises after a period of androgen withdrawal and represents the most advanced stage of the disease. CRPC is mediated by the reactivation of androgen receptor activity in the castrate patient. Androgen receptor is reactivated in CRPC by a variety of mechanisms, the breadth of which underscores the importance of androgen receptor for prostate cancer cell proliferation at all stages of the disease. Androgen receptor gene may be affected by the amplification of the locus on the X chromosome or by the activation of mutations. Androgen receptor protein may be phosphorylated by a variety of kinases to enhance its activity in the presence of subphysiologic concentrations of ligand. The cancer cells themselves may produce sufficient levels of androgenic steroids to sustain receptor activation. Androgen receptor activity may also be enhanced by the overexpression of coactivator proteins that allow the formation of the transcriptional complex after the androgen receptor binds to DNA. Lastly, androgen receptor mRNA may be subjected to alternative splicing that may generate ligand-independent truncated forms of activated androgen receptor protein. Thus CRPC cells reactivate androgen receptor as a critical pathway towards cancer progression.

Keywords Prostate cancer • Androgen receptor • Androgen • Mutation • Coactivator • p160 • Beta-catenin

E.P. Gelmann (✉)
Division of Hematology/Oncology, Herbert Irving
Comprehensive Cancer Center, Columbia University,
New York, NY, USA
e-mail: gelmanne@columbia.edu

The androgen receptor (AR) is a member of the nuclear hormone receptor family. Androgens are essential for prostate epithelial development and sustenance. Malignant prostate epithelium retains, to some degree, the dependence on AR that characterized the normal prostate epithelium from which it arose. Early in prostate cancer development, androgens activate the *TMPRSS2* gene promoter that is often recombined with the *ERG* transcription factor gene or, less frequently, other members of the ETS family to drive the invasiveness of the majority of prostate cancers [1, 2]. In advanced prostate cancer, androgen ablative therapy targets AR, but it is eventually overcome by AR reactivation in castration-resistant prostate cancer (CRPC). The reactivation of AR in CRPC occurs by a wide range of mechanisms. The molecular oncology of AR is the focus of this chapter.

Like the epithelium from which they arise, prostate cancer cells retain responsiveness to and dependence on androgens. It has been known for more than half a century that prostate cancer in most cases retains androgen responsiveness and undergoes regression in response to androgen deprivation [3, 4]. Over 80% of men with disseminated prostate cancer show some clinical response to androgen ablation. Still, there is no way to predict which patients will not respond or how long the responding patients will benefit from initial androgen deprivation. Androgen responsiveness in prostate cancer does not correlate with either the presence or the levels of androgen receptor in cancer tissues [5–10].

In nearly all instances, recurrent and metastatic prostate cancer escapes from the effects of androgen ablation and becomes castration-resistant. Preclinical models of castration resistance using both hormone-dependent cultured cells and tumor lines were analyzed using expression array analysis to determine gene expression changes common to a number of different hormone-independent derivative lines. It was surprising and paradigm-setting to find that the only expression change common to androgen independence of seven different cell lines and tumors was the increased expression of AR [11]. AR overexpression alone not only conferred androgen independence to cultured cells but also sensitized cells to picomolar concentrations of androgens and conferred AR agonism to the potent anti-androgen bicalutamide.

AR Structure

The three-dimensional structure of the AR ligand-binding domain is similar to that of other steroid hormone receptors. Ligand binding induces conformational changes that initiate translocation from the cytoplasm to the nucleus and also allows the AR to interact with coregulator proteins that mediate transcription initiated by AR binding to its cognate DNA sequences. The coactivators play a fundamental role in the activity of AR. Alterations in the structure or levels of coactivator proteins can therefore greatly impact AR transcriptional activity. Mutations in the AR, whether hereditary or sporadic, have been implicated in the development and growth of prostate cancer. Moreover, tumor suppressors, growth factors, and their receptors may also regulate the activity of AR [12–20].

The AR is located on the X chromosome at Xq11-12 [21, 22]. It is therefore a single-copy gene in males, allowing phenotypic expression of mutations without the influence of a wild-type codominant allele. Numerous spontaneous mutations of the human AR have been described, and the exploration of the effects of these mutations on AR activity has helped to elucidate the nature of the functional domains of the AR protein. Loss or attenuation of AR function results in complete or partial androgen insensitivity, respectively. Individuals who have complete androgen insensitivity syndrome are phenotypic, but sterile, females. Interestingly, they do not manifest sexual identity discordance, underscoring the fact that AR plays a role in the configuration of the male CNS as well as in morphologic development [23].

The AR gene consists of eight exons that encode a ~2,757-base pair open reading frame within a 10.6-kb mRNA [24–27]. Like the other members of the steroid hormone receptor family of genes, the exons of the AR gene code for functionally distinct regions of the protein that correspond to the exonic organization of other steroid hormone receptor genes suggesting a modular genetic composition that facilitated gene duplication and divergence during evolution. The AR genomic organization and location on the X chromosome is conserved in mammals and may reflect a developmentally significant association of AR with other syntenic genes [28]. The first exon codes for the N-terminal domain (NTD), which serves as the transcriptional regulatory region of the protein. Exons 2 and 3 code for the central DNA-binding domain. Exons 4–8 code for the C-terminal ligand-binding domain.

Segments of the AR gene have been conserved throughout evolution, implying that these regions are critical for the activity of the molecule. The DNA-binding domain is most highly conserved across species. Other regions of the gene striking in their degree of sequence conservation include much of the hinge region and the ligand-binding domain. A large number of conserved ligand-binding domain residues that are targets for mutations, which result in androgen insensitivity syndrome, are conserved from frog to man. The NTD is encoded by the first exon and does not demonstrate a high degree of sequence conservation, from frog to rodent to human, upstream of codon 539 in the human sequence. However, the sequence comparison of AR NTDs from primates reveals that codons 1–53 and 360–429 generate conserved protein segments across a broad evolutionary spectrum [29]. These regions are important for dimerization of human AR, and their genetic conservation reflects similarity in function for primate AR molecules.

Even though the AR ligand-binding domain shares only 20% sequence similarity with other steroid hormone receptors, the three-dimensional structure resembles that of other steroid hormone receptors [30–35]. Many steroid hormone receptor ligand-binding domains fold into 12 helices, three of which form a ligand-binding pocket. When an agonist is bound, helix 12 folds over the pocket to enclose the ligand. In the unbound state or in the presence of an antagonist, helix 12 is repositioned away from the pocket in such a way that the coactivator binding is impeded [32]. There is evidence to suggest that ligand-bound AR dimerizes in vivo, suggesting that the N-terminal region of AR is important for protein dimerization [36–38].

The NTD is the primary effector region of AR and plays a key role in transactivation. Deletion of the ligand-binding domain from AR results in a residual N-terminal fragment with transcriptional activity nearly equal to that of the ligand-bound, full-length protein, suggesting that the NTD is fully capable of initiating the assembly of the transcriptional complex, including binding to AR coactivators. The first 140 amino acids are not essential for transcriptional activity. Their deletion results in a receptor with nearly wild-type levels of activity. However, deletion of the regions between amino acids 210 and 337 markedly reduces the receptor activity [39].

The first exon contains a polymorphic region that influences the interindividual variation in AR activity and prostate cancer risk. The main cause of this variability lies in a CAG nucleotide triplet repeat that begins at codon 58 and extends for an average of 21 repeats [40]. The CAG repeat region encodes a polyglutamine region, similar to those found in other transcription factors such as CREB. This region is thought to mediate AR interactions with various coregulators [41]. Indeed, as the CAG repeat length increases, the interaction of AR with its coactivator ARA24 decreases [42]. Similarly, increased CAG length seems to diminish AR interaction with members of the p160 family of coactivators [43]. CAG repeat lengths are prone to variation because DNA polymerase is subject to slippage in the regions of multiple CAG nucleotide triplets. CAG repeat length in *AR* ranges from 14 to 35 repeats and varies with ethnicity. Variations in the repeat length impact AR transcriptional activity, prostate growth, and prostate cancer risk [44]. Ethnic differences have been noted in CAG repeat lengths, and these differences are inversely related to prostate cancer incidence [44, 45]. Shorter CAG length and increased incidence of prostate cancer has been demonstrated in diverse populations including Indian, Brazilian, and Mexican men [46–49], whereas longer CAG repeat length is associated with low prostate cancer incidence in Greenland [50].

In one instance of advanced prostate cancer, *AR* underwent insertional mutagenesis that interrupted the CAG repeat, effectively shortening it and increasing the AR transcriptional activity. This single example not only further underscores the importance of AR activation to prostate cancer progression but also shows the influence of CAG repeat length on AR activity [51]. Variations of CAG repeat lengths have been engineered in the *AR* and shown to regulate AR transcriptional activity in reporter assays [51]. Variations in CAG repeat length have also been engineered into transgenic mice that have been subjected to introduction of the human exon 1 to replace the murine exon 1. Shorter CAG repeat lengths have been shown to favor prostatic hyperplasia with advancing murine age [52].

Alterations of the Androgen Receptor in Prostate Cancer

AR Gene Amplification

It has been well established in a few studies that a common finding in patients with CRPC is the amplification of the *AR* gene that accounts for some instances of increased AR expression in tumor samples [53–56]. Since gene amplification requires continued selective pressure for the maintenance of the amplification, the finding is a compelling argument that AR overexpression is essential for some cases of CRPC. Interestingly, amplification of the *AR* gene is also an adaptive response to high-dose anti-androgen monotherapy, consistent with the in vitro findings that overexpression of a wild-type AR protein confers an agonistic response to bicalutamide [57]. *AR* gene amplification is associated with downstream overexpression of AR protein; however, AR overexpression is found in CRPC without *AR* gene amplification and thus may be achieved via alternative mechanisms [56].

AR Mutations

Androgen deprivation therapy, and particularly treatment with anti-androgens, may result in the selection of malignant cell clones with *AR* gene mutations [58, 59]. Primary prostate cancer may have a high background of clones with AR mutations available for selection in response to androgen deprivation [60]. *AR* mutations found in CRPC often affect the ligand-binding domain and alter the AR response to anti-androgens and may broaden the spectrum of ligand agonists conferring greater activity to adrenal androgens [61]. A number of investigators have detected *AR* mutations in prostate cancer tissue [58, 62–69]. Consistent with the notion of clonal selection, these *AR* mutations are very rare in patients with primary prostate cancer and are found with a higher frequency in patients with advanced disease [62].

The functional importance of *AR* mutations in CRPC is underscored by the finding that the mutations cluster in three regions of the molecule [17]. Mutations in the LBD affect the ligand-binding pocket and liberalize the spectrum of AR agonists to a wider range of steroid hormones and pharmaceutical anti-androgens [58, 61, 70]. *AR* mutations that affect the ligand-binding pocket, except for a single residue, are mutually exclusive of those that cause androgen insensitivity [30]. Mutation of methionine 740 to valine has been found in several individuals with complete or severe partial androgen insensitivity syndrome [71–75] and in prostate cancer mutated to isoleucine [76, 77].

AR mutations in CRPC also cluster in the region 874–910 that flanks the AF-2 domain, the region that affects the binding of p160 coactivator molecules to AR [78]. Mutations in the region of 874–900 affect the ligand-binding pocket and particularly allow anti-androgens to be recognized as agonists. Mutations that affect residues C-terminal to amino acid 880 may affect interactions with coactivators or subcellular localization of AR [79, 80]. Mutations are also found in the AR hinge region that borders the DNA-binding and ligand-binding domains [30, 81]. The hinge region appears to be targeted because it affects AR interactions with corepressors and thereby diminishes the efficacy of anti-androgens and may explain the sensitization of AR to ligand interactions in late-stage prostate cancer [81]. Just as steroid hormone receptors initiate transcriptional signals that have to be amplified by coactivators, the signals can be silenced by corepressors [82]. The hinge region of AR between the DNA binding and ligand-binding domains is frequently affected by mutations in prostate cancer. The mutation target region [668]QPIF[671] lies between the hinge and the ligand binding domain [17, 81, 83]. The four residues form a hydrophobic cleft that potentially mediates interactions with other proteins, perhaps corepressors. Deletion of the hinge region amino acids 628–646 results in significant activation of AR and marked enhancement of LXXLL-dependent ligand-dependent coactivation [84]. It is also possible that the hinge region may modulate N-terminal binding to the ligand binding domain via the FXXLF motif in the NTD.

Binding between the N-terminal and ligand-binding domains can interfere with p160 coactivator binding to the AF-2 groove of the ligand-binding domain and modulate the activity of the AR signaling complex [85].

All the reported *AR* mutations found in prostate cancer are catalogued in the Androgen Receptor Gene Mutations Database of the Lady Davis Institute for Medical Research. The URL for The Androgen Receptor Gene Mutations Database World Wide Web Server is http://www.mcgill.ca/androgendb/.

Posttranslational Modification of AR

AR activity can be enhanced by the HER family of kinases, which effect AR binding to DNA, AR stability, and interaction with the p160 coactivator TIF-2 [86, 87]. AR has not been shown to be a substrate of the HER kinases but rather is a target for phosphorylation by kinases activated downstream of the HER kinases. HER2 and 3 activation by heregulin activates ACK1, which directly affects AR activity [87, 88]. The inhibition of HER2 signaling decreases AR transcriptional activation [89], and ACK1 has been shown to phosphorylate AR in the NTD to enhance AR transcriptional activity [90]. HER kinase activation also results in the phosphorylation of AR at serine 578 in the DNA-binding domain. Loss The loss of serine 578 abrogates the effect of HER kinase on AR and alters the subcellular distribution of AR, demonstrating the importance of HER activity in AR regulation [91].

AR also interacts with and binds to the inner membrane tyrosine kinase SRC. In the cytoplasm, ligand-bound AR activates SRC via interaction with the AR N-terminal proline-rich domain. SRC, in turn, phosphorylates and activates the p85alpha subunit of PI3-kinase [92]. The interaction of AR and SRC also results in the phosphorylation of AR on tyrosine 534 in the NTD. SRC expression and levels of AR phosphorylated on tyrosine 534 are increased in CRPC. AR is activated by SRC phosphorylation, a modification that can facilitate the growth of prostate cancer xenografts in castrated mice [93]. Moreover, levels of SRC are increased in tissues from patients with CRPC.

AR transcripts have been shown to occur in various isoforms that result from alternative splicing events. Although these findings are to date restricted to cell lines, it has been shown that AR isoforms lacking the ligand-binding domain can be found in 22Rv1 cells and can drive transcription in a ligand-independent manner [94]. These findings are particularly important because if found in tumors, C-terminal truncated AR would be unaffected by anti-androgens and would be independent of all therapeutic measures that target ligand availability.

Ligand Availability

CRPC has been shown to overcome androgen deprivation by altering ligand availability through androgen synthesis by malignant epithelial cells. For example, in locally recurrent prostate cancer after androgen ablation, intracellular levels of dihydrotestosterone reach physiologic concentrations, theoretically providing sufficient ligand for the local activation of AR [95]. Tissues in CRPC have also been shown to increase the expression of genes coding for enzymes that convert adrenal steroids into androgens [96]. Moreover, the malignant cells of CRPC may activate more than one enzymatic pathway to synthesize androgens and are fully capable of converting two-carbon precursors to testosterone [97]. The potential of cancer cells to increase their own supply of ligand in CRPC argues for the application of drugs that inhibit adrenal steroidogenesis and androgen synthesis. These data explain, in part, the transient clinical effects of ketoconazole [98–100] and the early phase clinical effects of abiraterone acetate, a high-affinity inhibitor of cytochrome P450 CYP17 [101, 102].

AR Coregulators

AR interacts with hundreds of proteins that have the potential to act as coregulators to inhibit or enhance AR transcriptional activity. Variation in the expression or structure of these coregulators can greatly alter the transcriptional activity of AR and thereby affect the development of both the normal prostate and prostatic neoplasia.

The paradigmatic family of AR coactivators is the p160 family, a group of three 160 kDa proteins SRC-1, TIF-2, and SRC-3/AIB1, with substantial sequence homology. These proteins bind to the AR at a region called TAU-5 in the NTD as well as at AF-2 in the ligand-binding domain at a groove created by the rotation of helix 12 after ligand binding [103]. P160 family coactivators amplify the transcriptional signal initiated by AR binding to DNA and in doing so recruit secondary coactivators and regulatory proteins to the transcriptional complex. Overexpression of each of the p160 proteins has been observed in prostate cancer [104].

SRC-1 and TIF-2 overexpression have been demonstrated in androgen-insensitive prostate tumors as compared with androgen-sensitive tumors and BPH specimens [105]. SRC-1 is required for normal prostate growth, and it is overexpressed in CRPC. SRC-1 has been demonstrated to potentiate AR activity even at very low hormone levels [106]. SRC-1 interacts with AR at the LBD via LXXLL motifs. In addition, SRC-1 can exert its influence independently of the C-terminal LXXLL motifs by acting at a glutamine-rich region of the AR's C-terminal [107]. A second p160 coactivator, TIF-2, when overexpressed in prostate cancers is associated with early recurrence and a more aggressive clinical behavior [108]. High levels of AIB1/SRC-3 have been correlated with high tumor grade and stage. Overexpression of AIB1/SRC-3 has also been shown to be correlated with increased prostate cancer cell proliferation as well as decreased levels of apoptosis [109].

A number of other proteins that can potentiate AR transcription in vitro have been found to be overexpressed in prostate cancer. ARA-70 is a transcriptional coactivator that can interact with AR. ARA-70 is overexpressed in high-grade prostate cancer tissues and prostate cancer cell lines. ARA-70 interacts with AR via the N-terminal FXXLF domain and thereby can attenuate the inhibitory effects of anti-androgens [110]. Tip60 interacts with AR as well as ER and PR and is found in the nuclei of progressive and castration-resistant prostate cancer. Tip60 is upregulated as a response to androgen deprivation and accumulates in the nucleus [111]. Cdc25B is a member of the Cdc25 family of phosphatases. It activates cyclin-dependent kinases and enhances the transcriptional activity of the AR by binding directly to AR. Overexpression of Cdc25B is associated with poorly differentiated tumors as well as with high-grade disease [112]. CBP/p300 is involved in chromatin remodeling as well as the recruitment of TFIIB and TBP. A high level of expression is noted in advanced and castration-resistant prostate cancer [113]. ART27 is another AR-coactivating protein whose expression is altered in prostate cancer. It interacts with AR at the NTD. Normally found in prostate and breast tissue epithelium, ART27 expression is decreased in prostate cancer [114]. ARA55 enhances AR transactivation by binding to the C-terminal LIM domain [115]. PYK2 kinase targets ARA55 and thereby decreases interaction with AR. PYK2 expression levels decrease during prostate cancer progression thereby allowing a sustained interaction of ARA55 and AR [116].

The multifunction oncogene beta-catenin functions as an AR coactivator by interacting with the AR ligand-binding domain. The importance of beta-catenin in prostate cancer is suggested by the rare mutational activation in prostate cancer [117, 118]. A more common pathway toward beta-catenin activation in prostate cancer is via methylation of *APC*, the gene that codes for the colon cancer suppressor that complexes with beta-catenin in the cytoplasm and mediates phosphorylation and ubiquitination to modulate the intracellular levels of beta-catenin [119–121]. In addition, GSK3beta is inactivated in advanced prostate cancer [122]. GSK3beta is a key kinase for the beta-catenin NTD that activates ubiquitination on proteasomal degradation [123]. In advanced prostate cancer, calpain cleaves beta-catenin causing an N-terminal truncation. This is, potentially, another mechanism for beta-catenin activation during late stage disease [124]. Beta-catenin activates AR transcriptional activity, translocates AR to the nucleus, and shifts the ligand response curve to the left [125–128]. Beta-catenin interacts with the AF-2 domain of AR and forms a three-way complex with AR and TIF-2 as it also binds to TIF-2 [129, 130].

AR is negatively regulated by corepressor proteins that bind to AR to inhibit transcriptional activation when AR is located in the nucleus. SMRT and the closely related NcoR repress the AR by direct interaction with it. They also serve as competitors with the p160 coactivators [131]. Although some AR ligands activate binding to corepressors [132, 133], anti-androgens like bicalutamide mediate disruption of coactivator binding and do not appear to work by increasing corepressor binding [134]. Alteration of corepressor expression has not been reported in prostate cancer and does not appear to be a mechanism by which AR is activated in neoplastic prostate epithelial cells.

Summary

Prostate cancer cells depend on AR activity at all phases of tumor progression. Androgen deprivation therapy introduces a selective pressure that results in a wide range of genetic changes and biochemical modifications to restore sufficient AR activity for cell proliferation. More successful therapy for advanced prostate cancer may require combinations of treatments for patients with metastatic castration-sensitive disease to decrease the likelihood of development of castration-resistance. The availability of new higher affinity anti-androgens, more effective inhibitors of androgen synthesis, and new kinase inhibitors have the potential to achieve prolongation of control of prostate cancer proliferation and improved survival.

References

1. Tomlins SA, Rhodes DR, Perner S et al. Recurrent fusion of TMPRSS2 and ETS transcription factor genes in prostate cancer. Science 2005; 310(5748):644–648.
2. Tomlins SA, Laxman B, Varambally S et al. Role of the TMPRSS2-ERG gene fusion in prostate cancer. Neoplasia 2008; 10(2):177–188.
3. Huggins C, Stevens RE, Hodges CL. Studies on prostatic cancer II. The effect of castration on clinical patients with carcinoma of the prostate. Arch Surg 1941; 43:209.
4. Huggins C, Hodges CV. Studies on prostatic cancer; effect of castration, of estrogen and of androgen injection on serum phosphatases in metastatic carcinoma of the prostate. Cancer Res 1941; 1:293–297.
5. Sadi MV, Walsh PC, Barrack ER. Immunohistochemical study of androgen receptors in metastatic prostate cancer. Comparison of receptor content and response to hormonal therapy. Cancer 1991; 67:3057–3064.
6. Trachtenberg J, Walsh PC. Correlation of prostatic nuclear androgen receptor content with duration of response and survival following hormonal therapy in advanced prostatic cancer. J Urol 1982; 127(3):466–471.
7. Gonor SE, Lakey WH, McBlain WA. Relationship between concentrations of extractable and matrix-bound nuclear androgen receptor and clinical response to endocrine therapy for prostatic adenocarcinoma. J Urol 1984; 131(6):1196–1201.
8. Benson RC, Jr., Gorman PA, O'Brien PC, Holicky EL, Veneziale CM. Relationship between androgen receptor binding activity in human prostate cancer and clinical response to endocrine therapy. Cancer 1987; 59(9):1599–1606.
9. Rennie PS, Bruchovsky N, Goldenberg SL. Relationship of androgen receptors to the growth and regression of the prostate. Am J Clin Oncol 1988; 11:S13.

10. Castellanos JM, Galan A, Calvo MA, Schwartz S. Predicting response of prostatic carcinoma to endocrine therapy. Lancet 1982; 1(8269):448.

11. Chen CD, Welsbie DS, Tran C et al. Molecular determinants of resistance to antiandrogen therapy. Nat Med 2004; 10(1):33–39.

12. Roy AK, Lavrovsky Y, Song CS et al. Regulation of androgen action. Vitam Horm 1999; 55:309–352.

13. Gelmann EP. Androgen receptor mutations in prostate cancer. Cancer Treat Res 1996; 87:285–302.

14. Chang C, Saltzman A, Yeh S et al. Androgen receptor: an overview. Crit Rev Eukaryot Gene Expr 1995; 5(2): 97–125.

15. Lindzey J, Kumar MV, Grossman M, Young C, Tindall DJ. Molecular mechanisms of androgen action. Vitam Horm 1994; 49:383–432.

16. Quigley CA, De Bellis A, Marschke KB, el Awady MK, Wilson EM, French FS. Androgen receptor defects: historical, clinical, and molecular perspectives. Endocr Rev 1995; 16(3):271–321.

17. Buchanan G, Greenberg NM, Scher HI, Harris JM, Marshall VR, Tilley WD. Collocation of androgen receptor gene mutations in prostate cancer. Clin Cancer Res 2001; 7(5): 1273–1281.

18. Janne OA, Moilanen AM, Poukka H et al. Androgen-receptor-interacting nuclear proteins. Biochem Soc Trans 2000; 28(4):401–405.

19. Taplin ME, Ho SM. Clinical review 134: the endocrinology of prostate cancer. J Clin Endocrinol Metab 2001; 86(8): 3467–3477.

20. Bentel JM, Tilley WD. Androgen receptors in prostate cancer. J Endocrinol 1996; 151(1):1–11.

21. Lubahn DB, Joseph DR, Sullivan PM, Willard HF, French FS, Wilson EM. Cloning of human androgen receptor complementary DNA and localization to the X chromosome. Science 1988; 240(4850):327–330.

22. Brown CJ, Goss SJ, Lubahn DB et al. Androgen receptor locus on the human X chromosome: regional localization to Xq11-12 and description of a DNA polymorphism. Am J Hum Genet 1989; 44(2):264–269.

23. Wisniewski AB, Migeon CJ, Meyer-Bahlburg HF et al. Complete androgen insensitivity syndrome: long-term medical, surgical, and psychosexual outcome. J Clin Endocrinol Metab 2000; 85(8):2664–2669.

24. Lubahn DB, Brown TR, Simental JA et al. Sequence of the intron/exon junctions of the coding region of the human androgen receptor gene and identification of a point mutation in a family with complete androgen insensitivity. Proc Natl Acad Sci U S A 1989; 86(23):9534–9538.

25. Kuiper GG, Faber PW, van Rooij HC et al. Structural organization of the human androgen receptor gene. J Mol Endocrinol 1989; 2(3):R1–R4.

26. Faber PW, van Rooij HC, Schipper HJ, Brinkmann AO, Trapman J. Two different, overlapping pathways of transcription initiation are active on the TATA-less human androgen receptor promoter. The role of Sp1. J Biol Chem 1993; 268(13):9296–9301.

27. Tilley WD, Marcelli M, Wilson JD, McPhaul MJ. Characterization and expression of a cDNA encoding the human androgen receptor. Proc Natl Acad Sci U S A 1989; 86:327–331.

28. Spencer JA, Watson JM, Lubahn DB et al. The androgen receptor gene is located on a highly conserved region of the X chromosomes of marsupial and monotreme as well as eutherian mammals. J Hered 1991; 82(2):134–139.

29. Choong CS, Kemppainen JA, Wilson EM. Evolution of the primate androgen receptor: a structural basis for disease. J Mol Evol 1998; 47(3):334–342.

30. Matias PM, Donner P, Coelho R et al. Structural evidence for ligand specificity in the binding domain of the human androgen receptor. Implications for pathogenic gene mutations. J Biol Chem 2000; 275(34):26164–26171.

31. Sack JS, Kish KF, Wang C et al. Crystallographic structures of the ligand-binding domains of the androgen receptor and its T877A mutant complexed with the natural agonist dihydrotestosterone. Proc Natl Acad Sci U S A 2001; 98(9): 4904–4909.

32. Shiau AK, Barstad D, Loria PM et al. The structural basis of estrogen receptor/coactivator recognition and the antagonism of this interaction by tamoxifen. Cell 1998; 95(7):927–937.

33. Brzozowski AM, Pike AC, Dauter Z et al. Molecular basis of agonism and antagonism in the oestrogen receptor. Nature 1997; 389(6652):753–758.

34. Tanenbaum DM, Wang Y, Williams SP, Sigler PB. Crystallographic comparison of the estrogen and progesterone receptor's ligand binding domains. Proc Natl Acad Sci U S A 1998; 95(11):5998–6003.

35. Nolte RT, Wisely GB, Westin S et al. Ligand binding and co-activator assembly of the peroxisome proliferator- activated receptor-gamma. Nature 1998; 395(6698):137–143.

36. Wong CI, Zhou ZX, Sar M, Wilson EM. Steroid requirement for androgen receptor dimerization and DNA binding. Modulation by intramolecular interactions between the NH2-terminal and steroid-binding domains. J Biol Chem 1993; 268(25):19004–19012.

37. Langley E, Zhou ZX, Wilson EM. Evidence for an antiparallel orientation of the ligand-activated human androgen receptor dimer. J Biol Chem 1995; 270(50):29983–29990.

38. Liao M, Zhou Z, Wilson EM. Redox-dependent DNA binding of the purified androgen receptor: evidence for disulfide-linked androgen receptor dimers. Biochemistry 1999; 38(30):9718–9727.

39. Simental JA, Sar M, Lane MV, French FS, Wilson EM. Transcriptional activation and nuclear targeting signals of the human androgen receptor. J Biol Chem 1991; 266(1):510–518.

40. La Spada AR, Wilson EM, Lubahn DB, Harding AE, Fischbeck KH. Androgen receptor gene mutations in X-linked spinal and bulbar muscular atrophy. Nature 1991; 352(6330):77–79.

41. Heinlein CA, Chang C. Androgen receptor in prostate cancer. Endocr Rev 2004; 25(2):276–308.

42. Hsiao PW, Lin DL, Nakao R, Chang C. The linkage of Kennedy's neuron disease to ARA24, the first identified androgen receptor polyglutamine region-associated coactivator. J Biol Chem 1999; 274(29):20229–20234.

43. Irvine RA, Ma H, Yu MC, Ross RK, Stallcup MR, Coetzee GA. Inhibition of p160-mediated coactivation with increasing androgen receptor polyglutamine length. Hum Mol Genet 2000; 9(2):267–274.

44. Sartor O, Zheng Q, Eastham JA. Androgen receptor gene CAG repeat length varies in a race-specific fashion in men without prostate cancer. Urology 1999; 53(2):378–380.

45. Andersson P, Varenhorst E, Soderkvist P. Androgen receptor and vitamin D receptor gene polymorphisms and prostate cancer risk. Eur J Cancer 2006; 42(16):2833–2837.

46. Silva NB, Koff WJ, Biolchi V et al. Polymorphic CAG and GGC repeat lengths in the androgen receptor gene and prostate cancer risk: analysis of a Brazilian population. Cancer Invest 2008; 26(1):74–80.

47. Mittal RD, Mishra D, Mandhani AK. Role of an androgen receptor gene polymorphism in development of hormone refractory prostate cancer in Indian population. Asian Pac J Cancer Prev 2007; 8(2):275–278.

48. Patino-Garcia B, Arroyo C, Rangel-Villalobos H et al. Association between polymorphisms of the androgen and vitamin D receptor genes with prostate cancer risk in a Mexican population. Rev Invest Clin 2007; 59(1):25–31.

49. Krishnaswamy V, Kumarasamy T, Venkatesan V, Shroff S, Jayanth VR, Paul SF. South Indian men with reduced CAG repeat length in the androgen receptor gene have an increased risk of prostate cancer. J Hum Genet 2006; 51(3): 254–257.

50. Giwercman C, Giwercman A, Pedersen HS et al. Polymorphisms in genes regulating androgen activity among prostate cancer low-risk Inuit men and high-risk Scandinavians. Int J Androl 2008; 31(1):25–30.

51. Buchanan G, Yang M, Cheong A et al. Structural and functional consequences of glutamine tract variation in the androgen receptor. Hum Mol Genet 2004; 13(16): 1677–1692.

52. Robins DM, Albertelli MA, O'Mahony OA. Androgen receptor variants and prostate cancer in humanized AR mice. J Steroid Biochem Mol Biol 2008; 108(3–5): 230–236.

53. Visakorpi T, Hyytinen E, Koivisto P et al. In vivo amplification of the androgen receptor gene and progression of human prostate cancer. Nat Genet 1995; 9(4):401–406.

54. Koivisto P, Visakorpi T, Kallioniemi OP. Androgen receptor gene amplification: a novel molecular mechanism for endocrine therapy resistance in human prostate cancer. Scand J Clin Lab Invest Suppl 1996; 226:57–63.

55. Miyoshi Y, Uemura H, Fujinami K et al. Fluorescence in situ hybridization evaluation of c-myc and androgen receptor gene amplification and chromosomal anomalies in prostate cancer in Japanese patients. Prostate 2000; 43(3):225–232.

56. Linja MJ, Savinainen KJ, Saramaki OR, Tammela TL, Vessella RL, Visakorpi T. Amplification and overexpression of androgen receptor gene in hormone- refractory prostate cancer. Cancer Res 2001; 61(9):3550–3555.

57. Palmberg C, Koivisto P, Hyytinen E et al. Androgen receptor gene amplification in a recurrent prostate cancer after monotherapy with the nonsteroidal potent antiandrogen Casodex (bicalutamide) with a subsequent favorable response to maximal androgen blockade. Eur Urol 1997; 31(2):216–219.

58. Taplin ME, Bubley GJ, Shuster TD et al. Mutation of the androgen-receptor gene in metastatic androgen-independent prostate cancer. N Engl J Med 1995; 332(21):1393–1398.

59. Taplin ME, Bubley GJ, Ko YJ et al. Selection for androgen receptor mutations in prostate cancers treated with androgen antagonist. Cancer Res 1999; 59(11):2511–2515.

60. Tilley WD, Buchanan G, Hickey TE, Bentel JM. Mutations in the androgen receptor gene are associated with progression of human prostate cancer to androgen independence. Clin Cancer Res 1996; 2(2):277–285.

61. Tan J, Sharief Y, Hamil KG et al. Dehydroepiandrosterone activates mutant androgen receptors expressed in the androgen-dependent human prostate cancer xenograft CWR22 and LNCaP cells. Mol Endocrinol 1997; 11(4): 450–459.

62. Marcelli M, Ittmann M, Mariani S et al. Androgen receptor mutations in prostate cancer. Cancer Res 2000; 60(4): 944–949.

63. Barrack ER. Androgen receptor mutations in prostate cancer. Mt Sinai J Med 1996; 63(5–6):403–412.

64. Culig Z, Hobisch A, Hittmair A et al. Androgen receptor gene mutations in prostate cancer. Implications for disease progression and therapy. Drugs Aging 1997; 10(1):50–58.

65. Wang C, Uchida T. [Androgen receptor gene mutations in prostate cancer]. Nippon Hinyokika Gakkai Zasshi 1997; 88(5):550–556.

66. Suzuki H, Sato N, Watabe Y, Masai M, Seino S, Shimazaki J. Androgen receptor gene mutations in human prostate cancer. J Steroid Biochem Mol Biol 1993; 46(6):759–765.

67. Newmark JR, Hardy DO, Tonb DC et al. Androgen receptor gene mutations in human prostate cancer. Proc Natl Acad Sci U S A 1992; 89(14):6319–6323.

68. Wallen MJ, Linja M, Kaartinen K, Schleutker J, Visakorpi T. Androgen receptor gene mutations in hormone-refractory prostate cancer. J Pathol 1999; 189(4):559–563.

69. Castagnaro M, Yandell DW, Dockhorn-Dworniczak B, Wolfe HJ, Poremba C. [Androgen receptor gene mutations and p53 gene analysis in advanced prostate cancer]. Verh Dtsch Ges Pathol 1993; 77:119–123.

70. Veldscholte J, Voorhorst-Ogink MM, Bolt-de Vries J, van Rooij HC, Trapman J, Mulder E. Unusual specificity of the androgen receptor in the human prostate tumor cell line LNCaP: high affinity for progestagenic and estrogenic steroids. Biochim Biophys Acta 1990; 1052(1):187–194.

71. De BA, Quigley CA, Cariello NF et al. Single base mutations in the human androgen receptor gene causing complete androgen insensitivity: rapid detection by a modified denaturing gradient gel electrophoresis technique. Mol Endocrinol 1992; 6(11):1909–1920.

72. Jakubiczka S, Werder EA, Wieacker P. Point mutation in the steroid-binding domain of the androgen receptor gene in a family with complete androgen insensitivity syndrome (CAIS). Hum Genet 1992; 90(3):311–312.

73. Ahmed SF, Cheng A, Dovey L et al. Phenotypic features, androgen receptor binding, and mutational analysis in 278 clinical cases reported as androgen insensitivity syndrome. J Clin Endocrinol Metab 2000; 85(2):658–665.

74. Van YH, Lin JL, Huang SF, Luo CC, Hwang CS, Lo FS. Novel point mutations in complete androgen insensitivity syndrome with incomplete mullerian regression: two Taiwanese patients. Eur J Pediatr 2003; 162(11): 781–784.

75. Bouvattier C, Carel JC, Lecointre C et al. Postnatal changes of T, LH, and FSH in 46,XY infants with mutations in the AR gene. J Clin Endocrinol Metab 2002; 87(1):29–32.

76. Takahashi H, Furusato M, Allsbrook WC, Jr. et al. Prevalence of androgen receptor gene mutations in latent

prostatic carcinomas from Japanese men. Cancer Res 1995; 55(8):1621–1624.

77. Haapala K, Hyytinen ER, Roiha M et al. Androgen receptor alterations in prostate cancer relapsed during a combined androgen blockade by orchiectomy and bicalutamide. Lab Invest 2001; 81(12):1647–1651.

78. Gregory CW, Johnson RT, Jr., Mohler JL, French FS, Wilson EM. Androgen receptor stabilization in recurrent prostate cancer is associated with hypersensitivity to low androgen. Cancer Res 2001; 61(7):2892–2898.

79. Chen G, Wang X, Zhang S et al. Androgen receptor mutants detected in recurrent prostate cancer exhibit diverse functional characteristics. Prostate 2005; 63(4):395–406.

80. Jagla M, Feve M, Kessler P et al. A splicing variant of the androgen receptor detected in a metastatic prostate cancer exhibits exclusively cytoplasmic actions. Endocrinology 2007; 148(9):4334–4343

81. Buchanan G, Yang M, Harris JM et al. Mutations at the boundary of the hinge and ligand binding domain of the androgen receptor confer increased transactivation function. Mol Endocrinol 2001; 15(1):46–56.

82. Horwitz KB, Jackson TA, Bain DL, Richer JK, Takimoto GS, Tung L. Nuclear receptor coactivators and corepressors. Mol Endocrinol 1996; 10(10):1167–1177.

83. Greenberg NM, DeMayo F, Finegold MJ et al. Prostate cancer in a transgenic mouse. Proc Natl Acad Sci U S A 1995; 92(8):3439–3443.

84. Wang Q, Lu J, Yong EL. Ligand- and coactivator-mediated transactivation function (AF2) of the androgen receptor ligand-binding domain is inhibited by the cognate hinge region. J Biol Chem 2001; 276:7493–7499.

85. He B, Bowen NT, Minges JT, Wilson EM. Androgen-induced NH2- and COOH-terminal Interaction Inhibits p160 coactivator recruitment by activation function 2. J Biol Chem 2001; 276(45):42293–42301.

86. Gregory CW, Fei X, Ponguta LA et al. Epidermal growth factor increases coactivation of the androgen receptor in recurrent prostate cancer. J Biol Chem 2004; 279(8): 7119–7130.

87. Mellinghoff IK, Vivanco I, Kwon A, Tran C, Wongvipat J, Sawyers CL. HER2/neu kinase-dependent modulation of androgen receptor function through effects on DNA binding and stability. Cancer Cell 2004; 6(5):517–527.

88. Gregory CW, Whang YE, McCall W et al. Heregulin-induced activation of HER2 and HER3 increases androgen receptor transactivation and CWR-R1 human recurrent prostate cancer cell growth. Clin Cancer Res 2005; 11(5): 1704–1712.

89. Liu Y, Majumder S, McCall W et al. Inhibition of HER-2/neu kinase impairs androgen receptor recruitment to the androgen responsive enhancer. Cancer Res 2005; 65(8): 3404–3409.

90. Mahajan NP, Liu Y, Majumder S et al. Activated Cdc42-associated kinase Ack1 promotes prostate cancer progression via androgen receptor tyrosine phosphorylation. Proc Natl Acad Sci U S A 2007; 104(20):8438–8443.

91. Ponguta LA, Gregory CW, French FS, Wilson EM. Site specific androgen receptor serine phosphorylation linked to epidermal growth factor dependent growth of castration-recurrent prostate cancer. J Biol Chem 2008; 283(30): 20989–21001.

92. Sun M, Yang L, Feldman RI et al. Activation of phosphatidylinositol 3-kinase/Akt pathway by androgen through interaction of p85alpha, androgen receptor, and Src. J Biol Chem 2003; 278(44):42992–43000.

93. Guo Z, Dai B, Jiang T et al. Regulation of androgen receptor activity by tyrosine phosphorylation. Cancer Cell 2006; 10(4):309–319.

94. Dehm SM, Schmidt LJ, Heemers HV, Vessella RL, Tindall DJ. Splicing of a novel androgen receptor exon generates a constitutively active androgen receptor that mediates prostate cancer therapy resistance. Cancer Res 2008; 68(13):5469–5477.

95. Mohler JL, Gregory CW, Ford OH, III et al. The androgen axis in recurrent prostate cancer. Clin Cancer Res 2004; 10(2):440–448.

96. Stanbrough M, Bubley GJ, Ross K et al. Increased expression of genes converting adrenal androgens to testosterone in androgen-independent prostate cancer. Cancer Res 2006; 66(5):2815–2825.

97. Locke JA, Guns ES, Lubik AA et al. Androgen levels increase by intratumoral de novo steroidogenesis during progression of castration-resistant prostate cancer. Cancer Res 2008; 68(15):6407–6415.

98. Trachtenberg J, Halpern N, Pont A. Ketoconazole: a novel and rapid treatment for advanced prostatic cancer. J Urol 1983; 130(1):152–153.

99. Trachtenberg J, Pont A. Ketoconazole therapy for advanced prostate cancer. Lancet 1984; 2(8400):433–435.

100. Small EJ, Halabi S, Dawson NA et al. Antiandrogen withdrawal alone or in combination with ketoconazole in androgen-independent prostate cancer patients: a phase III trial (CALGB 9583). J Clin Oncol 2004; 22(6): 1025–1033.

101. Attard G, Reid AH, Yap TA et al. Phase I Clinical Trial of a Selective Inhibitor of CYP17, Abiraterone acetate, confirms that castration-resistant prostate cancer commonly remains hormone driven. J Clin Oncol 2008; 26(28): 4563–4571.

102. O'Donnell A, Judson I, Dowsett M et al. Hormonal impact of the 17alpha-hydroxylase/C(17,20)-lyase inhibitor abiraterone acetate (CB7630) in patients with prostate cancer. Br J Cancer 2004; 90(12):2317–2325.

103. Alen P, Claessens F, Verhoeven G, Rombauts W, Peeters B. The androgen receptor amino-terminal domain plays a key role in p160 coactivator-stimulated gene transcription. Mol Cell Biol 1999; 19(9):6085–6097.

104. Chmelar R, Buchanan G, Need EF, Tilley W, Greenberg NM. Androgen receptor coregulators and their involvement in the development and progression of prostate cancer. Int J Cancer 2007; 120(4):719–733.

105. Gregory CW, He B, Johnson RT et al. A mechanism for androgen receptor-mediated prostate cancer recurrence after androgen deprivation therapy. Cancer Res 2001; 61(11):4315–4319.

106. Agoulnik IU, Vaid A, Bingman WE, III et al. Role of SRC-1 in the promotion of prostate cancer cell growth and tumor progression. Cancer Res 2005; 65(17):7959–7967.

107. Bevan CL, Hoare S, Claessens F, Heery DM, Parker MG. The AF1 and AF2 domains of the androgen receptor interact with distinct regions of SRC1. Mol Cell Biol 1999; 19(12):8383–8392.

108. Agoulnik IU, Vaid A, Nakka M et al. Androgens modulate expression of transcription intermediary factor 2, an androgen receptor coactivator whose expression level correlates with early biochemical recurrence in prostate cancer. Cancer Res 2006; 66(21):10594–10602.

109. Zhou HJ, Yan J, Luo W et al. SRC-3 is required for prostate cancer cell proliferation and survival. Cancer Res 2005; 65(17):7976–7983.

110. Miyamoto H, Yeh S, Wilding G, Chang C. Promotion of agonist activity of antiandrogens by the androgen receptor coactivator, ARA70, in human prostate cancer DU145 cells. Proc Natl Acad Sci U S A 1998; 95(13):7379–7384.

111. Halkidou K, Gnanapragasam VJ, Mehta PB et al. Expression of Tip60, an androgen receptor coactivator, and its role in prostate cancer development. Oncogene 2003; 22(16): 2466–2477.

112. Ngan ES, Hashimoto Y, Ma ZQ, Tsai MJ, Tsai SY. Overexpression of Cdc25B, an androgen receptor coactivator, in prostate cancer. Oncogene 2003; 22(5):734–739.

113. Heemers HV, Sebo TJ, Debes JD et al. Androgen deprivation increases p300 expression in prostate cancer cells. Cancer Res 2007; 67(7):3422–3430.

114. Taneja SS, Ha S, Swenson NK et al. ART-27, an androgen receptor coactivator regulated in prostate development and cancer. J Biol Chem 2004; 279(14):13944–13952.

115. Fujimoto N, Yeh S, Kang HY et al. Cloning and characterization of androgen receptor coactivator, ARA55, in human prostate. J Biol Chem 1999; 274(12):8316–8321.

116. Wang X, Yang Y, Guo X et al. Suppression of androgen receptor transactivation by Pyk2 via interaction and phosphorylation of the ARA55 coregulator. J Biol Chem 2002; 277(18):15426–15431.

117. Voeller HJ, Truica CI, Gelmann EP. Beta-catenin mutations in human prostate cancer. Cancer Res 1998; 58(12): 2520–2523.

118. Chesire DR, Ewing CM, Sauvageot J, Bova GS, Isaacs WB. Detection and analysis of beta-catenin mutations in prostate cancer. Prostate 2000; 45(4):323–334.

119. Watanabe M, Kakiuchi H, Kato H et al. APC gene mutations in human prostate cancer. Jpn J Clin Oncol 1996; 26(2):77–81.

120. Gerstein AV, Almeida TA, Zhao G et al. APC/CTNNB1 (beta-catenin) pathway alterations in human prostate cancers. Genes Chromosomes Cancer 2002; 34(1):9–16.

121. Henrique R, Ribeiro FR, Fonseca D et al. High promoter methylation levels of APC predict poor prognosis in sextant biopsies from prostate cancer patients. Clin Cancer Res 2007; 13(20):6122–6129.

122. Mulholland DJ, Dedhar S, Wu H, Nelson CC. PTEN and GSK3beta: key regulators of progression to androgen-independent prostate cancer. Oncogene 2006; 25(3): 329–337.

123. Rubinfeld B, Albert I, Porfiri E, Fiol C, Munemitsu S, Polakis P. Binding of GSK3beta to the APC-beta-catenin complex and regulation of complex assembly. Science 1996; 272(5264):1023–1026.

124. Rios-Doria J, Kuefer R, Ethier SP, Day ML. Cleavage of beta-catenin by calpain in prostate and mammary tumor cells. Cancer Res 2004; 64(20):7237–7240.

125. Truica CI, Byers S, Gelmann EP. Beta-catenin affects androgen receptor transcriptional activity and ligand specificity. Cancer Res 2000; 60(17):4709–4713.

126. Yang F, Li X, Sharma M et al. Linking beta-catenin to androgen-signaling pathway. J Biol Chem 2002; 277(13): 11336–11344.

127. Mulholland DJ, Cheng H, Reid K, Rennie PS, Nelson CC. The androgen receptor can promote beta-catenin nuclear translocation independently of adenomatous polyposis coli. J Biol Chem 2002; 277(20):17933–17943.

128. Pawlowski JE, Ertel JR, Allen MP et al. Liganded androgen receptor interaction with beta-catenin: nuclear co-localization and modulation of transcriptional activity in neuronal cells. J Biol Chem 2002; 277(23):20702–20710.

129. Song LN, Herrell R, Byers S, Shah S, Wilson EM, Gelmann EP. Beta-catenin binds to the activation function 2 region of the androgen receptor and modulates the effects of the N-terminal domain and TIF2 on ligand-dependent transcription. Mol Cell Biol 2003; 23(5):1674–1687.

130. Song LN, Gelmann EP. Interaction of {beta}-Catenin and TIF2/GRIP1 in transcriptional activation by the androgen receptor. J Biol Chem 2005; 280(45):37853–37867.

131. Liao G, Chen LY, Zhang A et al. Regulation of androgen receptor activity by the nuclear receptor corepressor SMRT. J Biol Chem 2003; 278(7):5052–5061.

132. Song LN, Coghlan M, Gelmann EP. Antiandrogen effects of mifepristone on coactivator and corepressor interactions with the androgen receptor. Mol Endocrinol 2004; 18(1): 70–85.

133. Masiello D, Chen SY, Xu Y et al. Recruitment of beta-catenin by wild-type or mutant androgen receptors correlates with ligand-stimulated growth of prostate cancer cells. Mol Endocrinol 2004; 18(10):2388–2401.

134. Hodgson MC, Astapova I, Hollenberg AN, Balk SP. Activity of androgen receptor antagonist bicalutamide in prostate cancer cells is independent of NCoR and SMRT corepressors. Cancer Res 2007; 67(17):8388–8395.

Chapter 6
Androgen Receptor Antagonists

Howard C. Shen, Mary-Ellen Taplin, and Steven P. Balk

Abstract Androgen receptor (AR) antagonists used clinically include steroidal (cyproterone acetate) and nonsteroidal antagonists (bicalutamide, flutamide, and nilutamide), with the latter nonsteroidal compounds being the only ones in general use in the United States. AR antagonists are used as single agents or in conjunction with surgical or medical castration (combined androgen blockade) for the initial systemic treatment of prostate cancer (CaP). AR antagonists are somewhat less effective than castration but may be preferred in some patients due to potentially fewer side effects. Combined androgen blockade is more effective than castration alone based on rapid declines in serum prostate-specific antigen (PSA) levels and the lower nadir PSA levels, but this translates into only a very small survival advantage. Patients treated with single or combined therapies invariably relapse with CaP that has been termed castration-resistant prostate cancer (CRPC). Significantly, the AR is expressed at high levels and is transcriptionally active in most cases of CRPC, and a subset of these CRPC patients respond to AR antagonist treatment. However, these responses are generally partial and transient. Molecular mechanisms that contribute to AR reactivation in CRPC and impair the activity of AR antagonists are described in this chapter. Understanding these mechanisms is critical for the development of strategies to overcome resistance and for the generation of more effective AR antagonists.

Keywords Prostate cancer • Androgen receptor • Steroid • Steroid receptor • Testosterone • Dihydrotestosterone • Antagonist • Bicalutamide • Flutamide • Nilutamide

Steroidal and Nonsteroidal AR Antagonists

Androgen receptor (AR) antagonists used clinically for prostate cancer (CaP) include steroidal (cyproterone acetate) and nonsteroidal antagonists (flutamide, nilutamide, and bicalutamide), which all function as competitive inhibitors of AR binding to endogenous androgens (testosterone and dihydrotestosterone, DHT) (Fig. 6.1). The nonsteroidal compounds are the only ones that have been in general use in the United States, but cyproterone acetate has been used extensively in other countries. The disadvantages of steroidal antagonists include lack of specificity, with cyproterone acetate being an agonist for the progesterone receptor that can suppress gonadotropin release when used as a single agent [1]. Steroidal AR antagonists such as cyproterone acetate and mifepristone also have partial agonist activity, which may limit their ability to suppress AR activity [2].

The nonsteroidal AR antagonists in clinical use (flutamide, nilutamide, and bicalutamide) are all chemically related (substituted toluidides) [3, 4], and do not interact with other steroid receptors. Moreover, they function as relatively pure AR antagonists, although hydroxyflutamide (the active metabolite of flutamide) and nilutamide have some weak agonist activity at high concentrations. Flutamide is rapidly metabolized in vivo to hydroxyflutamide, which has about a tenfold higher affinity for AR compared to flutamide [4, 5]. Nilutamide is an analogue of

S.P. Balk (✉)
Department of Medicine, Beth Israel Deaconess Medical Center, Harvard Medical School, Boston, MA 02215, USA
e-mail: sbalk@bidmc.harvard.edu

W.D. Figg et al. (eds.), *Drug Management of Prostate Cancer*, DOI 10.1007/978-1-60327-829-4_6, © Springer Science+Business Media, LLC 2010

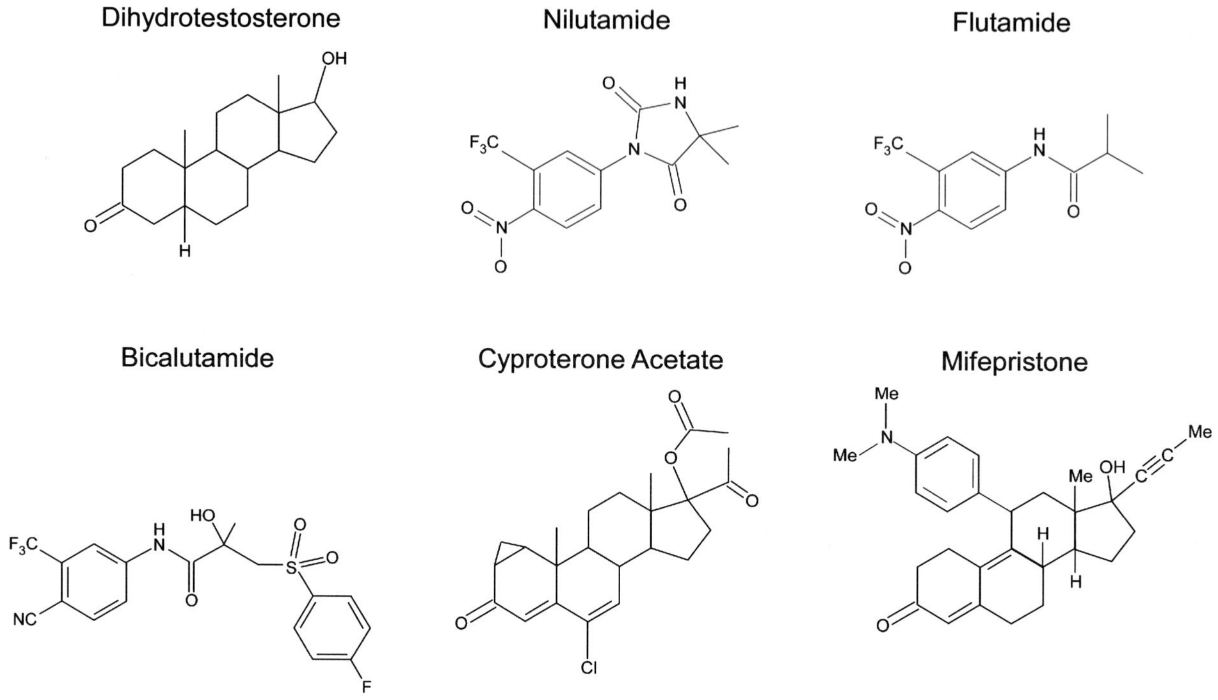

Dihydrotestosterone   Nilutamide   Flutamide

Bicalutamide   Cyproterone Acetate   Mifepristone

Fig. 6.1 Structures of DHT and AR antagonists

flutamide, and its affinity for AR is approximately the same as that of hydroxyflutamide [6]. Nilutamide has a longer half-life than flutamide; so it can be administered once per day (150–300 mg) as against the standard flutamide dose of 250 mg three times per day. The side effects of both drugs include diarrhea, nausea, and rarely hepatotoxicity, but nilutamide also frequently causes decreased darkness adaptation and rarely severe interstitial pneumonitis, which have limited its use [7]. Bicalutamide is administered as a mixture of two isomers, with the R-isomer having both the longest in vivo half-life and highest affinity for AR (about fourfold higher affinity than hydroxyflutamide) [8]. Due to its higher affinity, longer half-life (allowing once per day dosing of 50 mg), and more favorable side effect profile, bicalutamide has become the most commonly used AR antagonist. However, it should be emphasized that all of these compounds are still relatively weak AR antagonists, with the affinity of bicalutamide for the AR being ~50-fold lower than that of DHT in direct radioactive ligand competition binding assays [9]. Moreover, in cellular transcription assays, ~1,000-fold excess of bicalutamide is required to inhibit AR activation by DHT [10].

Mechanisms of AR Antagonist Action

AR Activation by Agonist Binding

The AR is a steroid receptor member of the large nuclear receptor superfamily. Similar to other steroid/nuclear receptors, the AR has an N-terminal domain (NTD) that mediates transcriptional activity, a C-terminal domain that binds androgen and can also stimulate transcription (ligand binding domain, LBD), a central domain that mediates sequence-specific DNA binding (DNA binding domain, DBD), and a hinge region between the DBD and LBD that regulates AR nuclear localization and degradation [11]. In contrast to other steroid/nuclear receptors, the AR NTD is larger and makes a major contribution to transcriptional activity through recruitment of multiple coactivator proteins.

The overall structure of steroid receptor LBDs, with 12 α-helices, and the way their structures are altered by ligand binding are very similar. In the absence of ligand, the AR associates with heat shock protein 90 (Hsp90) and a complex of additional chaperone proteins, which maintain AR in a conformation that permits ligand binding. Binding of agonist ligands (testosterone or DHT) shifts the position of the most C-terminal helix (helix 12), which moves towards a surface generated by helices 3–5. This movement of helix 12 has two consequences: First, it caps the steroid binding pocket to prevent the release of the bound testosterone or DHT, resulting in a slow off rate for agonist binding and a very high overall binding affinity. Second, helices 3–5, and 12 combine to generate a hydrophobic cleft (the coactivator binding site) that can bind transcriptional coactivator proteins via leucine-X-X-leucine-leucine (LXXLL) motif containing peptides. Multiple copies of the LXXLL motif (also termed nuclear receptor boxes or NR boxes) are found in the p160 family of coactivator proteins (SRC-1–3) and in several other proteins that contribute to the transcriptional activity. The agonist-liganded AR then binds as a dimer to specific DNA sequences in androgen-regulated genes (termed androgen responsive elements or AREs), where it recruits multiple coactivator and chromatin modifying proteins and ultimately RNA polymerase II, resulting in gene expression.

A further unique feature of AR is that its coactivator binding site, generated by helices 3–5, and 12, has a relatively low affinity for the LXXLL motifs found in most coactivator proteins. Instead, the AR coactivator binding site is specialized for binding to an LXXLL-like motif in the NTD (amino acids 23–27, FQNLF), and this interaction between the AR NTD and LBD further stabilizes helix 12 in the agonist position and ligand binding [12–15]. As a result of this reduced affinity of the AR LBD for LXXLL motif peptides, the AR NTD plays a more substantial role in the recruitment of transcriptional coactivator proteins (including the p160 coactivators that can interact with both the AR NTD and LBD).

Structural Changes in AR Mediated by Antagonist Binding

All characterized steroidal and nonsteroidal AR antagonists bind to the steroid binding pocket in the LBD and function as competitive inhibitors of androgen binding. Significantly, crystal structures of the wild-type AR bound to antagonists have not yet been successfully generated. However, certain mutations in the AR LBD can convert AR antagonists into agonists, and

crystal structures of these antagonist-liganded mutant AR LBDs have been obtained [16–20]. Moreover, crystal structures of other steroid receptors bound to antagonists can be used to model AR. Overall, these studies reveal two general mechanisms by which antagonists may inhibit AR transcriptional activity.

One mechanism is by distortion of the ligand-binding pocket. Binding of hydroxyflutamide (HF, the active metabolite of flutamide) forces repositioning of a threonine residue at codon 877 in the ligand-binding pocket. This is presumed to distort the LBD, preventing the movement of helix 12 into the agonist position and the generation of the coactivator binding site. Indeed, the HF liganded AR LBD does not bind to LXXLL motif containing coactivators and does not interact with the FQNLF peptide in the AR NTD. A threonine to alanine mutation in codon 877 can generate increased space to accommodate HF binding, so the T877A mutant AR is strongly stimulated by HF (but not by bicalutamide). Significantly, this T877A mutation is found with increased frequency in CRPC patients who were treated initially with flutamide [21] (see below). Nilutamide and cyproterone acetate appear to function in a manner similar to HF by distorting the ligand binding pocket, and their agonist activity is enhanced by T877A and related mutations.

Bicalutamide still inhibits the T877A mutant AR, but an AR with a tryptophan 741 to leucine mutation is strongly stimulated by bicalutamide. This W741L mutation has also been identified in patients treated with bicalutamide and in LNCaP cells adapted to grow in the presence of bicalutamide [22, 23]. The crystal structure of the bicalutamide-liganded W741L mutant AR LBD indicates that bicalutamide makes direct contact with this residue, and likely forces tryptophan (in the wild-type AR) to move into a position where it directly or indirectly prevents the appropriate positioning of helix 12 [24] (Fig. 6.2). As mentioned above for HF, the bicalutamide-liganded wild-type AR LBD cannot effectively recruit coactivator proteins or mediate binding of the AR NTD [10].

A second mechanism of antagonism is best exemplified by the tamoxifen and raloxifene liganded ERα. Rather than distorting the steroid binding pocket, crystal structures of the tamoxifen- and raloxifene-liganded ERα show that bulky side groups of these drugs stick out from the ligand-binding pocket and directly block the surface that would be occupied by helix 12 in response to agonists, forcing helix 12 into

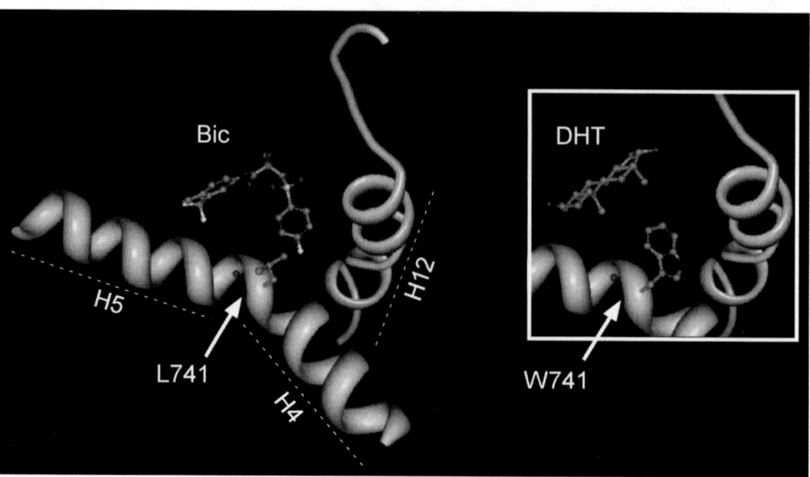

Fig. 6.2 Structure of bicalutamide-liganded W741L mutant AR versus DHT-liganded wild-type AR. The substitution of leucine for tryptophan at residue 741 allows bicalutamide to bind and helix 12 to fold into the agonist position. In contrast, based on the positioning of tryptophan in the wild-type DHT-liganded AR (*inset*), it appears that bicalutamide binding to the wild-type AR would force the repositioning of tryptophan 741 and either distort helix 4 or directly interfere with helix 12

alternative nonagonist positions [25, 26]. As a result, the LXXLL motif-binding cleft is not generated, and the ERα does not effectively recruit coactivator proteins. With respect to AR, this is the likely mechanism for antagonism by mifepristone, which is also an antagonist for the glucocorticoid and progesterone receptors [27], and for a recently synthesized AR antagonist [28].

As noted above, an important consequence of agonist-induced positioning of helix 12 is that it caps the ligand-binding pocket, which prevents ligand dissociation and thereby increases the affinity for agonist ligands. In contrast, it is presumed that the alternative positioning of helix 12 in response to antagonists does not stabilize antagonist binding, resulting in a more rapid dissociation rate and lower overall affinity for the antagonist. Significantly, this fundamental difference in agonist- versus antagonist-induced positioning of helix 12 may limit the ability to develop potent competitive antagonists for testosterone and DHT.

Role of Transcriptional Corepressors in AR Antagonist Action

In the absence of ligand, nonsteroidal nuclear receptors such as thyroid and retinoid receptors repress transcription by recruiting the corepressor proteins NCoR and SMRT, which are associated with histone deacetylase 3. Binding of these corepressor proteins is mediated by extended LXXLL-like motifs (L-X-X-I/H-I-X-X-X-L/I), termed corepressor nuclear receptor boxes (CoRNR boxes), which are located in the C-terminal half of NCoR and SMRT. The positioning of helix 12 away from helices 3 to 5 in unliganded nuclear receptors opens the LXXLL site to accommodate these larger CoRNR boxes, which make three helical turns (versus two turns for LXXLL motifs). While the nonsteroidal nuclear receptors bind DNA in the absence of ligand and actively repress transcription via NCoR and SMRT recruitment, DNA binding by steroid receptors is generally ligand-dependent and mediated physiologically by agonist ligands. Nonetheless, certain steroid hormone receptor antagonists (or partial agonists) can stimulate DNA binding and recruitment of NCoR or SMRT. This appears to contribute to the action of the ERα antagonists tamoxifen and raloxifene. As noted above, the crystal structures of the tamoxifen- and raloxifene-liganded ERα show that the side groups of these drugs force alternative nonagonist positions for helix 12 [25, 26]. In addition to impairing recruitment of coactivator proteins, this repositioning of helix 12 allows corepressor binding. Significantly, the tissue-selective activities of these drugs (antagonists in breast cancer and agonists in bone and other tissues) appear to reflect the relative levels of transcriptional coactivators versus corepressors in the respective tissues [29].

Biochemical studies of mifepristone similarly indicate that its antagonist activity against the glucocorticoid and progesterone receptors as well as AR is enhanced by the recruitment of NCoR or SMRT [30–34].

In contrast to other steroid receptors, the agonist-liganded AR interacts with NCoR and SMRT [35–37]. The interaction between AR and these corepressors is complex as NCoR and SMRT interact with both the AR LBD (via CoRNR boxes) and the AR NTD (via direct interactions and indirectly through an adaptor protein, TAB2) (see below) [34, 36, 38, 39]. Moreover, RNAi approaches have shown that NCoR and SMRT function at physiological levels as negative regulators of androgen stimulated AR transcriptional activity [34, 40, 41]. AR recruitment of NCoR, as assessed by chromatin immunoprecipitation (ChIP), is increased by AR antagonists or partial agonists including bicalutamide, hydroxyflutamide, and cyproterone acetate, although mifepristone appears to mediate more robust NCoR/SMRT recruitment [33, 34]. Consistent with NCoR/SMRT recruitment, downregulation of these corepressors by RNAi or other mechanisms can increase the agonist activity of AR antagonists such as hydroxyflutamide that have partial agonist activity [34, 40, 42–45]. Loss of NCoR/SMRT may also stimulate the agonist activity of the bicalutamide-liganded AR, though additional factors may be required to augment coactivator activity (see below).

Clinical Applications of AR Antagonists in CaP

AR antagonists are used as single agents or in conjunction with suppression of testicular androgen synthesis (surgical castration or medical castration by administration of an LHRH superagonist) for the initial systemic treatment of CaP. AR antagonists are also used in CaP that recurs after initial castration therapy. These recurrent tumors have been termed hormone refractory, androgen-independent, or castration-resistant prostate cancers (CRPC), the latter being the currently preferred term as it does not have mechanistic implications. However, as outlined below, the efficacy of AR antagonists in each of these settings and how their use may be optimized remain as important questions.

AR Antagonist Monotherapy in Previously Untreated Patients

Flutamide (with or without finasteride) and nilutamide as single agents have efficacy in previously untreated CaP but have not been directly compared to castration in clinical trials and are not commonly prescribed as monotherapy. Bicalutamide at a standard dose (50 mg/day) is less effective than castration, and at a higher dose (150 mg/day) it was less effective than castration in terms of survival in men with metastatic CaP [46]. In contrast, bicalutamide at 150 mg/day appears to be equivalent to castration in terms of time to progression and overall mortality in previously untreated men with nonmetastatic locally advanced disease [47, 48]. Another trial compared initial bicalutamide monotherapy (150 mg/day) and castration at disease progression with up front combined goserelin plus flutamide and found no difference in disease-specific or overall mortality [49]. However, an unexplained increase in overall mortality was observed in a subgroup that was treated only with bicalutamide. Further studies of 150 mg/day bicalutamide versus primary therapy (radical prostatectomy, radiation, or watchful waiting) in men with early stage CaP showed no improvement in progression-free survival for the bicalutamide group, and a small increase in nonprostate-specific mortality was observed in the bicalutamide versus watchful waiting group [50]. Bicalutamide monotherapy has not been approved by the U.S. Food and Drug Administration for use in CaP but is commonly prescribed outside the U.S.

While AR antagonists as single agents appear inferior to castration, particularly in men with more advanced CaP, they have advantages with respect to side effects. Recent studies have clearly established the negative metabolic consequences of castration, which include weight gain, increased cardiovascular mortality, bone and muscle loss, and glucose intolerance [51, 52]. In contrast, these effects are not observed in patients treated with single agent nonsteroidal antagonists [53, 54]. This likely reflects the differences in effects on steroid hormone levels, with testosterone and estradiol being decreased in response to castration versus modestly increased in patients treated with nonsteroidal AR antagonists (GnRH levels are decreased by cyproterone acetate due to its progestin activity). In some patients, the maintained or increased sex steroid levels after treatment with nonsteroidal AR antagonists, possibly in conjunction with lower CNS levels of these drugs, also results in less loss of libido and sexual function compared to castration.

Combined Castration and AR Antagonist Therapy (Combined Androgen Blockade, CAB)

The pioneering work of Huggins and others showed that bilateral surgical adrenalectomy or hypophysectomy to ablate adrenal androgen production resulted in objective responses in about one-third of patients and pain relief in more than two-third of them. This surgical approach to ablate adrenal androgens was later replaced by medical adrenalectomy with aminoglutethimide or ketoconazole (both suppress adrenal androgen synthesis), which yielded similar results. While most responses to suppression or ablation of adrenal androgen production in CRPC were partial and transient, they suggested that adrenal androgens were providing some stimulus for CRPC and that blocking adrenal androgens at an earlier stage may be beneficial. This led to a series of clinical trials that compared castration alone (orchiectomy or LHRH superagonist monotherapy) versus castration plus an AR antagonist (flutamide, bicalutamide, cyproterone acetate, or nilutamide) to block AR stimulation by residual adrenal androgens (combined androgen blockade, CAB).

Although the combined therapies resulted in more rapid responses and lower nadir PSA levels, the results of the largest trial and meta-analyses of the multiple other trials showed that the addition of AR antagonists caused only a very small (approximately 2%) improvement in survival [55, 56]. Importantly, the conclusion that can be drawn from these studies is that the available AR antagonists do not have substantial activity against the tumor cells that survive castration and emerge as CRPC. Consistent with this conclusion, the majority of CRPC that occur after orchiectomy or LHRH superagonist monotherapy do not respond to secondary treatments with AR antagonists, including high dose therapy (150–200 mg/day) with bicalutamide (see below) [57–59]. The efficacy of CAB will need to be readdressed as more effective AR antagonists or other approaches to suppress AR activity are developed (see below).

AR Antagonist Withdrawal Responses

Responses to the withdrawal of nonsteroidal AR antagonists were first observed when flutamide was discontinued in patients who relapsed after combined castration plus flutamide treatment [60, 61], and have since been documented for withdrawal of bicalutamide and nilutamide [62–65]. In a recent multi-institutional prospective trial, withdrawal responses (>50% decline in PSA) were observed in 24, 13, and 25% of patients after discontinuing flutamide, bicalutamide, and nilutamide, respectively [66]. Median progression-free survival was only 3 months, but prolonged responses (>1 year) were observed in 19% of responders. Longer duration of AR antagonist use was a predictor of response and progression-free survival.

The molecular basis for these withdrawal responses remains unclear but likely reflects multiple adaptations by the tumor cells that can enhance the partial agonist activities of these antagonists, including mutations in the AR LBD (see below). Interestingly, two studies found that withdrawal responses could be enhanced by suppression of adrenal androgen synthesis, suggesting that adrenal androgens (or intratumoral synthesized androgens, see below) are stimulating all or a subset of tumor cells in these patients after AR antagonist withdrawal [67, 68]. However, a randomized trial comparing anti-androgen withdrawal combined with adrenal androgen suppression (ketoconazole/hydrocortisone) to sequential anti-androgen withdrawal followed by adrenal androgen suppression at progression demonstrated no significant clinical benefits [68].

AR Antagonists in CRPC

AR and AR-regulated genes are still expressed at high levels in CRPC, indicating that AR transcriptional activity is reactivated in these tumors and that AR remains a therapeutic target [69–73]. Consistent with this conclusion, patients with CRPC who were not treated with an AR antagonist during their initial androgen deprivation therapy may respond to treatment with an AR antagonist (or to a switch to another AR antagonist), though response rates (>50% PSA decline) are generally low (15–40%) and transient (3–6 months) [58, 59, 74, 75]. Understanding why AR antagonists do not substantially enhance responses to castration therapy in the initial therapy of CaP and why these drugs are relatively ineffective in CRPC is clearly critical for the development of more effective AR antagonists. Therefore, the section below outlines mechanisms that may contribute to their loss of function in CRPC.

Mechanism Mediating AR Reactivation and Resistance to AR Antagonists in CRPC

Increased AR Expression

AR mRNA is consistently increased in CRPC (though protein levels may be more variable) with AR gene amplification in approximately one-third of cases [70, 72, 73, 76, 77]. Increased AR protein would presumably amplify residual AR activity and may enhance the agonist activity of bicalutamide by unclear mechanisms [78]. A recent study investigated bicalutamide resistance in C4–2 cells, which are derived from a LNCaP xenograft that relapsed after castration. Bicalutamide did not have AR agonist activity in these cells, but it was unable to inhibit basal AR NTD transcriptional activity, suggesting that uncoupling of the NTD from inhibition by the LBD (by unclear mechanisms) may contribute to bicalutamide resistance in CRPC [79].

Expression of Antagonist Activated Mutant ARs

AR mutations identified in CRPC can enhance AR activation by weak androgens, other steroid hormones, or AR antagonists [77, 80]. While the overall frequency of AR mutations in patients treated with castration alone was low [22], mutant ARs that were stimulated by hydroxyflutamide were more frequent (~one-third of cases) in patients who relapsed after combined androgen blockade with flutamide, indicating that there is positive selection for these mutations [21]. Moreover, these flutamide-activated mutant ARs are still inhibited by bicalutamide, and patients who relapse with CRPC after combined castration plus flutamide therapy have increased responses to bicalutamide [21,

58, 59]. A mutant AR (W741C) that is activated by bicalutamide has also been found in patients treated with bicalutamide [22] and in LNCaP CaP cells adapted to grow in the presence of bicalutamide [23].

Increased Intratumoral Androgen Synthesis

Direct measurements of intraprostatic androgens in castrated men with locally recurrent CRPC have shown that levels are increased compared to those in prostate soon after castration and are not significantly lower than levels prior to castration, indicating that increased testosterone uptake or synthesis by tumor cells may be a mechanism for reactivation of AR activity [71, 81, 82]. Moreover, a recent study has found that testosterone levels in metastatic CRPC samples are actually higher than in prostate from eugonadal men, despite castrate levels of serum androgens [73]. Gene expression studies in CRPC have revealed increased levels of multiple enzymes that mediate synthesis of weak androgens (DHEA and androstenedione) from cholesterol (including CYP17A), and enzymes mediating synthesis of testosterone and DHT from weak androgens [70, 72, 73, 83]. Importantly, the efficacy of AR antagonists, which are weak competitive inhibitors of testosterone and DHT binding, would clearly be impaired by high levels of intracellular androgens. The synthesis of weak androgens (by the adrenals and, presumably, the tumor cells) can be suppressed by CYP17A inhibitors including ketoconazole and by a more potent inhibitor, abiraterone, which is currently in phase III clinical trials [84]. Therefore, it will be of interest to determine whether the efficacy of AR antagonists can be enhanced by these or other inhibitors of androgen synthesis.

Altered Expression of Transcriptional Coactivator Versus Corepressor Proteins

Data from several groups indicate that expression of transcriptional coactivator proteins is increased in CRPC, which would increase residual AR activity and may enhance partial agonist activity of AR antagonists [85, 86]. With respect to corepressors, NCoR and SMRT are recruited as part of a complex containing HDAC3, TBL1, TBLR1, and TAB2 [45, 87–90]. TAB2 phosphorylation by MEKK1 in response to inflammatory signals has been shown to result in loss of the NCoR/HDAC3 complex from the AR and has also been reported to convert bicalutamide to an agonist [45, 91]. Using RNAi approaches, we have failed to detect bicalutamide agonist activity in response to NCoR or SMRT downregulation [41], but loss of NCoR via the MEKK1/TAB2 mechanism versus NCoR downregulation by siRNA may result in functionally distinct complexes, with MEKK1 possibly having additional effects that enhance coactivator recruitment by the bicalutamide-liganded AR. In any case, further analyses of links between inflammation and AR antagonist resistance are clearly warranted.

Enhanced Responses to Low Androgen Levels Mediated by Activation of Kinase Signaling Pathways

Studies in cell culture and xenografts indicate that CaP cells can adapt to markedly enhance their responses to low (subnanomolar) androgen concentrations, which would presumably increase their resistance to weak competitive AR antagonists. This AR hypersensitivity may occur in response to activation of certain kinases, including protein kinase A, ErbB2, Ras, c-Src, Cdk1, and the PI3 kinase/Akt pathway. The molecular basis for AR activation by these kinases is unclear but may include direct phosphorylation of AR or coactivator proteins. Further studies are needed to determine the extent to which these pathways contribute to AR activation and antagonist resistance in CRPC.

New AR Antagonists and Future Directions

While it may be possible to enhance the efficacy of available AR antagonists by targeting one or more of the mechanisms outlined above, it seems clear that there is a need for new AR antagonists that are more potent or function by novel mechanisms. BMS 641988 represents a chemically novel class of nonsteroidal AR

antagonists [92]. This compound is ~tenfold more potent than bicalutamide and is currently in phase I evaluation. MDV3100 is a nonsteroidal AR antagonist that functions by a novel mechanism (blocking nuclear transport), and it is about to enter phase III testing. Additional promising approaches are the development of antagonists that enhance AR degradation [93] or recruitment of corepressor proteins [33, 34, 94].

References

1. Isurugi K, Fukutani K, Ishida H, Hosoi Y. Endocrine effects of cyproterone acetate in patients with prostatic cancer. J Urol 1980; 123(2):180–183.
2. Kemppainen JA, Lane MV, Sar M, Wilson EM. Androgen receptor phosphorylation, turnover, nuclear transport, and transcriptional activation. Specificity for steroids and anti-hormones. J Biol Chem 1992; 267(2):968–974.
3. Gao W, Kim J, Dalton JT. Pharmacokinetics and pharmacodynamics of nonsteroidal androgen receptor ligands. Pharm Res 2006; 23(8):1641–1658.
4. Yin D, He Y, Perera MA, Hong SS, Marhefka C, Stourman N et al. Key structural features of nonsteroidal ligands for binding and activation of the androgen receptor. Mol Pharmacol 2003; 63(1):211–223.
5. Schulz M, Schmoldt A, Donn F, Becker H. The pharmacokinetics of flutamide and its major metabolites after a single oral dose and during chronic treatment. Eur J Clin Pharmacol 1988; 34(6):633–636.
6. Creaven PJ, Pendyala L, Tremblay D. Pharmacokinetics and metabolism of nilutamide. Urology 1991; 37(Suppl 2):13–19.
7. Janknegt RA, Abbou CC, Bartoletti R, Bernstein-Hahn L, Bracken B, Brisset JM et al. Orchiectomy and nilutamide or placebo as treatment of metastatic prostatic cancer in a multinational double-blind randomized trial. J Urol 1993; 149(1):77–82.
8. Mukherjee A, Kirkovsky L, Yao XT, Yates RC, Miller DD, Dalton JT. Enantioselective binding of Casodex to the androgen receptor. Xenobiotica 1996; 26(2):117–122.
9. Furr BJ, Tucker H. The preclinical development of bicalutamide: pharmacodynamics and mechanism of action. Urology 1996; 47(Suppl 1A):13–25.
10. Masiello D, Cheng S, Bubley GJ, Lu ML, Balk SP. Bicalutamide functions as an androgen receptor antagonist by assembly of a transcriptionally inactive receptor. J Biol Chem 2002; 277(29):26321–26326.
11. Gelmann EP. Molecular biology of the androgen receptor. J Clin Oncol 2002; 20(13):3001–3015.
12. He B, Gampe RT, Jr., Kole AJ, Hnat AT, Stanley TB, An G et al. Structural basis for androgen receptor interdomain and coactivator interactions suggests a transition in nuclear receptor activation function dominance. Mol Cell 2004; 16(3):425–438.
13. Hur E, Pfaff SJ, Payne ES, Gron H, Buehrer BM, Fletterick RJ. Recognition and accommodation at the androgen receptor coactivator binding interface. PLoS Biol 2004; 2(9):E274.

14. Estebanez-Perpina E, Moore JM, Mar E, Delgado-Rodrigues E, Nguyen P, Baxter JD et al. The molecular mechanisms of coactivator utilization in ligand-dependent transactivation by the androgen receptor. J Biol Chem 2005; 280(9):8060–8068.

15. He B, Kemppainen JA, Wilson EM. FXXLF and WXXLF sequences mediate the NH2-terminal interaction with the ligand binding domain of the androgen receptor. J Biol Chem 2000; 275(30):22986–22994.

16. Matias PM, Donner P, Coelho R, Thomaz M, Peixoto C, Macedo S et al. Structural evidence for ligand specificity in the binding domain of the human androgen receptor. Implications for pathogenic gene mutations. J Biol Chem 2000; 275(34):26164–26171.

17. Sack JS, Kish KF, Wang C, Attar RM, Kiefer SE, An Y et al. Crystallographic structures of the ligand-binding domains of the androgen receptor and its T877A mutant complexed with the natural agonist dihydrotestosterone. Proc Natl Acad Sci U S A 2001; 98(9):4904–4909.

18. Marhefka CA, Moore BM, Bishop TC, Kirkovsky L, Mukherjee A, Dalton JT et al. Homology modeling using multiple molecular dynamics simulations and docking studies of the human androgen receptor ligand binding domain bound to testosterone and nonsteroidal ligands. J Med Chem 2001; 44(11):1729–1740.

19. Bohl CE, Miller DD, Chen J, Bell CE, Dalton JT. Structural basis for accommodation of nonsteroidal ligands in the androgen receptor. J Biol Chem 2005; 280(45):37747–37754.

20. Bohl CE, Wu Z, Miller DD, Bell CE, Dalton JT. Crystal structure of the T877A human androgen receptor ligand-binding domain complexed to cyproterone acetate provides insight for ligand-induced conformational changes and structure-based drug design. J Biol Chem 2007; 282(18):13648–13655.

21. Taplin ME, Bubley GJ, Ko YJ, Small EJ, Upton M, Rajeshkumar B et al. Selection for androgen receptor mutations in prostate cancers treated with androgen antagonist. Cancer Res 1999; 59(11):2511–2515.

22. Taplin ME, Rajeshkumar B, Halabi S, Werner CP, Woda BA, Picus J et al. Androgen receptor mutations in androgen-independent prostate cancer: Cancer and Leukemia Group B Study 9663. J Clin Oncol 2003; 21(14):2673–2678.

23. Hara T, Miyazaki J, Araki H, Yamaoka M, Kanzaki N, Kusaka M et al. Novel mutations of androgen receptor: a possible mechanism of bicalutamide withdrawal syndrome. Cancer Res 2003; 63(1):149–153.

24. Bohl CE, Gao W, Miller DD, Bell CE, Dalton JT. Structural basis for antagonism and resistance of bicalutamide in prostate cancer. Proc Natl Acad Sci U S A 2005; 102(17):6201–6206.

25. Brzozowski AM, Pike AC, Dauter Z, Hubbard RE, Bonn T, Engstrom O et al. Molecular basis of agonism and antagonism in the oestrogen receptor. Nature 1997; 389(6652):753–758.

26. Shiau AK, Barstad D, Loria PM, Cheng L, Kushner PJ, Agard DA et al. The structural basis of estrogen receptor/coactivator recognition and the antagonism of this interaction by tamoxifen. Cell 1998; 95(7):927–937.

27. Cadepond F, Ulmann A, Baulieu EE. RU486 (mifepristone): mechanisms of action and clinical uses. Annu Rev Med 1997; 48:129–156.

28. Cantin L, Faucher F, Couture JF, Jesus-Tran KP, Legrand P, Ciobanu LC et al. Structural characterization of the human androgen receptor ligand-binding domain complexed with EM5744, a rationally designed steroidal ligand bearing a bulky chain directed toward helix 12. J Biol Chem 2007; 282(42):30910–30919.

29. Shang Y, Brown M. Molecular determinants for the tissue specificity of SERMs. Science 2002; 295(5564):2465–2468.

30. Jackson TA, Richer JK, Bain DL, Takimoto GS, Tung L, Horwitz KB. The partial agonist activity of antagonist-occupied steroid receptors is controlled by a novel hinge domain-binding coactivator L7/SPA and the corepressors N-CoR or SMRT. Mol Endocrinol 1997; 11(6):693–705.

31. Schulz M, Eggert M, Baniahmad A, Dostert A, Heinzel T, Renkawitz R. RU486-induced glucocorticoid receptor agonism is controlled by the receptor N terminus and by corepressor binding. J Biol Chem 2002; 277(29):26238–26243.

32. Wagner BL, Norris JD, Knotts TA, Weigel NL, McDonnell DP. The nuclear corepressors NCoR and SMRT are key regulators of both ligand- and 8-bromo-cyclic AMP-dependent transcriptional activity of the human progesterone receptor. Mol Cell Biol 1998; 18(3):1369–1378.

33. Song LN, Coghlan M, Gelmann EP. Antiandrogen effects of mifepristone on coactivator and corepressor interactions with the androgen receptor. Mol Endocrinol 2004; 18(1):70–85.

34. Hodgson MC, Astapova I, Cheng S, Lee LJ, Verhoeven MC, Choi E et al. The androgen receptor recruits nuclear receptor CoRepressor (N-CoR) in the presence of mifepristone via its N and C termini revealing a novel molecular mechanism for androgen receptor antagonists. J Biol Chem 2005; 280(8):6511–6519.

35. Cheng S, Brzostek S, Lee SR, Hollenberg AN, Balk SP. Inhibition of the dihydrotestosterone-activated androgen receptor by nuclear receptor corepressor. Mol Endocrinol 2002; 16(7):1492–1501.

36. Dotzlaw H, Moehren U, Mink S, Cato AC, Iniguez Lluhi JA, Baniahmad A. The amino terminus of the human AR is target for corepressor action and antihormone agonism. Mol Endocrinol 2002; 16(4):661–673.

37. Liao G, Chen LY, Zhang A, Godavarthy A, Xia F, Ghosh JC et al. Regulation of androgen receptor activity by the nuclear receptor corepressor SMRT. J Biol Chem 2003; 278(7):5052–5061.

38. Dotzlaw H, Papaioannou M, Moehren U, Claessens F, Baniahmad A. Agonist-antagonist induced coactivator and corepressor interplay on the human androgen receptor. Mol Cell Endocrinol 2003; 213(1):79–85.

39. Wu Y, Kawate H, Ohnaka K, Nawata H, Takayanagi R. Nuclear compartmentalization of N-CoR and its interactions with steroid receptors. Mol Cell Biol 2006; 26(17):6633–6655.

40. Yoon HG, Wong J. The corepressors SMRT and N-CoR are involved in agonist- and antagonist-regulated transcription by androgen receptor. Mol Endocrinol 2005; 20(5):1048–1060.

41. Hodgson MC, Astapova I, Hollenberg AN, Balk SP. Activity of androgen receptor antagonist bicalutamide in prostate cancer cells is independent of NCoR and SMRT corepressors. Cancer Res 2007; 67(17):8388–8395.

42. Shang Y, Myers M, Brown M. Formation of the androgen receptor transcription complex. Mol Cell 2002; 9(3):601–610.

43. Kang Z, Janne OA, Palvimo JJ. Coregulator recruitment and histone modifications in transcriptional regulation by the androgen receptor. Mol Endocrinol 2004; 18(11):2633–2648.

44. Berrevoets CA, Umar A, Trapman J, Brinkmann AO. Differential modulation of androgen receptor transcriptional activity by the nuclear receptor corepressor (N-CoR). Biochem J 2004; 379(Pt 3):731–738.

45. Zhu P, Baek SH, Bourk EM, Ohgi KA, Garcia-Bassets I, Sanjo H et al. Macrophage/cancer cell interactions mediate hormone resistance by a nuclear receptor derepression pathway. Cell 2006; 124(3):615–629.

46. Tyrrell CJ, Kaisary AV, Iversen P, Anderson JB, Baert L, Tammela T et al. A randomised comparison of 'Casodex' (bicalutamide) 150 mg monotherapy versus castration in the treatment of metastatic and locally advanced prostate cancer. Eur Urol 1998; 33(5):447–456.

47. Iversen P, Tyrrell CJ, Kaisary AV, Anderson JB, van Poppel H, Tammela TL et al. Bicalutamide monotherapy compared with castration in patients with nonmetastatic locally advanced prostate cancer: 6.3 years of followup. J Urol 2000; 164(5):1579–1582.

48. Iversen P, Tyrrell CJ, Kaisary AV, Anderson JB, Baert L, Tammela T et al. Casodex (bicalutamide) 150-mg monotherapy compared with castration in patients with previously untreated nonmetastatic prostate cancer: results from two multicenter randomized trials at a median follow-up of 4 years. Urology 1998; 51(3):389–396.

49. Boccardo F, Barichello M, Battaglia M, Carmignani G, Comeri G, Ferraris V et al. Bicalutamide monotherapy versus flutamide plus goserelin in prostate cancer: updated results of a multicentric trial. Eur Urol 2002; 42(5):481–490.

50. McLeod DG, Iversen P, See WA, Morris T, Armstrong J, Wirth MP. Bicalutamide 150 mg plus standard care vs standard care alone for early prostate cancer. BJU Int 2006; 97(2):247–254.

51. Yannucci J, Manola J, Garnick MB, Bhat G, Bubley GJ. The effect of androgen deprivation therapy on fasting serum lipid and glucose parameters. J Urol 2006; 176(2):520–525.

52. Keating NL, O'Malley AJ, Smith MR. Diabetes and cardiovascular disease during androgen deprivation therapy for prostate cancer. J Clin Oncol 2006; 24(27):4448–4456.

53. Sieber PR, Keiller DL, Kahnoski RJ, Gallo J, McFadden S. Bicalutamide 150 mg maintains bone mineral density during monotherapy for localized or locally advanced prostate cancer. J Urol 2004; 171(6 Pt 1):2272–2276, quiz.

54. Smith MR, Goode M, Zietman AL, McGovern FJ, Lee H, Finkelstein JS. Bicalutamide monotherapy versus leuprolide monotherapy for prostate cancer: effects on bone mineral density and body composition. J Clin Oncol 2004; 22(13):2546–2553.

55. Eisenberger MA, Blumenstein BA, Crawford ED, Miller G, McLeod DG, Loehrer PJ et al. Bilateral orchiectomy with or without flutamide for metastatic prostate cancer. N Engl J Med 1998; 339(15):1036–1042.

56. Prostate Cancer Trialists' Collaborative Group. Maximum androgen blockade in advanced prostate cancer: an overview of the randomised trials. Lancet 2000; 355(9214):1491–1498.

57. Fowler JE, Jr., Pandey P, Seaver LE, Feliz TP. Prostate specific antigen after gonadal androgen withdrawal and deferred flutamide treatment. J Urol 1995; 154(2 Pt 1):448–453.

58. Scher HI, Liebertz C, Kelly WK, Mazumdar M, Brett C, Schwartz L et al. Bicalutamide for advanced prostate cancer: the natural versus treated history of disease. J Clin Oncol 1997; 15(8):2928–2938.

59. Joyce R, Fenton MA, Rode P, Constantine M, Gaynes L, Kolvenbag G et al. High dose bicalutamide for androgen independent prostate cancer: effect of prior hormonal therapy. J Urol 1998; 159(1):149–153.

60. Kelly WK, Scher HI. Prostate specific antigen decline after antiandrogen withdrawal: the flutamide withdrawal syndrome. J Urol 1993; 149(3):607–609.

61. Dupont A, Gomez JL, Cusan L, Koutsilieris M, Labrie F. Response to flutamide withdrawal in advanced prostate cancer in progression under combination therapy. J Urol 1993; 150(3):908–913.

62. Small EJ, Carroll PR. Prostate-specific antigen decline after casodex withdrawal: evidence for an antiandrogen withdrawal syndrome. Urology 1994; 43(3):408–410.

63. Nieh PT. Withdrawal phenomenon with the antiandrogen casodex. J Urol 1995; 153(3 Pt 2):1070–1072.

64. Schellhammer PF, Venner P, Haas GP, Small EJ, Nieh PT, Seabaugh DR et al. Prostate specific antigen decreases after withdrawal of antiandrogen therapy with bicalutamide or flutamide in patients receiving combined androgen blockade. J Urol 1997; 157(5):1731–1735.

65. Huan SD, Gerridzen RG, Yau JC, Stewart DJ. Antiandrogen withdrawal syndrome with nilutamide. Urology 1997; 49(4):632–634.

66. Sartor AO, Tangen CM, Hussain MH, Eisenberger MA, Parab M, Fontana JA et al. Antiandrogen withdrawal in castrate-refractory prostate cancer: a Southwest Oncology Group trial (SWOG 9426). Cancer 2008; 112(11):2393–2400.

67. Sartor O, Cooper M, Weinberger M, Headlee D, Thibault A, Tompkins A et al. Surprising activity of flutamide withdrawal, when combined with aminoglutethimide, in treatment of "hormone-refractory" prostate cancer. J Natl Cancer Inst 1994; 86(3):222–227.

68. Small EJ, Halabi S, Dawson NA, Stadler WM, Rini BI, Picus J et al. Antiandrogen withdrawal alone or in combination with ketoconazole in androgen-independent prostate cancer patients: a phase III trial (CALGB 9583). J Clin Oncol 2004; 22(6):1025–1033.

69. van der Kwast TH, Schalken J, Ruizeveld de Winter JA, van Vroonhoven CC, Mulder E, Boersma W et al. Androgen receptors in endocrine-therapy-resistant human prostate cancer. Int J Cancer 1991; 48(2):189–193.

70. Holzbeierlein J, Lal P, LaTulippe E, Smith A, Satagopan J, Zhang L et al. Gene expression analysis of human prostate carcinoma during hormonal therapy identifies androgen-responsive genes and mechanisms of therapy resistance. Am J Pathol 2004; 164(1):217–227.

71. Mohler JL, Gregory CW, Ford OH, III, Kim D, Weaver CM, Petrusz P et al. The androgen axis in recurrent prostate cancer. Clin Cancer Res 2004; 10(2):440–448.

72. Stanbrough M, Bubley GJ, Ross K, Golub TR, Rubin MA, Penning TM et al. Increased expression of genes converting adrenal androgens to testosterone in androgen-independent prostate cancer. Cancer Res 2006; 66(5):2815–2825.

73. Montgomery RB, Mostaghel EA, Vessella R, Hess DL, Kalhorn TF, Higano CS et al. Maintenance of intratumoral androgens in metastatic prostate cancer: a mechanism for castration-resistant tumor growth. Cancer Res 2008; 68(11):4447–4454.

74. Nakabayashi M, Regan MM, Lifsey D, Kantoff PW, Taplin ME, Sartor O et al. Efficacy of nilutamide as secondary

hormonal therapy in androgen-independent prostate cancer. BJU Int 2005; 96(6):783–786.

75. Suzuki H, Okihara K, Miyake H, Fujisawa M, Miyoshi S, Matsumoto T et al. Alternative nonsteroidal antiandrogen therapy for advanced prostate cancer that relapsed after initial maximum androgen blockade. J Urol 2008; 180(3):921–927.

76. Visakorpi T, Hyytinen E, Koivisto P, Tanner M, Keinanen R, Palmberg C et al. In vivo amplification of the androgen receptor gene and progression of human prostate cancer. Nat Genet 1995; 9(4):401–406.

77. Taplin ME, Bubley GJ, Shuster TD, Frantz ME, Spooner AE, Ogata GK et al. Mutation of the androgen-receptor gene in metastatic androgen-independent prostate cancer. N Engl J Med 1995; 332(21):1393–1398.

78. Chen CD, Welsbie DS, Tran C, Baek SH, Chen R, Vessella R et al. Molecular determinants of resistance to antiandrogen therapy. Nat Med 2004; 10(1):33–39.

79. Dehm SM, Tindall DJ. Ligand-independent androgen receptor activity is activation function-2-independent and resistant to antiandrogens in androgen refractory prostate cancer cells. J Biol Chem 2006; 281(38):27882–27893.

80. Fenton MA, Shuster TD, Fertig AM, Taplin ME, Kolvenbag G, Bubley GJ et al. Functional characterization of mutant androgen receptors from androgen-independent prostate cancer. Clin Cancer Res 1997; 3(8):1383–1388.

81. Geller J, Albert JD, Nachtsheim DA, Loza D. Comparison of prostatic cancer tissue dihydrotestosterone levels at the time of relapse following orchiectomy or estrogen therapy. J Urol 1984; 132(4):693–696.

82. Titus MA, Schell MJ, Lih FB, Tomer KB, Mohler JL. Testosterone and dihydrotestosterone tissue levels in recurrent prostate cancer. Clin Cancer Res 2005; 11(13):4653–4657.

83. Ettinger SL, Sobel R, Whitmore TG, Akbari M, Bradley DR, Gleave ME et al. Dysregulation of sterol response element-binding proteins and downstream effectors in prostate cancer during progression to androgen independence. Cancer Res 2004; 64(6):2212–2221.

84. Attard G, Reid AH, Yap TA, Raynaud F, Dowsett M, Settatree S et al. Phase I clinical trial of a selective inhibitor of CYP17, abiraterone acetate, confirms that castration-resistant prostate cancer commonly remains hormone driven. J Clin Oncol 2008; 26(28):4563–4571.

85. Gregory CW, He B, Johnson RT, Ford OH, Mohler JL, French FS et al. A mechanism for androgen receptor-mediated prostate cancer recurrence after androgen deprivation therapy. Cancer Res 2001; 61(11):4315–4319.

86. Agoulnik IU, Vaid A, Nakka M, Alvarado M, Bingman WE, III, Erdem H et al. Androgens modulate expression of transcription intermediary factor 2, an androgen receptor coactivator whose expression level correlates with early biochemical recurrence in prostate cancer. Cancer Res 2006; 66(21):10594–10602.

87. Yoon HG, Chan DW, Huang ZQ, Li J, Fondell JD, Qin J et al. Purification and functional characterization of the human N-CoR complex: the roles of HDAC3, TBL1 and TBLR1. EMBO J 2003; 22(6):1336–1346.

88. Guenther MG, Lane WS, Fischle W, Verdin E, Lazar MA, Shiekhattar R. A core SMRT corepressor complex containing HDAC3 and TBL1, a WD40-repeat protein linked to deafness. Genes Dev 2000; 14(9):1048–1057.

89. Baek SH, Ohgi KA, Rose DW, Koo EH, Glass CK, Rosenfeld MG. Exchange of N-CoR corepressor and Tip60 coactivator complexes links gene expression by NF-kappaB and beta-amyloid precursor protein. Cell 2002; 110(1):55–67.

90. Perissi V, Aggarwal A, Glass CK, Rose DW, Rosenfeld MG. A corepressor/coactivator exchange complex required for transcriptional activation by nuclear receptors and other regulated transcription factors. Cell 2004; 116(4):511–526.

91. Baek SH, Ohgi KA, Nelson CA, Welsbie D, Chen C, Sawyers CL et al. Ligand-specific allosteric regulation of coactivator functions of androgen receptor in prostate cancer cells. Proc Natl Acad Sci U S A 2006; 103(9):3100–3105.

92. Salvati ME, Balog A, Wei DD, Pickering D, Attar RM, Geng J et al. Identification of a novel class of androgen receptor antagonists based on the bicyclic-1H-isoindole-1,3(2H)-dione nucleus. Bioorg Med Chem Lett 2005; 15(2):389–393.

93. Schayowitz A, Sabnis G, Njar VC, Brodie AM. Synergistic effect of a novel antiandrogen, VN/124-1, and signal transduction inhibitors in prostate cancer progression to hormone independence in vitro. Mol Cancer Ther 2008; 7(1):121–132.

94. Taplin ME, Manola J, Oh WK, Kantoff PW, Bubley GJ, Smith M et al. A phase II study of mifepristone (RU-486) in castration-resistant prostate cancer, with a correlative assessment of androgen-related hormones. BJU Int 2008; 101(9):1084–1089.

Chapter 7
5-Alpha Reductase Inhibitors in Prostate Cancer

Zoran Culig

Abstract Androgenic effects in prostate cancer cells depend on the synthesis and metabolism of hormones and the presence of androgen receptor. 5-alpha reductase isoenzymes I and II differ in chromosomal localization, pH optimum, enzyme kinetics, and expression in benign and malignant prostate tissue. In prostate cancer tissues, there is an increased expression of the isoenzyme type I. The possibilities for pharmacological intervention include drug(s) that inhibit both isoforms such as dutasteride or extract from *Serenoa repens* or type II inhibitors such as finasteride. 5-alpha reductase inhibitors are used in benign prostate hyperplasia therapy, and it has been postulated that they may also be beneficial in preventive strategies for prostate cancer. Due to its dual effect on 5-alpha reductase inhibition, dutasteride may be preferred over finasteride for prostate cancer prevention. Data from large clinical studies have indicated that these inhibitors reduce the risk of prostate cancer; however, there are concerns that should be discussed. Importantly, there may be an increased number of high-grade Gleason tumors in patients treated with finasteride.

Keywords 5-alpha reductase • Dutasteride • Finasteride • Izoenzyme • Prostate cancer

Z. Culig (✉)
Department of Urology, Innsbruck Medical University, Innsbruck, Austria
e-mail: zoran.culig@1-med.ac.at

Introduction

Prostate cancer (CaP) dependency on androgenic stimulation has been well known since the early work of Huggins and Hodges in the twentieth century. Therapies for advanced prostate cancer are therefore based on inhibition of androgenic stimulation but are palliative only. A number of paracrine and autocrine factors that stimulate the growth of CaP have been identified, and some novel experimental therapies have been considered in combination with antiandrogen treatment. The two most important androgenic steroids are testosterone and dihydrotestosterone (DHT). They both bind to the androgen receptor (AR). Conventional nonsteroidal antiandrogens, such as hydroxyflutamide and bicalutamide, are effective for a certain time period and cause a temporary control of tumor growth. It was shown that these two antiandrogens may act as agonists under certain conditions [1, 2]. In particular, a prolonged treatment with an antiandrogen may lead to appearance of receptor mutations. If mutant ARs are stimulated by antiandrogens, one could understand that the tumor growth is paradoxically promoted by the drug. It should be kept in mind that AR expression and transcriptional activity may increase during long-term androgen ablation. The data obtained in several laboratories indicate that the inhibition of the ligand–receptor axis of AR may be reasonable in a subgroup of patients who present with a late stage tumor [3, 4]. On the other hand, there is experimental evidence showing the role of the AR in maintaining differentiation function of the prostate gland. Prostate-specific antigen (PSA) is thus induced by some nonsteroidal agents such as interleukin-6, phenylbutyrate, and phenylacetate [5, 6]. Current therapies cannot unfortunately distinguish between the inhibition of proliferation and differentiation mediated by the AR. In this chapter, there is a focus on

W.D. Figg et al. (eds.), *Drug Management of Prostate Cancer*,
DOI 10.1007/978-1-60327-829-4_7, © Springer Science+Business Media, LLC 2010

therapeutic inhibition of the androgen–AR axis by interfering with production of the ligand DHT.

Androgens and Androgen Receptor

There is a major difference between testosterone and its derivative DHT in the binding affinity for the AR. It has been shown that the binding affinity of testosterone is about one-third of that of DHT. Consequently, higher concentrations of testosterone are required to achieve the same effect. In many in vitro experiments, the synthetic androgens such as methyltrienolone (R1881) or mibolerone are used because of their low metabolic rate in comparison with natural androgens. Binding of androgens to the receptor leads to receptor translocation to the nucleus where the ligand–receptor complex is recruited onto DNA sequences of promoters of target genes. Importantly, testosterone and DHT regulate the proliferation in a biphasic manner thus stimulating cellular growth at lower concentrations. It is known that this effect is mostly mediated through stimulation of cyclin-dependent kinases and cyclins [7]. At higher androgen concentrations, the inhibitors of cell cycle such as p27 or p21 are induced. There is a growing body of evidence clearly showing that AR-associated coactivators are required for optimal action of androgens. The knowledge on coactivators whose expression has increased in prostate cancer is being improved recently. It is, however, not known whether there are preferential coactivators for DHT and testosterone in benign and malignant prostate cells. Some of the coactivators are being considered targets for therapy because of their high expression in CaP and promotion of agonistic activities of antiandrogens and stimulation of proliferation and migration [8, 9]. Interestingly, it was shown that the transcriptional integrator p300 may even replace the AR in induction of expression of specific genes in prostate cancer cells [10].

Conversion of Testosterone to DHT: 5-Alpha Reductase

The 5-alpha reductase enzyme, which is membrane-associated and NAPDH-dependent, exists in two isoforms in the human body: type I (SRD5A1), which is expressed in the liver and skin, and type II (SRD5A2), which is predominant in the prostate [11]. Chromosomal localization of these two isoforms differs; while the gene encoding the type I 5-alpha reductase is located on chromosome 5, the gene for the 5-alpha reductase II is situated on chromosome 2. The two isoforms do have a dissimilar homology and enzyme kinetics. The pH optimum for the isoenzyme I is between 6 and 8 and for the isoenzyme II between 5 and 6. The type II isoform has a higher affinity for testosterone than the type I isoform. 5-alpha reductase type I requires a higher steroid substrate concentration to achieve a half maximal rate of DHT production.

In the organs of the genitourinary system, the 5-alpha reductase I isoenzyme is expressed in preputial skin, whereas stromal cells in the seminal vesicle are type II-positive. A clinical syndrome of 5-alpha reductase deficiency is not associated with the type I isoenzyme. A genetic mutation of the type II 5-alpha reductase was discovered in a male population of the Dominican Republic [12]. Due to this somatic mutation, affected subjects present with ambiguous genitalia at birth and rudimentary prostate. Partial virilization is sometimes observed in males during puberty because of an increased expression of the type I enzyme. Defects in virilization were also reported in male monkeys that were treated with an inhibitor of type II 5-alpha reductase. In individuals with 5-alpha reductase II mutations, there is no development of benign prostate hyperplasia (BPH) or prostate cancer. In the prostate gland, 5-alpha reductase type II was detected in both epithelial and stromal cells.

The Role of 5-Alpha Reductase in the Nonmalignant Disease of the Prostate

Androgens regulate vasculogenesis in both benign and malignant prostate tissue. The underlying mechanism involves upregulation of vascular endothelial growth factor [13]. Since BPH is characterized by increased blood flow, the inhibitors of 5-alpha reductase may provide some relief in this disorder. In addition, the inhibitors of 5-alpha reductase could be used for prophylaxis of BPH complications. However, it is generally accepted that these drugs should not be used in individuals who have severe BPH symptoms [14]. If the medication is discontinued, the symptoms usually reappear.

5-Alpha Reductase and Cancer

With the development of specific anti-5-alpha reductase antibodies, it has become possible to perform isotype-specific immunohistochemical and Western blot analyses. In general, these studies yielded the consensus that the relationship between the enzyme isoforms I and II may change in prostate tumor development and carcinogenesis. Moreover, it was confirmed by steroid 5-alpha reductase in vitro assays that the activity of 5-alpha reductase I increases in prostate cancer [15]. Thus, the isoform I may become, for reasons which are not completely clear, the predominant isoform in high-grade prostate intraepithelial neoplasia and malignancy. It has been speculated that under conditions in which the hypoxia-inducible factor 1 alpha is elevated, the promoter of carboanhydrase 9, a tumor-associated transmembrane enzyme that influences intracellular pH towards increased activity of the isoenzyme type I, becomes more active. Since Mohler's group demonstrated that the intraprostatic androgens are present at sufficient levels to stimulate growth of recurrent tumors, the presence of the 5-alpha reductase in clinical specimens is clinically relevant [16]. Testosterone levels of 3.75 pmol/g tissue were measured in recurrent tumors, whereas its content in androgen-stimulated benign prostate was 2.75 pmol/g. When 5-alpha reductase was compared between different grades of localized prostate tumors by immunohistochemistry, it was shown, however, that there is an increase of either 5-alpha reductase isoenzyme with a higher Gleason grade [17]. It is also interesting that Habib and associates reported the loss of both 5-alpha reductase isoforms in metastatic lymph node and bone lesions of CaP [18]. This finding is important and undoubtedly leads to some novel questions related to the generation of androgens in the metastatic lesions of CaP. In prostate cancer, there is either the presence of AR in metastatic lesions or its absence due to epigenetic changes in the promoter of the gene [19, 20].

Somatic 5-alpha reductase mutations may occur in prostate cancer tissue. Makriadis and associates reported that such mutations could be detected in about two third of CaP patients [21]. These mutations may lead to either increased or decreased activity of the enzyme, or they may not change its activity. The mutations with increased 5-alpha reductase activity appear to be more common than those with an opposite effect. The presence of 5-alpha reductase mutations should be taken into consideration when discussing the responsiveness of individual patients to therapy with 5-alpha reductase inhibitors. Most mutations of the coding region of the 5-alpha reductase gene occurred early in prostate cancer development. A49T mutation of the 5-alpha reductase gene has increased the risk of African-American men by 7.2-fold and of men of Hispanic origin in Los Angeles by 3.6-fold [22]. The higher risk may be due to an increased conversion of testosterone into DHT.

5-Alpha Reductase Inhibitors

5-alpha reductase inhibitors lead, in general, to inhibition of DHT serum concentration, whereas the testosterone serum levels are elevated. Intraprostatic levels of DHT, however, remain significantly lower after treatment with an 5-alpha reductase inhibitor. Pharmacological inhibitors of 5-alpha reductase discussed in the chapter are finasteride and dutasteride. There is no specific 5-alpha reductase type I isoform inhibitor available in the market. The first compound is a product of Merck that was developed earlier and inhibits the type II isoform. Several years after the development of finasteride, GlaxoSmithKline developed dutasteride, a drug that inhibits both enzyme isoforms and causes a stronger inhibition of intraprostatic DHT expression. Dutasteride is approved at a dosage of 0.5 mg/day orally for the treatment of BPH. A higher percentage of primary cultures of prostate cancer cells was inhibited by dutasteride than finasteride [23]. Dutasteride was found to exert a more potent effect on the H rat prostate Dunning tumor that contains increased levels of the type I enzyme. In preclinical research with LNCaP xenografts, the effects of finasteride and dutasteride were compared by Xu and associates [24]. They reported a double advantage for dutasteride, causing an inhibition of xenograft growth that is more effective than that caused by castration alone. The effect of dutasteride was also more pronounced than that of finasteride. Dutasteride has been also identified as a molecule that inhibits enzyme fatty acid synthase that is overexpressed in CaP and correlates with a poor prognosis. The genes involved in metabolism and catalytic activity are strongly influenced by treatment with dutasteride in vitro [25]. Dutasteride also upregulated the expression of caspases 3 and 7 and genes involved in the pro-apoptotic pathway of FasL/tumor necrosis factor alpha. Thus, experimental data have indicated that dual 5-alpha reductase inhibitor(s) may be more appropriate for prevention and/or therapy than a single type inhibitor. Since the treatment with dutasteride will not eliminate all androgenic actions in prostate cancer, the addition of an antiandrogen to a therapy regimen may be appropriate. Finasteride, in combination with intermittent androgen withdrawal, improved survival of mice bearing LNCaP tumor [26]. On the other hand, it was found that finasteride has a favorable effect on the Bcl-2/Bax ratio and also decreases Bcl-x. The same authors showed that finasteride increases the effect on caspase 3, thus confirming induction of apoptosis. In other studies, it was reported that finasteride may prevent the progression of rat prostate cancer to macroscopic disease [27].

Clinical Studies with 5-Alpha Reductase Inhibitors in Prostate Cancer

Different study endpoints have been considered in clinical studies with 5-alpha reductase inhibitors. Some investigators follow a decrease in serum PSA parameters. This section focuses on the proposed role of finasteride in prevention of prostate cancer and discusses the reasons for the controversial findings reported. In an early clinical study, finasteride treatment over 6 weeks was associated with a decrease in PSA in individuals who did not present with a positive bone scan [28]. Similar findings were obtained in another study in which the most notable response was that of PSA [29]. However, it should be kept in mind that PSA is not a useful endpoint for a study with finasteride since it is known that finasteride itself has a negative regulatory effect on PSA. Finasteride inhibits complex formation between steroid receptor-binding consensus and nuclear proteins as a consequence of AR expression inhibition [30]. In this context, it is worthwhile to note that the phytotherapeutic agent *Serenoa repens* has an effect on 5-alpha reductase inhibition in the growth of prostate cancer cell lines without affecting PSA protein expression [31]. Thus, *Serenoa repens*, a dual 5-alpha reductase inhibitor, does not interfere with expression or transcriptional activity of the AR. Prostate cancer cells treated with *Serenoa repens* show accumulation of lipids in the cytoplasm and damage of mitochondrial and nuclear membranes. However, it should be pointed out that the strong effects of *Serenoa repens* were not observed by all researchers and may be cell context-dependent. In addition to inhibition of 5-alpha reductase, alternative mechanisms such as anti-inflammatory action by which *Serenoa repens* inhibits tumor growth are being discussed.

In much larger studies, such as Prostate Cancer Prevention Trial (PCPT) study, medical therapy of prostate symptoms (MTOPS), and the phase IIIa program for dutasteride, the focus was on (a) treatment of BPH and (b) prevention of cancer development (Table 7.1). Male individuals with high levels of PSA (>10 ng/ml) were excluded from the studies because of the likelihood of the presence of prostate cancer. At present, it is rather difficult to distinguish between clinically indolent and significant cancers detected in large prevention studies, especially if the Gleason score is intermediate. Considerable effort has been taken to better distinguish between these two groups on the basis of genomic and proteomic analyses; however, there are remarkable differences between the results reported from different centers.

Table 7.1 Large clinical studies with 5-alpha reductase inhibitors in prostate diseases

Study	Number of subjects	End of the study	Effect on cancer incidence	Higher gleason score
PCPT	1,300	Yes	Yes	Yes
MTOPS	18,882	Yes		
IIIa for dutasteride	1,908	Yes		
Reduce	8,000	No		

In the MTOPS study, which was designed to assess the effects of finasteride alone or in combination with the blocker of alpha 1-adrenoreceptor doxazosine, more than 1,300 men participated [32]. It was evident that the percentage of prostate cancer-positive biopsies decreased in patients who were treated with finasteride. It was found that finasteride treatment had provided beneficial effects on BPH symptoms. One of the issues that cause controversies in discussions on the impact of finasteride treatment for prostate cancer is an increasing number of tumors detected with a higher Gleason score (i.e., 7–10) [33]. In the dutasteride study, there was no evidence for increased risk of high Gleason score cancer following inhibition of 5-alpha reductase. There is a concern that most studies cited in this paragraph are more relevant to BPH rather than cancer biology, and the results regarding cancer histology could not be accepted with confidence.

The largest number of patients ($n = 18,882$ subjects) in a single study was recruited in the PCPT study performed between 1994 and 2004 [34]. The study subjects had normal digital rectal examination and serum PSA level lower than 3 ng/ml. The patients were randomized to take either finasteride or placebo. The difference in the cancer prevalence between 24.4% (placebo group) and 18.4% (finasteride group) was found to be statistically significant. Considering the clinical stage, most of the tumors detected in the study were T1 and T2. In the finasteride group, most tumors were less likely to be bilateral. At the same time, the percentage of high Gleason score tumors (7–10) was 37% after finasteride treatment in contrast to 22% in the placebo group. However, the validity of these results was questioned because of a fewer number of biopsies performed in the group of patients who received finasteride. Other arguments against the causative role of finasteride include the lack of divergence over time, increase in PSA levels in patients receiving placebo only, and lack of assessment of prostate cancer status in men treated with finasteride. An "effect" of finasteride on the increase in the percentage of high-grade tumors might, in fact, be masked by a decrease in the percentage of low-grade tumors. For the REDUCE trial, 8,000 individuals with increased risk of prostate cancer development have been selected on the basis of clinical evaluation and biopsy [35]. The running time of the REDUCE study is 4 years, and the study is international, multi-centered, randomized, double-blinded, and placebo-controlled.

Both finasteride and dutasteride have an impact on reduction of prostate volume. Thus, the detection of prostate cancer may, in fact, increase since the tumors might be easily diagnosed due to a smaller volume of the prostate [36]. Dutasteride was applied in combination with bicalutamide prior to brachytherapy, and it was show to display an inhibitory effect on prostate volume comparable to that caused by luteinizing hormone-releasing hormone [37].

Histologically, the effects of 5-alpha reductase inhibitors in prostate caused changes similar to those caused by androgen ablation therapy [38]. However, they were milder compared to those caused by androgen withdrawal. Signs of atrophy and involution, existence of smaller nuclei and nucleoli, increased apoptosis, and reduced density of microvessels were seen. There is a consensus that Gleason grading could, therefore, not be appropriately determined after prostate cancer treatment, with either anti-androgens or 5-alpha reductase inhibitors. At present, there are several novel molecules proposed to be used as markers for prostate cancer. They may be used in further studies with finasteride as well.

Some additional effects of finasteride treatment in prostate cancer may include impaired sexual function in these men, and in rare cases, disturbances such as depression or neurotoxicity.

In summary, although there is some clinical evidence supporting the use of 5-alpha reductase inhibitors in prostate cancer prevention, several additional studies seem to be justified. Further studies may be designed also with the aim of including information on the preventive effects of finasteride or dutasteride in ethnic groups with different levels of prostate cancer risk. The effectiveness of finasteride or dutasteride may be compared with that of some other agents being currently used such as selenium or resveratrol.

References

1. Veldscholte J, Ris-Stalpers C, Kuiper GG, Jenster G, Berrevoets C, Claassen E, et al. A mutation in the ligand binding domain of the androgen receptor of human LNCaP cells affects steroid binding characteristics and response to anti-androgens. Biochem Biophys Res Commun 1998;173: 534–40.
2. Hara T, Miyazaki J, Araki H, Yamaoka M, Kanzaki N, Kusaka M, et al. Novel mutations of androgen receptor: a

possible mechanism of bicalutamide withdrawal syndrome. Cancer Res 2003;63:149–53.

3. Kokontsi J, Takakura K, Hay N, Liao S. Increased androgen receptor activity and altered c-myc expression in prostate cancer cells after long-term androgen deprivation. Cancer Res 1994;54:1566–73.

4. Culig Z, Hoffmann J, Erdel M, Eder IE, Hobisch A, Hittmair A, et al. Switch from antagonist to agonist of the androgen receptor blocker bicalutamide is associated with prostate tumour progression in a new model system. Br J Cancer 1999;81:242–51.

5. Hobisch A, Eder IE, Putz T, Horninger W, Bartsch G, Klocker H, et al. Interleukin-6 regulates prostate-specific protein expression in prostate carcinoma cells by activation of the androgen receptor. Cancer Res 1998;58:4640–5.

6. Sadar MD, Gleave ME. Ligand-independent activation of the androgen receptor by the differentiation agent butyrate in human prostate cancer cells. Cancer Res 2000;60:5825–31.

7. Lu S, Tsai SY, Tsai MJ. Regulation of androgen-dependent prostatic cancer cell growth: androgen regulation of CDK2, CDK4, and CKI p16 genes. Cancer Res 1997;57:4511–6.

8. Yan J, Erdem H, Li R, Cai Y, Ayala G, Ittmann M, et al. Steroid receptor coactivator-3/AIB1 promotes cell migration and invasiveness through focal adhesion turnover and matrix metalloproteinase expression. Cancer Res 2008;68:5460–8.

9. Comuzzi B, Lambrinidis L, Rogatsch H, Godoy-Tundidor S, Knezevic N, Krhen I, et al. The transcriptional co-activator cAMP response element-binding protein-binding protein is expressed in prostate cancer and enhances androgen- and anti-androgen-induced receptor function. Am J Pathol 2003;162:233–41.

10. Debes JD, Comuzzi B, Schmidt LJ, Dehm SM, Culig Z, Tindall DJ. p300 regulates androgen receptor-independent expression of prostate-specific antigen in prostate cancer cells treated chronically with interleukin-6. Cancer Res 2005; 65:5965–73.

11. Steers WD. 5alpha-reductase activity in the prostate. Urology 2001;58:17–24.

12. Cai LQ, Zhu YS, Katz MD, Herrera C, Baez J, de Fillo-Ricart M, et al. 5-alpha-reductase-2 gene mutations in the Dominican republic. Clin Endocrinol Metab. 199;81:1730–5.

13. Joseph IB, Nelson JB, Denmeade SR, Isaacs JT. Androgens regulate vascular endothelial growth factor content in normal and malignant prostatic tissue. Clin Cancer Res 1997;3: 2507–11.

14. O'Leary MP, Roehrborn C, Andriole G, Nickel C, Boyle P, Höfner K. Improvements in benign prostatic hyperplasia-specific quality of life with dutasteride, the novel dual 5alpha-reductase inhibitor. BJU Int 2003;92:262–6.

15. Titus MA, Gregory CW, Ford 3rd OH, Schell MJ, Maygarden SJ, Mohler JL. Steroid 5alpha-reductase isozymes I and II in recurrent prostate cancer. Clin Cancer Res 2005;11:4365–71.

16. Titus MA, Schell MJ, Lih FB, Tomer KB, Mohler JL. Testosterone and dihydrotestosterone tissue levels in recurrent prostate cancer. Clin Cancer Res 2005;11:4653–7.

17. Thomas LN, Douglas RC, Lazier CB, Gupta R, Norman RW, Murphy PR, et al. Levels of 5alpha-reductase type 1 and type 2 are increased in localized high grade compared to low grade prostate cancer. J Urol 2008;179:147–51.

18. Habib FK, Ross M, Bayne CW, Bollina P, Grigor K, Chapman K. The loss of 5alpha-reductase type I and type II

19. Hobisch A, Culig Z, Radmayr C, Bartsch G, Klocker H, Hittmair A. Distant metastases from prostatic carcinoma express androgen receptor protein. Cancer Res 1995;55: 3068–72.

20. Kinoshita H, Shi Y, Sandefur C, Meisner LF, Chang C, Choon A, et al. Methylation of the androgen receptor minimal promoter silences transcription in human prostate cancer. Cancer Res 2000;60:3623–30.

21. Makridakis N, Akalu A, Reichardt JK. Identification and characterization of somatic steroid 5alpha-reductase (SRD5A2) mutations in human prostate cancer tissue. Oncogene 2004;23:7399–405.

22. Makridakis NM, Ross RK, Pike MC, Crocitto LE, Kolonel LN, Pearce CL, et al. Association of mis-sense subtitution in SRD5A2 gene with prostate cancer in African-American and Hispanic men in Los Angeles. USA Lancet 1999; 354:975–8.

23. Festuccia C, Gravina GL, Muzi P, Pomante R, Angelucci A, Vicentini C, et al. Effects of dutasteride on prostate carcinoma primary cultures: a comparative study with finasteride and MK386. J Urol 2008;180:367–72.

24. Xu Y, Dalrymple SL, Becker RE, Denmeade SR, Isaacs JT. Pharmacologic basis for the enhanced efficacy of dutasteride against prostatic cancers. Clin Cancer Res 2006;12:4072–9.

25. Schmidt LJ, Murillo H, Tindall DJ. Gene expression in prostate cancer cells treated with the dual 5-alpha-reductase inhibitor dutasteride. J Androl 2004;25:944–53.

26. Eggener SE, Stern JA, Jain PM, Oram S, Ai J, Cai X, et al. Enhancement of intermittent androgen ablation by "off-cycle" maintenance with finasteride in LNCaP prostate cancer xenograft model. Prostate 2006;66:495–502.

27. Tsukamoto S, Akaza H, Onozawa M, Shirai T, Ideyama A. A five-alpha reductase inhibitor or an antiandrogen prevents the progression of microscopic prostate carcinoma to macroscopic carcinoma in rats. Cancer 1998;82:531–7.

28. Presti JC, Fair WR, Andriole G, Sogani PC, Seidmon EJ, Ferguson D. Multicenter, randomized, double-blind, placebo controlled study to investigate the effect of finasteride (MK-906) on stage D prostate cancer. J Urol 1992;148:1201.

29. Andriole G, Lieber M, Smith J, Soloway M, Schroeder F, Kadmon D. Treatment with finasteride following radical prostatectomy for prostate cancer. Urology 1995;45:491–7.

30. Wang LG, Liu XM, Kreis W, Budman DR. Down-regulation of prostate-specific antigen expression by finasteride through inhibition of complex formation between androgen receptor and steroid receptor-binding consensus in the promoter of the PSA gene in LNCaP cells. Cancer Res 1997;57:714–9.

31. Habib FK, Ross M, Ho CK, Lyons V, Chapman K. *Serenoa repens* (Permixon) inhibits the 5alpha-reductase activity of human prostate cancer cell lines without interfering with PSA expression. Int J Cancer 2005;114:190–4.

32. Klotz L, Saad F, PCPT-MTOPS Consensus Panel. PCPT, MTOPS and the use of 5ARIs: a Canadian consensus regarding implications for clinical practice. Can Urol Assoc J 2007;1:17–21.

33. Lucia MS, Epstein JI, Goodman PJ, Darke AK, Reuter VE, Civantos F, et al. Finasteride and high-grade prostate cancer in the Prostate Cancer Prevention Trial. J Natl Cancer Inst 2007;99:1375–83.

34. Goodman PJ, Tangen CM, Crowley JJ, Carlin SM, Ryan A, Coltman Jr CA, et al. Implementation of the prostate cancer prevention trial control. Clin Trials 2004;25:203–22.

35. Gommella LG. Chemoprevention using dutasteride: the REDUCE trial. Curr Opin Urol 2005;15:29–32.

36. McConnell JD, Bruskewitz R, Walsh P, Andriole G, Lieber M, Holtgrewe HL, et al. The effect of finasteride on the risk of acute urinary retention and the need for surgical treatment among men with benign prostatic hyperplasia. Finasteride long-term efficacy and safety study group. N Engl J Med 1998;338:557–63.

37. Merrick GS, Butler WM, Wallner KE, Galbreath RW, Allen ZA, Kurko B. Efficacy of neoadjuvant bicalutamide and dutasteride as a cytoreductive regimen before prostate brachytherapy. Urology 2006;68:116–20.

38. Rubin MA, Kantoff PW. Effect of finasteride on risk of prostate cancer: how little we really know. J Cell Biochem 2004;91:478–82.

Chapter 8
Adrenal Androgen Synthesis Inhibitor Therapies in Castration-Resistant Prostate Cancer

Terence W. Friedlander and Charles J. Ryan

Abstract It is well recognized that the vast majority of prostate cancers rely on testosterone for growth. Even after medical or surgical castration, a significant number of men will unfortunately experience disease progression manifested as an increasing prostate-specific antigen (PSA) or objective tumor growth. Left untreated, castration-resistant prostate cancer (CRPC) is uniformly fatal. It causes close to 30,000 deaths annually in the United States, with most men living only 2–4 years from the time castration resistance develops. In recent years, research has shown that despite castration resistance these tumors still retain sensitivity to low levels of circulating testosterone and other androgens. By inhibiting androgen synthesis, targeted adrenal androgen synthesis inhibitors slow the growth of castration-resistant tumors. The major agents in use today include corticosteroids, ketoconazole, aminoglutethimide, estrogens and progestins, as well as the novel CYP17 inhibitors abiraterone acetate, TAK-700 and TOK-001. The following article reviews the clinical data supporting the use of each of these adrenal androgen synthesis inhibitors in advanced prostate cancer, including the dosing, schedules, and common side effects.

Keywords Secondary hormonal therapy • Adrenal androgens • Androgen-independent prostate cancer • Hormone refractory prostate cancer • Phase I clinical trial • Pharmacokinetics

C.J. Ryan (✉)
Department of Medicine,
University of California San Francisco,
San Francisco, CA, USA
e-mail: ryanc@medicine.ucsf.edu

Introduction

For over 60 years, it has been recognized that testosterone plays a critical role in promoting the growth of adenocarcinoma of the prostate. Huggins and Hodges received the 1967 Nobel Prize for their discovery that surgical or medical castration could produce a striking regression of metastatic prostate cancer (CaP) and improve bone pain, lower urinary tract symptoms, and quality of life [1, 2]. Since then, hormonal suppression therapy has become the mainstay of treatment for men with metastatic prostate cancer at diagnosis or for men with rising PSA or recurrent CaP after definitive surgery or radiation. As surgical castration has become a less popular option in recent years, there has been growing interest in agents that can effectively deprive the growing tumor of androgenic stimulation.

In the United States, there currently exist three major anti-hormonal classes of agents to suppress the growth of prostate cancer. These include the GnRH or LHRH analogs leuprolide, goserelin, histrelin, degarelix, and triptorelin, the androgen receptor antagonists flutamide, bicalutamide, and nilutamide, and lastly the inhibitors of adrenal androgen synthesis, a heterogeneous group including corticosteroids, ketoconazole, and aminoglutethimide. More recently, abiraterone acetate, a specific inhibitor of 17 alpha-hydroxylase-17, 20-lyase (CYP17), has generated significant interest in clinical studies and is currently being evaluated in phase III studies. Two other inhibitors of CYP17, TAK-700 and TOK-001 have also begun early phase clinical testing. Estrogens may also be included in the category of androgen synthesis inhibitors, though they exert effects both in the adrenal gland as well as directly in the prostate cancer cell.

Given the wide array of agents available to treat patients with advanced prostate cancer, (defined as

W.D. Figg et al. (eds.), *Drug Management of Prostate Cancer*,
DOI 10.1007/978-1-60327-829-4_8, © Springer Science+Business Media, LLC 2010

metastatic disease at diagnosis, or a rising PSA, or recurrent disease after definitive surgery/radiation) the choice of initial, second-line, and in many cases third- and fourth-line agents can be confusing to the practitioner. Particularly, when and where should adrenal androgen synthesis inhibitors be used? How effective are they at slowing the growth of prostate cancer? What are the major side effects of these therapies? To answer these questions, a review of the role of androgens in promoting the growth of prostate cancer will be helpful.

The Role of Androgens

It has been long recognized that androgenic stimulation is the major factor promoting the growth and the malignant transformation of prostatic tissue. Androgens are a group of chemically related 19-carbon steroid hormones produced in the adrenal cortex, testis, and ovaries; all are derived from cholesterol, a common precursor. Androgens exert their effect on prostate cell primarily via interaction with the androgen receptor (AR); this interaction promotes growth and cell division, while at the same time inhibits apoptosis. Among the androgens, testosterone and its derivative dihydrotestosterone (DHT) are the most potent in terms of prostate tumorigenesis and growth stimulus, though androgens arising from the adrenal gland such as androstenedione, dehydroepiandrostenedione (DHEA), and DHEA-sulfate are capable of binding to and activating the AR [3]. It is important to remember that approximately 95% of all circulating testosterone is derived from the testes; the remainder is produced by the adrenal cortex. Thus, therapies targeting the adrenal glands can have an important role in further suppressing testosterone secretion.

Initial Therapy for Advanced Prostate Cancer: Orchiectomy and GnRH/LHRH Analogs

The fact that prostate cancer is uniquely sensitive to androgenic stimulation provides a clear rationale for anti-hormonal therapy to slow the growth of prostate cancer. Androgen deprivation therapy (ADT) is the initial treatment of choice for advanced prostate cancer and aims to

inhibit signals for growth and development provided by androgens and, in particular, by testosterone. ADT was traditionally accomplished via either bilateral surgical orchiectomy or the use of estrogens, particularly diethylstilbestrol (DES). While clinical trials proved DES to be as effective as orchiectomy in slowing tumor growth, the significant cardiovascular and thromboembolic toxicity associated with DES spurred the development and use of relatively less toxic GnRH/LHRH analogs. These agents markedly reduce circulating testosterone levels and induce state of castration, with fewer side effects than DES. The development and use of GnRH/LHRH analogs has since obviated the use of DES as a frontline therapy.

GnRH/LHRH therapy and orchiectomy can markedly improve bony pain in up to 90% of patients with metastatic disease and can significantly slow objective tumor growth and PSA rise. A meta-analysis of ten trials encompassing 1,908 patients showed equivalence in overall survival between these two modalities [4]. Furthermore, several studies have demonstrated that ADT concurrent with or adjuvant to local therapies such as radiation or radical prostatectomy can improve disease-specific survival [5]. Guidelines issued by the American Society of Clinical Oncology currently recommend surgical castration or the use of a GnRH/LHRH analog as the initial treatment for advanced prostate cancer [6].

An important aspect of LHRH therapy is that testosterone levels decline by approximately 90%, leaving a small amount in the circulation that would be capable of stimulating a tumor that is hypersensitive to these low levels.

Second-Line Therapies for Advanced Prostate Cancer: Anti-Androgens and Anti-androgen-Withdrawal

The vast majority of patients with advanced prostate cancer treated initially with ADT in the form of LHRH agonist-based therapy will respond with a significant decrease in serum PSA and a reduction in radiographically evident disease. Despite this benefit, castration-resistant prostate cancer is likely to develop within a range of 18–24 months in most patients [7].

Moderate incremental benefit can be achieved with either the immediate or deferred addition of oral anti-androgens such as flutamide, bicalutamide, or nilutamide, in what is termed combined androgen blockade

(CAB). The addition of anti-androgens results in clinical response and improvement in quality of life in a majority of men; however, there is little data to suggest any overall survival benefit. With progression of disease and amplification (see below) of the androgen receptor (AR), the receptor may be paradoxically activated [8], and thus withdrawal of anti-androgens (anti-androgen withdrawal or AAWD) has, in some cases, resulted in a short-lived PSA decline and an improvement in clinical symptoms [9, 10]. After AAWD, some patients will benefit from using a second, or even third anti-androgen; the likelihood of response to second-line anti-androgen is generally higher if the patient exhibited a PSA decline with AAWD [11].

Progressive Disease: Mechanisms

Persistent AR signaling is widely recognized to be a common molecular event underlying disease progression despite castrate levels of testosterone (commonly defined as serum testosterone <50 ng/ml) and is referred to as castration-resistant prostate cancer or CRPC. This signaling occurs through multiple mechanisms, including amplification of the AR itself, increased sensitivity of the AR to low levels of circulating androgens produced by the adrenal context or by the tumor itself, or by increased sensitivity of the AR to nonandrogen stimulators such as epidermal growth factor, insulin-like growth factor-1, and keratinocyte growth factor [3]. Taken together, these data suggest that the combination of persistent and alternative androgens coupled with a tumor that is hypersensitive to androgen stimulation play a major role in the development of tumor progression in the castrate state.

Adrenal Androgen Synthesis Inhibitors

While many of the mechanisms discussed here play a role in promoting growth in the castrate environment, it has become clear that despite castration resistance, CRPC still remains responsive to "secondary" hormonal manipulation. This was recognized early, and clinical trials using surgical adrenalectomy for advanced prostate cancer clearly showed that tumor growth can be slowed by decreasing circulating testosterone and nontestosterone androgens [12]. The understanding of the stimulatory effect of these nontesticular androgens on CRPC provides the rationale for the ongoing use and development of inhibitors of adrenal androgen synthesis.

Broadly defined, several agents are available that exert inhibitory effects on the interaction of adrenal androgens and the AR, including corticosteroids, the antifungal agent ketoconazole, estrogenic compounds such as DES, the rarely used drug aminoglutethimide, and more recently, abiraterone acetate, TAK-700, and TOK-001. The common thread linking all of these agents is their net effect on decreasing androgen synthesis by the adrenal cortex, either through direct inhibition of enzymes involved in androgen synthesis (ketoconazole, aminoglutethimide, abiraterone acetate, TAK-700, and TOK-001) or through feedback inhibition of the hypothalamic/pituitary axis (corticosteroids and estrogens). Each of these agents is variably effective at slowing down prostate tumor growth, and each carries its own side effects and toxicities.

Adrenalectomy

Bilateral surgical adrenalectomy was demonstrated to have a clear antitumor effect in the 1940s [12, 13]. Due to the high morbidity of surgery, the need for lifelong corticosteroid replacement, and better outcomes with medical approaches, its use has been largely abandoned in favor of medical therapies that more directly target adrenal androgen biosynthesis pathways.

Corticosteroids

Corticosteroids function in a wide range of physiologic systems and are involved in the regulation of blood pressure, inflammation, the systemic immune response, serum electrolytes, and in protein and carbohydrate metabolism. Like the androgens, they are all synthesized in the adrenal cortex from the common precursor cholesterol.

Corticosteroid production is regulated by a complex feedback loop involving the hypothalamus, pituitary gland, and the adrenal glands. Exogenous use of corticosteroids causes a disruption in this hypothalamic–pituitary–adrenal axis; high levels of circulating corticosteroids cause a decrease in coticotropin-releasing hormone (CRH) secretion by the hypothalamus. This leads to decreased secretion of corticotropin (ACTH) by the pituitary gland. Low circulating ACTH levels then lead to adrenal cortical atrophy and reduction in endogenous corticosteroid production. A side effect of this adrenal atrophy is a decrease in endogenous androgen production, making corticosteroid therapy a potential tool for treatment of advanced prostate cancer.

Besides inhibiting tumor growth by indirectly downregulating adrenal androgen production, corticosteroids may directly inhibit tumor growth through disruption of intracellular signaling pathways and suppression of tumor lymphangiogenesis [14–17]. While not yet fully characterized, this direct cytotoxicity likely exerts a modest effect in suppressing tumor growth in CRPC. As single agents, corticosteroids have been tested in multiple clinical trials in men with CRPC. In one study, 37 patients with CRPC were treated with daily oral prednisone at doses of 7.5–10 mg. After one month of therapy, improvements in quality of life were noted in 38% of patients, and in 19% of patients, the effect was maintained for a median of 4 months [18]. Similar results have been noted in other small studies, with PSA decreases of >50% reported in anywhere from 16 to 61% of patients. The two largest randomized trials incorporating corticosteroid-only control arms showed a 22 and 16% response rates respectively [19, 20]. Median duration of response in many of these studies was short, in the order of 4 months. Small studies have suggested that dexamethasone may be the most potent of the corticosteroids, with data suggesting that 0.75 mg of dexamethasone given orally three times a day may have higher antitumor activity than prednisone or hydrocortisone [21]. Taken together, the data from clinical trials using single-agent corticosteroids as therapy for prostate cancer show that they have, at best, modest activity in the disease. One possible explanation of the mechanism of resistance to or lack of activity of corticosteroids may come from the peripheral conversion of exogenous glucocorticoids into androgens or androgen precursors, which then stimulate tumor growth.

The systemic side effects of glucocorticoids generally limit high-dose or long-term therapy. They include hypertension, hyperglycemia, hypercholesterolemia, immune suppression, osteoporosis, cataract development, weight gain, anxiety and mood instability, and others. Careful attention should be paid to the discontinuation of therapy as abrupt cessation of long-term therapy can lead to corticosteroid withdrawal and precipitate an Addisonian crisis.

Despite their modest activity as single-agent therapy, corticosteroids still play significant role in palliation of bony pain attributable to metastatic disease. In low doses, they are frequently used to supplement other adrenolytic therapies such as ketoconazole or abiraterone acetate and can additionally help palliate nausea and other side effects of chemotherapy. More importantly, corticosteroids, particularly prednisone, have consistently been used as a control arm in clinical trials of chemotherapies for prostate cancer. Phase III studies of mitoxantrone/prednisone vs. prednisone, satraplatin/prednisone vs. prednisone, and now abiraterone/prednisone vs. prednisone attest the widespread recognition that corticosteroids exert some benefit to patients with CRPC, likely, in part, due to their ability to decrease adrenal androgen synthesis.

Aminoglutethimide

Aminoglutethimide was one of the first recognized orally available nonsteroidal inhibitors of adrenal androgen synthesis. Aminoglutethimide blocks the first step in adrenal hormone synthesis via inhibition of CYP11A1 (P450 side-chain cleavage enzyme), an enzyme that forms pregnenolone from cholesterol (Fig. 8.1). At higher doses, aminoglutethimide is also an inhibitor of CYP11B1 (3-beta hydroxylase) and CYP19 (aromatase) (Table 8.1).

Clinical data supporting the effectiveness of aminoglutethimide show that approximately half of the patients achieve an 80% decline in PSA level when aminoglutethimide is administered concomitantly with replacement dose hydrocortisone along with flutamide withdrawal [22]. Another similar study showed a greater than 50% PSA decrease in 37% of patients with CRPC treated with 1,000 mg aminoglutethimide daily and 40 mg hydrocortisone daily with a median duration of response of 9 months and median survival of 23 months. A more recent phase III randomized controlled trial comparing vinorelbine plus hydrocortisone vs. hydrocortisone alone in which individual centers could choose to add aminoglutethimide to hydrocortisone failed to demonstrate improvement with aminoglutethimide in either group [23].

Aminoglutethimide is dosed 250 mg orally three times daily for 3 weeks and then increased to four times daily. Due to its inhibition of glucocorticoid synthesis, it is usually given with either prednisone or an equivalent glucocorticoid. The use of aminoglutethimide has been largely

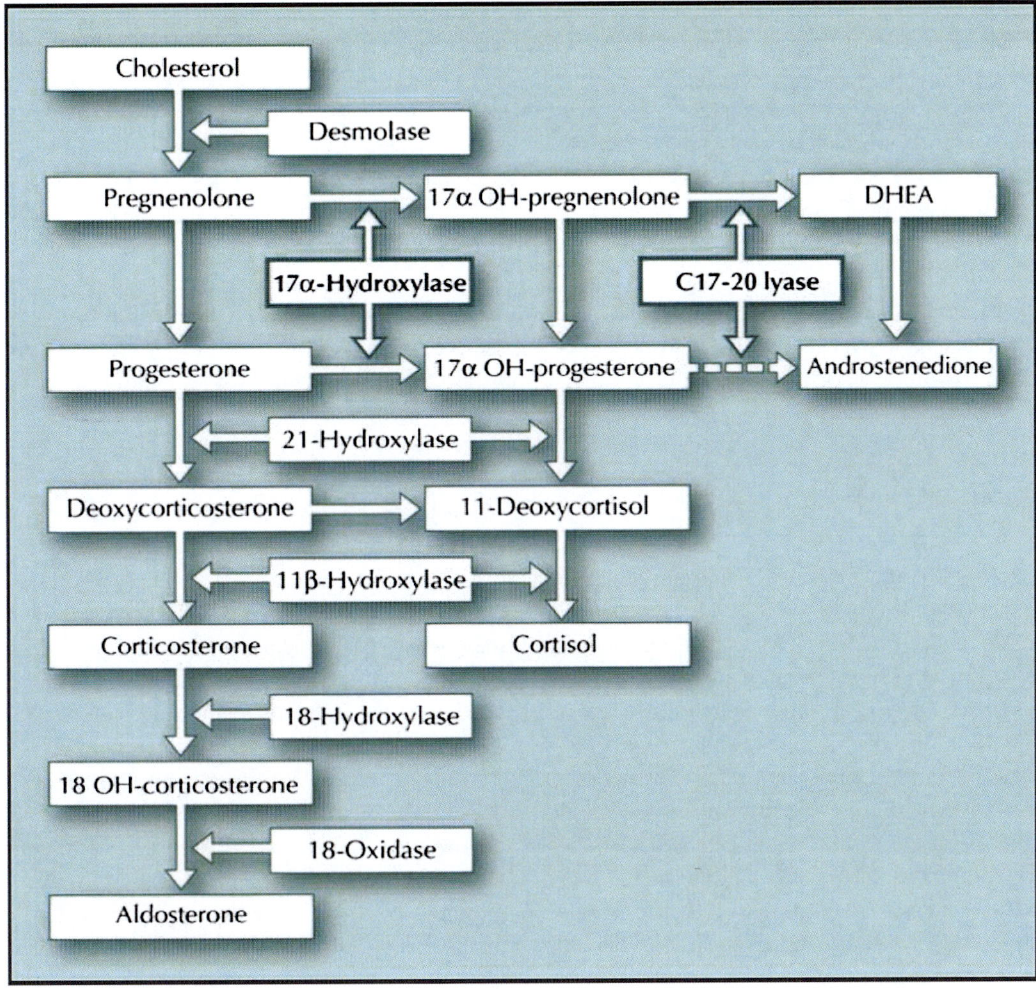

Fig. 8.1 Adrenal androgen synthesis cascade. *Black highlighted boxes* represent enzymes inhibited by abiraterone acetate. *DHEA*, dehydroepiandrosterone

Table 8.1 Adrenolytic agents that act through direct inhibition of enzymes involved in androgen synthesis

Agent	Major toxological target and inhibition coefficent (nM)	Minor toxological targets and selected inhibition coeffcents (nM)	Clinical effect	Side effects
Ketaconazole	CYP51 (430), CYP11B1 (127), CYP11B2 (67)	CYP11A1, CYPA4 (72), CYP19 (2,000), CYP17 (2,380)	Decrease in androgen, corticosteroid, & mineralocorticoid synthesis	Nausea, vomiting, diarrhea, hepatitis, adrenal insufficiency, rash pruritis, impotence, photosensitivity, breast tenderness or enlargement, headache
Abiraterone acetate	CYP17 (72)	CYP11A1 (1,608), CYP11B1 (1751), CYP11B2 (2,704)	Decrease in androgen & corticosteroid synthesis	Hypertension, fatigue, hepatitis, anorexia, edema, adrenal insufficiency, hypokalemia
Aminoglutethimide	CYP11A1 (~20,000)	CYP11B1, CYP19 (600)	Decrease in androgen, corticosteroid, & mineralocorticoid synthesis	Lethargy, drowsiness, rash, anorexia, nausea, vomiting, dizziness, adrenal insufficiency, hypotension, headache

superseded by ketoconazole, which can achieve a similar effect in decreasing circulating androgens but has been shown to be more effective in preventing tumor growth in clinical trials and is moderately less toxic. Aminoglutethimide, nonetheless, remains an alternative for patients who have either failed or are unable to tolerate ketoconazole, abiraterone, estrogens, or chemotherapy, and are not interested in a clinical trial. The side effects associated with aminoglutethimide are relatively mild and are usually limited to rashes, lethargy, somnolence, adrenal dysfunction, hypothyroidism, LFT and thyroid abnormalities, and occasional nausea and vomiting.

Ketoconazole

Ketoconazole is a synthetic oral imidazole antifungal, first developed and marketed in the 1970s. Like all members of the imidazole antifungal class, it was designed to disrupt fungal cell membrane function via inhibition of the synthesis of ergosterol, a critical component of the fungal cell membrane. Ketoconazole specifically inhibits CYP51A (cytochrome P450 14a-demethylase), an enzyme which catalyzes ergosterol synthesis from lanosterol. The net effect of ketoconazole in the fungal cell is depletion of ergosterol from the membrane, leading to altered membrane fluidity, altered signaling, increased permeability, and inhibition of growth and replication [24]. Of all the imidazole antifungals, ketoconazole has the highest affinity for mammalian cytochrome p450 enzymes. Thus, humans taking ketoconazole experience inhibition of CYP51A and, with varying degrees of potency, CYP11A1, CYP11B1, CYP11B2, CYP17, and CYP19, leading to a marked decrease in adrenal functioning [25].

The use of ketoconazole impairs the adrenal gland's ability to synthesize adequate levels of glucocorticoids, mineralocorticoids, and androgens. This relatively toxic side effect was recognized early and spurred the development of newer imidazole antifungals (fluconazole, itraconazole) with less affinity for mammalian cytochrome p450 enzymes. This same mechanism has been exploited, however, as a means to decrease circulating androgens in patients with CRPC.

Recent studies have shown that ketoconazole clearly has activity in CRPC. In a pilot study, 20 patients with progressive disease despite combined androgen blockade were treated with ketoconazole 400 mg TID orally and hydrocortisone while undergoing AAWD. Eleven of these patients (55%)

experienced a >50% decrease in PSA, with a median duration of response of 8.5 months [26]. When studied after AAWD, high-dose ketoconazole resulted in a PSA decrease of >50% in 30 of 48 (62.5%) evaluable patients. In this study, 48% of patients exhibited a >80% decrease in PSA [27]. Low-dose ketoconazole (200 mg tid orally) was subsequently studied prospectively in 28 patients. This dose was found to be well tolerated, and a PSA decrease of >50% was seen in 46% of patients. The median time of response based on PSA values was >30 weeks. At the time of progression, 16 patients were subsequently treated with high-dose (400 mg tid orally) ketoconazole, but there was no patient response [28].

Based on the results of previous studies, a randomized phase III trial of AAWD alone or in combination with high-dose ketoconazole, with replacement doses of hydrocortisone, was undertaken and reported in 2004 [29]. In this study, the proportion of PSA response in those who underwent AAWD alone was 10% compared to 32% in the combination arm ($p<0.001$). Fourteen percent of patients treated with ketoconazole and AAWD experienced objective responses compared with 7% of subjects who underwent AAWD alone. Because of the high proportion of patients randomized to AAWD who ultimately crossed over to therapy with ketoconazole, an overall survival difference was not detected in this study. Nevertheless, a critical observation that emerged from this study was that patients who had experienced a 50% decline in PSA while on ketoconazole showed a survival of 41 months, compared to 13 months in those who had not (p<0.001). Similarly, subsequent analysis showed that patients with high baseline circulating androstenedione levels are more likely to benefit from therapy with ketoconazole than patients with low circulating androstenedione levels, leading to the hypothesis that potential responders could be prospectively identified by determination of baseline circulating androgen levels. A similar observation from this study is that most patients who develop sustained responses to ketoconazole have "early" PSA declines within 3 months of initiating therapy, giving physicians a rationale for discontinuing therapy if no PSA response is seen at 3 months [30]. Taken together, these data suggest that ketoconazole is an active drug in a substantial proportion of patients with progressive disease on an anti-androgen and may be considered an acceptable secondary hormonal agent in this clinical context.

Ketoconazole is dosed at 400 mg orally three times a day and is given with replacement hydrocortisone, usually 5-10 mg orally twice a day. Common side effects include nausea, vomiting, diarrhea, and elevations in hepatic transammonases; other side effects include rash/pruritis, impotence, photosensitivity, breast tenderness or enlargement, or headache. Close attention should be paid to possible drug-drug interactions, as well as to the development of adrenal insufficiency even with corticosteroid replacement; stress-dose steroids should be considered in the event of serious illness.

Abiraterone Acetate

The development of a novel targeted androgen synthesis inhibitor, abiraterone acetate, has renewed interest in using secondary hormonal agents in the management of CRPC. Abiraterone acetate is an orally available prodrug of abiraterone, an inhibitor of CYP17 (17alpha-hydroxylase/C17,20-lyase). In contrast to the nonselective nature of ketoconazole, abiraterone acetate was developed as a highly selective, highly potent, irreversible inhibitor of CYP17, an enzyme that catalyzes key steps in the synthetic pathway of adrenal androgens (see Fig. 8.1). Preclinical animal studies of abiraterone acetate showed significant reduction in testosterone levels, as well as reductions in prostate, seminal vesicle, and testicular size. Phase I testing has shown that abiraterone acetate suppresses testosterone and DHEA-S levels, and causes increases in plasma ACTH, 11-deoxycorticosterone, and corticosterone, consistent with upregulation of "upstream" signals.

The effect of abiraterone acetate on PSA was evident in the Phase I testing in the United States, with a >50% decline in PSA after 3 months occurring in 12 of 25 patients completing the initial 28 days of treatment [31]. Additionally, seven of the 16 patients who had received prior ketoconazole showed a >50% PSA response. A similar trial in the United Kingdom showed a >50% decline in PSA in 57% of men, with five out of eight patients with measurable disease at the outset of therapy experiencing partial tumor shrinkage [32].

A Phase II study conducted in the UK showed that 60% of chemotherapy-naïve men with CRPC experienced a >50% decline in PSA, and eight out of 15 men with bone metastases experienced a partial response [33]. Median time to progression (TTP) was approximately 8 months. Addition of dexamethasone 0.5 mg daily suppressed ACTH and reversed resistance in six out of 18 patients. Another Phase II trial using abiraterone acetate for patients with CRPC and progression after

docetaxel-based chemotherapy confirmed many of the Phase I findings [34]. In this study, 41% of patients experienced >50% decline in PSA from baseline after 12 weeks of treatment. Additionally, 24% experienced radiologic partial response or stable disease. This study serves as a proof of the principle that patients who experience disease progression despite docetaxel-based chemotherapy may continue to derive benefit from the additional androgen blockade, thus forming the basis for the ongoing Phase III studies.

The major side effects associated with abiraterone are due to inhibition of CYP17. This inhibition leads to a reduction in cortisol and androgen levels; however, it does not affect circulating mineralocorticoid levels (as CYP17 is not required for mineralocorticoid synthesis). The reduction in circulating corticosteroid levels caused by abiraterone leads to upregulation of ACTH secretion by the hypothalamic–pituitary axis. This, in turn, stimulates further mineralocorticoid synthesis; the major clinical effect of this excess mineralocorticoid secretion is hypertension and hypokalemia. The administration of low-dose corticosteroids can suppress ACTH secretion and improve hypertension in these patients. Anti-aldosterone agents such as spironolactone may be effective, as well, in treating the hypertension induced by abiraterone acetate; however, they are generally avoided as they may stimulate the AR [32]. Other common side effects of abiraterone include fatigue, transammonitis, anorexia, and edema. Partly due to the fact that replacement corticosteroids are given with abiraterone acetate, adrenal insufficiency is not commonly associated with abiraterone acetate use. Abiraterone acetate is dosed at 1,000 mg orally daily with prednisone 5 mg orally twice-daily in the current Phase III trials.

While abiraterone acetate has shown much promise in early testing, the optimal timing or use of abiraterone among the many therapies that exist for prostate cancer has still not been established. Should it be used in combination with LHRH analogues? What is the efficacy of this agent in patients who have received prior therapy with ketoconazole? Should it be used by itself as a secondary hormonal agent? Should it be used before, after, or concurrently with chemotherapy? While a series of studies are underway to explore these questions, evidence indicates that patients who previously received either ketoconazole or DES therapy benefit from abiraterone acetate therapy, suggesting that the mechanism of action and resistance to these therapies may be nonoverlapping [31].

Based on the evidence of activity in men who have previously received chemotherapy, a multicentered, multinational, double-blinded, randomized, placebo-controlled, Phase III study is currently underway to evaluate abiraterone acetate in this setting. The primary endpoint of the study is overall survival. If positive, this study would be the first to demonstrate a true survival benefit to secondary hormonal therapy, though it may not address the issue of the optimal timing of the use of this agent. To test the efficacy of abiraterone before chemotherapy, a similar multicentered, double-blinded, randomized, placebo-controlled Phase III study is also underway in men with metastatic CRPC who have not yet received chemotherapy, with overall survival as the primary endpoint.

Alternative CYP17 Inhibitors

Two different CYP17 inhibitors, TAK-700 and TOK-001, are similar to abiraterone acetate in their method of action and are currently in early stage clinical development.

TAK-700, an orally available, selective CYP17 inhibitor, has shown efficacy and tolerability in a Phase I/II study [35]. In Phase I testing TAK-700 was shown to be safe at doses of 400-600 mg BID when administered with prednisone 5 mg BID, with 4 out of 26 patients (15.4%) experiencing ≥ Grade 3 fatigue or nausea. Testosterone and DHEA-S levels significantly decreased, and all patients treated at doses ≥300 mg had PSA declines. Of the 14 patients who received TAK-700 ≥300 mg and for ≥3 cycles, 11 (85%) had PSA reductions ≥50% and 4 (31%) had PSA reductions ≥90%.

TOK-001 is a similar small molecule inhibitor of CYP17, however the compound also has AR antagonistic properties, and in preclinical models has been shown to decrease AR levels in prostate tumors. Phase I/II clinical trials to test clinical safety and efficacy began in 2010.

Estrogens and Progestins

Estrogens are structurally related steroid hormones derived from androstenedione and testosterone; their synthesis is catalyzed by CYP19 (aromatase). While the majority of circulating estrogens in women are produced in the ovaries, in both sexes the adrenal gland has the ability produce estrone and estradiol either directly from androstenedione or from conversion from testosterone. Similarly, CYP19 can convert circulating precursors to estrogens in peripheral tissues.

Exogenous estrogen administration is thought to disrupt the hypothalamic–pituitary–adrenal axis by causing a decrease in LHRH synthesis and a concomitant decrease in circulating testosterone and DHEA-S levels [36]. While estrogen receptors are known to be expressed in prostate carcinoma, whether estrogen administration has a direct role in promoting tumor growth and spread is not known.

Diethylstilbestrol (DES) is an inexpensive synthetic estrogen that has been in use since 1965 and has been the most widely studied estrogenic agent in prostate cancer. Although phase III trials showed DES to be equivalent to orchiectomy as frontline therapy for hormone-sensitive prostate cancer, its excessive cardiovascular and thromboembolic toxicity, as well as the advent of the less toxic GnRH/LHRH analogs, have made it an unacceptable first-line agent in prostate cancer.

In the advanced setting, DES has shown modest efficacy in several studies. In a phase II trial of men with CRPC, 43% had a significant PSA response when treated with DES 1 mg orally daily, with only one out 21 patients experiencing a thromboembolic complication (deep venous thrombosis) [37]. In another study, 21% of patients had a >50% decline in PSA in response to DES 3 mg daily plus 2 mg warfarin [38]. A third study randomly assigned subjects to DES 3 mg orally daily with low dose warfarin or to PC-SPES, an herbal supplement withdrawn from the market. PSA declines of >50% were observed in 24% of patients receiving DES [39]. Median response duration in this trial was 3.8 months for DES with a median time to progression of 2.9 months. Response rates to DES have varied in other studies between 15 and 33%. Taken together, the data suggest that estrogen agonists have some activity in patients with CRPC, though there is no likelihood of a significant dose response effect with DES [40].

Other synthetic estrogenic compounds such as the conjugated estrogens, ethinyl estradiol and chlorotrianisene have been evaluated in the treatment for CRPC; however, they have neither demonstrated significantly more activity nor shown significantly less toxicity, compared to DES. Recent testing has shown that transdermal estradiol administration can induce castrate levels of circulating testosterone and result in PSA responses; however, it is unclear at present whether this mode of administration will be more efficacious or less toxic than DES [41]. Estramustine, a synthetic estrogen conjugated to a nitrogen mustard, has little activity as a single agent but may have significant activity when combined with taxane-based chemotherapy [42].

Because of an association with vaginal clear cell carcinoma and other reproductive abnormalities in females exposed to DES in utero, DES is no longer directly marketed in the US but must be obtained through a dedicated pharmacy. When prescribed, it is usually given with low dose warfarin (2–3 mg orally per day) to mitigate the prothrombotic risk.

Side effects of all estrogens include increased risk of myocardial infarction, stroke, venous thrombosis/pulmonary embolism, other cardiovascular events, nausea, vomiting, weight gain, and edema. There is clear evidence, however, that estrogens improve bone density, and thus these agents may be a reasonable choice for men with severe osteoporosis. Gynecomastia induced by estrogens may be decreased by prophylactic irradiation of the breasts.

Progestins

Progestational agents such as megestrol and medroxyprogesterone acetate, while lacking the toxicity of the estrogens, have shown limited efficacy in prostate cancer. Megesterol acetate is thought to suppress LHRH, to lower testosterone, to block the conversion of testosterone to DHT, as well as to contribute to AR blockade. Only 10–15% of patients receiving megesterol in clinical studies have had >50% PSA declines, with no observed differences between low dose (160 mg/day) and high-dose (640 mg/day) groups [43, 44]. Despite this limited activity, the progestins may have a role in palliation of bony pain when corticosteroids are contraindicated.

Conclusion

The inhibitors of adrenal androgen synthesis comprise a diverse group including corticosteroids, ketoconazole, aminoglutethimide, estrogenic and progestin compounds such as DES, megestrol, medroxyprogesterone acetate and more recently, abiraterone acetate, TAK-700, and TOK-001. The common thread linking these agents is their net effect on decreasing androgen synthesis by the adrenal glands. From large clinical studies, it is clear that secondary hormonal manipulations are effective at depriving CRPC of growth signals. More recent evidence has emerged that they can be effective even after tumors have developed resistance to chemotherapy. Of all the therapies discussed here, abiraterone acetate is the most promising new adrenolytic agent, and the results of the current phase III studies are eagerly anticipated. Continued research will help to develop novel hormonal strategies to slow the growth of advanced prostate cancer.

References

1. Huggins C, Hodges CV. Studies on prostatic cancer: I. The effect of castration, of estrogen and of androgen injection on serum phosphatases in metastatic carcinoma of the prostate. 1941. J Urol 2002;168:9–12.
2. Huggins C. Effect of orchiectomy and irradiation on cancer of the prostate. Ann Surg 1942;115:1192–200.
3. Small EJ, Ryan CJ. The case for secondary hormonal therapies in the chemotherapy age. J Urol 2006;176:S66–71.
4. Seidenfeld J, Samson DJ, Hasselblad V et al. Single-therapy androgen suppression in men with advanced prostate cancer: a systematic review and meta-analysis. Ann Intern Med 2000;132:566–77.
5. Roach M, 3rd, Izaguirre A. Goserelin acetate in combination with radiotherapy for prostate cancer. Expert Opin Pharmacother 2007;8:257–64.
6. Loblaw DA, Mendelson DS, Talcott JA et al. American Society of Clinical Oncology recommendations for the initial hormonal management of androgen-sensitive metastatic, recurrent, or progressive prostate cancer. J Clin Oncol 2004;22:2927–41.
7. Janknegt RA, Abbou CC, Bartoletti R et al. Orchiectomy and nilutamide or placebo as treatment of metastatic prostatic cancer in a multinational double-blind randomized trial. J Urol 1993;149:77–82; discussion 3.
8. Chen CD, Welsbie DS, Tran C et al. Molecular determinants of resistance to antiandrogen therapy. Nat Med 2004;10:33–9.
9. Kelly WK, Scher HI. Prostate specific antigen decline after antiandrogen withdrawal: the flutamide withdrawal syndrome. J Urol 1993;149:607–9.
10. Schellhammer PF, Venner P, Haas GP et al. Prostate specific antigen decreases after withdrawal of antiandrogen therapy with bicalutamide or flutamide in patients receiving combined androgen blockade. J Urol 1997;157:1731–5.
11. Kassouf W, Tanguay S, Aprikian AG. Nilutamide as second line hormone therapy for prostate cancer after androgen ablation fails. J Urol 2003;169:1742–4.
12. Bhanalaph T, Varkarakis MJ, Murphy GP. Current status of bilateral adrenalectomy or advanced prostatic carcinoma. Ann Surg 1974;179:17–23.
13. Huggins C, Bergenstal DM. Inhibition of human mammary and prostatic cancers by adrenalectomy. Cancer Res 1952;12:134–41.
14. Fakih M, Johnson CS, Trump DL. Glucocorticoids and treatment of prostate cancer: a preclinical and clinical review. Urology 2002;60:553–61.

15. Nishimura K, Nonomura N, Satoh E et al. Potential mechanism for the effects of dexamethasone on growth of androgen-independent prostate cancer. J Natl Cancer Inst 2001;93:1739–46.

16. Yano A, Fujii Y, Iwai A, Kageyama Y, Kihara K. Glucocorticoids suppress tumor angiogenesis and in vivo growth of prostate cancer cells. Clin Cancer Res 2006;12:3003–9.

17. Yano A, Fujii Y, Iwai A, Kawakami S, Kageyama Y, Kihara K. Glucocorticoids suppress tumor lymphangiogenesis of prostate cancer cells. Clin Cancer Res 2006;12:6012–7.

18. Tannock IF, Osoba D, Stockler MR et al. Chemotherapy with mitoxantrone plus prednisone or prednisone alone for symptomatic hormone-resistant prostate cancer: a Canadian randomized trial with palliative end points. J Clin Oncol 1996;14:1756–64.

19. Kantoff PW, Halabi S, Conaway M et al. Hydrocortisone with or without mitoxantrone in men with hormone-refractory prostate cancer: results of the cancer and leukemia group B 9182 study. J Clin Oncol 1999;17:2506–13.

20. Small EJ, Meyer M, Marshall ME et al. Suramin therapy for patients with symptomatic hormone-refractory prostate cancer: results of a randomized phase III trial comparing suramin plus hydrocortisone to placebo plus hydrocortisone. J Clin Oncol 2000;18:1440–50.

21. Storlie JA, Buckner JC, Wiseman GA, Burch PA, Hartmann LC, Richardson RL. Prostate specific antigen levels and clinical response to low dose dexamethasone for hormone-refractory metastatic prostate carcinoma. Cancer 1995;76:96–100.

22. Sartor O, Cooper M, Weinberger M et al. Surprising activity of flutamide withdrawal, when combined with aminoglutethimide, in treatment of "hormone-refractory" prostate cancer. J Natl Cancer Inst 1994;86:222–7.

23. Abratt RP, Brune D, Dimopoulos MA et al. Randomised phase III study of intravenous vinorelbine plus hormone therapy versus hormone therapy alone in hormone-refractory prostate cancer. Ann Oncol 2004;15:1613–21.

24. Como JA, Dismukes WE. Oral azole drugs as systemic antifungal therapy. N Engl J Med 1994;330:263–72.

25. Lamberts SW, Bons EG, Bruining HA, de Jong FH. Differential effects of the imidazole derivatives etomidate, ketoconazole and miconazole and of metyrapone on the secretion of cortisol and its precursors by human adrenocortical cells. J Pharmacol Exp Ther 1987;240:259–64.

26. Small EJ, Baron A, Bok R. Simultaneous antiandrogen withdrawal and treatment with ketoconazole and hydrocortisone in patients with advanced prostate carcinoma. Cancer 1997;80:1755–9.

27. Small EJ, Baron AD, Fippin L, Apodaca D. Ketoconazole retains activity in advanced prostate cancer patients with progression despite flutamide withdrawal. J Urol 1997;157:1204–7.

28. Harris KA, Weinberg V, Bok RA, Kakefuda M, Small EJ. Low dose ketoconazole with replacement doses of hydrocortisone in patients with progressive androgen independent prostate cancer. J Urol 2002;168:542–5.

29. Rini BI, Halabi S, Taylor J, Small EJ, Schilsky RL. Cancer and Leukemia Group B 90206: a randomized phase III trial of interferon-alpha or interferon-alpha plus anti-vascular endothelial growth factor antibody (bevacizumab) in metastatic renal cell carcinoma. Clin Cancer Res 2004;10:2584–6.

30. Ryan CJ, Halabi S, Ou SS, Vogelzang NJ, Kantoff P, Small EJ. Adrenal androgen levels as predictors of outcome in prostate cancer patients treated with ketoconazole plus anti-androgen withdrawal: results from a cancer and leukemia group B study. Clin Cancer Res 2007;13:2030–7.

31. Ryan C, Rosenberg JR, Lin A, Valiente A, Kim J, Small EJ. Phase I evaluation of abiraterone acetate (CB7630), a 17 alpha hydroxylase C17,20-Lyase inhibitor in androgen-independent prostate cancer (AiPC). ASCO Annual Meeting Proceedings J Clin Oncol 2007;25:5064.

32. Attard G, Reid AH, Yap TA et al. Phase I clinical trial of a selective inhibitor of CYP17, abiraterone acetate, confirms that castration-resistant prostate cancer commonly remains hormone driven. J Clin Oncol 2008;26:4563–71.

33. De Bono JGA, Reid AH, Parker C, Dowsett M, Mollife R, Yap TA, Molina A, Lee G, Dearnaley D. Anti-tumor activity of abiraterone acetate (AA), a CYP17 inhibitor of androgen synthesis, in chemotherapy naive and docetaxel pre-treated castration resistant prostate cancer (CRPC). ASCO Annual Meeting Proceedings J Clin Oncol 2008;26:5005.

34. Danila DDER, Morris MJ, Slovin SF, Schwartz LH, Farmer K, Anand A, Haqq C, Fleisher M, Scher HI. Abiraterone acetate and prednisone in patients (Pts) with progressive metastatic castration resistant prostate cancer (CRPC) after failure of docetaxel-based chemotherapy. ASCO Annual Meeting Proceedings J Clin Oncol 2008;26:5019.

35. Dreicer R, Agus DB, MacVicar GR et al. Safety, pharmacokinetics, and efficacy of TAK-700 in castration-resistant, metastatic prostate cancer: a phase I/II, open-label study. In Proceedings of the 2010 American Society of Clinical Oncology Genitourinary Cancers Symposium; 2010 Mar 5–7; San Francisco. ASCO; 2010. Abstract 103.

36. Kitahara S, Umeda H, Yano M et al. Effects of intravenous administration of high dose-diethylstilbestrol diphosphate on serum hormonal levels in patients with hormone-refractory prostate cancer. Endocr J 1999;46:659–64.

37. Smith DC, Redman BG, Flaherty LE, Li L, Strawderman M, Pienta KJ. A phase II trial of oral diethylstilbesterol as a second-line hormonal agent in advanced prostate cancer. Urology 1998;52:257–60.

38. Small EJ, Frohlich MW, Bok R et al. Prospective trial of the herbal supplement PC-SPES in patients with progressive prostate cancer. J Clin Oncol 2000;18:3595–603.

39. Oh WK, Kantoff PW, Weinberg V et al. Prospective, multicenter, randomized phase II trial of the herbal supplement, PC-SPES, and diethylstilbestrol in patients with androgen-independent prostate cancer. J Clin Oncol 2004;22:3705–12.

40. Lam JS, Leppert JT, Vemulapalli SN, Shvarts O, Belldegrun AS. Secondary hormonal therapy for advanced prostate cancer. J Urol 2006;175:27–34.

41. Langley RE, Godsland IF, Kynaston H et al. Early hormonal data from a multicentre phase II trial using transdermal oestrogen patches as first-line hormonal therapy in patients with locally advanced or metastatic prostate cancer. BJU Int 2008;102:442–5.

42. Hudes G, Einhorn L, Ross E et al. Vinblastine versus vinblastine plus oral estramustine phosphate for patients with hormone-refractory prostate cancer: a hoosier oncology group and fox chase network phase III trial. J Clin Oncol 1999;17:3160–6.

43. Osborn JL, Smith DC, Trump DL. Megestrol acetate in the treatment of hormone refractory prostate cancer. Am J Clin Oncol 1997;20:308–10.

44. Dawson NA, Conaway M, Halabi S et al. A randomized study comparing standard versus moderately high dose megestrol acetate for patients with advanced prostate carcinoma: cancer and leukemia group B study 9181. Cancer 2000;88:825–34.

Chapter 9
Androgen Deprivation Therapy

Nima Sharifi

Abstract Androgen deprivation therapy (ADT) is the upfront systemic therapy for advanced prostate cancer. ADT is administered medically or through surgical castration, and it suppresses serum testosterone levels. Furthermore, ADT may be given alone or in combination with an androgen receptor antagonist. Adverse effects include hot flashes, sexual dysfunction, increased risk of fracture, metabolic syndrome and increased risk of cardiovascular events. The timing of administration of early versus late ADT is still contentious and under active debate. Intermittent ADT may be an alternative to continuous testosterone depletion; although intermittent therapy decreases adverse effects, the comparative efficacy of each is still under active study. The study of germline genetic determinants in response to ADT is in its early phase. However, these studies have the potential to allow for patient selection for the type and timing of ADT.

Keywords Androgen deprivation therapy • Androgens • Prostate cancer • Testosterone

Introduction

Survival and proliferation of prostate cancer is entirely dependent on the availability of androgens and expression of the androgen receptor (AR). The testes are the primary source of androgens and release testosterone into systemic circulation [1]. Once serum testosterone reaches prostatic tissue, it is converted into dihydrotestosterone, the chief and most potent natural ligand and stimulus for AR [2, 3]. The molecular basis of signaling through the AR transcription factor is discussed in further detail in Chap. 5 and is beyond the scope of this section. The near-ubiquitous expression of AR in prostate cancer cases provides the foundation for the efficacy of androgen deprivation therapy (ADT) as the frontline treatment for advanced prostate cancer. ADT is defined herein as androgen depletion with medical or surgical castration. The beneficial effects of ADT with surgical castration and the administration of estrogens were first noted by Huggins and Hodges in 1941 [4]. Although the science behind the understanding of hormonal therapy has made remarkable progress, the efficacy of standard hormonal therapy for metastatic prostate cancer has not changed significantly for over nearly 70 years. However, recent investigations into the timing and context of ADT, progress with novel agents in clinical trials, and a better understanding of the predisposition of some patients to castration-resistance promise the development of a standard of care that will deliver improved survival and better outcomes for prostate cancer patients.

Androgen Deprivation Therapy

ADT, in current practice, is administered through medical or surgical castration [5]. Surgical castration with orchiectomy is generally a low surgical risk procedure [6]. However, it is not favored by many men, given the psychological impact and the availability of a medical alternative. Medical castration is attained with the administration of gonadotropin-releasing hormone agonists (GnRH-As). Leuprolide acetate and

N. Sharifi (✉)
Division of Hematology/Oncology, University of Texas
Southwestern Medical Center, Dallas, TX, USA
e-mail: nima.sharifi@utsouthwestern.edu

W.D. Figg et al. (eds.), *Drug Management of Prostate Cancer*,
DOI 10.1007/978-1-60327-829-4_9, © Springer Science+Business Media, LLC 2010

goserelin acetate are two commonly used GnRH-As that are equally effective for the induction of medical castration [7]. The hypothalamus releases endogenous GnRH in a pulsatile manner and its corresponding receptor is expressed in the anterior pituitary [8]. GnRH receptor stimulation induces the release of luteinizing hormone (LH) from the anterior pituitary into the systemic circulation, which then acts upon the testes to induce testosterone secretion. The stimulatory effect of GnRH on LH release from the anterior pituitary is dependent on the pulsatile nature of GnRH secretion. Therefore, continuous stimulation of the anterior pituitary by administration of exogenous GnRH-As effectively inhibits LH release, which, in turn, suppresses testosterone release from the testes (Fig. 9.1) [6, 9].

Although GnRH-As generally lead to castrate levels of serum testosterone by 3 weeks after starting therapy, the initiation of drug administration leads to an initial stimulatory effect on the pituitary and generates a testosterone surge. A GnRH-A induced surge may lead to a twofold increase in testosterone, become evident from 2–3 days after initiation of therapy, and last up to 20 days [10]. This surge of androgens induces a growth-stimulatory effect on prostate cancer cells and may lead to a detrimental "flare" reaction in patients who have metastatic disease, which can increase bone pain at sites of metastasis. Furthermore, patients with vertebral metastases may develop spinal cord compression; those at risk may develop urinary obstruction, and cardiovascular events may occur due to hypercoagulability [11]. Concomitant administration of an AR antagonist with the initiation of GnRH-A and continuation for 2–4 weeks will block the effects of the testosterone surge and the "flare" reaction that follows [12]. The testosterone surge may also be avoided by the use of GnRH antagonists as an alternative to agonists [10].

Serum testosterone levels less than 50 ng/dL (1.7 nmol/L) are generally accepted as being in the range of castration [13]. However, the current understanding of AR- and androgen-signaling-dependent growth of prostate cancer [1, 14, 15] dictates that men should achieve a testosterone level as low as possible to optimize therapy. Most men will attain a testosterone level below 20 ng/dL (0.7 nmol/L), which has also been suggested as an alternative lower level that should be achieved for optimal therapy [16].

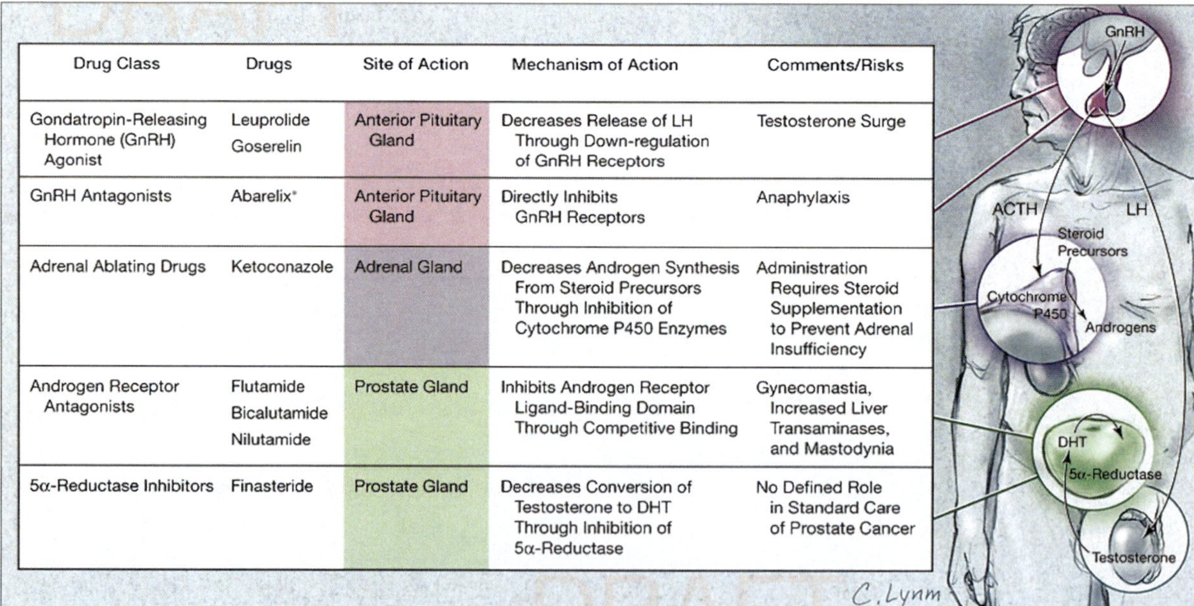

Drug Class	Drugs	Site of Action	Mechanism of Action	Comments/Risks
Gondatropin-Releasing Hormone (GnRH) Agonist	Leuprolide Goserelin	Anterior Pituitary Gland	Decreases Release of LH Through Down-regulation of GnRH Receptors	Testosterone Surge
GnRH Antagonists	Abarelix*	Anterior Pituitary Gland	Directly Inhibits GnRH Receptors	Anaphylaxis
Adrenal Ablating Drugs	Ketoconazole	Adrenal Gland	Decreases Androgen Synthesis From Steroid Precursors Through Inhibition of Cytochrome P450 Enzymes	Administration Requires Steroid Supplementation to Prevent Adrenal Insufficiency
Androgen Receptor Antagonists	Flutamide Bicalutamide Nilutamide	Prostate Gland	Inhibits Androgen Receptor Ligand-Binding Domain Through Competitive Binding	Gynecomastia, Increased Liver Transaminases, and Mastodynia
5α-Reductase Inhibitors	Finasteride	Prostate Gland	Decreases Conversion of Testosterone to DHT Through Inhibition of 5α-Reductase	No Defined Role in Standard Care of Prostate Cancer

Fig. 9.1 Hormonal interventions and endocrine axis in prostate cancer. DHT indicates dihydrotestosterone and LH, luteinizing hormone. Asterisk indicates that it is no longer available for new patients in the United States. Illustration based on the original concept by Lydia Kibiuk. Reprinted from [5]. Copyright ©2005 American Medical Association. All rights reserved

Timing of ADT

While considering the initiation of any form of therapy, the relative balance of risks and benefits must be weighed. These risks and predispositions to adverse events must be similarly considered before the commencement of ADT. The risks of ADT include hot flashes [17], osteoporosis with an increased risk of fracture [18], the metabolic syndrome [19, 20], sexual dysfunction [21], and an increased risk of cardiovascular events [22]. The potential benefit of early ADT is that treatment is initiated with a lower tumor burden, with a correspondingly lower number of cells that have the capacity for being resistant to therapy. Early ADT can be defined in several clinical contexts, including (1) metastatic disease before symptoms arise, (2) biochemical recurrence after local therapy with prostate-specific antigen (PSA) rise without evidence of metastatic disease, (3) watchful waiting for patients with local disease who are not candidates for local therapy, and (4) pelvic lymph node involvement at radical prostatectomy. In addressing the debate between early and late ADT in the metastatic setting, the Medical Research Council conducted a randomized trial of immediate ADT versus deferred treatment until an indication arose for 934 men with locally advanced or asymptomatic metastatic prostate cancer [23]. Men in the immediate ADT arm had a lower probability of death from prostate cancer (62% vs. 71%; $P=0.001$) and lower rates of extraskeletal metastasis (7.9% vs. 11.8%; $P<0.05$), pathological fracture (2.3% vs. 4.5%; not statistically significant), ureteral obstruction (7.0% vs. 11.8%; $P<0.025$), and spinal cord compression (1.9% vs. 4.9%; $P<0.025$). Although outcomes were more favorable in the immediate ADT arm, a weakness of this study is that 29 men in the deferred ADT arm died without treatment with ADT.

Pelvic lymph node involvement without bone metastasis for men who have had surgical removal of the prostate is another clinical context of early ADT. Messing et al. [24, 25] completed a randomized clinical trial of immediate adjuvant ADT versus observation of men who underwent radical prostatectomy and were found to have disease involving the pelvic lymph nodes. A significantly higher proportion of men who were randomized to observation died compared to men in the immediate ADT arm with a median follow-up of 10 years (51% vs. 28%; $P=0.025$). This suggests the possibility that early ADT with lower, minimal tumor burden may provide a treatment advantage.

Three recent randomized clinical trials of early versus deferred ADT have been completed in the setting of men who were not candidates for local therapy or who did not get local therapy because of the presence of pelvic lymph node involvement. EORTC 30846 included 302 patients with node positive disease and showed a trend for increased survival with early ADT [26]. However, this study was underpowered and the survival difference was not statistically significant. The SAKK 08/88 study enrolled 197 patients who were not candidates for local therapy and showed a non-statistically significant difference in deaths due to prostate cancer ($P=0.09$) in the immediate ADT group versus the deferred ADT group (76% vs. 63%), with no difference in median overall survival (5.2 vs. 4.4 years; $P=0.96$) [27]. EORTC 30891, which enrolled 985 patients who were not candidates for local therapy, did show an increase in overall survival for patients treated with immediate ADT, with an overall survival hazard ratio of 1.25, 95% CI, 1.05–1.48 [28]. Perplexingly, this difference seemed to be due to non-prostate cancer related deaths. One fourth of the men in the deferred ADT arm died without ever requiring ADT. A large population-based cohort study involving 19,271 men who did not receive definitive local therapy found that primary ADT is not associated with improved survival [29], and similar to EORTC 30891, men with lower risk cancer treated with early ADT may have a worse cancer-specific survival.

Yet another clinical scenario is that of patients who have a PSA recurrence only, after failure of surgery or radiation for the treatment of localized disease. A single-institution study of men with PSA recurrence only after radical prostatectomy suggests that these men have a relatively indolent history, with a median actuarial time to metastasis of 8 years after PSA recurrence [30]. However, about half of the men in this study with a Gleason score of 8–10 who had a biochemical recurrence within 2 years were free of metastasis at 3 years. The shorter time to metastasis in patients with high Gleason scores suggests that a subgroup of men with biochemical recurrence who have a more aggressive clinical course may potentially benefit from early treatment. Nonetheless, there are no data from prospective randomized clinical trials to guide the treatment of men with PSA recurrence after the failure of local therapy. Furthermore, the 2007 American Society of

Table 9.1 2007 updated American society of clinical oncology practice guidelines for initial hormonal management of androgen-sensitive metastatic, recurrent, or progressive prostate cancer

Question	Recommendation
What are the standard initial treatment options?	Bilateral orchiectomy or GnRH agonist
Are AR antagonists as effective as orchiectomy or GnRH agonist?	Nonsteroidal antiandrogen monotherapy, but not steroidal antiandrogen monotherapy may be discussed as an alternative
Is combined androgen blockade better than androgen deprivation therapy alone?	Combined androgen blockage should be considered as an alternative
Does early androgen deprivation therapy lead to better outcomes than deferred androgen deprivation?	There is no overall survival advantage for early androgen deprivation therapy, and hence, the panel cannot strongly recommend early treatment
Is there a role for intermittent androgen deprivation therapy?	There are insufficient data to recommend use of intermittent androgen deprivation outside clinical trials

Clinical Oncology Practice Panel does not make a strong recommendation for the institution of early ADT for patients with metastatic or progressive prostate cancer (Table 9.1) [31].

Androgen Deprivation Therapy, AR Antagonist, or Both?

In principle, two ways of preventing stimulation of AR-mediated growth are to deplete levels of the ligand or directly block AR with competitive antagonists. Bicalutamide, nilutamide, and flutamide are three nonsteroidal AR antagonists in clinical use [5]. Although there is, without question, a mechanistic difference between these two methods of blocking androgen function, comparisons of ADT versus monotherapy with nonsteroidal anti-androgens do not show a significant difference in overall survival [32]. However, nonsteroidal anti-androgens may have a more desirable side-effect profile than ADT. ASCO practice guidelines suggest that nonsteroidal anti-androgen monotherapy may be discussed as an alternative to ADT [33].

The concomitant use of ADT and therapy with AR antagonists to both suppress testicular androgen production and directly antagonize AR at the level of the tumor is termed combined androgen blockade (CAB). Numerous clinical trials have compared the utility of ADT alone versus CAB. A meta-analysis of 27 randomized trials comparing ADT with CAB shows that there is a 2–3% 5-year survival benefit with the use of CAB [34]. However, this benefit is limited to the use of nonsteroidal antiandrogens, and it was found that the sum total of the data on CAB with the steroidal

anti-androgen, cyproterone acetate, suggested less favorable outcomes. A recent study of GnRH-A versus CAB in Japanese men showed a significantly improved overall survival (63.4% vs. 75.3%; $P=0.0425$) at a median follow-up of over 5 years [35]. The survival benefit of CAB with nonsteroidal anti-androgens comes at a significant cost, which amounts to a price of $1 million per quality-adjusted life-year [33]. However, the most recent ASCO practice guidelines suggest that CAB should be considered as an alternative to ADT alone [31]. Although numerous well-conducted randomized trials have been done to compare ADT with CAB and the benefit of CAB has been analyzed with varying methods, the issue of CAB is almost certain to become once again unsettled. Novel and more potent AR antagonists are in early clinical trials [36–38], and as these agents undergo further clinical development, the issue of the utility of CAB with these new agents will undoubtedly be revisited. Furthermore, the development of new and more potent agents that inhibit androgen synthesis, such as abiraterone acetate [39], offer the opportunity to apply these agents at earlier stages, along with ADT. If these agents provide benefit when given concomitantly along with ADT, they may serve to redefine the meaning of CAB.

Intermittent Androgen Deprivation

An alternative to continuous ADT with GnRH-A is intermittent androgen deprivation by alternating between periods of testosterone depletion and testosterone recovery. Such an approach is feasible, and testosterone recovery for limited periods of time may allow the patient to enjoy a lessening of adverse effects associated with ADT [40]. A randomized prospective study of intermittent versus continuous CAB with GnRH-A plus bicalutamide was conducted with 335 patients with disease involving lymph nodes or distant metastasis [41]. Off treatment periods were greater than 40% in the intermittent ADT arm, and this was associated with more favorable sexual activity. There was no significant difference in median time to death between the two treatment arms ($P = 0.658$). SWOG 9346 is an ongoing trial of 1,345 men with metastatic prostate cancer who received induction ADT with GnRH-A and bicalutamide for 7 months [42]. 965 men who achieved a PSA level of 4 ng/mL or less have been randomized to continuous ADT or intermittent ADT. While this study is ongoing and the outcomes with continuous versus intermittent ADT have yet to be determined, it is clear that PSA nadir is a strong predictor of survival. PSA nadirs of <0.2, <4, and >4 ng/mL are associated with median survival times of 75, 44, and 13 months [42]. Thus, PSA nadirs after induction ADT may eventually be used to select patients for a specific therapy [43]. However, the final results of this trial are awaited before determining the exact utility of this prognostic value.

Genetic Determinants of Response to Androgen Deprivation

Prostate cancer is a heterogeneous disease, and variables attributable to a specific patient take part in determining the course of the disease and the response to therapy. The response and response duration to ADT is tremendously variable. Ultimately, it would be desirable to administer hormonal therapy that is tailored for a patient and the specific molecular features of an individual prostate tumor. It is clear that after ADT is administered for metastatic prostate cancer, the evolution of the tumor into castration-resistant disease involves the reactivation of AR [15, 44]. However, it is difficult to apply the delineation of these somatic genetic or epigenetic changes that occur within the tumor to prognosticate response or response duration to ADT. In contrast, defining germline genetic polymorphisms that bear some responsibility in determining the response to ADT may have utility in stratifying patients in terms of the likelihood of response [45]. One would suspect that germline genetic factors would play some part in defining the response to ADT, and there is recent evidence to suggest that this is indeed the case. One study examined polymorphisms associated with 20 genes that are implicated in androgen metabolism in 529 patients who underwent ADT for advanced prostate cancer [46]. Three single nucleotide polymorphisms (SNP) that are associated with genes involved in androgen metabolism were found to be associated with the duration of response to ADT. These SNPs were found upstream of or within the introns of these genes and therefore are not known protein coding sequences. The significance of these polymorphisms may be an involvement in the regulation of gene expression. The first gene is *CYP19A1*, which encodes for aromatase, which converts testosterone to estradiol [47]. The second gene is *HSD3B1*, which is involved in the generation of androstenedione and testosterone from adrenal precursors [48]. The third gene is *HSD17B4*, which regulates the interconversion of active to inactive androgens and estrogens [49].

A second study of 68 patients began with the observation that a testosterone transporter has protein coding SNPs that confer changes in cellular testosterone uptake activity [50]. The *SLCO1B3* gene encodes for the OATP1B3 transporter protein and has two amino acid-changing SNPs that are in complete linkage disequilibrium. It is important to note that the *SLCO1B3* SNPs associated with increased testosterone uptake are found more frequently in African-Americans compared to Caucasians [51] and that because of the small numbers, the analysis in this study on duration of response to ADT was limited to Caucasian patients. OATP1B3 is overexpressed in prostate cancer compared to benign prostate [50]. Patients with advanced prostate cancer treated with ADT, who have one or two germline copies of the more active OATP1B3 transporter, have a shorter time to castration resistance compared to patients who have two copies of the less-active transporter [52].

Both of these studies that suggest germline polymorphisms of genes involved in androgen metabolism and transport influence of the response duration to ADT, require confirmation in independent patient cohorts. If confirmed, such data can be used not only to determine the likelihood of response to ADT, but also to tease out a subset of patients who would benefit from early hormonal therapy tailored to their specific germline. For example, the patients who have more active testosterone import activity may be the ones who specifically benefit from CAB with upfront AR antagonist because they have higher intracellular testosterone concentrations despite castrate levels of serum testosterone.

Conclusions

ADT with medical or surgical castration is the mainstay of the treatment of advanced prostate cancer. There may be a small benefit of CAB with the use of nonsteroidal AR antagonists, and this method may also be considered. However, AR antagonists with increased AR binding affinity and potency are in early clinical trials and may redefine the role of CAB. The debate on administering early vs. late ADT for advanced prostate cancer continues. Although there is no data for the use of ADT in patients with biochemical relapse after local therapy, the rationale for delaying ADT for patients with asymptomatic metastatic disease is more tenuous and may only be considered for select patients with careful monitoring for disease progression. Although there is data to support the use of intermittent androgen deprivation for patients with advanced disease, a large ongoing trial is poised to provide more definitive results and may also identify those patients who are appropriate candidates for this alternative to continuous ADT. The study of germline genetic polymorphisms in the androgen pathway that contribute to determining the response to ADT is just beginning. Future directions should lead to the matching of a patient's molecular features and other prognostic factors with a specific type and timing of hormonal therapy to optimize the benefits and minimize adverse effects of treatment.

References

1. McPhaul MJ. Mechanisms of prostate cancer progression to androgen independence. Best Pract Res Clin Endocrinol Metab 2008;22:373–88.
2. Bruchovsky N, Wilson JD. The intranuclear binding of testosterone and 5-alpha-androstan-17-beta-ol-3-one by rat prostate. J Biol Chem 1968;243:5953–60.
3. Russell DW, Wilson JD. Steroid 5 alpha-reductase: two genes/two enzymes. Annu Rev Biochem 1994;63:25–61.
4. Huggins C, Hodges CV. Studies on prostate cancer, I: the effect of estrogen and of androgen injection on serum phosphatases in metastatic carcinoma of the prostate. Cancer Res 1941;1:293–7.
5. Sharifi N, Gulley JL, Dahut WL. Androgen deprivation therapy for prostate cancer. JAMA 2005;294:238–44.
6. McLeod DG. Hormonal therapy: historical perspective to future directions. Urology 2003;61:3–7.
7. Fujii Y, Yonese J, Kawakami S, Yamamoto S, Okubo Y, Fukui I. Equivalent and sufficient effects of leuprolide acetate and goserelin acetate to suppress serum testosterone levels in patients with prostate cancer. BJU Int 2008;101:1096–100.
8. Engel JB, Schally AV. Drug insight: clinical use of agonists and antagonists of luteinizing-hormone-releasing hormone. Nat Clin Pract Endocrinol Metab 2007;3:157–67.
9. Limonta P, Montagnani MM, Moretti RM. LHRH analogues as anticancer agents: pituitary and extrapituitary sites of action. Expert Opin Investig Drugs 2001;10:709–20.
10. van Poppel H, Nilsson S. Testosterone surge: rationale for gonadotropin-releasing hormone blockers? Urology 2008;71:1001–6.
11. Bubley GJ. Is the flare phenomenon clinically significant? Urology 2001;58:5–9.
12. Kuhn JM, Billebaud T, Navratil H, et al. Prevention of the transient adverse effects of a gonadotropin-releasing hormone analogue (buserelin) in metastatic prostatic carcinoma by administration of an antiandrogen (nilutamide). N Engl J Med 1989;321:413–8.
13. Bubley GJ, Carducci M, Dahut W, et al. Eligibility and response guidelines for phase II clinical trials in androgen-independent prostate cancer: recommendations from the Prostate-Specific Antigen Working Group. J Clin Oncol 1999;17:3461–7.
14. Tomlins SA, Mehra R, Rhodes DR, et al. Integrative molecular concept modeling of prostate cancer progression. Nat Genet 2007;39:41–51.
15. Gelmann EP. Molecular biology of the androgen receptor. J Clin Oncol 2002;20:3001–15.
16. Oefelein MG, Feng A, Scolieri MJ, Ricchiutti D, Resnick MI. Reassessment of the definition of castrate levels of testosterone: implications for clinical decision making. Urology 2000;56:1021–4.
17. Holzbeierlein JM, McLaughlin MD, Thrasher JB. Complications of androgen deprivation therapy for prostate cancer. Curr Opin Urol 2004;14:177–83.
18. Shahinian VB, Kuo YF, Freeman JL, Goodwin JS. Risk of fracture after androgen deprivation for prostate cancer. N Engl J Med 2005;352:154–64.
19. Smith MR. Androgen deprivation therapy for prostate cancer: new concepts and concerns. Curr Opin Endocrinol Diabetes Obes 2007;14:247–54.
20. Higano C. Androgen deprivation therapy: monitoring and managing the complications. Hematol Oncol Clin North Am 2006;20:909–23.
21. Fowler FJ, Jr., McNaughton CM, Walker CE, Elliott DB, Barry MJ. The impact of androgen deprivation on quality of life after radical prostatectomy for prostate carcinoma. Cancer 2002;95:287–95.
22. Shahani S, Braga-Basaria M, Basaria S. Androgen deprivation therapy in prostate cancer and metabolic risk for atherosclerosis. J Clin Endocrinol Metab 2008;93:2042–9.
23. The Medical Research Council Prostate Cancer Working Party Investigators Group. Immediate versus deferred treatment for advanced prostatic cancer: initial results of the Medical Research Council Trial. Br J Urol 1997;79:235–46.
24. Messing EM, Manola J, Sarosdy M, Wilding G, Crawford ED, Trump D. Immediate hormonal therapy compared with observation after radical prostatectomy and pelvic lymphadenectomy in men with node-positive prostate cancer. N Engl J Med 1999;341:1781–8.
25. Messing EM, Manola J, Sarosdy M, Wilding G, Crawford ED, Trump D. Immediate hormonal therapy compared with

observation after radical prostatectomy and pelvic lymphadenoectomy in men with node-positive prostate cancer: results at 10 years of EST 3886. In: American Urological Association meeting. Chicago, IL; 2003.

26. Schroder FH, Kurth KH, Fossa SD, et al. Early versus delayed endocrine treatment of pN1-3 M0 prostate cancer without local treatment of the primary tumor: results of European organisation for the research and treatment of Cancer 30846 – a phase III study. J Urol 2004;172:923–7.

27. Studer UE, Hauri D, Hanselmann S, et al. Immediate versus deferred hormonal treatment for patients with prostate cancer who are not suitable for curative local treatment: results of the randomized trial SAKK 08/88. J Clin Oncol 2004;22:4109–18.

28. Studer UE, Whelan P, Albrecht W, et al. Immediate or deferred androgen deprivation for patients with prostate cancer not suitable for local treatment with curative intent: European organisation for research and treatment of cancer (EORTC) trial 30891. J Clin Oncol 2006;24:1868–76.

29. Lu-Yao GL, Albertsen PC, Moore DF, et al. Survival following primary androgen deprivation therapy among men with localized prostate cancer. JAMA 2008;300:173–81.

30. Pound CR, Partin AW, Eisenberger MA, Chan DW, Pearson JD, Walsh PC. Natural history of progression after PSA elevation following radical prostatectomy. JAMA 1999;281:1591–7.

31. Loblaw DA, Virgo KS, Nam R, et al. Initial hormonal management of androgen-sensitive metastatic, recurrent, or progressive prostate cancer: 2006 update of an American society of clinical oncology practice guideline. J Clin Oncol 2007;25:1596–605.

32. Seidenfeld J, Samson DJ, Hasselblad V, et al. Single-therapy androgen suppression in men with advanced prostate cancer: a systematic review and meta-analysis. Ann Intern Med 2000;132:566–77.

33. Loblaw DA, Mendelson DS, Talcott JA, et al. American society of clinical oncology recommendations for the initial hormonal management of androgen-sensitive metastatic, recurrent, or progressive prostate cancer. J Clin Oncol 2004;22:2927–41.

34. Prostate Cancer Trialists' Collaborative Group. Maximum androgen blockade in advanced prostate cancer: an overview of the randomised trials. Lancet 2000;355:1491–8.

35. Akaza H, Hinotsu S, Usami M, et al. Extended analyses: Combined androgen blockade (CAB) therapy with bicalutamide vs. leuteinizing hormone-releasing hormone agonist (LHRHa) monotherapy in Japanese men with untreated advanced prostate cancer. In: American society of clinical oncology Annual Meeting. Chicago, IL; 2008.

36. Scher HI, Beer TM, Higano CS, et al. Antitumor activity of MDV3100 in castration-resistant prostate cancer: a phase 1-2 study. Lancet 2010;375:1437–46.

37. Taplin ME. Drug insight: role of the androgen receptor in the development and progression of prostate cancer. Nat Clin Pract Oncol 2007;4:236–44.

38. Sharifi N, Dahut WL, Figg WD. Secondary hormonal therapy for prostate cancer: what lies on the horizon? BJU Int 2008;101:271–4.

39. Hsieh AC, Ryan CJ. Novel concepts in androgen receptor blockade. Cancer J 2008;14:11–4.

40. Bhandari MS, Crook J, Hussain M. Should intermittent androgen deprivation be used in routine clinical practice? J Clin Oncol 2005;23:8212–8.

41. Miller K, Steiner U, Lingnau A, et al. Randomised prospective study of intermittent versus continuous androgen suppression in advanced prostate cancer. In: American society of clinical oncology Annual Meeting. Chicago, IL; 2007.

42. Hussain M, Tangen CM, Higano C, et al. Absolute prostate-specific antigen value after androgen deprivation is a strong independent predictor of survival in new metastatic prostate cancer: data from Southwest Oncology Group Trial 9346 (INT-0162). J Clin Oncol 2006;24:3984–90.

43. Heidenreich A, Aus G, Bolla M, et al. EAU guidelines on prostate cancer. Eur Urol 2008;53:68–80.

44. Mostaghel EA, Montgomery RB, Lin DW. The basic biochemistry and molecular events of hormone therapy. Curr Urol Rep 2007;8:224–32.

45. Sharifi N, Dahut W, Figg WD. The genetics of castration-resistant prostate cancer: What can the germline tell us? Clin Cancer Res 2008;14:4691–3.

46. Ross RW, Oh WK, Xie W, et al. Inherited variation in the androgen pathway is associated with the efficacy of androgen-deprivation therapy in men with prostate cancer. J Clin Oncol 2008;26:842–7.

47. Modugno F, Weissfeld JL, Trump DL, et al. Allelic variants of aromatase and the androgen and estrogen receptors: toward a multigenic model of prostate cancer risk. Clin Cancer Res 2001;7:3092–6.

48. Evaul K, Li R, Papari-Zareei M, Auchus RJ, and Sharifi N. 3β-hydroxysteroid dehydrogenase is a possible pharmacological target in the treatment of castration-resistant prostate cancer. Endocrinology. 2010. In press.

49. de Launoit Y, Adamski J. Unique multifunctional HSD17B4 gene product: 17beta-hydroxysteroid dehydrogenase 4 and D-3-hydroxyacyl-coenzyme A dehydrogenase/hydratase involved in Zellweger syndrome. J Mol Endocrinol 1999;22:227–40.

50. Hamada A, Sissung T, Price DK, et al. Effect of SLCO1B3 haplotype on testosterone transport and clinical outcome in caucasian patients with androgen-independent prostatic cancer. Clin Cancer Res 2008;14:3312–8.

51. Smith NF, Marsh S, Scott-Horton TJ, et al. Variants in the SLCO1B3 gene: interethnic distribution and association with paclitaxel pharmacokinetics. Clin Pharmacol Ther 2007;81:76–82.

52. Sharifi N, Hamada A, Sissung T, et al. A polymorphism in a transporter of testosterone is a determinant of androgen independence in prostate cancer. BJU Int 2008;102:617–621.

Chapter 10
Pharmacogenetics of the Androgen Metabolic Pathway

Francine Zanchetta Coelho Marques and Juergen K.V. Reichardt

Abstract Androgens are steroid hormones responsible for the development, growth, and maintenance of masculine characteristics, including the prostate. It has been known for decades that they are very important in the development and progression of prostate cancer (CaP). The most common treatment for CaP is based on androgen deprivation therapy. There are preventive strategies that seem to act on the same pathway, such as finasteride, dutasteride, selenium, and vitamin E. Various genes in androgen synthesis and metabolism have been studied in relation to the predisposition and progression of CaP, such as several members of the steroid 5α-reductase (SRD5A), 3β-hydroxysteroid dehydrogenase (HSD3B), and 17β-hydroxysteroid dehydrogenase (HSD17B) families, androgen receptor (AR), cytochrome P450 17 (CYP17), and cytochrome P450 19A1 (CYP19A1). However, most of them have not been biochemically evaluated, or the studies are contradictory. For example, the expression reports about CYP19A1 indicate positive and negative results for both benign and carcinogen prostate. There is a need for extensive research in response to prostate carcinoma prevention as well as treatment. Studies have shown that other genes, such as the solute carrier organic anion transporter 1B3 (SLCO1B3), and gene fusions may be involved in CaP personalized medicine, but the results are inconclusive since the number of reports is small, and there is a lack of replication in larger samples. Pharmacogenetics is the key to future medicine, especially for cancer and personalized medicine. More investigations should be done to evaluate the role of these genes in prostate cancer biochemistry, prevention, progression, development, and treatment.

Keywords Multifactorial disease • Prostate cancer • Androgen • Treatment • Prevention • Pharmacogenomics

Androgens and Prostate Cancer

Androgens are steroid hormones that are widely accepted to be responsible for the development, growth, and maintenance of the prostate (Fig. 10.1). Although they can be formed by peripheral tissues, such as skin and prostate, the adrenal gland and the testes are fundamentally responsible for their production in males. The pathway comprising the formation of androgens is well described (Fig. 10.1). Testosterone, the major male androgen in circulation, and dihydrotestosterone (DHT), the principal androgen in tissues and the most potent one, are the two most important androgens in adult men. They both bind to the androgen receptor (AR), which mediates the physiologic effects of androgens by binding to specific DNA sequences that influence the transcription of androgen-responsive genes (for review, see [1]). DHT has a higher binding affinity for AR and induces transcriptional activity 2–10 times more than testosterone [2]. The importance of these hormones in male sexual differentiation is supported by the clinical observation that the deficiency of steroid 5α-reductase (SRD5A) or 17β-hydroxysteroid dehydrogenase (HSD17B) can lead to male pseudohermaphroditism (for review, see [3]).

J.K.V. Reichardt (✉)
Plunkett Chair of Molecular Biology (Medicine),
The University of Sydney, Sydney, NSW, Australia
e-mail: jreichardt@med.usyd.edu.au

W.D. Figg et al. (eds.), *Drug Management of Prostate Cancer*,
DOI 10.1007/978-1-60327-829-4_10, © Springer Science+Business Media, LLC 2010

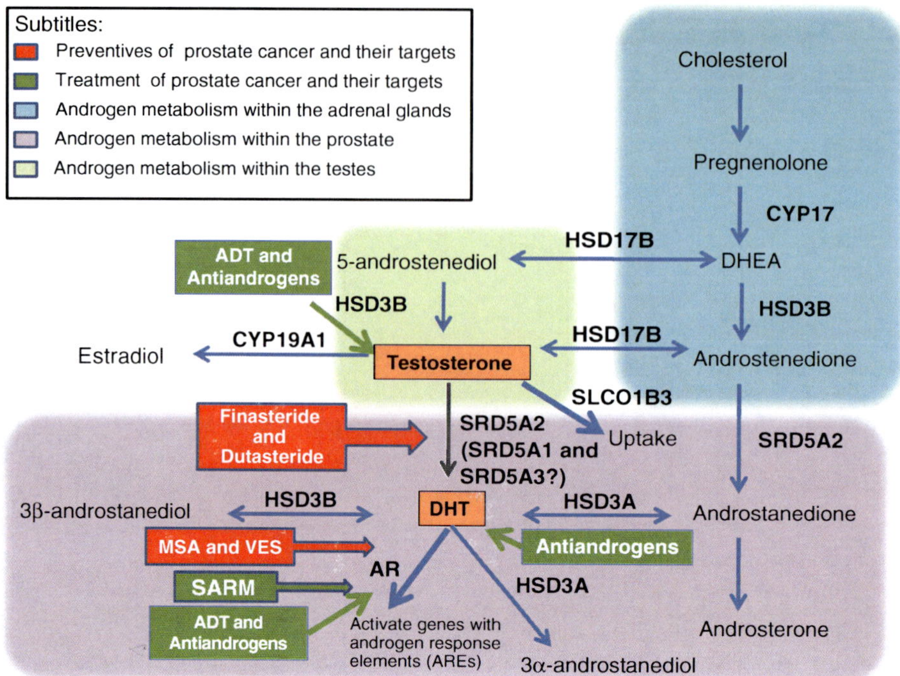

Fig. 10.1 Biosynthesis and metabolism of androgens and target genes for prostate cancer prevention and treatment. Genes involved in the androgen pathway are in bold. They are discussed in the text. *AR* androgen receptor, *CYP* cythocrome P450, *DHEA* dehydroepiandrosterone, *DHT* dihydrotestosterone, *HSD* hydroxysteroid dehydrogenase, *MES* methylseleninic acid, *SARM* selective AR modulators, *SLCO1B3* solute carrier organic anion transporter family member 1B3, *SRD5A* steroid 5α-reductase (type I, II, or III), *VES* α-tocopheryl succinate (vitamin E)

Prostate cancer (CaP) is the most common cancer diagnosis in males and is highly prevalent in many countries [4, 5]. Androgens are very important to CaP development and progression. It was observed that the prostate atrophies with withdrawal of androgenic hormones, and eunuchoid individuals do not develop the disease [6]. In an animal model, early castration testified to significantly reduce prostate tumor growth [7]. Also an in vitro model showed that there is a molecular mechanism of androgen action in cell cycle regulation and growth in prostate carcinoma [8]. Moreover, androgen deprivation therapy (ADT) is the most common and efficient therapy currently in use for metastic CaP (for review, see [9]).

In this chapter, we will review significant polymorphisms, especially single nucleotide polymorphisms (SNPs), found in various androgen metabolic genes, and we will evaluate their contribution to CaP chemoprevention and treatment.

Prostate Cancer and Androgen Therapy and Prevention

Treatment of Prostate Cancer

Several different treatments for metastatic CaP are currently available, such as androgen ablation therapy, estrogen therapy, and steroidal and nonsteroidal antiandrogens (for review, see [10]). We will review here those that are involved in the androgen metabolism and are already in use therapeutically in CaP patients. Since the early 1940s, ADT has been the main treatment for metastatic CaP, first reported with the removal of the prostate [11]. Nowadays, chemical treatment is the most popular choice, with the use of gonadotropin-releasing hormone (GnRH) agonists (for review, see [9]). Other medications called antiandrogens, such as flutamide, bicalutamide, nilutamide (nonsteroidal antiandrogens), and cyproterone acetate (steroidal antiandrogens), block the action of androgens within CaP cells [10] (see Fig. 10.1). They inhibit the binding of testosterone and DHT to specific receptors in tumor cells.

Prevention of Prostate Cancer

Diverse substances have been studied as potential chemopreventives for CaP. Here, we will review only the ones that are in phase III trials or for which trials have been concluded and shown substantial effects. For more information about prevention of CaP, see Chap. 31 of this book.

Finasteride is a potent SRD5A type II inhibitor [12, 13] utilized in the prevention of prostate cancer. A large 7-year study called the Prostate Cancer Prevention Trial (PCPT) showed that men who had regular doses of finasteride had a decreased risk of CaP by 24.8% [14]. It was observed, however, that the same group had a higher incidence of high-grade CaP compared with placebo [14]. Interestingly and importantly, this original finding has recently become controversial [15, 16]. Finasteride, in the meantime, seems to facilitate the detection of CaP and to inhibit low-grade cancers instead of increasing their rates [15, 16]. Avoiding DHT synthesis through SRD5A2 inhibition could be a useful strategy to delay or prevent the initiation of CaP. Until now, finasteride is the only agent proven to be efficient in the reduction of prostate carcinoma in a randomized and placebo-controlled phase III study [17].

Dutasteride is another SRD5A inhibitor, and it acts on both type I and type II enzymes [18, 19]. It is antiandrogenic and promotes cell death in CaP cells [20, 21]. The results of a 4-year study called Reduction by Dutasteride of Prostate Cancer Events (REDUCE), a phase III trial, were disclosed in 2008 [22].

Methylseleninic acid (MSA) seems to modulate the expression of diverse androgen-regulated genes and suppress AR and prostate-specific antigen (PSA) expressions [23, 24] and inhibit the growth of CaP in vivo [24]. In the same way, a stereoisomer of vitamin E, α-tocopheryl succinate (VES), has shown to suppress AR expression [25]. The Selenium and vitamin E Cancer Prevention Trial (SELECT) examines MSA and VES [26] in relation to CaP prevention. The results of the SELECT trial are discussed in Chap. 31.

Genes and Polymorphisms in the Androgen Pathway in Prostate Cancer

Diverse genes involved in the androgen pathway (see Fig. 10.1) have been analyzed in relation to the risk of CaP. Here we will evaluate the ones relevant to the pharmacogenetics analysis.

Androgen Receptor

The *AR* gene (located in Xq11.2-q12) is a steroid-binding transcription factor that regulates prostate cellular proliferation and differentiation [27] (Table 10.1). It is the main gene studied in CaP risk as it is involved in the regulation of diverse genes of cell regulation and binds to both DHT and testosterone. The AR gene comprises eight exons that encode four functional domains. The amino-terminal transactivation domain (exon 1), which is the transcriptional regulatory region of the protein and regulates the expression of target genes, is highly polymorphic. The DNA-binding domain is coded by exons 2 and 3, while exons 4–8 code to a hinge region and a carboxyl-terminal ligand-binding domain [27]. The transactivation domain, which regulates the expression of target genes and represents 60% of the entire protein, is highly polymorphic [28]. Irrespective of how current CaP treatments affect the levels of circulating androgens, the most important factor determining the success or failure of the treatment is the AR protein [29]. Moreover, the development of selective AR modulators (SARM), such as pyrazolines, is also promising as a CaP treatment [29]. Consequently, a complete understanding of the AR is necessary in the search for new approaches in the prevention and treatment of prostate cancer [29]. It was shown by immunohistochemistry of CaP tissues that AR is upregulated in high-grade or advanced disease [30].

More than 600 somatic mutations have been reported for the *AR* gene; of those, about 85, most of them in advanced grades, have been described in CaP (for review, see [29]). Many of these mutations could change the affinity for ligands and increase transcriptional activity [29]. The most noteworthy polymorphisms are a $(CAG)_n$ (coding for polyglutamine) and a $(GGN)_n$ (coding for glycine) triplet repeats in exon 1

Table 10.1 Variants of the androgen receptor gene, reported functional effects and association studies with prostate cancer

AR variant	Reported functional effects	Association studies
$(CAG)_n$	Structurally altered protein with reduced transcriptional activity [31]	Positive but small association with short repeats in meta-analysis [32]
$(GGN)_n$	Structurally altered protein [31]	Positive but small association with short repeats in meta-analysis [32]
E211E	None	Contradictory [38]
Q640Stop	C-terminal truncated AR [31]	Associated with low risk of metastatic CaP [96]
L701H	Reduced affinity to DHT but increased to glucocorticoids [23]	None
R726L	Change transactivational specificity of the AR [31]	Contradictory [38]
A748T	Decreased stability [31]	None
T877A	Enlarged ligand specificity [31]	None

AR androgen receptor, *DHT* dyhydrotestosterone, *CaP* prostate cancer

(see Table 10.1). Both are expected to produce structurally altered proteins (for review, see [31]). A meta-analysis showed that shorter repeats of both polymorphisms may increase the risk of CaP, although these increased risks appear to be very small [32]. More recent investigations about the role of these trinucleotides in CaP predisposition are also contradictory (for review, see [33]). Perhaps they could be in linkage disequilibrium (LD) with other important regions of the gene [32]. Although diverse polymorphisms have been analyzed in this gene in relation to CaP risk (see Table 10.1), none of them have conclusive results, mostly because of the difference between ethnicities. Meta-analysis and larger studies regarding population stratification should help to elucidate the role of the AR gene in prostate carcinoma development and progression. Most of them have functional effects in the protein and may be involved in an altered response to treatment. Detailed analysis about the biology of the AR in CaP is discussed in Chap. 5 of this book.

The Steroid 5α-Reductase Family

The three SRD5A isozymes are apparently expressed in different tissues. Type I is mostly expressed in non-reproductive tissues including skin and liver [34, 35] and type II predominantly in the male reproductive tissues such as seminal vesicles, epididymis, and prostate [34, 35]. The type III (or 2L) enzyme, which was described more recently, seems to work like type I [36].

Diverse studies have shown that SRD5A1 expression is increased in cancer tissue [36–39], while expression and activity are decreased for SRD5A2 [36, 37, 40–42]. A study of immunostaining in CaP tissue of nontreated patients reported that both enzymes were increased in high versus low-grade tumors [38]. These results suggest that SRD5A1 might be more important in CaP progression and development than originally thought. Like the other genes of the family, SRD5A3 might produce DHT, and its expression seems to be increased in CaP [36].

Several polymorphisms in the *SRD5A2* gene (located in band 2p23) have been extensively studied in terms of CaP risk (for review, see [33]) (Table 10.2). The most commonly analyzed polymorphism is a nonsynonymous SNP in exon 1, A49T, an alanine to threonine substitution (first reported by [43] in the Hawaii–Los-Angeles Multiethnic Cohort – MEC), which is believed to increase the levels of enzyme activity about fivefold [44]. Diverse studies have evaluated this polymorphism in relation to CaP, and the results are contradictory (for review, see [45]). However, the updated analysis of a larger MEC sample (6,000 controls vs. 6,000 patients) did not show any positive association between A49T and CaP risk in four ethnic groups [46]. Different genotyping techniques were utilized, and that apparently explains the discrepancy between these and previous results [46]. Moreover, meta-analyses support very small association and little effect of this polymorphism with CaP [45, 46]. The low frequency of the polymorphic T allele (1%) also implies that the public health impact would be low [46]. This case highlights the importance

Table 10.2 Variants of the steroid 5α-hydroxylase (*SRD5A2*) gene, reported functional effects, association study and pharmacogenetic variation with prostate cancer risk

SRD5A2 variants	Somatic or constitutional DNA	Reported functional effects	Association studies	Pharmacogenetic variation [a]
V3I in exon 1 [87, 88]	Somatic [87, 88]	Increased enzyme activity [87, 88]	None	Increased sensitivity to finasteride, decreased sensitivity to dutasteride [87, 88]
C5R in exon 1 [44]	Constitutional [44]	Almost the same [44]	None	Almost same sensitivity to finasteride and dutasteride 1,3
P30L in exon 1 [44]	Constitutional [44]	Decreased enzyme activity [44]	None	Decreased sensitivity to finasteride 1,3
P48R in exon 1 [44]	Constitutional [44]	Decreased enzyme activity [44]	None	Increased sensitivity to finasteride [44, 87]
A49T in exon 1 [44]	Constitutional [87] and somatic [44, 87, 88]	Increased enzyme activity [44, 87, 88]	Negative meta-analyses [45, 46] and large sample [46]	Decreased sensitivity to finasteride, increased sensitivity to dutasteride [44, 87, 88]
A51T in exon 1 [44]	Constitutional [44]	Slightly decreased in activity [44]	None	Slightly increased sensitivity to finasteride, slightly decreased sensitivity to dutasteride [44, 87]
V63M in exon 1 [87, 88]	Somatic [87, 88]	Slightly decreased in activity [87, 88]	None	Increased sensitivity to finasteride, decreased sensitivity to dutasteride [87, 88]
V89L in exon 14	Constitutional [44, 47]	Decreased enzyme activity [44, 47]	Negative meta-analysis [45], LL associated with CaP in large sample [49]	Decreased sensitivity to finasteride, increased sensitivity to dutasteride [44, 87]
F118L in exon 2 [87, 88]	Somatic [87, 88]	Increased enzyme activity [87, 88]	None	Increased sensitivity to finasteride and dutasteride [87, 88]
G183D in exon 4 [87, 88]	Somatic [87, 88]	Slightly decreased in activity [87, 88]	None	Increased sensitivity to finasteride [87, 88]
T187M in exon 4 [44]	Constitutional [44]	Decreased enzyme activity [44]	None	Slightly decreased for both finasteride and dutasteride [44, 87]
V189L in exon 4 [87, 88]	Somatic [87, 88]	Decreased enzyme activity [87, 88]	None	Decreased sensitivity to finasteride, slightly decreased to dutasteride [87, 88]
G191E in exon 4 [87, 88]	Somatic [87, 88]	Decreased enzyme activity [87, 88]	None	Increased sensitivity to finasteride, slightly decreased to dutasteride [87, 88]
F194L in exon 4 [44]	Constitutional [44]	Increased enzyme activity [44]	None	Increased sensitivity to finasteride [44, 87]
L221P in exon 4 [87, 88]	Somatic [87, 88]	Decreased enzyme activity [87, 88]	None	Almost same sensitivity to finasteride, slightly increased to dutasteride [87, 88]
L226P in exon 4 [87, 88]	Somatic [87, 88]	Slightly decreased in activity [87, 88]	None	Decreased sensitivity to finasteride, increased sensitivity to dutasteride [87, 88]
R227Q in exon 4 [44]	Constitutional [44]	Decreased enzyme activity [44]	Negative [97, 98]	Decreased sensitivity to finasteride, increased sensitivity to dutasteride [44, 87]
F234L in exon 4 [44]	Constitutional [44]	Decreased enzyme activity [44]	None	Decreased sensitivity to finasteride, increased sensitivity to dutasteride [44, 87]
A248V in exon 5 [87, 88]	Somatic [87, 88]	Increased enzyme activity [87, 88]	None	Decreased sensitivity to finasteride, increased sensitivity to dutasteride [87, 88]
(TA)$_n$ in 5'UTR	Constitutional [48]	None	Negative meta-analysis [45]	None

[a]The pharmacogenetic variation was compared to wild type

of experimental replications and very large samples in association studies in multifactorial diseases and the severe control quality of the results.

Other polymorphisms in *SRD5A2* gene have been evaluated (see Table 10.2), such as the missense SNP V89L (a valine to leucine substitution), which reduces SRD5A2 activity in vitro [47] and a $(TA)_n$ dinucleotide repeat located in the 3′ untranslated region after exon 5 [48]. Both, however, were not associated with CaP in meta-analyses [45]. Nevertheless, more recently an investigation evaluated 803 CaP cases and 802 controls in relation to the V89L SNP and found that the L/L genotype was associated with increased risk of the disease and also higher aggressiveness [49]. The association with the low-activity variant corroborates with the PCPT findings with long-term exposition of finasteride and inhibition of SRD5A2 [49]. SRD5A1 (5p15) and SRD5A3 (4q12) polymorphisms have not been studied until now in relation to prostate carcinoma. Probably in the future, more researchers will approach these genes, as their role in CaP development and progression is emerging.

Aromatase (CYP19A1)

The aromatase enzyme, encoded by *CYP19A1* gene (15q21.1), is a critical regulator of the balance between androgens and estrogens and contributes to circulating and tissue levels of these hormones in the prostate (see Fig. 10.1). Aromatase inhibitors work to block the production of estradiol, widely used in breast cancer treatment, they are another possibility for CaP treatment (for review, see [50]), which suggests that intraprostatic estradiol might contribute to the disease [51]. However, phase II trials using aromatase inhibitors, such as anastrozole and tetrozole, did not present satisfactory results as a CaP treatment [52, 53].

The analyses of mRNA in various tissues showed that aromatase transcripts are tissue-specifically regulated, with differential splice patterns in the prostate [54]. The results of expression of this enzyme in benign or carcinogen prostate are unfortunately contradictory [51, 55, 56]. Few studies have evaluated polymorphisms in this gene and their relation to CaP risk (Table 10.3). More than seven repeats of a tetranucleotide repeat $(TTTA)_n$ in intron 4 were associated with decreased survival in men with metastatic CaP [57]. The repeat alleles of 171 and 187 bp in size were associated with

CaP patients in another study as well [58]. However, other studies were not able to observe any association between this tetranucleotide repeat and CaP risk [59, 60]. Another polymorphism analyzed was the SNP R264C (a C to T substitution in exon 7), with positive reports [61, 62], which yielded negative results as well [59, 63].

Other Genes

Various genes have been approached in the androgen metabolism in relation to CaP risk [33]. However, their role in the disease is not as well comprehended as the other genes discussed above. These genes have been rapidly reviewed in this section (see Table 10.3).

The cytochrome P450 17 (*CYP17*) gene (10q24.3) encodes for the enzyme P450c 17α-hydroxylase (see Fig. 10.1). The 5′ untranslated promoter region of the gene contains a substitution of T for a C (A1 and A2 alleles) [64]. Although diverse studies were done and the results were often conflicting, a meta-analysis of 12 case-control studies suggests that the C/C genotype is unlikely to be a major risk factor for sporadic CaP on a wide population base, especially in men of European descent (see Table 10.3) [65]. This result is supported by recent analyses in large samples [60, 66, 67]. There is a controversy on whether this polymorphism would increase the expression levels of the gene, creating an additional Sp1-binding site in the promoter [64, 68]. Moreover, the levels of serum hormone in men seemed not to correlate with the genotype of this polymorphism [66, 67, 69]. However, Sp1, Sp3, and NF-1C binding sites are essential transcriptional factors for the expression of CYP17 gene [70].

The enzyme 3β-hydroxysteroid dehydrogenase (HSD3B) is responsible for the inactivation of DHT in steroid target tissues (see Fig. 10.1). The *HSD3B* gene family is composed of two genes and five pseudogenes, which are all located in chromosome band 1p13.1. The type I and type II enzymes are differentially expressed [71]. HSD3B2 expression was observed to be increased in androgen-independent CaP [72]. This would increase androstenedione levels, which could generate substrate for conversion into testosterone [72]. Diverse polymorphisms in *HSD3B1* and *HSD3B2* genes have been described and evaluated in CaP (see Table 10.3) [73, 74], and help to explain the racial and ethnic variations in the risk [73]. However, there is a general lack

Table 10.3 Genes in the androgen pathway involved in prostate cancer development and progression

Gene name	Polymorphism studied	Expression in CaP	Association to CaP risk	Relevance to pharmacogenetic
CYP17	T for C in the 5′UTR (A2 allele)	Inconclusive results for the gene expression in CaP[a]	Negative meta-analysis [65]	None
CYP19A1	A/C SNP 5 kb upstream the gene (rs1870050)	Inconclusive results for aromatase expression in CaP[a]	None	rs1870050 was associated with TTP during ADT [94][a]
	(TTTA)$_n$ repeat in intron 4		Inconclusive[a]	Aromatase inhibitors were unsuccessful used as a CaP treatment[a]
	R264C in exon 7 (C/T)		Inconclusive[a]	None
HSD3B1	L338L (C/T) in exon 3	None	Both SNPs associated with tumor aggressiveness [59]	Associated with TTP during ADT [94][a]
	N367T (A/C) in exon 4		Weak association with CaP risk [74]	None
HSB3B2	(TG)$_n$ (TA)$_n$ (CA)$_n$ repeat in exon 3	Gene is overexpressed in androgen-independent CaP [72]	Inconclusive[a]	None
	C7519G in the 3′UTR		Effect in association with L338L of HSD3B1 [74]	None
HSD17B1	26 Polymorphisms studied	None	Negative large study [75]	Overexpression in dutasteride-treated cells [89][a]
HSD17B3	G289S (G/A) in exon 11	Gene is overexpressed in high-grade CaP [76]	Associated with increase risk in Caucasians [99]	Overexpression in dutasteride-treated cells [89][a]
HSD17B4	Intronic SNP (C/G) (rs7737181)	Gene is overexpressed in high-grade CaP [76]	None	Associated with TTP during ADT [94][a]
SLCO1B3	S112A (T/G) in exon 3 M233I (G/A) in exon 6	Gene is overexpressed in CaP and it is dependent of the genotype; variants are less active than wild type [79]	Both polymorphisms are in LD; haplotype of homozygous to variants is associated with better survival of CaP patients [79]	Presence of T (wild type) associated with shorter time to androgen independence [95][a]

CaP prostate cancer, *LD* linkage disequilibrium, *TTP* time to progression, *ADT* androgen deprivation therapy

[a]See text for more details

of biochemical analysis for these genes and polymorphisms.

The *HSD17* gene family catalyzes the interconversions between 17β-hydroxysteroids and 17-ketosteroids (see Fig. 10.1). Although polymorphisms in the *HSD17B1* gene (located in 17q12-q21), including S3131G, have been described as a predisposition factor to CaP [59], any polymorphism of the 26 analyzed could be associated with the disease in a very large ethnically mixed sample (8,301 CaP cases vs. 9,373 controls) (see Table 10.3) [75]. Different analyses for ethnicity were done to make sure that the negative associations were not due to population stratification [75]. The *HSD17B3* gene (9q22) encodes the testicular (or type III) enzyme (see Fig. 10.1). Polymorphisms in this gene (Table 10.3) might increase the output of testosterone, which can directly or indirectly activate

AR through DHT, by potentially increasing the predisposition to CaP. The expression of *HSD17B3* and *HSD17B4* (5q2) genes were increased in high-grade CaP microdissections from radical prostatectomy samples [76]. These results are consistent with the overexpression of HSD17B4 at both mRNA and protein levels accompanied by increased enzymatic activity reported earlier [77]. Nevertheless, there is a need for the study of polymorphisms and their biochemical effects on these genes to evaluate if they are associated with increased risk of CaP.

The organic anion transporter OATP1B3 involved in the uptake of steroid anions, such as estradiol-17β-glucuronide, DHEA-3-sulfate, estrone-3-sulfate [78], and testosterone [79], is encoded by the solute carrier organic anion transporter 1B3 (*SLCO1B3*) gene [80]. This enzyme is considered to be important for drug elimination and pharmacokinetics, which could contribute to interindividual variability in drug response [78]. Two major SNPs are described in different populations: S112A in exon 3 and M233I in exon 6, which are in complete LD [81]. SLCO1B3 is overexpressed in CaP [79] (see Table 10.3). Testosterone transport by OATP1B3 appears to be dependent on its genotype, the haplotype for the homozygous to the variant of both SNPs being less active in comparison to the normal [79]. In preclinical data, the same haplotype is associated with better survival in CaP patients; however, no difference was observed in relation to Gleason score [79].

Gene Fusions

In the last few years, several gene rearrangements have been described in patients with CaP. First, an androgen-responsive gene called fused transcription factor gene (TMPRSS2) was described in prostate carcinomas with an overexpression of the erythroblast transformation specific (ETS) transcription factor ERG, which regulates other genes' activity [82]. Following that, diverse studies have confirmed their high levels in CaP patients (for review, see [83]), and other gene fusions, not so common, were also described (for review, see [84]). One of the new genes involved was kallikrein 2 (KLK2) [85] which, like PSA (also known as KLK3), is an androgen-induction and prostate-specific expressed gene [86]. The prostate cancer gene fusions are generally characterized by 5′ genomic regulatory elements, most of them controlled by androgen and fused to members of transcription factors that contribute to the overexpression of oncogenic transcription factors [83]. Studies with larger samples will be useful to identify specific clinical subtypes and different types of personalized medicine. Perhaps in the near future, these gene fusions will be utilized as biomarkers and as therapeutic targets to prostate cancer therapy.

Pharmacogenetics of Prostate Cancer

Pharmacogenetic variation of different 5α-reductase inhibitors has been analyzed in the *SRD5A2* gene [44, 87, 88]. In a first study, ten single and three double constitutional amino acid substitutions were identified and biochemically characterized [44] (see Table 10.2). Substantial pharmacogenetic variation was observed for finasteride, dutasteride, and PNU-157706 when incubated with the enzyme variants, and it was most pronounced with finasteride, especially for the mutants P30L, A49T, V89L, R227Q, F234L, and V89L-F234L (increased activity), and for P48R and F194L (decreased activity) [44] (see Table 10.2). Furthermore, SRD5A2 somatic mutations in human CaP tissue were identified [44] and characterized in relation to finasteride and dutasteride [87, 88]. Dutasteride proved to be more efficient as an inhibitor in vitro than finasteride in most variants [87, 88]. However, the efficacy of both drugs was dependent on the genotype of SRD5A2 [87, 88] (see Table 10.2). For example, the P30L and A49T mutants seemed to have a better response to dutasteride than finasteride, while F194L and P48R displayed higher affinity for the latter [88] (see Table 10.2). The treatment with dutasteride is expected to be more efficient in the reduction of the enzyme activity in vivo than that with finasteride [88]. The results of these studies might help in the development of personalized medicine, including personalized prevention, for prostate cancer. Depending on the results of the REDUCT trial, the selection between finasteride and dutasteride as a preventive of CaP would be based on the genotype of SRD5A2.

The expression of SRD5A1 and SRD5A2 was tested in different normal and CaP cell lines of rat and human treated with finasteride and dutasteride [39]. In androgenic-responsive prostatic cancer (Dunning R-3327H) rats, the use of dutasteride, but not finasteride, inhibited CaP growth [39]. In BALB/c nude mice, daily oral treatment with finasteride was effective in inhibiting the growth of androgen-responsive human CaP cell line (LNCaP) xenografts; however, the results were not as clearcut as with dutasteride [39]. Dutasteride also enhanced in vivo therapeutic efficacy of castration [39]. This study shows that the inhibition of SRD5A1 and SRD5A2 by themselves is not enough to inhibit tumor growth, but it can be used as an additive to anti-androgen therapy.

The expression profile of 190 genes related to the androgen pathway was analyzed in nonresponsive (DU145) human CaP and LNCaP cell lines to evaluate the effects of dutasteride treatment [89]. The effect of dutasteride showed to be time-dependent and killed both cell lines at elevated doses [89]. A differential regulation of gene expression by dutasteride in LNCaP cells was observed [89]. Diverse genes were overexpressed in dutasteride-treated cells, including genes encoding proteins in androgen biosynthesis and metabolism (such as HSD17B1, HSD17B3, CYP11B2), signal transduction (ERBB2, VCAM, SOS1), androgen receptor and AR coregulators (AR, CCND1) (according to [90]), while androgen-regulated genes (ARGs) (such as KLK3, KLK2, DHCR24) were underexpressed [89]. Microarray data analysis was confirmed by quantitative real-time PCR assay [89]. The upregulation of the AR is a response to the decreased levels of DHT of the LNCaP cells when treated with dutasteride [89]. No differential gene expression was observed on DU145 cell line in dutasteride-treated cells because AR is required by cells to respond to this substance [39]. These findings show that AR-dependent cells treated with dutasteride decrease intracellular DHT concentration despite the active pathways that control androgen-independent growth [89].

The transcriptional response of LNCaP to MSA was investigated, and 951 genes, including cell-cycleregulators and androgen-regulated genes, with altered expression were identified [91]. The expression of AR and PSA at both mRNA and protein levels were decreased [91]. These results were confirmed in different human cell lines (LNCaP, LAPC-4, CWR22Rv1, LNCaP-C81, and LNCaP-LN3) where a decrease in AR and PSA expression was observed, independent of the AR genotypes or sensitivity to androgen-stimulated growth [92]. Diverse AR-regulated genes implicated in prostate carcinogenesis (PSA, KLK2, ABCC4, DHCR24, and GUCY1A3) were inhibited by MSA, but this could be attenuated by the overexpression of AR [92]. MSA seems to reduce AR availability by blocking AR transcription. In conjunction, these results indicate that MSA may protect against CaP by modulating the expression of AR and AR-regulated genes.

A positive association between men with PCP and presence of the A allele in a 10 kb upstream substitution of the AR gene was observed when patients who received hormonal therapy as primary treatment at diagnosis were assessed [93]. There was no correlation between this polymorphism and other variables, such as Gleason score [93]. It is possible that AR genotypes may affect the response to hormonal treatment and CaP death [93]. Recently, 529 advanced prostate cancer patients treated with ADT (orchiectomy or luteinizing hormone-releasing therapy with or without antiandrogen)

were genotyped for 129 polymorphisms (SNPs and microsatellite repeats) in 20 genes in the androgen synthesis and metabolism [94]. Three polymorphisms showed positive association with time to progression (TTP) during ADT in the *CYP19A1* (a SNP 5 kb upstream of the gene), *HSD3B1* (a SNP 13 kb upstream of the gene), and *HSD17B4* (an intronic SNP) genes [94]. Progression was described as two proven increases in PSA levels or initiation of secondary hormonal therapy for rising PSA [94]. Individuals homozygous for *HSD17B4* (C/C) presented lower PSA values at ADT initiation than the other genotypes. Patients who carried more than one of these polymorphisms presented a better response to the treatment (34 months) compared to the ones with any favorable alleles (11.8 months) [94]. On this basis, the efficacy of ADT was hypothesized to be improved by drugs that inhibit or increase these targets [94]. These polymorphisms, however, were not evaluated in relation to their functional enzymatic consequences.

Also the genotypes of the *SLCO1B3* gene were evaluated in 68 Caucasian patients with advanced CaP in relation to the interval of ADT to androgen independence [95]. These patients enrolled in a clinical trial using ketoconazole with or without alendronate or in a clinical trial of docetaxel with or without thalidomide [95]. The presence of the wild-type allele (T) of S112A polymorphism was associated with a shorter time to androgen independence in both ADT with metastatic disease and biochemical failure with no metastatic disease [95]. This association was confirmed even in combined analysis of the two groups stratified by stage [95]. These findings, if replicated, can have potential implications in the evaluation of response to hormonal therapy.

Conclusions

Nowadays, many genes are recognized to be involved in CaP progression and development. Detailed knowledge of polymorphisms and biochemical variation of these genes has implications for the identification of presymptomatic but at-risk men and the development and selection of drugs to treat the cancer in a personalized manner or even prevent the disease in an individualized fashion.

Despite the accumulating knowledge of polymorphisms in genes in the androgen pathway, their biochemical characterization, and their relation to CaP, there is a lack in pharmacogenetic studies of most drugs currently in use. The few reports available at the moment have to be replicated in independent and larger samples. New targets for CaP prevention and treatment, such as SRD5A1 and the gene fusions, are available for investigation, but their effects in the disease are not totally understood yet.

In summary, we have reviewed here the DNA variation in prostate cancer candidate genes in the androgen pathway and pharmacogenetic studies available at the moment. Molecular research in chemoprevention and therapy of CaP might lead to impressive pharmacological advances in the next few years.

Acknowledgment JKVR is a Medical Foundation Fellow at the University of Sydney. The work in his laboratory is also supported in part by NCI grant P01 CA108964 (project 1 to JKVR).

References

1. Balk SP, Knudsen KE. AR, the cell cycle, and prostate cancer. Nucl Recept Signal 2008;6:e001.
2. Wright AS, Douglas RC, Thomas LN, Lazier CB, Rittmaster RS. Androgen-induced regrowth in the castrated rat ventral prostate: role of 5alpha-reductase. Endocrinology 1999;140: 4509–15.
3. Luu-The V, Bélanger A, Labrie F. Androgen biosynthetic pathways in the human prostate. Best Pract Res Clin Endocrinol Metab 2008;22:207–21.
4. Australian Institute of Health and Welfare. Australia's health 2008. Canberra: AIHW; 2008. Cat. no. AUS 99.
5. American Cancer Society. Cancer facts & figures 2008. Atlanta: American Cancer Society; 2008.
6. Wu CP, Gu FL. The prostate in eunuchs. Prog Clin Biol Res 1991;370:249–55.
7. Eng MH, Charles LG, Ross BD, Chrisp CE, Pienta KJ, Greenberg NM, et al. Early castration reduces prostatic carcinogenesis in transgenic mice. Urology 1999;54:1112–9.
8. Lu S, Tsai SY, Tsai MJ. Regulation of androgen-dependent prostatic cancer cell growth: androgen regulation of CDK2, CDK4, and CKI p16 genes. Cancer Res 1997;57:4511–6.
9. Loblaw DA, Virgo KS, Nam R, Somerfield MR, Ben-Josef E, Mendelson DS, et al. Initial hormonal management of androgen-sensitive metastatic, recurrent, or progressive prostate cancer: 2006 update of an American Society of Clinical Oncology practice guideline. J Clin Oncol 2007;25: 1596–605.
10. Damber JE, Aus G. Prostate cancer. Lancet 2008;371: 1710–21.
11. Huggins C. Effect of orchiectomy and irradiation on cancer of the prostate. Ann Surg 1942;115:1192–200.
12. Carlin JR, Höglund P, Eriksson LO, Christofalo P, Gregoire SL, Taylor AM, et al. Disposition and pharmacokinetics of [^{14}C]finasteride after oral administration in humans. Drug Metab Dispos 1992;20:48–55.
13. Tian G, Mook Jr RA, Moss ML, Frye SV. Mechanism of time-dependent inhibition of 5 alpha-reductases by delta 1-4-azasteroids: toward perfection of rates of time-dependent inhibition by using ligand-binding energies. Biochemistry 1995;34:13453–9.
14. Thompson IM, Goodman PJ, Tangen CM, Lucia MS, Miller GJ, Ford LG, et al. The influence of finasteride on the development of prostate cancer. N Engl J Med 2003;349: 215–24.
15. Lucia MS, Epstein JI, Goodman PJ, Darke AK, Reuter VE, Civantos F, et al. Finasteride and high-grade prostate cancer in the Prostate Cancer Prevention Trial. J Natl Cancer Inst 2007;99:1375–83.
16. Thompson IM, Tangen CM, Goodman PJ, Lucia MS, Parnes HL, Lippman SM, et al. Finasteride improves the sensitivity of digital rectal examination for prostate cancer detection. J Urol 2007;177:1749–52.
17. Canby-Hagino E, Hernandez J, Brand TC, Thompson I. Looking back at PCPT: looking forward to new paradigms in prostate cancer screening and prevention. Eur Urol 2007; 51:27–33.
18. Evans HC, Goa KL. Dutasteride. Drugs Aging 2003;20: 905–16.
19. Clark RV, Hermann DJ, Cunningham GR, Wilson TH, Morrill BB, Hobbs S. Marked suppression of dihydrotestosterone in men with benign prostatic hyperplasia by dutasteride, a dual 5alpha-reductase inhibitor. J Clin Endocrinol Metab 2004;89:2179–84.
20. Lazier CB, Thomas LN, Douglas RC, Vessey JP, Rittmaster RS. Dutasteride, the dual 5alpha-reductase inhibitor, inhibits androgen action and promotes cell death in the LNCaP prostate cancer cell line. Prostate 2004;58:130–44.
21. Maria McCrohan A, Morrissey C, O'Keane C, Mulligan N, Watson C, Smith J, et al. Effects of the dual 5 alpha-reductase inhibitor dutasteride on apoptosis in primary cultures of prostate cancer epithelial cells and cell lines. Cancer 2006; 106:2743–52.
22. Musquera M, Fleshner NE, Finelli A, Zlotta AR. The REDUCE trial: chemoprevention in prostate cancer using a dual 5alpha-reductase inhibitor, dutasteride. Expert Rev Anticancer Ther 2008;8:1073–9.
23. Zhao XY, Malloy PJ, Krishnan AV, Swami S, Navone NM, Peehl DM, et al. Glucocorticoids can promote androgen-independent growth of prostate cancer cells through a mutated androgen receptor. Nat Med 2000;6:703–6.
24. Lee SO, Yeon Chun J, Nadiminty N, Trump DL, Ip C, Dong Y, et al. Monomethylated selenium inhibits growth of LNCaP human prostate cancer xenograft accompanied by a decrease in the expression of androgen receptor and prostate-specific antigen (PSA). Prostate 2006;66:1070–5.
25. Zhang Y, Ni J, Messing EM, Chang E, Yang CR, Yeh S. Vitamin E succinate inhibits the function of androgen receptor and the expression of prostate-specific antigen in prostate cancer cells. Proc Natl Acad Sci U S A 2002; 99:7408–13.
26. Klein EA. Selenium and vitamin E cancer prevention trial. Ann N Y Acad Sci 2004;1031:234–41.
27. Gelmann EP. Molecular biology of the androgen receptor. J Clin Oncol 2002;20:3001–15.

28. Dehm SM, Tindall DJ. Androgen receptor structural and functional elements: role and regulation in prostate cancer. Mol Endocrinol 2007;21:2855–63.

29. Sarvis JA, Thompson IM. Androgens and prevention of prostate cancer. Curr Opin Endocrinol Diabetes Obes 2008;15:271–7.

30. Wako K, Kawasaki T, Yamana K, Suzuki K, Jiang S, Umezu H, et al. Expression of androgen receptor through androgen-converting enzymes is associated with biological aggressiveness in prostate cancer. J Clin Pathol 2008;61:448–54.

31. Singh AS, Chau CH, Price DK, Figg WD. Mechanisms of disease: polymorphisms of androgen regulatory genes in the development of prostate cancer. Nat Clin Pract Urol 2005; 2:101–7.

32. Zeegers MP, Kiemeney LA, Nieder AM, Ostrer H. How strong is the association between CAG and GGN repeat length polymorphisms in the androgen receptor gene and prostate cancer risk? Cancer Epidemiol Biomarkers Prev 2004;13:1765–71.

33. D'Amico F, Biancolella M, Margiotti K, Reichardt JK, Novelli G. Genomic biomarkers, androgen pathway and prostate cancer. Pharmacogenomics 2007;8:645–61.

34. Normington K, Russell DW. Tissue distribution and kinetic characteristics of rat steroid 5 alpha-reductase isozymes. Evidence for distinct physiological functions. J Biol Chem 1992;267:19548–54.

35. Thigpen AE, Silver RI, Guileyardo JM, Casey ML, McConnell JD, Russell DW. Tissue distribution and ontogeny of steroid 5 alpha-reductase isozyme expression. J Clin Invest 1993;92:903–10.

36. Uemura M, Tamura K, Chung S, Honma S, Okuyama A, Nakamura Y, et al. Novel 5 alpha-steroid reductase (SRD5A3, type-3) is overexpressed in hormone-refractory prostate cancer. Cancer Sci 2008;99:81–6.

37. Thomas LN, Lazier CB, Gupta R, Norman RW, Troyer DA, O'Brien SP, et al. Differential alterations in 5alpha-reductase type 1 and type 2 levels during development and progression of prostate cancer. Prostate 2005;63:231–9.

38. Thomas LN, Douglas RC, Lazier CB, Gupta R, Norman RW, Murphy PR, et al. Levels of 5alpha-reductase type 1 and type 2 are increased in localized high grade compared to low grade prostate cancer. J Urol 2008;179:147–51.

39. Xu Y, Dalrymple SL, Becker RE, Denmeade SR, Isaacs JT. Pharmacologic basis for the enhanced efficacy of dutasteride against prostatic cancers. Clin Cancer Res 2006;12:4072–9.

40. Söderström T, Wadelius M, Andersson SO, Johansson JE, Johansson S, Granath F, et al. 5alpha-reductase 2 polymorphisms as risk factors in prostate cancer. Pharmacogenetics 2002;12:307–12.

41. Luo J, Dunn TA, Ewing CM, Walsh PC, Isaacs WB. Decreased gene expression of steroid 5 alpha-reductase 2 in human prostate cancer: implications for finasteride therapy of prostate carcinoma. Prostate 2003;57:134–9.

42. Titus MA, Gregory CW, Ford OH, Schell MJ, Maygarden SJ, Mohler JL. Steroid 5alpha-reductase isozymes I and II in recurrent prostate cancer. Clin Cancer Res 2005;11: 4365–71.

43. Makridakis NM, Ross RK, Pike MC, Crocitto LE, Kolonel LN, Pearce CL, et al. Association of mis-sense substitution in SRD5A2 gene with prostate cancer in African-American and Hispanic men in Los Angeles, USA. Lancet 1999;354:975–8.

44. Makridakis NM, di Salle E, Reichardt JK. Biochemical and pharmacogenetic dissection of human steroid 5 alpha-reductase type II. Pharmacogenetics 2000;10:407–13.

45. Ntais C, Polycarpou A, Ioannidis JP. SRD5A2 gene polymorphisms and the risk of prostate cancer: a meta-analysis. Cancer Epidemiol Biomarkers Prev 2003;12:618–24.

46. Pearce CL, Van Den Berg DJ, Makridakis N, Reichardt JK, Ross RK, Pike MC, et al. No association between the SRD5A2 Gene A49T missense variant and prostate cancer risk: lessons learned. Hum Mol Genet 2008;17(16): 2456–61.

47. Makridakis N, Ross RK, Pike MC, Chang L, Stanczyk FZ, Kolonel LN, et al. A prevalent missense substitution that modulates activity of prostatic steroid 5alpha-reductase. Cancer Res 1997;57:1020–2.

48. Davis DL, Russell DW. Unusual length polymorphism in human steroid 5 alpha-reductase type 2 gene (SRD5A2). Hum Mol Genet 1993;2:820.

49. Cussenot O, Azzouzi AR, Nicolaiew N, Mangin P, Cormier L, Fournier G, et al. Low-activity V89L variant in SRD5A2 is associated with aggressive prostate cancer risk: an explanation for the adverse effects observed in chemoprevention trials using 5-alpha-reductase inhibitors. Eur Urol 2007;52: 1082–7.

50. Prins GS, Korach KS. The role of estrogens and estrogen receptors in normal prostate growth and disease. Steroids 2008;73:233–44.

51. Ellem SJ, Schmitt JF, Pedersen JS, Frydenberg M, Risbridger GP. Local aromatase expression in human prostate is altered in malignancy. J Clin Endocrinol Metab 2004;89:2434–41.

52. Santen RJ, Petroni GR, Fisch MJ, Myers CE, Theodorescu D, Cohen RB. Use of the aromatase inhibitor anastrozole in the treatment of patients with advanced prostate carcinoma. Cancer 2001;92:2095–101.

53. Smith MR, Kaufman D, George D, Oh WK, Kazanis M, Manola J, et al. Selective aromatase inhibition for patients with androgen-independent prostate carcinoma. Cancer 2002;95:1864–8.

54. Harada N, Utsumi T, Takagi Y. Tissue-specific expression of the human aromatase cytochrome P-450 gene by alternative use of multiple exons 1 and promoters, and switching of tissue-specific exons 1 in carcinogenesis. Proc Natl Acad Sci U S A 1993;90:11312–6.

55. Hiramatsu M, Maehara I, Ozaki M, Harada N, Orikasa S, Sasano H. Aromatase in hyperplasia and carcinoma of the human prostate. Prostate 1997;31:118–24.

56. Negri-Cesi P, Poletti A, Colciago A, Magni P, Martini P, Motta M. Presence of 5alpha-reductase isozymes and aromatase in human prostate cancer cells and in benign prostate hyperplastic tissue. Prostate 1998;34:283–91.

57. Tsuchiya N, Wang L, Suzuki H, Segawa T, Fukuda H, Narita S, et al. Impact of IGF-I and CYP19 gene polymorphisms on the survival of patients with metastatic prostate cancer. J Clin Oncol 2006;24:1982–9.

58. Latil AG, Azzouzi R, Cancel GS, Guillaume EC, Cochan-Priollet B, Berthon PL, et al. Prostate carcinoma risk and allelic variants of genes involved in androgen biosynthesis and metabolism pathways. Cancer 2001;92:1130–7.

59. Cunningham JM, Hebbring SJ, McDonnell SK, Cicek MS, Christensen GB, Wang L, et al. Evaluation of genetic variations in the androgen and estrogen metabolic pathways as

risk factors for sporadic and familial prostate cancer. Cancer Epidemiol Biomarkers Prev 2007;16:969–78.

60. Dos Santos RM, de Jesus CM, Filho JC, Trindade JC, de Camargo JL, Rainho CA, et al. PSA and androgen-related gene (AR, CYP17, and CYP19) polymorphisms and the risk of adenocarcinoma at prostate biopsy. DNA Cell Biol 2008;27(9):497–503.

61. Modugno F, Weissfeld JL, Trump DL, Zmuda JM, Shea P, Cauley JA, et al. Allelic variants of aromatase and the androgen and estrogen receptors: toward a multigenic model of prostate cancer risk. Clin Cancer Res 2001;7:3092–6.

62. Onsory K, Sobti RC, Al-Badran AI, Watanabe M, Shiraishi T, Krishan A, et al. Hormone receptor-related gene polymorphisms and prostate cancer risk in North Indian population. Mol Cell Biochem 2008;314:25–35.

63. Sarma AV, Dunn RL, Lange LA, Ray A, Wang Y, Lange EM, et al. Genetic polymorphisms in CYP17, CYP3A4, CYP19A1, SRD5A2, IGF-1, and IGFBP-3 and prostate cancer risk in African-American men: the Flint Men's Health Study. Prostate 2008;68:296–305.

64. Carey AH, Waterworth D, Patel K, White D, Little J, Novelli P, et al. Polycystic ovaries and premature male pattern baldness are associated with one allele of the steroid metabolism gene CYP17. Hum Mol Genet 1994;3:1873–6.

65. Ntais C, Polycarpou A, Ioannidis JP. Association of the CYP17 gene polymorphism with the risk of prostate cancer: a meta-analysis. Cancer Epidemiol Biomarkers Prev 2003;12:120–6.

66. Setiawan VW, Schumacher FR, Haiman CA, et al. CYP17 genetic variation and risk of breast and prostate cancer from the National Cancer Institute Breast and Prostate Cancer Cohort Consortium (BPC3). Cancer Epidemiol Biomarkers Prev 2007;16:2237–46.

67. Severi G, Hayes VM, Tesoriero AA, Southey MC, Hoang HN, Padilla EJ, et al. The rs743572 common variant in the promoter of CYP17A1 is not associated with prostate cancer risk or circulating hormonal levels. BJU Int 2008;101: 492–6.

68. Nedelcheva Kristensen V, Haraldsen EK, Anderson KB, Lønning PE, Erikstein B, Kåresen R, et al. CYP17 and breast cancer risk: the polymorphism in the 5' flanking area of the gene does not influence binding to Sp-1. Cancer Res 1999;59:2825–8.

69. Wang JQ, Gu X, Chen JC, Sun XQ, Mu HT, Wei ZH, et al. Association between polymorphism of CYP17 gene and serum hormone concentrations in aged men. Zhonghua Nan Ke Xue 2005;11:442–4.

70. Lin CJ, Martens JW, Miller WL. NF-1C, Sp1, and Sp3 are essential for transcription of the human gene for P450c17 (steroid 17alpha-hydroxylase/17,20 lyase) in human adrenal NCI-H295A cells. Mol Endocrinol 2001;15:1277–93.

71. Rhéaume E, Lachance Y, Zhao HF, Breton N, Dumont M, de Launoit Y, et al. Structure and expression of a new complementary DNA encoding the almost exclusive 3 beta-hydroxysteroid dehydrogenase/delta 5-delta 4-isomerase in human adrenals and gonads. Mol Endocrinol 1991;5: 1147–57.

72. Stanbrough M, Bubley GJ, Ross K, Golub TR, Rubin MA, Penning TM, et al. Increased expression of genes converting adrenal androgens to testosterone in androgen-independent prostate cancer. Cancer Res 2006;66:2815–25.

73. Devgan SA, Henderson BE, Yu MC, Shi CY, Pike MC, Ross RK, et al. Genetic variation of 3 beta-hydroxysteroid dehydrogenase type II in three racial/ethnic groups: implications for prostate cancer risk. Prostate 1997;33:9–12.

74. Chang BL, Zheng SL, Hawkins GA, Isaacs SD, Wiley KE, Turner A, et al. Joint effect of HSD3B1 and HSD3B2 genes is associated with hereditary and sporadic prostate cancer susceptibility. Cancer Res 2002;62:1784–9.

75. Kraft P, Pharoah P, Chanock SJ, et al. Genetic variation in the HSD17B1 gene and risk of prostate cancer. PLoS Genet 2005;1:68.

76. True L, Coleman I, Hawley S, Huang CY, Gifford D, Coleman R, et al. A molecular correlate to the Gleason grading system for prostate adenocarcinoma. Proc Natl Acad Sci U S A 2006;103:10991–6.

77. Zha S, Ferdinandusse S, Hicks JL, Denis S, Dunn TA, Wanders RJ, et al. Peroxisomal branched chain fatty acid beta-oxidation pathway is upregulated in prostate cancer. Prostate 2005;63:316–23.

78. Smith NF, Figg WD, Sparreboom A. Role of the liver-specific transporters OATP1B1 and OATP1B3 in governing drug elimination. Expert Opin Drug Metab Toxicol 2005;1: 429–45.

79. Hamada A, Sissung T, Price DK, Danesi R, Chau CH, Sharifi N, et al. Effect of SLCO1B3 haplotype on testosterone transport and clinical outcome in Caucasian patients with androgen-independent prostatic cancer. Clin Cancer Res 2008;14: 3312–8.

80. König J, Cui Y, Nies AT, Keppler D. Localization and genomic organization of a new hepatocellular organic anion transporting polypeptide. J Biol Chem 2000;275:23161–8.

81. Smith NF, Marsh S, Scott-Horton TJ, Hamada A, Mielke S, Mross K, et al. Variants in the SLCO1B3 gene: interethnic distribution and association with paclitaxel pharmacokinetics. Clin Pharmacol Ther 2007;81:76–82.

82. Tomlins SA, Rhodes DR, Perner S, Dhanasekaran SM, Mehra R, Sun XW, et al. Recurrent fusion of TMPRSS2 and ETS transcription factor genes in prostate cancer. Science 2005;310:644–8.

83. Kumar-Sinha C, Tomlins SA, Chinnaiyan AM. Recurrent gene fusions in prostate cancer. Nat Rev Cancer 2008; 8:497–511.

84. Attard G, Ang JE, Olmos D, De-Bono JS. Dissecting prostate carcinogenesis through ETS gene rearrangement studies: implications for anticancer drug development. J Clin Pathol 2008;61:891–6.

85. Hermans KG, Bressers AA, van der Korput HA, Dits NF, Jenster G, Trapman J. Two unique novel prostate-specific and androgen-regulated fusion partners of ETV4 in prostate cancer. Cancer Res 2008;68:3094–8.

86. Riegman PH, Vlietstra RJ, van der Korput HA, Romijn JC, Trapman J. Identification and androgen-regulated expression of two major human glandular kallikrein-1 (hGK-1) mRNA species. Mol Cell Endocrinol 1991;76:181–90.

87. Makridakis N, Akalu A, Reichardt JK. Identification and characterization of somatic steroid 5alpha-reductase (SRD5A2) mutations in human prostate cancer tissue. Oncogene 2004; 23:7399–405.

88. Makridakis N, Reichardt JK. Pharmacogenetic analysis of human steroid 5 alpha reductase type II: comparison of finasteride and dutasteride. J Mol Endocrinol 2005;34:617–23.

89. Biancolella M, Valentini A, Minella D, Vecchione L, D'Amico F, Chillemi G, et al. Effects of dutasteride on the expression of genes related to androgen metabolism and related pathway in human prostate cancer cell lines. Invest New Drugs 2007;25:491–7.

90. Schmidt LJ, Murillo H, Tindall DJ. Gene expression in prostate cancer cells treated with the dual 5 alpha-reductase inhibitor dutasteride. J Androl 2004;25:944–53.

91. Zhao H, Whitfield ML, Xu T, Botstein D, Brooks JD. Diverse effects of methylseleninic acid on the transcriptional program of human prostate cancer cells. Mol Biol Cell 2004; 15:506–19.

92. Dong Y, Zhang H, Gao AC, Marshall JR, Ip C. Androgen receptor signaling intensity is a key factor in determining the sensitivity of prostate cancer cells to selenium inhibition of growth and cancer-specific biomarkers. Mol Cancer Ther 2005;4:1047–55.

93. Lindström S, Adami HO, Bälter KA, Xu J, Zheng SL, Stattin P, et al. Inherited variation in hormone-regulating genes and prostate cancer survival. Clin Cancer Res 2007;13: 5156–61.

94. Ross RW, Oh WK, Xie W, Pomerantz M, Nakabayashi M, Sartor O, et al. Inherited variation in the androgen pathway is associated with the efficacy of androgen-deprivation therapy in men with prostate cancer. J Clin Oncol 2008;26: 842–7.

95. Sharifi N, Hamada A, Sissung T, Danesi R, Venzon D, Baum C, et al. A polymorphism in a transporter of testosterone is a determinant of androgen independence in prostate cancer. BJU Int 2008;102(5):617–21.

96. Hayes VM, Severi G, Eggleton SA, Padilla EJ, Southey MC, Sutherland RL, et al. The E211 G>A androgen receptor polymorphism is associated with a decreased risk of metastatic prostate cancer and androgenetic alopecia. Cancer Epidemiol Biomarkers Prev 2005;14:993–6.

97. Hsing AW, Chen C, Chokkalingam AP, Gao YT, Dightman DA, Nguyen HT, et al. Polymorphic markers in the SRD5A2 gene and prostate cancer risk: a population-based case-control study. Cancer Epidemiol Biomarkers Prev 2001;10: 1077–82.

98. Giwercman C, Giwercman A, Pedersen HS, Toft G, Lundin K, Bonde JP, et al. Polymorphisms in genes regulating androgen activity among prostate cancer low-risk Inuit men and high-risk Scandinavians. Int J Androl 2008;31:25–30.

99. Margiotti K, Kim E, Pearce CL, Spera E, Novelli G, Reichardt JK. Association of the G289S single nucleotide polymorphism in the HSD17B3 gene with prostate cancer in Italian men. Prostate 2002;53:65–8.

Part II
Chemotherapy

Chapter 11
Mitoxantrone

Patricia Halterman, Nicholas J. Vogelzang, Alireza Farabishahadel, and Oscar B. Goodman Jr.

Abstract Mitoxantrone (dihydroxyanthracenedione, DHAD) is an anthracenedione derivative developed in the 1970s in an effort to find a less cardiotoxic doxorubicin derivative. Although the exact mechanism of action remains unclear, mitoxantrone intercalates between base pairs of the DNA double helix, resulting in cross links, strand breaks, and inhibition of nucleic acid synthesis. Early studies with mitoxantrone demonstrated a low potential for drug–drug interactions, other than a significantly increased risk of infection when administered concomitantly with live vaccines. Currently, there are five black box warnings described in the US package insert. Initially approved in 1987 for treatment of acute non-lymphocytic leukemia (ANLL – now AML) in adults, mitoxantrone was approved in 1996 for use in combination with corticosteroids as initial chemotherapy for the treatment of patients with pain related to advanced castration-resistant prostate cancer (CRPC). For this indication, the recommended dosage is 12–14 mg/m^2 every 3 weeks, as a 30-min intravenous infusion. In multiple large randomized studies, mitoxantrone plus prednisone was shown to reduce pain and increase quality of life for patients with CRPC, though it does not extend survival. Subsequent to the approval of docetaxel as a treatment for CRPC, mitoxantrone has primarily been used as a second-line therapy.

Keywords Mitoxantrone • DHAD • Prostate cancer • CRPC • Salvage therapy

Introduction

Mitoxantrone is an anthracenedione derivative developed in the 1970s, a discovery of the synthetic chemistry program at the Medicinal Research Division of the American Cyanamid Company [1]. Development began with a molecule predicted to favor intercalation with double-stranded DNA. From this original class of compounds with immunomodulatory effects and significant activity against murine tumors, mitoxantrone was selected for further development based on its potency and excellent tumor activity. Mitoxantrone is cytotoxic to both proliferating and nonproliferating cells.

Since its initial approval in 1987 for treatment of acute nonlymphocytic leukemia (ANLL – now AML) in adults, mitoxantrone continues to demonstrate efficacy in treatment of recurrent AML. When used in combination with cytarabine, response rate has been reported at 50–60% in first relapse [2] and at 55% when utilizing the MEC regimen (mitoxantrone, etoposide, and cytarabine) [3]. Mitoxantrone was approved in 1996 for use in combination with corticosteroids as initial chemotherapy for the treatment of patients with pain related to advanced castration-resistant prostate cancer (CRPC) [4].

Mechanism of Action

Mitoxantrone is an analog of the anthracyclines which intercalates DNA. Although the exact mechanism of action remains unclear, mitoxantrone intercalates between base pairs of the DNA double helix, resulting in cross links, strand breaks, and inhibition of nucleic acid

P. Halterman (✉)
Clinical Pharmacy, Nevada Cancer Institute, Las Vegas, NV, USA
e-mail: phalterman@nvcancer.org

W.D. Figg et al. (eds.), *Drug Management of Prostate Cancer*,
DOI 10.1007/978-1-60327-829-4_11, © Springer Science+Business Media, LLC 2010

synthesis. Upon binding to nucleic acids, it inhibits DNA and RNA synthesis by template disordering and steric obstruction [5]. Additionally, replication is decreased by binding to DNA topoisomerase II and seems to inhibit the incorporation of uridine into RNA and thymidine into DNA [6], leading to protein-linked DNA breaks. Again, because of these multiple mechanisms of action, mitoxantrone is active throughout the entire cell cycle.

Pharmacological Considerations

The pharmacokinetic parameters of mitoxantrone are best described by an open three-compartment model [7] as follows.

Distribution

In the concentration range of 26–455 ng/mL, protein binding is 78%. Binding is independent of concentration and is unaffected by phenytoin, doxorubicin, methotrexate, prednisone, heparin, or aspirin [8]. Mitoxantrone distributes into a deep tissue compartment from which it is slowly released, as evidenced by prolonged plasma terminal phase half-life, extremely large volume of distribution, and the relatively large amount (>15% of administered dose) retained in tissue at ~35 days postdose [9]. The distribution half-life is 1.1–3.1 h, mean α half-life is 6–12 min, and mean β half-life is 1.1–3.1 h [8–10]. The volume of distribution is greater than 1,000 L/m^2 and has been reported at 1,382–3,792 L, specifically. This has also been reported as 14 L/kg in patients with normal hepatic function. In patients with hepatic disease, this drops to 11 L/kg [7, 8].

Metabolism

Mitoxantrone undergoes extensive metabolism, mostly in the liver, to two inactive metabolites, a monocarboxylic acid derivative and a dicarboxylic acid derivative. Again, neither of these metabolites are cytocidal. Abnormal liver function leads to decreased rates of total body mitoxantrone clearance [11], suggesting a possible need for dose reduction in patients with severe hepatic impairment. Although reported AUCs in patients with severe hepatic impairment or third spacing are more than threefolds of that of patients with normal hepatic function, no definitive dose reductions have been established.

Excretion

Renal clearance of mitoxantrone has been reported in the range of 26.2–70 mL/min [7–9]. Within five days of administration, 11% or less of the drug is recovered in the urine. Of this, 65% is excreted unchanged. Because of this minimal renal excretion, it is unlikely that dose adjustments would be needed in patients with renal impairment. 18.3% of the drug is excreted via the biliary tract, and most importantly, 25% is recovered in the feces. The terminal elimination half-life has been reported from 23 to 215 h and is significantly increased with hepatic impairment or third spacing.

Mitoxantrone is extensively bound to tissues; therefore, neither the therapeutic nor the toxic effects would be lessened by hemodialysis or peritoneal dialysis [8].

Drug Interactions

Early studies with mitoxantrone demonstrated a low potential for drug–drug interactions, other than a significantly increased risk of infection when administered concomitantly with live vaccines. Administration of live vaccines to patients who are immunocompromised by chemotherapeutic agents has resulted in severe and sometimes fatal infections [12, 13]. Live virus and bacterial vaccines should not be administered to patients undergoing immunosuppressive chemotherapy. At least a 3 month washout period should elapse between discontinuation of chemotherapy and vaccination with a live vaccine (Table 11.1) [13]. Patients with hormone-dependent tumors should be instructed to avoid black cohosh and dong quai [14].

Safety and Precautions

In early single-agent studies, the most commonly reported adverse reactions for mitoxantrone were nausea and vomiting or stomatitis. Patients infrequently

Table 11.1 Live vaccines

Bacillus of Calmette and Guerin (BCG) vaccine
Measles virus vaccine
Mumps virus vaccine
Poliovirus vaccine
Rotavirus vaccine
Rubella virus vaccine
Smallpox vaccine
Typhoid vaccine
Varicella virus vaccine
Yellow fever vaccine

encountered diarrhea, abdominal pain and constipation, mild irritation at the site of infusion, shortness of breath, infection, lethargy, weakness, and fatigue. A small number of patients reported altered taste or nail changes. Overall, the adverse reaction profile for mitoxantrone was found to be superior to that of doxorubicin [15].

Currently, there are five black box warnings described in the US package insert [6]: (1) Mitoxantrone should be administered under the supervision of a physician experienced in the use of cytotoxic chemotherapy agents. Mitoxantrone is considered a high-alert medication by the Institute for Safe Medication Practices (ISMP), and may cause significant harm if medication errors occur [16]. Dosage should be reduced in patients with impaired hepatobiliary function. Safety and efficacy in children has not been established yet. (2) Mitoxantrone should be given slowly into a freely flowing intravenous infusion. It must never be given subcutaneously, intramuscularly, or intra-arterially. Severe local tissue damage may occur if there is extravasation during administration. Mitoxantrone is not for intrathecal use. Severe injury with permanent sequelae can result from intrathecal administration. (3) Except for the treatment of acute nonlymphocytic leukemia, mitoxantrone generally should not be administered to patients with baseline neutrophil counts less than 1,500 cells/mm³. In order to monitor the occurrence of bone marrow suppression, primarily neutropenia, which may be severe and result in infection, it is recommended that frequent peripheral blood cell counts be performed on all patients receiving mitoxantrone. (4) Use of mitoxantrone has been associated with cardiotoxicity. Cardiotoxicity can occur at any time during mitoxantrone therapy, and the risk increases with cumulative dose. Congestive heart failure (CHF), potentially fatal, may occur either during therapy with mitoxantrone or months to years after termination of therapy. All patients should be carefully assessed for cardiac signs and symptoms by history and physical examination prior to start of mitoxantrone therapy. Baseline evaluation of left ventricular ejection fraction (LVEF) by echocardiogram or multigated radionuclide angiography (MUGA) should be performed prior to initiation of therapy. Patients with a baseline LVEF less than 50% generally should not be treated with mitoxantrone. LVEF should be reevaluated by echocardiogram or MUGA periodically during therapy. Additional doses of mitoxantrone should not be administered to patients who have experienced either a drop in LVEF to below 50% or a clinically significant reduction in LVEF during treatment with mitoxantrone. Patients generally should not receive a cumulative dose greater than 140 mg/m². In cancer patients, the risk of symptomatic congestive heart failure (CHF) was estimated to be 2.6% for patients receiving up to a cumulative dose of 140 mg/m². Presence or history of cardiovascular disease, prior or concomitant radiotherapy to the mediastinal/pericardial area, previous therapy with other anthracyclines or anthracenediones, or concomitant use of other cardiotoxic drugs may increase the risk of cardiac toxicity; however, cardiac toxicity with mitoxantrone may occur whether or not cardiac risk factors are present. (5) Secondary acute myelogenous leukemia (AML) has been reported in patients treated with mitoxantrone. Postmarketing cases of secondary AML have also been reported. In 1,774 patients with breast cancer who received mitoxantrone concomitantly with other cytotoxic agents and radiotherapy, the cumulative risk of developing treatment-related AML, was estimated as 1.1% and 1.6% at 5 and 10 years, respectively. Secondary acute myelogenous leukemia (AML) has also been reported in cancer patients treated with anthracyclines, and mitoxantrone, an anthracenedione, is a related drug. The occurrence of refractory secondary leukemia is more common when anthracyclines are given in combination with DNA-damaging antineoplastic agents, when patients have been heavily pretreated with cytotoxic drugs, or when doses of anthracyclines have been escalated. Similar risk factors should be anticipated with mitoxantrone [17]. Most recently, AML incidence was reported at 0.6% for high-risk prostate cancer patients undergoing adjuvant chemotherapy with mitoxantrone. This is similar to the rates of AML reported in breast cancer patients treated with mitoxantrone [18]. Other characteristics of leukemias linked to treatment with topoisomerase II inhibitors are a latency period of approximately 2 years and balanced chromosomal aberrations [19]. Many of these leukemias have translocations involving the 11q23 band, though inv [17] and t [15–17] abnormalities are also seen [20].

In addition to these warnings, adverse reactions that have been reported to date in greater than 10% of patients are as follows: central nervous system (CNS): pain, fatigue, weakness, fever, and headache; dermatologic: alopecia and nail bed changes; endocrine/metabolic: amenorrhea, menstrual disorder, and hyperglycemia; gastrointestinal (GI): abdominal pain, anorexia, nausea, constipation, diarrhea, GI bleeding, mucositis, stomatitis, dyspepsia, vomiting, and weight gain/loss; genitourinary (GU): abnormal urine and urinary tract infection; hematologic: neutropenia, leukopenia, lymphopenia, anemia, thrombocytopenia, and petechiae/bruising; hepatic: increased liver function tests (LFTs); renal: increased creatinine/BUN and hematuria; respiratory: cough, dyspnea, and upper respiratory tract infections; and miscellaneous: fungal infections and sepsis. An additional 1–10% of patients experienced the following: central nervous system (CNS): chills, anxiety, depression, and seizures; dermatologic: cellulitis; endocrine/metabolic: hypocalcemia, hypokalemia, hyponatremia, and mennorhagia; gastrointestinal (GI): aphthosis; genitourinary (GU): impotence and sterility; hematologic: hemorrhage; hepatic: jaundice; neuromuscular: back pain, myalgia, and arthralgia; ocular: conjunctivitis and blurred vision; renal: renal failure and proteinuria; respiratory: rhinitis, sinusitis, and pneumonia; and miscellaneous: diaphoresis [14].

Incidence of these adverse reactions varies based on treatment and dose administered. Although it is not a clinically significant toxicity, patients should be counseled that mitoxantrone may cause urine, tears, saliva, sweat, and the whites of the eyes to have a blue-green tinge for 24 h postinfusion [17].

Mitoxantrone is classified as a Pregnancy Category D. When administered during pregnancy, it can cause fetal harm in humans. Animal studies have shown delayed fetal development, fetal external anomalies, and neonatal abnormalities [16]. The risk to the fetus from semen of the male is unknown.

Symptoms of overdose include leukopenia, tachycardia, and marrow hypoplasia. There is no known antidote available [14].

Dosing and Administration

The dose of mitoxantrone for CRPC is 12–14 mg/m^2 administered intravenously (IV) every 3 weeks as a 30-min intravenous infusion, in combination with a corticosteroid [21, 22]. Mitoxantrone should not be administered by intra-arterial, subcutaneous, intramuscular, or intrathecal routes. Diluted solutions of mitoxantrone should be infused into free-flowing normal saline (NS) or 5% dextrose in water solution (D5W). Because mitoxantrone is a known vesicant, care should be taken to avoid extravasation or any contact with the skin, eyes, or mucosa. Infusion should be stopped immediately if extravasation occurs, and the site should be monitored for signs of necrosis or phlebitis that may require medical attention [8–15, 17]. Therapy should not be initiated in patients with baseline neutrophil counts less than 1,500 cells/mm^3 [14].

Cumulative Dose Limits

Similar to doxorubicin, mitoxantrone has been associated with cardiomyopathy when cumulative doses reach 80–120 mg/m^2 or if administered for periods exceeding 9–12 months. Caution should be exercised when approaching either of these limits [23, 24].

Dosage in Renal Impairment

As only small amounts (~7%) are excreted unchanged into the urine, dosing adjustments are not necessary in renal impairment [25].

Dosage in Hepatic Impairment

Mitoxantrone clearance is significantly reduced in patients with severe hepatic impairment or third spacing, and terminal half-life is doubled. Though a reduction in dosage is advised [25], no specific dose adjustments are suggested.

Efficacy

Mitoxantrone was approved in 1996 for use in combination with corticosteroids as initial chemotherapy for the treatment of patients with pain related to CRPC [4]. In multiple large randomized studies, mitoxantrone plus prednisone was shown to reduce pain and increase quality of life for patients with CRPC, though it does not extend survival [26, 27]. Subsequent to the approval of docetaxel as treatment for CRPC, mitoxantrone has primarily been used as a second-line therapy.

Place in Therapy

In the natural history of prostate cancer, CRPC occurs during the final 2–3 years of life [28]. Initial treatment of metastatic disease by orchiectomy, which is the patient-preferred treatment in Europe; or by therapy with drugs that decrease androgen stimulation, the patient-preferred treatment in the United States [29]; can relieve symptoms related to pelvic node and bone metastases in approximately 75% of patients, but all patients eventually progress to castration-resistant disease. Although many of these patients are elderly with significant comorbidities and increased potential for toxicity, cytotoxic chemotherapy has been shown to significantly prolong survival in men with CRPC [21, 22, 26, 30].

Prostate cancer was largely considered resistant to chemotherapy until the mid-1990s when mitoxantrone plus prednisone (MP) was shown to provide palliation for patients with CRPC [21]. To date, three drugs – docetaxel, estramustine, and mitoxantrone – have been approved by the FDA for first-line treatment of CRPC (See Table 11.2). Mitoxantrone is indicated in combination with steroids as initial chemotherapy for palliation of pain related to advanced CRPC. Mitoxantrone and prednisone have nearly twice the response of prednisone alone with significantly more durable responses [31]. As a single agent, mitoxantrone has palliative activity and is well tolerated in elderly patients [8, 32].

In 2004, a large trial TAX327,comparing mitoxantrone to docetaxel in castration-resistant prostate cancer, randomized patients to receive docetaxel 75 mg/m^2 administered every 3 weeks, docetaxel 30 mg/m^2 administered weekly for 5 of 6 weeks, or mitoxantrone 12 mg/m^2 every 3 weeks, each with prednisone 5 mg orally twice daily.

Table 11.2 Trials of mitoxantrone in castration resistant prostate cancer (CRPC) [26, 27, 32–35]

Publication year	Author	Number of patients	Setting	Study results
2004	Tannock (TAX327)	1,006	Mitoxantrone/prednisone (MP) vs. weekly (D1P) or Q3 weekly docetaxel (D3P) with prednisone as first-line chemotherapy in CRPC	Median overall survival was 19.2 months in the D3P arm (95% CI, 17.5–21.3), 17.8 months in the D1P arm (95% CI, 16.2–19.2) and 16.3 months in the MP arm (95% CI, 14.3–17.9) respectively.
2004	Petrylak (SWOG 99–16)	770	Docetaxel/estramustine vs. mitoxantrone/prednisone as first-line chemotherapy in CRPC	Median overall survival was prolonged in the docetaxel/estramustine group compared to mitoxantrone/prednisone – 17.5 months vs. 15.6 months ($P=0.02$)
2006	Michels	68	Mitoxantrone vs. docetaxel in either sequence for CRPC	Front-line docetaxel prolonged median overall survival compared to front-line Mitoxantrone – 22 months (95% CI, 17.2–26.8) vs. 15 months (95% CI, 10.4–19.6)
2006	Hart	78	Irofulven/prednisone (IP) vs. Irofulven/capecitabine (IC) vs. mitoxantrone/prednisone (MP) as second-line chemotherapy for CRPC	TTP 2.1 months (IP and IC) vs. 1.1 months (MP)
2007	Rosenberg	82	Ixabepilone vs. mitoxantrone/prednisone in CRPC progressing through first-line chemotherapy	Median overall survival 10.4 months for ixabepilone arm vs. 9.8 months for mitoxantrone arm

On the basis of this study's findings, the FDA approved docetaxel in combination with prednisone for treatment of CRPC. Updated survival analysis of the study confirmed that survival is significantly increased in patients receiving docetaxel plus prednisone every 3 weeks compared to those receiving mitoxantrone plus prednisone. The difference in median overall survival time is now reported at 2.9 months ($P=0.004$, HR=0.79).

Treatment with weekly docetaxel, however, did not lead to an increase in overall survival, and patients on this arm of the trial were more likely to experience deterioration in quality of life due to disease progression or increased toxicities. In general, patients with visceral disease, pain, poorer performance status, and higher baseline PSA had shorter survival times.

Treatment with docetaxel and estramustine has also demonstrated a survival advantage over the combination of mitoxantrone and prednisone. In addition to TAX327, a second pivotal trial in 2004, SWOG 99–16 randomly assigned patients to either 280 mg estramustine orally three times daily 1 h before or 2 h after meals on days 1–5 plus docetaxel 60 mg/m^2 on day 2 or mitoxantrone 12 mg/m^2 on day 1 plus prednisone 5 mg twice daily. After intent-to-treat analysis, median survival was 17.5 months among the patients assigned to estramustine and docetaxel and 15.6 months among the patients assigned to mitoxantrone and prednisone ($P=0.02$); the corresponding hazard ratio for death was 0.8 [27]. Again the trade-off was an increased incidence of adverse events in the estramustine and docetaxel arm, specifically cardiovascular and gastrointestinal events, though these were not associated with either an increased rate of treatment discontinuation or treatment-related deaths [27, 28].

Patients who progress after first-line chemotherapy have limited treatment options, none of which are FDA-approved. In fact, it has been reported that less than half of men with CRPC will receive a second-line therapy [33]. In 2006, a study of 68 men with CRPC evaluated the sequencing of first- and second-line treatment with docetaxel and mitoxantrone. This study favored initial treatment with docetaxel, and although second-line docetaxel lead to a higher PSA response than second-line mitoxantrone (38% vs. 12%, $P=0.012$), both docetaxel and mitoxantrone have limited tolerability in the second-line setting, with significant rates of treatment-related adverse events, dose reductions, dose delays, or discontinuation of therapy (64% and 46% of patients, respectively) [34]. For patients with taxane-refractory CRPC, defined as progression during or within 60 days of cessation of taxane therapy, mitoxantrone with prednisone 5 mg twice daily has been shown to have modest activity as a second-line agent. Elevated lactate dehydrogenase and the presence of visceral metastases are both poor prognostic indicators in the second-line setting. Patients experiencing a PSA response to prior therapy were 7–8 times more likely to respond to second-line treatment, and patients who have had no response to taxanes are unlikely to have a response to mitoxantrone [32]. For this population of men who are candidates for second-line chemotherapy, investigational agents should be considered.

Conclusions

Systemic chemotherapy should be reserved only for patients with metastatic CRPC unless under study in clinical trials. Mitoxantrone plus prednisone was shown to reduce pain and increase quality of life for patients with CRPC, though it does not extend survival. Subsequent to the approval of docetaxel as treatment for CRPC, mitoxantrone has primarily been used as a second-line therapy. In addition to the discovery of newer agents to be used both in first- and second-line chemotherapy, important decisions regarding the direction of future clinical trials in prostate cancer remain, specifically the endpoints that are most beneficial to the patient and/or valid to the scientific community. Although survival remains the conventional FDA-preferred endpoint, with surrogate markers of progression-free survival and the related time to progression, future clinical trials of patients with CRPC must also take into consideration the clinical experience of patients (pain and other quality of life measures) and the utility of parameters such as PSA measurements and circulating tumor cells to predict survival. Treatment decisions must be individualized based on tumor characteristics, efficacy data, toxicity profile, convenience of scheduling, and impact on quality of life, as well as survival statistics.

References

1. White RJ, Durr FE. Development of mitoxantrone. Invest New Drugs 1985;3:85–93.
2. Paciucci PA, Dutcher JP, Cuttner J, Strauman JJ, Wiernik PH, Holland JF. Mitoxantrone and ara-C in previously treated patients with acute myelogenous leukemia. Leukemia 1987; 1:565–7.

3. Spadea A, Petti MC, Fazi P et al. Mitoxantrone, etoposide and intermediate-dose Ara-C (MEC): an effective regimen for poor risk acute myeloid leukemia. Leukemia 1993;7: 549–52.

4. U.S. Food and Drug Administration Center for Drug Evaluation and Research Approval Summary for Mitoxantrone. (Accessed May 6, 2008, at www.accessdata.fda.gov/scripts/ cder/onctools/summary.cfm?ID=91).

5. Lown JW, Hanstock CC, Bradley RD, Scraba DG. Interactions of the antitumor agents mitoxantrone and bisantrene with deoxyribonucleic acids studied by electron microscopy. Mol Pharmacol 1984;25:178–84.

6. Tewey KM, Rowe TC, Yang L, Halligan BD, Liu LF. Adriamycin-induced DNA damage mediated by mammalian DNA topoisomerase II. Science 1984;226:466–8.

7. Ehninger G, Proksch B, Heinzel G, Schiller E, Weible KH, Woodward DL. The pharmacokinetics and metabolism of mitoxantrone in man. Invest New Drugs 1985;3:109–16.

8. Mitoxantrone. In: Micromedex Healthcare Series: Thomson Health Care; 2008.

9. Alberts DS, Peng YM, Bowden GT, Dalton WS, Mackel C. Pharmacology of mitoxantrone: mode of action and pharmacokinetics. Invest New Drugs 1985;3:101–7.

10. Van Belle SJ, de Planque MM, Smith IE et al. Pharmacokinetics of mitoxantrone in humans following single-agent infusion or intra-arterial injection therapy or combined-agent infusion therapy. Cancer Chemother Pharmacol 1986;18:27–32.

11. Savaraj N, Lu K, Manuel V, Loo TL. Pharmacology of mitoxantrone in cancer patients. Cancer Chemother Pharmacol 1982;8:113–7.

12. Rosenbaum EH, Cohen RA, Glatstein HR. Vaccination of a patient receiving immunosuppressive therapy for lymphosarcoma. JAMA 1966;198:737–40.

13. Kroger AT, Atkinson WL, Marcuse EK, Pickering LK. General recommendations on immunization: recommendations of the Advisory Committee on Immunization Practices (ACIP). MMWR Recomm Rep 2006;55:1–48.

14. Lacy CF ed. Drug Information Handbook. 16 ed. Hudson, OH: Lexi-Comp. 2008.

15. Posner LE, Dukart G, Goldberg J, Bernstein T, Cartwright K. Mitoxantrone: an overview of safety and toxicity. Invest New Drugs 1985;3:123–32.

16. ISMP's List of High Alert Medications. 2008. (Accessed June 13, 2008, at http://www.ismp.org/Tools/highalert medications.pdf.)

17. Novantrone (mitoxantrone) Package Insert. In. Melville, NY: OSI Oncology; 2008.

18. Flaig TW, Tangen CM, Hussain MH et al. Randomization reveals unexpected acute leukemias in Southwest Oncology Group prostate cancer trial. J Clin Oncol 2008;26:1532–6.

19. Pedersen-Bjergaard J, Rowley JD. The balanced and the unbalanced chromosome aberrations of acute myeloid leukemia may develop in different ways and may contribute differently to malignant transformation. Blood 1994;83:2780–6.

20. Pedersen-Bjergaard J, Andersen MK, Johansson B. Balanced chromosome aberrations in leukemias following chemotherapy with DNA-topoisomerase II inhibitors. J Clin Oncol 1998;16:1897–8.

21. Tannock IF, Osoba D, Stockler MR et al. Chemotherapy with mitoxantrone plus prednisone or prednisone alone for symptomatic hormone-resistant prostate cancer: a Canadian randomized trial with palliative end points. J Clin Oncol 1996;14:1756–64.

22. Kantoff PW, Halabi S, Conaway M et al. Hydrocortisone with or without mitoxantrone in men with hormone-refractory prostate cancer: results of the cancer and leukemia group B 9182 study. J Clin Oncol 1999;17: 2506–13.

23. Coleman RE, Maisey MN, Knight RK, Rubens RD. Mitoxantrone in advanced breast cancer – a phase II study with special attention to cardiotoxicity. Eur J Cancer Clin Oncol 1984;20:771–6.

24. Stuart-Harris R, Pearson M, Smith IE, Olsen EG. Cardiotoxicity associated with mitoxantrone. Lancet 1984;2: 219–20.

25. Savaraj N, Lu K, Valdivieso M et al. Clinical kinetics of 1,4-dihydroxy-5,8-bis [(2-[(2-hydroxyethyl) amino] ethyl] amino-9, 10-anthracenedione. Clin Pharmacol Ther 1982;31: 312–6.

26. Tannock IF, de Wit R, Berry WR et al. Docetaxel plus prednisone or mitoxantrone plus prednisone for advanced prostate cancer. N Engl J Med 2004;351:1502–12.

27. Petrylak DP, Tangen CM, Hussain MH et al. Docetaxel and estramustine compared with mitoxantrone and prednisone for advanced refractory prostate cancer. N Engl J Med 2004;351:1513–20.

28. Hussain M, Petrylak D, Fisher E, Tangen C, Crawford D. Docetaxel (Taxotere) and estramustine versus mitoxantrone and prednisone for hormone-refractory prostate cancer: scientific basis and design of Southwest Oncology Group Study 9916. Semin Oncol 1999;26:55–60.

29. Kolesar J. Oncology pharmacy preparatory review course – prostate cancer In: Pharmacy ACoC, editor. Oncology Pharmacy Preparatory Review Course; 2006; Fort Lauderdale, Florida: American College of Clinical Pharmacy; 2006. p. 203–22.

30. Berthold DR, Pond GR, Soban F, de Wit R, Eisenberger M, Tannock IF. Docetaxel plus prednisone or mitoxantrone plus prednisone for advanced prostate cancer: updated survival in the TAX 327 study. J Clin Oncol 2008;26:242–5.

31. Osoba D, Tannock IF, Ernst DS, Neville AJ. Health-related quality of life in men with metastatic prostate cancer treated with prednisone alone or mitoxantrone and prednisone. J Clin Oncol 1999;17:1654–63.

32. Rosenberg JE, Weinberg VK, Kelly WK et al. Activity of second-line chemotherapy in docetaxel-refractory hormone-refractory prostate cancer patients: randomized phase 2 study of ixabepilone or mitoxantrone and prednisone. Cancer 2007;110:556–63.

33. Garmey EG, Sartor O, Halabi S, Vogelzang NJ. Second-line chemotherapy for advanced hormone-refractory prostate cancer. Clin Adv Hematol Oncol 2008;6:118–22, 27–32.

34. Michels J, Montemurro T, Murray N, Kollmannsberger C, Nguyen Chi K. First- and second-line chemotherapy with docetaxel or mitoxantrone in patients with hormone-refractory prostate cancer: does sequence matter? Cancer 2006;106:1041–6.

35. Hart L, Ciuleanu T, Hainsworth J et al. Randomized Phase 11 Trial of irofulven (IROF)/prednisone(P), IROF/ Capecitabine(C)/P or mitoxantrone (M)/P in docetaxel pretreated hormone refractory prostate cancer (HRPC) patients. J clin Oncol 2006;24(18S pt):Abstract 14513.

Chapter 12
Docetaxel

Courtney K. Phillips and Daniel P. Petrylak

Abstract Despite the widespread use of prostate-specific antigen (PSA) for prostate cancer screening, many patients still present with or develop evidence of progressive, metastatic, or recurrent disease. First-line treatment for these patients has long been androgen deprivation therapy (ADT). Initial ADT usually consists of medical or surgical castration, but these agents fail in a median of 18–24 months, as patients develop castration-resistant prostate cancer (CRPC). Treatment options at this point in disease progression traditionally provided palliation only. Secondary hormonal manipulations can produce PSA responses, and the standard chemotherapy combination of mitoxantrone and prednisone can ameliorate symptoms but neither approach ever produced better survival than prednisone alone. Docetaxel-based chemotherapy is the first treatment regimen demonstrated to increase survival in patients with CRPC. The exact timing of treatment in the spectrum of CRPC and duration of docetaxel therapy remains controversial. This chapter reviews the use of docetaxel in prostate cancer, discusses the optimal timing of chemotherapy, and highlights the future directions in taxane-combination therapy involving novel investigational uses.

Keywords Docetaxel • Chemotherapy • Survival • Castration-resistant prostate cancer

Introduction

Approximately 186,320 were diagnosed with prostate cancer in the USA in 2008, and another 28,660 men died of their disease, making prostate cancer the most common malignancy in men and the second leading cause of cancer-related deaths in men [1]. Due to prostate-specific antigen (PSA) screening, the vast majority of patients are diagnosed while the disease is still clinically localized. These patients have a number of therapeutic options available depending on risk factors and life expectancy, including radical prostatectomy (open, laparoscopic, or robotic), external beam radiation with or without androgen deprivation, brachytherapy, active surveillance, and watchful waiting. Additionally, ablative technologies, such as high-intensity focused ultrasound (HIFU) and cryoablation, are being utilized in select patients at specialty centers.

Despite the widespread use of PSA screening, many patients still present with or develop evidence of progressive, metastatic, or recurrent disease. First-line treatment for these patients has long been androgen deprivation therapy (ADT). Initial ADT usually consists of medical or surgical castration [2], but these agents fail in a median of 18–24 months, as patients develop castration-resistant prostate cancer (CRPC) [3]. Treatment options at this point in disease progression traditionally provided palliation only. Secondary hormonal manipulations can produce PSA responses, and the standard chemotherapy combination of mitoxantrone and prednisone can ameliorate symptoms but neither approach ever produced better survival than prednisone alone [4, 5]. Two randomized trials published in 2004 demonstrated that docetaxel therapy improved survival in men with CRPC, changing

D.P. Petrylak (✉)
Division of Medical Oncology, Columbia University Medical Center, New York, NY

W.D. Figg et al. (eds.), *Drug Management of Prostate Cancer*,
DOI 10.1007/978-1-60327-829-4_12, © Springer Science+Business Media, LLC 2010

the paradigm that chemotherapy is both toxic and ineffective. This chapter reviews the use of docetaxel in prostate cancer and reviews novel investigational uses.

Initial Studies of Taxane-Based Therapy in Prostate Cancer

Paclitaxel, derived from the bark of the Pacific yew tree (*Taxus brevifolia*) stabilizes microtubules and prevents depolymerization, resulting in cell cycle arrest in $\sigma_2 m$ [6–8]. Early clinical studies utilizing paclitaxel in advanced, drug-resistant ovarian, breast, and non-small cell lung cancers demonstrated promising activity [9]. Initial trials utilizing single-agent paclitaxel for CRPC, however, did not demonstrate significant efficacy. In an ECOG phase II trial, paclitaxel was administered every 3 weeks to 23 patients with bidimensionally measurable CRPC [10]. Of the 23 patients, only 21 were evaluable due to two early trial deaths. There were no patients who experienced a complete response and only one patient experienced a 9-month partial response. Of the remaining 20 patients, 11 had stable disease, whereas another 9 patients progressed despite treatment. Overall median survival was only 9 months, with two deaths from drug toxicity. Though the authors acknowledge that their inclusion criteria selected patients with extremely advanced and aggressive disease, these results initially discouraged further investigation of taxanes in CRPC.

Despite initial poor single-agent activity, attempts to utilize paclitaxel for CRPC were revisited when preclinical studies demonstrated that the addition of estramustine to paclitaxel or vinblastine resulted in increased anticancer activity in vitro [11, 12]. The results of three clinical trials utilizing estramustine and vinblastine showed PSA response rates of 34–54% and a 31% partial response rate [13–15]. Phase I dose escalation studies examining the efficacy of the paclitaxel-estramustine combination utilized a 96-h continuous infusion of paclitaxel with daily oral estramustine [16]. Using the established dose of 120 mg/m² of paclitaxel, phase II studies utilizing the 96-h infusion strategy showed greater activity with the drug combination than with either single agent alone [10, 17]. Another phase I study of weekly paclitaxel established the maximal tolerated dose (MTD) of paclitaxel at 60–107 mg/m²; however, the estramustine used in this protocol produced

a 33% rate of discontinuation of therapy due to thrombotic or gastrointestinal toxicity [18].

Docetaxel, synthesized from the rapidly renewable leaves of the *Taxus baccata* tree, also possesses potent antimitotic activity [19–21]. When compared to paclitaxel, docetaxel has significantly longer absorption coupled with slower efflux [22]. It is clinically active against several malignancies including anthracycline-resistant advanced breast cancer, non-small cell lung cancer, ovarian cancer, and pancreatic cancer. The dose-limiting toxicity of docetaxel is neutropenia, and side effects such as fluid retention can be adequately managed with steroid premedication. An additional benefit is that, unlike paclitaxel, docetaxel does not need to be administered in cremophor.

Preclinical studies revealed that in vitro, docetaxel was cytotoxic to androgen-dependent LnCAP cells as well as androgen-independent PC-3, and DU145 cells. Docetaxel also appeared to be more active than paclitaxel and could be effectively combined with other agents [23, 24]. This compelling evidence laid enough groundwork to justify clinical trials examining the efficacy of docetaxel for CRPC. In stark contrast to the ECOG single-agent paclitaxel study, a single-agent docetaxel study showed significant activity in CRPC [25]. In this study, 35 patients received a median of six doses of docetaxel administered at 75 mg/m² every 3 weeks. A total of 20% of patients experienced a PSA decrease of greater than 80%, while 46% had >50% decrease in PSA. Of the 25 patients with measurable disease, there was one complete response, three near complete responses, and three partial responses with a median response rate of 9 months. The overall survival was 27 months.

Phase I studies demonstrated that estramustine could be combined with docetaxel. A study by Petrylak et al. combined estramustine 280-mg PO TID for 5 days with escalating doses of docetaxel. The recommended phase II dose of docetaxel combined with estramustine was 70 mg/m² as in minimally pretreated patients and 60 mg/m² in extensively pretreated patients [26]. The dose-limiting toxicities were primarily hematologic. There was a 63% overall rate of ≥50% PSA decline while 28% of the patients with bidimensionally measurable disease experienced a partial response to treatment. The median survival was of 22.8 months, with 21% of patients surviving more than 30 months. Kreis and colleagues' phase I study of docetaxel and estramustine also established 70 mg/m² as the MTD for phase II studies [27]. In this study, 82% of patients experienced a PSA decrease of more than 50% and there was one soft tissue partial response. A phase II study at Columbia University Medical Center treated 31 chemotherapy naïve patients with estramustine three times daily on days 1–5 of a 21-day cycle along with docetaxel 70 mg/m^2 on day 2 [28]. The most serious side effects were vascular and included three deep venous thromboses. The most commonly observed grade 3 and 4 adverse events were neutropenia and fatigue. At the time of publication 18 of the phase II patients were evaluable for response. Of these, 84% had PSA declines of ≥50% while 61% had PSA declines of more than 75%. These results were supported by a phase II study in the CALGB (Cancer and Leukemia Group B) combining docetaxel, estramustine, and hydrocortisone [29]. In this study, there was a 3% complete response rate and a 20% partial response rate. A total of 69% of patients experienced a ≥50% decline in PSA while 54% had a decrease of 75% or more, all with manageable toxicity. These studies provided the rationale for evaluating single-agent and combination docetaxel therapy in two large phase III studies.

TAX 327

TAX 327 was an international, randomized, open-label phase III study comparing two schedules of docetaxel plus prednisone to mitoxantrone plus prednisone for the treatment of metastatic CRPC [30]. To qualify for inclusion, patients were required to have evidence of disease progression while on ADT and were not permitted to have received prior radioisotope treatment. Patients who had received any chemotherapy other than estramustine and corticosteroids were also excluded, and all patients were withdrawn from antiandrogens. Patients were randomized to one of three arms. The first group (D3P) received docetaxel 75 mg/m^2 every 3 weeks with prednisone 5 mg twice daily (up to ten cycles); the second group (D1P) received docetaxel 30 mg/m^2 weekly with prednisone 5 mg twice daily (up to five cycles of 6 weeks each); and the third group (MP) received mitoxantrone 12 mg/m^2 every 3 weeks with prednisone 5 mg twice daily (up to ten cycles). The primary endpoint of this study was overall survival while secondary endpoints included serum PSA decrease

of at least 50%, objective tumor response, improvement in quality of life scores, and decrease in pain.

A total of 1,006 patients were randomized into the study. Baseline characteristics between the groups were similar. In the initial 2004 report, the median follow-up was 20.8 months for patients receiving docetaxel every 3 weeks, and 20.7 months for patients in the other two groups. Overall median survival was 18.9 months for D3P patients, which differed significantly from the 16.5-month survival seen in the MP arm ($p = 0.009$). There was no significant difference in survival between MP and D1P patients (median survival 17.4 months, $p = 0.36$). A multivariate analysis revealed that visceral involvement, high baseline alkaline phosphatase, anemia and, on post-hoc analysis, Gleason grade 8–10 were negative prognostic factors.

Pain reduction occurred more frequently in the D3P arm than the MP arm (35% vs. 22%, respectively, $p = 0.01$). Thirty-one percent of patients in the weekly docetaxel group reported palliation of pain symptoms; this was not significantly different from either of the other two groups. Both docetaxel arms had significantly higher rates of PSA response (45% for the D3P group, 48% for the D1P group; $p < 0.001$) than the mitoxantrone arm (32%). Neither the median duration of PSA response (7.7–8.2 months) nor the change in volume of soft tissue disease varied significantly between any of the groups.

Only 815 patients could be evaluated for quality of life changes because the FACT-P questionnaire was not available in all patients' languages. In this intent-to-treat analysis, a quality of life response was defined as a 16-point improvement from baseline on two surveys administered at least 3 weeks apart. Only 13% of MP patients reported quality of life response. This was significantly less than both the D3P and D1P arms, in which 22% ($p = 0.009$) and 23% ($p = 0.005$) of patients, respectively, reported improvements. In a subset analysis, patients receiving docetaxel exhibited the greatest improvement in factors directly related to the prostate.

The overall incidence of grade 3 and 4 neutropenia was low for all three study arms: the incidence was higher in the D3P group (3%) than the D1P group (0%) and the mitoxantrone group (0.9%). Two patients died of sepsis: one in a docetaxel group and one in the mitoxantrone group. No patients received concomitant colony stimulating factors. Deterioration of cardiac function was significantly higher in the mitoxantrone group; however, patients receiving docetaxel on either schedule had higher rates of one or more serious adverse events (26% and 29%, respectively) than patients receiving mitoxantrone (20%). Despite this, three of the five deaths, which were likely to be treatment related, were in the mitoxantrone group.

In October 2006, a follow-up survival analysis was performed [31]. Median survival times were not significantly different from the initial report, and D3P continued to demonstrate a survival benefit over mitoxantrone-based therapies ($p=0.004$). Median survival times were 19.2 months in the D3P arm, 17.8 months in the D1P arm, and 16.3 months in the MP arm. Three-year survival rates were significantly higher in DP1-treated patients (17.2%) than in mitoxantrone-treated patients (12.8%) ($p=0.005$). A subset analysis showed that this survival benefit persisted in men both above and below the age of 65 years, as well as those who did and did not have baseline pain symptoms and those who had baseline PSA's above and below the median PSA value of 115 ng/ml.

An additional analysis of patients who crossed over from docetaxel-based treatment to mitoxantrone-based treatment and vice versa was also reported [32]. There were 89 D3P patients and 76 D1P patients who crossed over to the MP group. Another 68 patients crossed over from mitoxantrone-based therapy to docetaxel-based therapies, schedules of which were varied and/or unspecified. Though there were no significant differences in performance status between groups in the initial study, men who crossed over from docetaxel to mitoxantrone had lower Karnofsky performance scores, higher pain scores, and higher serum alkaline phosphatase and PSA levels than patients crossing from mitoxantrone to docetaxel. The median follow-up after cross over was 11 months, and the median survival for patients crossing in either direction was 10 months. PSA data after cross over was available for 96 patients. After cross over, 9.8, 22.2, and 28% of patients starting in the D3P, D1P, and MP group, respectively, experienced a 50% or greater reduction in PSA. Any degree of PSA reduction was experienced in 34, 37, and 72% of patients, respectively; however, the overall median PSA progression-free survival (PFS) was brief (3.2, 3.7, and 5.9 months, respectively). The authors did not find a correlation between response to first-line chemotherapy and response to second-line chemotherapy though they acknowledged that their sample sizes were too small for such an analysis. A phase II study examining men given D3P after progression on mitoxantrone and prednisone has since been reported [33]. Though small, this study reported that more than 60% of men

had a reduction in pain and 57% of men experienced a PSA decrease of at least 50%. Median PFS was 5 months, and median overall survival was 15 months.

One of the more puzzling outcomes of TAX 327 was the discrepancy seen between the D3P and D1P administration schedules. It is known that docetaxel clearance is affected by liver function, body surface area, age, and CYP3A4 function [34], and, consistent with the TAX 327 results, it has been found that weekly administration schedules often have lower rates of adverse events, particularly myelosuppression [35]. What is important to remember, however, about the TAX 327 trial, is that the study was not powered or designed to compare the D3P and D1P arms. As such, it is impossible to compare the two to each other [36]. Despite the fact that weekly docetaxel did not result in increased survival, there was a significant improvement in quality of life, pain response and PSA response over mitoxantrone-based therapies.

SWOG 99-16

SWOG Intergroup protocol 99-16 (SWOG 99-16) was a multicenter, randomized, nonblinded clinical trial published at the same time as TAX 327 [37]. Based on the synergistic anticancer effects of estramustine and docetaxel in vitro [24], as well as phase I and II trials examining docetaxel in men [28], SWOG 99-16 was designed to compare docetaxel and estramustine (DE) with mitoxantrone and prednisone (MP). Both regimens were administered in 21-day cycles. Estramustine 280 mg was given three times a day on days 1–5; 60 mg/m^2 of docetaxel was given on day 2 with dexamethasone pretreatment. Patients recruited after January 15, 2001 also received warfarin (2 mg daily) and aspirin 325 mg daily, after a report showed that this regimen would decrease thrombotic events. Patients in the MP arm received 12 mg/m^2 of mitoxantrone on day 1 and prednisone 5 mg twice daily. Doses were escalated to 70 mg/m^2 of docetaxel or 14 mg/m^2 of mitoxantrone if there were no grade 3 or 4 adverse events in the first cycle. Patients were eligible for inclusion in this study if they had biochemical or radiologic progression of metastatic CRPC. As with the TAX 327 study, patients who had received radioisotopes were ineligible, and antiandrogens were discontinued. Patients were, however, still eligible if they had received one prior systemic therapy as long as that therapy was stopped more than 4 weeks prior and did not include estramustine, anthracyclines, mitoxantrone, or taxanes. The primary endpoint of SWOG 99-16 was overall survival while PFS, objective response rates, and PSA decreases of 50% or more were secondary endpoints. A total of 770 patients were enrolled into this study; 96 patients were subsequently found to be ineligible, primarily due to inadequate antiandrogen withdrawal. The baseline characteristics of the 674 eligible patients were similar in all study arms. Patients were followed for a median of 32 months. In that time, 64% of the patients in the DE group and 70% of the patients in the MP group died. In an intent-to-treat analysis, the median survival for docetaxel patients was significantly longer than mitoxantrone patients (17.5 months vs. 15.6 months, $p = 0.02$). The median time to progression was significantly longer in the DE group (6.3 months) than in the MP group (3.2 months, $p < 0.001$). Additionally, while 50% of patients receiving docetaxel had PSA decreases of at least 50%, only 27% of patients receiving mitoxantrone exhibited this decrease ($p < 0.001$). There was no significant difference in measurable disease response.

Over the course of the study, docetaxel resulted in significantly higher rates of neutropenic fevers, cardiovascular events, nausea and vomiting, metabolic alterations, and neurologic events. There were no significant differences in rates of grade 3–5 neutropenia between the groups. There were eight deaths attributed to docetaxel treatment and four related to mitoxantrone.

Quality of life and pain scores for patients in SWOG 99-16 were reported in 2006 [38]. SWOG 99-16 utilized the McGill Pain Questionnaire's Present Pain Intensity scale as well as the European Organization for Research and Treatment of Cancer Core Quality of Life Questionnaire C30. Unlike TAX 327, there were no significant differences in pain or quality of life scores between the two SWOG 99-16 study arms.

Clinical Implications of TAX 327 and SWOG 99-16

SWOG 99-16 and TAX 327 were the first trials to demonstrate the survival benefit of taxane-based chemotherapy for CRPC. Though it remains unclear why weekly docetaxel did not result in the same survival benefit as docetaxel administered every 3 weeks, it is clear that therapy with docetaxel represents a significant improvement over mitoxantrone-based therapy. What

remains unclear, however, is whether docetaxel is more effective when administered with prednisone or estramustine. The agent administered with docetaxel may impact pain and quality of life more than the docetaxel itself, explaining the discrepancy between the two trials, and a direct comparison of SWOG 99-16 and TAX 327 has too many confounding factors to be valid [39]. Today, a clinical trial comparing estramustine and prednisone is unlikely to be conducted because agents less toxic than estramustine have been introduced in the interim. Additionally, because patients both with and without pain and measurable disease were included, it is not yet clear at what point in disease progression patients are most likely to benefit from taxane-based therapy. Only when more specific markers of response become available can optimal treatment timing be studied.

Optimal Timing of Chemotherapy

While the utility of docetaxel for CRPC is clear, the point in disease progression that it should be administered is controversial. Because SWOG 99-16 and TAX 327 included both symptomatic and asymptomatic patients, the question of the optimal timing of chemotherapy administration was not addressed by either study. There are two main questions that arise regarding the appropriate timing of cytotoxic therapy. First, can cytotoxic therapy prevent or delay the progression from androgen-sensitive prostate cancer to CRPC? And secondly, should cytotoxic chemotherapy be administered as soon as there is evidence of CRPC or once disease becomes symptomatic? [3].

To date, the evidence supporting the hypothesis that cytotoxic therapy can prevent the development of CRPC is primarily preclinical. Whether hormone insensitive cells exist prior to androgen ablation or develop soon thereafter is unclear. What is apparent is that soon after ADT is initiated, cells resistant to apoptosis become predominant. The molecular mechanisms behind this are thought to be largely regulated by the ratios of bax, a proapoptotic protein, and bcl-2, an antiapoptotic protein [40]. In rat castration models, it has been shown that immediately after androgen deprivation, the ratio of bax to bcl-2 increases, favoring apoptosis [41]. A few days later, however, this ratio rapidly reverses implying that cells resistant to apoptosis are increasing in number. In LnCaP xenograft models, mice that received paclitaxel and castration simultaneously fared better than those that received sequential therapy [42]. Mice in this study that were castrated after cytotoxic therapy had much poorer outcomes. This is in contrast to an SCID mouse line injected with LnCaP cells; the mice receiving docetaxel prior to castration developed the smallest tumors [43]. To date, there has been only one human study done to address this question [44]. In 2005, Hussain and colleagues published their experience administering docetaxel every 3 weeks (up to six cycles) to 39 men who had experienced a biochemical recurrence after primary therapy. Of the men enrolled, 32 initially had PSA-only recurrence while the remaining 7 also had clinical evidence of metastasis. All of these men had noncastrate testosterone levels. All men received docetaxel and 33 went on to receive 4–12 months of complete androgen blockade with subsequent peripheral androgen blockade. After treatment with docetaxel, the median PSA was 5.7 ng/ml and 48.5% had a ≥50% decrease in PSA while 20% had a ≥75% decrease. With total androgen blockade, all patients achieved completely castrate levels of testosterone with a median PSA of 0.1 ng/ml. After peripheral androgen blockade, PSA remained at 0.1 ng/ml. Median time from end of treatment to the last follow-up for the 33 patients who had received androgen ablation was 26 months. After a median of 2.3 months, 28 of the 33 men's PSA rose to a median of 0.41 ng/ml, whereas 5 others remained at a stable 0.1 ng/ml. Three of these five patients had started off with clinical evidence of metastatic disease.

Contrary to the body of work done on androgen-dependent prostate cancer, there has been little research done to determine the optimal timing of docetaxel in CRPC. Generally speaking, cytotoxic therapy can be initiated when the PSA first rises on ADT, when radiologic evidence of metastatic disease develops, or when patients become symptomatic. The vast majority of chemotherapy trials have included both symptomatic and asymptomatic patients as well as those with bone metastasis only and bidimensionally measurable disease. A small phase III trial conducted by Berry and coworkers examined the impact of mitoxantrone and prednisone vs. prednisone alone in patients with asymptomatic CRPC [45]. Though the addition of mitoxantrone in these patients increased median time to progression and the percent of patients achieving a PSA response, mitoxantrone did not result in an overall survival benefit and the impact of early treatment could not be assessed. About 19% of the patients enrolled in

SWOG 99-16 and 21% of the patients enrolled in TAX 327 had asymptomatic CRPC without evidence of metastasis [3, 27, 30]. A subgroup analysis of asymptomatic TAX 327 patients revealed that these patients derived the same survival benefit from docetaxel as the group overall [46, 47]. When Oudard and coworkers retrospectively examined patients with metastatic CRPC who had received chemotherapy, they did find a significant difference in survival between patients with PSA doubling times above and below 45 days [48]. Patients with metastatic disease, however, are a very heterogeneous group, and it still remains unclear which patients within this subgroup may derive the most benefit from early cytotoxic intervention.

Future Directions in Taxane-Combination Therapy

Antiangiogenesis Agents

It has long been known that tumors cannot proliferate without developing neovasculature to support this growth [49]. Angiogenesis has therefore been an attractive target of antitumor therapies. Early on in taxane studies, it was noted that the taxanes have direct effects on angiogenesis as well. In 2001, Sweeney and colleagues reported that docetaxel inhibited the growth of human umbilical vein endothelial cells (HUVEC) [50]. This inhibition was temporized when vascular endothelial growth factor (VEGF) or basic fibroblast growth factor (bFGF) was added to the HUVEC culture medium. The effect of VEGF and bFGF was reversed by a soluble recombinant human monoclonal antibody to VEGF (rhuMAb-VEGF). Similar results were found in in vivo Matrigel models: docetaxel was able to directly inhibit angiogenesis, and while this effect was abrogated by the addition of VEGF and bFGF, rhuMAb-VEGF was able to restore antiangiogenesis activity.

This study, along with others demonstrating that cyclophosphamide, vinblastine, paclitaxel, and docetaxel have antiangiogenic properties in vivo, sets the stage for clinical trials combining targeted antiangiogenic agents with these cytotoxic agents [51]. Moreover, the correlation of elevated serum levels of VEGF with poor prognosis in men with CRPC further justified targeting angiogenesis in these patients. Monoclonal antibodies, which bind VEGF, are currently under evaluation in combination with docetaxel chemotherapy in men with CRPC. Picus et al. treated 79 men with CRPC with docetaxel 70 mg/m^2 every 3 weeks, estramustine 280-mg PO TID for 5 days, and bevacizumab 15 mg/kg day 2 [25]. The 23-month median survival reported in this study supported the design of a phase III study in the CALGB comparing docetaxel 75 mg/m^2 every 3 weeks, prednisone 5-mg PO twice daily, and bevacizumab 15 mg/kg IV on day 1 every 3 weeks with docetaxel combined with prednisone. A second trial evaluated the combination of bevacizumab and docetaxel in patients who exhibited disease progression on docetaxel. This phase II study of heavily pretreated patients administered bevacizumab 10 mg/kg and docetaxel 60 mg/m^2 every 3 weeks [52]. All of the 20 patients had bone metastasis and 8 had bidimensionally measurable disease. Of those treated, 11 (55%) exhibited major PSA responses and 3 had objective responses. Of the 11 patients exhibiting major PSA responses, 4 had not had any PSA response to docetaxel alone. Aflibercept (VEGF Trap), a protein constructed to include the extracellular domains of human VEGF receptor 1 and 2 fused to the constant region (Fc) of human IgG1 antibody, functions as a soluble decoy receptor that effectively binds VEGF-A. The VENICE trial, employing a similar design to the CALGB study, compares docetaxel combined with prednisone and aflibercept 6 mg/kg IV to docetaxel and prednisone. It is designed to detect an improvement in median survival from 19 to 23 months.

Immunomodulators (IMiDs), such as thalidomide and lenolidamide, are currently being evaluated in combination with docetaxel. In addition to antiangiogenic effects, IMiDs also possess immunomodulatory and anti-inflammatory activity. Preclinical studies have demonstrated that lenalidomide both alone and in combination with docetaxel significantly increases apoptosis in PC-3 cells [53]. A phase I study looking at low-dose metronomic therapy combination of docetaxel and thalidomide concluded that the MTD was thalidomide 100 mg twice daily and docetaxel 25 mg/m^2 weekly [54]. To further evaluate this combination, a randomized phase II study designed by Figg et al. compared weekly docetaxel to the combination of docetaxel and thalidomide. Although the primary endpoint of this trial was to evaluate the increase in toxicity of adding thalidomide to docetaxel, and not to detect a survival difference, the reported median survival of 28.9 months for docetaxel combined with thalidomide is the highest median survival reported for a phase II study to date.

More recently, another phase II trial evaluated the combination of thalidomide 200 mg daily, docetaxel 75 mg/m^2 every 3 weeks, and bevacizumab 15 mg/kg every 3 weeks [55]. All 60 patients were chemotherapy naïve. A total of 41 patients experienced PSA declines of >80%, and 51 patients had PSA declines of >50%. In patients with measurable disease, there were 2 complete responses, 18 partial responses, 11 stable diseases, and 1 progressive disease for an overall response rate of 63%. The estimated PFS was 18.2 months. Five patients experienced febrile neutropenia, five experienced syncope, three had gastrointestinal perforation or fistula formation, three developed thrombosis, and two had grade 3 bleeding.

Sorafenib and sunitinib are multi-tyrosine kinase inhibitors that act on pathways, which regulate cell division, survival, and apoptosis. Their antiangiogenic properties come from their affinity for VEGF receptors. Though both drugs are already approved and indicated for other solid malignancies, testing of these agents in prostate cancer has just begun. Sunitinib alone and in combination has been shown to inhibit growth in both DU-145 and PC-3 prostate cancer xenografts [56, 57]. In a preliminary report of an ongoing phase II study of sunitinib, docetaxel, and prednisone in patients with metastatic CRPC, 5 of the 18 evaluable patients have discontinued the study [58]. Thus far, there is a 50% PSA response rate, and 39% of the patients with measurable disease have had partial responses. An additional 54% have stable disease. Currently, phase II studies are also underway examining the efficacy of docetaxel and sorafenib, while sunitinib is being studied as first-line chemotherapy in combination with prednisone and docetaxel and as second-line chemotherapy after progression on docetaxel [59].

Calcitriol Combination Therapy

Calcitriol (1,25-dihydrocholecalciferol, 1,25(OH)$_2$-D$_3$) is a biologically active form of vitamin D with known activity against a number of malignancies. Preclinical studies have demonstrated that calcitriol is able to inhibit the mitogenesis of prostate cancer cell lines, and combination studies performed in vitro and in vivo have confirmed that it enhances the antitumor effects of paclitaxel [60–62]. Though relatively safe, the dose-limiting toxicity of calcitriol is hypercalcemia. A formulation of calcitriol, DN-101, has been created to overcome this limitation. DN-101 is designed to be administered in pulsed weekly doses, which prevents much of its adverse affects. After a single institution phase II trial demonstrated promising results using weekly pulsed calcitriol and docetaxel [63], a second double-blinded, randomized trial, the Androgen Insensitive Prostate Cancer Study of Calcitriol Enhancing Taxotere (ASCENT) trial was conducted [64]. This study compared treatment with docetaxel and placebo with docetaxel and DN-101. The primary endpoint of the trial was proportion of patients experiencing at least a 50% reduction in serum PSA. Overall survival, decrease in measurable disease, safety, and tolerability as well as PSA, tumor, and clinical PFS were secondary outcomes. The median follow-up was 18.3 months. There was no significant difference between the two groups in primary endpoint ($p=0.16$), skeletal morbidity-free survival ($p=0.13$), or measurable disease ($p=0.51$). A survival analysis performed after adjusting for differences in hemoglobin and ECOG performance status, however, demonstrated that patients receiving docetaxel and DN-101 had an improvement in survival when compared to the docetaxel placebo group ($p=0.04$). At the time of analysis, median survival in the placebo group was 16.4 months, and median survival in the DN-101 group, though not met, was estimated to be 24.5 months. Additionally, gastrointestinal toxicity and incidence of deep venous thrombosis (DVT) was significantly lower in the DN-101 arm (9.6% vs. 2.4% and 7.2% vs. 1.5%, respectively). The difference in the incidence of DVT, while not fully understood, is potentially due to reductions in the procoagulant known as tissue factor [39]. ASCENT II, a phase III study comparing D3P to weekly docetaxel combined with DN-101/ D1P, was terminated early due to an increased death rate observed on the experimental arm. Since these findings have yet to be presented or published, the reason for the increased death rate is unknown.

Bone-Targeted Therapies

Osteoblastic bone metastases are a devastating hallmark of prostate cancer. Because bone metastases and the resulting symptoms have a deleterious impact on quality of life and result in serious complications, bone-targeted therapies have garnered tremendous interest, particularly in combination with docetaxel. The endothelin axis is a signaling cascade pivotal to a number of processes including mitogenesis, pain, survival, vasoconstriction, and bone homeostasis [65, 66]. Ligand binding to one of the endothelin receptors ($ET_{A(alpha)}$ or $ET_{B(beta)}$) results in bone-matrix formation as well as proliferation, invasion, and evasion of apoptosis. One of the bone-targeted agents most actively being studied is atrasentan. Atrasentan is an orally bioavailable inhibitor of endothelin ligand-$1_{A(alpha)}$ (ET-$1_{A(alpha)}$). In preclinical and clinical trials, atrasentan has been shown to downregulate bone formation, mitosis, angiogenesis, and pain signaling [67]. Atrasentan has been studied as a single agent in several studies. The M96-594 trial compared two doses of atrasentan (10 mg and 2.5 mg) to placebo. Although atrasentan resulted in a significant improvement in time to progression and survival when compared to placebo, when an intent-to-treat analysis was performed, this difference was no longer observed [68]. There were, however, promising improvements in serum alkaline phosphatase and PSA. A follow-up study, M00-211, was performed comparing 10 mg of atrasentan to placebo in men with CRPC and asymptomatic metastatic disease. While there was no significant difference in time to disease progression in the two arms, the subset of men with bone metastasis only disease did experience a significant improvement in serum parameters and quality of life measurements. Since then, preclinical studies have supported the combined use of atrasentan and docetaxel [69], and a phase I/II study has demonstrated its safety in humans. A trial is currently being conducted in SWOG comparing docetaxel and prednisone to docetaxel, prednisone, and atrasentan [39].

Like atrasentan and the endothelin axis, RANK (receptor activator of NF-κB) ligand and the osteoprotegerin pathway, first garnered interest because of its role in bone homeostasis. This axis was soon recognized to be pivotal in inflammation and the development of metastases. In 2007, Luo and coworkers demonstrated that a mutation, which prevented phosphorylation of the inhibitor of NF-κB kinase α (IκB kinase α or IKKα), increased the sequestration and destruction of NF-κB. Clinically, this mutation delayed and prevented the development of prostate cancer metastases via maspin, a known metastasis suppressor [70, 71]. When the RANK ligand inhibitor osteoprotegerin-Fc was coadministered with docetaxel to murine bone metastasis cancer models, survival time was significantly increased and skeletal tumor burden was significantly decreased [72]. A clinical study is underway comparing denosumab (a RANK ligand inhibitor) and zoledronic acid for the treatment of patients with CaP metastases to the bone [59].

Bortezomib is a dipeptide boronic acid, which also acts on the NF-κB pathway [73]. At the molecular level, bortezomib reversibly inhibits the 26S proteosome, which is responsible for destroying IκB kinase α. Like docetaxel, bortezomib can also downregulate bcl-2 expression. However, unlike docetaxel, bortezomib arrests cells in G1 and G2, whereas docetaxel-treated cells arrest at σ_2m [73, 74]. In vivo, the combination of bortezomib and docetaxel has been shown to alter bcl-2 and bcl-xL expression and sensitize cell lines to radiation. In phase I and II trials, single-agent bortezomib has had effect on CRPC [75, 76]. Subsequently, a phase I/II study demonstrated that, in combination with 40 mg/m^2 docetaxel, 1.6 mg/m^2 of bortezomib was safe and tolerable and demonstrated antitumor activity [73].

Vaccine-Taxane Therapy

Vaccine-based therapies are one of the most promising, but technically challenging, classes of agents. The theoretical advantage of vaccine therapy is that the use of the body's own immune system may potentially avoid many of the side effects caused by chemotherapy. Logistically, however, the identification and creation of effective vaccines has been difficult. Antigens must be identified and expressed in a quantity adequate to mount an immune response. The vaccine must be delivered in such a way that it comes in contact with the antigen, and this response must be maintained but cannot incite other more toxic reactions. Several vaccines have been created and tested in malignant diseases. Among these are the carbohydrate and glycoprotein vaccines, which use "self" antigens, such as PSA, MUC-1, and PSMA, to induce a T-cell response directed against the tumor. These vaccines, however, often produce a limited response. Recombinant virus vaccines are much more immunogenic. Recombinant fowlpox expressing PSA (rF-PSA) and recombinant *Vaccinia virus* expressing PSA (rV-PSA) were studied in a randomized phase II study (E7897) in the adjuvant setting after patients were treated for clinically localized disease [77]. Patients were vaccinated four times with one of the two vaccines in varying sequences. Patients receiving one rV-PSA vaccination followed by three vaccinations of rF-PSA, in a "vaccinia prime – avipox boost" strategy, had a significant increase in PSA PFS, supporting the importance of chronology in vaccine administration. In an update of this study after a median of 50 months of follow-up, patients in the prime-boost arm experienced an 18.2 month median time to progression while patients in the other two arms (three rF-PSA vaccinations vs. three rF-PSA vaccinations followed by a single rV-PSA vaccination) progressed at a median of 9.2 and 9.1 months, respectively [78].

Inciting T-cell immune reactions is a complex process requiring initial antigen presentation via the MHC molecule. A second co-stimulatory molecule, such as B7.1, presented by an antigen-presenting cell (APC) is also required. Because of this, a phase II study in metastatic CRPC patients utilizing a prime-boost vaccination scheme coadministered with a recombinant virus expressing a co-stimulatory molecule was performed [79]. This regimen was compared to another arm receiving the same vaccinations and docetaxel. Twenty-eight patients were ultimately randomized into this study and no patient receiving vaccinations only experienced more than a grade 2 toxicity. PSA-specific T cells were upregulated 3.33-fold in both study arms as determined by ELISPOT assay. Interestingly, the immune response did not remain antigen specific. T cells recognizing other prostate cancer specific antigens were also identified after vaccination. Serum PSA declines were modest in both scope and degree (3/14 patients in the vaccine only arm and 6/14 in the vaccine/docetaxel arm). Although the study was not powered to detect differences in PFS, patients receiving only vaccine had a median PFS of 1.8 months, while patients receiving combination therapy had a median PFS of 3.2 months. Thus, as newer vaccines are developed, the use of docetaxel is likely to continue, especially because unlike other chemotherapy agents, such as cyclophosphamide, docetaxel does not inhibit the function of T-regulatory cells but does enhance CD8+ response to CD3 binding [80]. Since prolonged activation of the immune system may result from vaccines, the sequence of chemotherapy and immunotherapy must be considered in clinical trial design.

Docetaxel and Prostatectomy

Though there are many treatment options for men diagnosed with localized prostate cancer, the vast majority undergo surgical resection or radiation; despite the fact that the disease is localized at the time of presentation, approximately 30–40% of patients undergoing prostatectomy will have a PSA recurrence within 10 years of surgery [81]. There have been multiple studies examining the effect of both neoadjuvant and adjuvant treatments on outcomes; however, to date, this approach is considered investigational [82–85].

Several phase I/II studies have looked at the safety of docetaxel alone or in combination as neoadjuvant treatment for patients with high-risk prostate cancer undergoing prostatectomy [86–90]. Though docetaxel dosing schedules and the duration of treatment have varied, these studies have found that neoadjuvant docetaxel is safe and well tolerated and does not result in any additional surgical complications. All studies demonstrated a certain degree of preoperative PSA reduction though there were few to no complete pathologic responses noted after prostatectomy. To date, the largest study published has been a multi-institutional phase II study, which coadministered docetaxel ($35\ \text{mg/m}^2$ weekly for 6 out of 8 weeks for three doses) with combined androgen deprivation prior to prostatectomy [91]. A total of 72 high-risk patients were treated though four did not complete the protocol due to toxicity (two hypersensitivity reactions and two pneumonitides). Ultimately 64 patients underwent prostatectomy after completing neoadjuvant treatment. There were two postoperative complications: one postoperative myocardial infarction and one DVT. On pathology, four patients had regional lymph node involvement, and 275 had positive margins. Two patients were downstaged to pT0. At a median follow-up of 42.7 months, 30% of patients had a PSA recurrence; median PSA recurrence-free survival (RFS) had not yet been met at the time of publication. Though, on univariate analysis, Gleason score and pathologic stage were associated with PSA RFS, while on multivariate analysis, only Gleason score remained significant. Three patients died of their disease, two of whom had positive nodes at the time of surgery. A phase III, multi-institutional study, PUNCH (Preoperative Use of Neoadjuvant ChemoHormonal Therapy, CALGB 90203) by the Cancer and Leukemia Group B is currently underway and is comparing the impact of neoadjuvant docetaxel and estramustine vs. prostatectomy alone on 5-year PSA RFS [92].

Although several studies have examined the effect of adjuvant radiation and ADT in prostatectomy patients, there is a marked paucity of adjuvant chemotherapy studies despite the known success of adjuvant treatments for non-small cell lung cancer, colon cancer, and breast cancer. Lack of these studies is not due to lack of trial initiation; SWOG 9921 was closed in 2007 after three patients treated with mitoxantrone developed leukemia. TAX 3501 was a study comparing immediate and delayed ADT and six cycles of docetaxel (given every 3 weeks) after prostatectomy. This study, which randomized a total of 228 patients, was closed due to slow accrual [93]. A phase II pilot study, which treated 77 men with six weekly cycles of adjuvant docetaxel, recently reported a 26% grade 3 toxicity rate and a 4% grade 4 toxicity rate [94]. With a median follow-up of 29.2 months, there was a 60.5% rate of progression and a median PFS of 15.7 months. A total of seven patients died with four deaths due to prostate cancer. While these results are interesting, clearly randomized trials are needed. Currently, the VA Cooperative Studies Program Study 553 is the only phase III adjuvant taxane-based chemotherapy study accruing [95].

Docetaxel and Radiation Therapy

Patients with high-risk localized prostate cancer, who are ineligible or do not desire prostatectomy, most often undergo external beam radiation therapy (EBRT). EBRT is routinely administered with both neoadjuvant and adjuvant ADT. Even prior to demonstrating docetaxel's efficacy in prostate cancer, interest in combining taxanes with radiation for other malignancies was evident. These studies largely stemmed from the fact that both docetaxel and EBRT induce cell cycle arrest and apoptosis in the G2 and M phases, and consistent with the hypothesis, preclinical data did suggest that docetaxel may sensitize tissues to the effects of radiation. In murine mammary carcinoma xenograft models, administration of docetaxel 48 h prior to a single dose of radiation enhanced tumor response to radiation by a factor of 2.33 [96]. The effect on normal tissues was minimal.

In humans with localized high-risk disease, a phase I trial of weekly docetaxel administered concomitantly with a total of 70.2 Gy of radiation (fractionated 1.8 Gy daily) demonstrated that 20 mg/m² of docetaxel was the MTD for docetaxel administered with EBRT [97]. The dose-limiting toxicity in this study was grade 3 diarrhea. Four years later, phase I/II data were published [98]. Twenty men were enrolled, 17 of whom were also receiving ADT. The most frequent toxicities were grade 2 diarrhea, fatigue, urinary frequency, and constipation. There were no hematologic toxicities greater than grade 1, and only three patients experienced an interruption in treatment (two for dehydration and one for a nonsteroidal anti-inflammatory drug-induced gastrointestinal bleed). At a median follow-up of 11.7 months, the rate of PFS was 85%.

A third pilot study has since examined the feasibility of aggressive multimodal therapy after prostatectomy [99]. Twenty-eight high-risk prostate cancer patients underwent prostatectomy followed by six cycles of combination chemotherapy (either docetaxel and estramustine or docetaxel and carboplatin), followed by 5 years of ADT. Patients who had pT4 disease or more than one positive margin also received EBRT after chemotherapy. In this study, 20 patients received docetaxel and estramustine while 8 received docetaxel and carboplatin; 7 of the patients also received EBRT. The most frequent major toxicity was grade 3–4 neutropenia in 65% and edema in 30%. Of the patients receiving estramustine, 25% developed DVTs. At a mean follow-up of 31 months, no patient experienced a PSA recurrence, and 93% were free of disease progression. Interestingly, there were two deaths in the cohort, both of whom died of prostate cancer, but neither of whom had PSA relapse. The Radiation Therapy Oncology Group (RTOG) is currently enrolling patients into a randomized phase III study (RTOG 0521), which will compare patients treated with ADT and EBRT to patients receiving six cycles of docetaxel prednisone after EBRT and ADT [100].

Conclusions

Docetaxel-based chemotherapy is the first treatment regimen demonstrated to increase survival in patients with CRPC. The exact timing of treatment in the spectrum of CRPC and duration of docetaxel therapy remains controversial. Ongoing studies are evaluating the optimal combination of docetaxel with targeted therapy to improve survival. Aggressive accrual into randomized, controlled trials should be encouraged in patients with CRPC.

References

1. Jemal A, Siegel R, Ward E, et al. Cancer statistics, 2008. CA: Cancer J Clin 2008;58(2):71–96.
2. Loblaw DA, Virgo KS, Nam R, et al. Initial hormonal management of androgen-sensitive metastatic, recurrent, or progressive prostate cancer: 2006 update of an American Society of Clinical Oncology practice guideline. J Clin Oncol 2007;25(12):1596–605.
3. Lucas A, Petrylak DP. The case for early chemotherapy for the treatment of metastatic disease. J Urol 2006;176(6 Pt 2): S72–5.
4. Kantoff PW, Halabi S, Conaway M, et al. Hydrocortisone with or without mitoxantrone in men with hormone-refractory prostate cancer: results of the cancer and leukemia group B 9182 study. J Clin Oncol 1999;17(8):2506–13.
5. Tannock IF, Osoba D, Stockler MR, et al. Chemotherapy with mitoxantrone plus prednisone or prednisone alone for symptomatic hormone-resistant prostate cancer: a Canadian randomized trial with palliative end points. J Clin Oncol 1996;14(6):1756–64.
6. Parness J, Horwitz SB. Taxol binds to polymerized tubulin in vitro. J Cell Biol 1981;91(2 Pt 1):479–87.
7. Schiff PB, Fant J, Horwitz SB. Promotion of microtubule assembly in vitro by taxol. Nature 1979;277(5698):665–7.
8. Schiff PB, Horwitz SB. Taxol stabilizes microtubules in mouse fibroblast cells. Proc Natl Acad Sci USA 1980;77(3): 1561–5.
9. Foa R, Norton L, Seidman AD. Taxol (paclitaxel): a novel anti-microtubule agent with remarkable anti-neoplastic activity. Int J Clin Lab Res 1994;24(1):6–14.
10. Roth BJ, Yeap BY, Wilding G, Kasimis B, McLeod D, Loehrer PJ. Taxol in advanced, hormone-refractory carcinoma of the prostate. A phase II trial of the Eastern Cooperative Oncology Group. Cancer 1993;72(8):2457–60.
11. Tew KD, Glusker JP, Hartley-Asp B, Hudes G, Speicher LA. Preclinical and clinical perspectives on the use of estramustine as an antimitotic drug. Pharmcol Ther 1992;56(3):323–39.
12. Speicher LA, Barone L, Tew KD. Combined antimicrotubule activity of estramustine and taxol in human prostatic carcinoma cell lines. Cancer Res 1992;52(16):4433–40.
13. Haas N, Roth B, Garay C, et al. Phase I trial of weekly paclitaxel plus oral estramustine phosphate in patients with hormone-refractory prostate cancer. Urology 2001;58(1):59–64.
14. Seidman AD, Scher HI, Petrylak D, Dershaw DD, Curley T. Estramustine and vinblastine: use of prostate specific antigen as a clinical trial end point for hormone refractory prostatic cancer. J Urol 1992;147(3 Pt 2):931–4.

15. Hudes GR, Greenberg R, Krigel RL, et al. Phase II study of estramustine and vinblastine, two microtubule inhibitors, in hormone-refractory prostate cancer. J Clin Oncol 1992;10(11):1754–61.

16. Hudes GR, Obasaju C, Chapman A, Gallo J, McAleer C, Greenberg R. Phase I study of paclitaxel and estramustine: preliminary activity in hormone-refractory prostate cancer. Semin Oncol 1995;22(3 Suppl 6):6–11.

17. Hudes GR, Nathan F, Khater C, et al. Phase II trial of 96-hour paclitaxel plus oral estramustine phosphate in metastatic hormone-refractory prostate cancer. J Clin Oncol 1997;15(9):3156–63.

18. Ringel I, Horwitz SB. Studies with RP 56976 (taxotere): a semisynthetic analogue of taxol. J Natl Cancer Inst 1991;83(4):288–91.

19. Vidensek N, Lim P, Campbell A, Carlson C. Taxol content in bark, wood, root, leaf, twig, and seedling from several Taxus species. J Nat Prod1990;53(6):1609–10.

20. Bissery MC, Guenard D, Gueritte-Voegelein F, Lavelle F. Experimental antitumor activity of taxotere (RP 56976, NSC 628503), a taxol analogue. Cancer Res 1991;51(18):4845–52.

21. Vogel M, Hilsenbeck SG, Depenbrock H, et al. Preclinical activity of taxotere (RP 56976, NSC 628503) against freshly explanted clonogenic human tumour cells: comparison with taxol and conventional antineoplastic agents. Eur J Cancer 1993;29A(14):2009–14.

22. Lavelle F, Bissery MC, Combeau C, Riou JF, Vrignaud P, Andre S. Preclinical evaluation of docetaxel (Taxotere). Semin Oncol 1995;22(2 Suppl 4):3–16.

23. Budman DR, Calabro A, Kreis W. Synergistic and antagonistic combinations of drugs in human prostate cancer cell lines in vitro. Anticancer Drugs 2002;13(10):1011–6.

24. Kreis W, Budman DR, Calabro A. Unique synergism or antagonism of combinations of chemotherapeutic and hormonal agents in human prostate cancer cell lines. Br J Urol 1997;79(2):196–202.

25. Picus J, Schultz M. Docetaxel (Taxotere) as monotherapy in the treatment of hormone-refractory prostate cancer: preliminary results. Semin Oncol 1999;26(5 Suppl 17):14–8.

26. Petrylak DP, Macarthur RB, O'Connor J, et al. Phase I trial of docetaxel with estramustine in androgen-independent prostate cancer. J Clin Oncol 1999;17(3):958–67.

27. Kreis W, Budman DR, Fetten J, Gonzales AL, Barile B, Vinciguerra V. Phase I trial of the combination of daily estramustine phosphate and intermittent docetaxel in patients with metastatic hormone refractory prostate carcinoma. Ann Oncol 1999;10(1):33–8.

28. Petrylak DP, Macarthur R, O'Connor J, et al. Phase I/II studies of docetaxel (Taxotere) combined with estramustine in men with hormone-refractory prostate cancer. Semin Oncol 1999;26(5 Suppl 17):28–33.

29. Savarese D, Taplin ME, Halabi S, Hars V, Kreis W, Vogelzang N. A phase II study of docetaxel (Taxotere), estramustine, and low-dose hydrocortisone in men with hormone-refractory prostate cancer: preliminary results of cancer and leukemia group B Trial 9780. Semin Oncol 1999;26(5 Suppl 17):39–44.

30. Tannock IF, de Wit R, Berry WR, et al. Docetaxel plus prednisone or mitoxantrone plus prednisone for advanced prostate cancer. New Engl J Med 2004;351(15):1502–12.

31. Berthold DR, Pond GR, Soban F, de Wit R, Eisenberger M, Tannock IF. Docetaxel plus prednisone or mitoxantrone plus prednisone for advanced prostate cancer: updated survival in the TAX 327 study. J Clin Oncol 2008;26(2):242–5.

32. Berthold DR, Pond GR, de Wit R, Eisenberger M, Tannock IF. Survival and PSA response of patients in the TAX 327 study who crossed over to receive docetaxel after mitoxantrone or vice versa. Ann Oncol 2008;19(10):1749–53.

33. Saad F, Ruether D, Ernst S, et al. The Canadian Uro-Oncology Group multicentre phase II study of docetaxel administered every 3 weeks with prednisone in men with metastatic hormone-refractory prostate cancer progressing after mitoxantrone/prednisone. BJU Int 2008;102(5):551–5.

34. Slaviero KA, Clarke SJ, McLachlan AJ, Blair EY, Rivory LP. Population pharmacokinetics of weekly docetaxel in patients with advanced cancer. Br J Clin Pharmacol 2004;57(1):44–53.

35. Hainsworth JD. Practical aspects of weekly docetaxel administration schedules. Oncologist 2004;9(5):538–45.

36. Petrylak DP. Chemotherapy for androgen-independent prostate cancer. World J Urol 2005;23(1):10–3.

37. Petrylak DP, Tangen CM, Hussain MH, et al. Docetaxel and estramustine compared with mitoxantrone and prednisone for advanced refractory prostate cancer. New Engl J Med 2004;351(15):1513–20.

38. Berry DL, Moinpour CM, Jiang CS, et al. Quality of life and pain in advanced stage prostate cancer: results of a Southwest Oncology Group randomized trial comparing docetaxel and estramustine to mitoxantrone and prednisone. J Clin Oncol 2006;24(18):2828–35.

39. Petrylak DP. New paradigms for advanced prostate cancer. Rev Urol 2007;9(Suppl 2):S3–12.

40. Oltvai ZN, Milliman CL, Korsmeyer SJ. Bcl-2 heterodimerizes in vivo with a conserved homolog, Bax, that accelerates programmed cell death. Cell 1993;74(4):609–19.

41. Perlman H, Zhang X, Chen MW, Walsh K, Buttyan R. An elevated bax/bcl-2 ratio corresponds with the onset of prostate epithelial cell apoptosis. Cell Death Differ 1999;6(1):48–54.

42. Eigl BJ, Eggener SE, Baybik J, et al. Timing is everything: preclinical evidence supporting simultaneous rather than sequential chemohormonal therapy for prostate cancer. Clin Cancer Res 2005;11(13):4905–11.

43. Tang Y, Khan MA, Goloubeva O, et al. Docetaxel followed by castration improves outcomes in LNCaP prostate cancer-bearing severe combined immunodeficient mice. Clin Cancer Res 2006;12(1):169–74.

44. Hussain A, Dawson N, Amin P, et al. Docetaxel followed by hormone therapy in men experiencing increasing prostate-specific antigen after primary local treatments for prostate cancer. J Clin Oncol 2005;23(12):2789–96.

45. Berry W, Dakhil S, Modiano M, Gregurich M, Asmar L. Phase III study of mitoxantrone plus low dose prednisone versus low dose prednisone alone in patients with asymptomatic hormone refractory prostate cancer. J Urol 2002;168(6):2439–43.

46. Hamberg P, Verhagen PC, de Wit R. When to start cytotoxic therapy in asymptomatic patients with hormone refractory prostate cancer? Eur J Cancer 2008;44(9):1193–7.

47. Armstrong AJ, Garrett-Mayer ES, Yang YC, de Wit R, Tannock IF, Eisenberger M. A contemporary prognostic

nomogram for men with hormone-refractory metastatic prostate cancer: a TAX327 study analysis. Clin Cancer Res 2007;13(21):6396–403.

48. Oudard S, Banu E, Scotte F, et al. Prostate-specific antigen doubling time before onset of chemotherapy as a predictor of survival for hormone-refractory prostate cancer patients. Ann Oncol 2007;18(11):1828–33.

49. Folkman J. Tumor angiogenesis: therapeutic implications. New Engl J Med 1971;285(21):1182–6.

50. Sweeney CJ, Miller KD, Sissons SE, et al. The antiangiogenic property of docetaxel is synergistic with a recombinant humanized monoclonal antibody against vascular endothelial growth factor or 2-methoxyestradiol but antagonized by endothelial growth factors. Cancer Res 2001;61(8):3369–72.

51. Gasparini G, Longo R, Fanelli M, Teicher BA. Combination of antiangiogenic therapy with other anticancer therapies: results, challenges, and open questions. J Clin Oncol 2005;23(6):1295–311.

52. Di Lorenzo G, Figg WD, Fossa SD, et al. Combination of bevacizumab and docetaxel in docetaxel-pretreated hormone-refractory prostate cancer: a phase 2 study. Eur Urol 2008;54(5):1089–94.

53. Zhu D, Corral LG, Fleming YW, Stein B. Immunomodulatory drugs Revlimid® (lenalidomide) and CC-4047 induce apoptosis of both hematological and solid tumor cells through NK cell activation. Cancer Immunol Immunother 2008;57(12):1849–59.

54. Sanborn SL, Cooney MM, Dowlati A, et al. Phase I trial of docetaxel and thalidomide: a regimen based on metronomic therapeutic principles. Invest New Drugs 2008;26(4):355–62.

55. Ning Y, Arlen P, Fulley J, et al. Phase II trial of thalidomide (T), bevacizumab (Bv), and docetaxel (DOC) in patients (pts) with metastatic castration-refractory prostate cancer (mCRPC). J Clin Oncol 2008;26:abstr 5000.

56. Cumashi A, Tinari N, Rossi C, et al. Sunitinib malate (SU-11248) alone or in combination with low-dose docetaxel inhibits the growth of DU-145 prostate cancer xenografts. Cancer Lett 2008;270(2):229–33.

57. Guerin O, Formento P, Lo Nigro C, et al. Supra-additive antitumor effect of sunitinib malate (SU11248, Sutent) combined with docetaxel. A new therapeutic perspective in hormone refractory prostate cancer. J Cancer Res Clin Oncol 2008;134(1):51–7.

58. George D, Liu G, Wilding G, et al. Sunitinib in combination with docetaxel and prednisone in patients with metastatic hormone refractor prostate cancer (mHRPC) – preliminary results. J Clin Oncol 2008;26:abstr 5131.

59. ClinicalTrials.gov. Accessed 2008, at http://www.clinicaltrials.gov

60. Wang YR, Wigington DP, Strugnell SA, Knutson JC. Growth inhibition of cancer cells by an active metabolite of a novel vitamin D prodrug. Anticancer Res 2005;25(6B):4333–9.

61. Blutt SE, Polek TC, Stewart LV, Kattan MW, Weigel NL. A calcitriol analogue, EB1089, inhibits the growth of LNCaP tumors in nude mice. Cancer Res 2000;60(4):779–82.

62. Hershberger PA, Yu WD, Modzelewski RA, Rueger RM, Johnson CS, Trump DL. Calcitriol (1,25-dihydroxycholecalciferol) enhances paclitaxel antitumor activity in vitro and in vivo and accelerates paclitaxel-induced apoptosis. Clin Cancer Res 2001;7(4):1043–51.

63. Beer TM, Hough KM, Garzotto M, Lowe BA, Henner WD. Weekly high-dose calcitriol and docetaxel in advanced prostate cancer. Semin Oncol 2001;28(4 Suppl 15):49–55.

64. Beer TM, Ryan CW, Venner PM, et al. Double-blinded randomized study of high-dose calcitriol plus docetaxel compared with placebo plus docetaxel in androgen-independent prostate cancer: a report from the ASCENT Investigators. J Clin Oncol 2007;25(6):669–74.

65. Bagnato A, Rosano L. The endothelin axis in cancer. Int J Biochem Cell Biol 2008;40(8):1443–51.

66. Carducci MA, Jimeno A. Targeting bone metastasis in prostate cancer with endothelin receptor antagonists. Clin Cancer Res 2006;12(20 Pt 2):6296s–300s.

67. Jimeno A, Carducci M. Atrasentan: a novel and rationally designed therapeutic alternative in the management of cancer. Expert Rev Anticancer Ther 2005;5(3):419–27.

68. Carducci MA, Padley RJ, Breul J, et al. Effect of endothelin-A receptor blockade with atrasentan on tumor progression in men with hormone-refractory prostate cancer: a randomized, phase II, placebo-controlled trial. J Clin Oncol 2003;21(4):679–89.

69. Banerjee S, Hussain M, Wang Z, et al. In vitro and in vivo molecular evidence for better therapeutic efficacy of ABT-627 and taxotere combination in prostate cancer. Cancer Res 2007;67(8):3818–26.

70. Zou Z, Anisowicz A, Hendrix MJ, et al. Maspin, a serpin with tumor-suppressing activity in human mammary epithelial cells. Science 1994;263(5146):526-9.

71. Luo JL, Tan W, Ricono JM, et al. Nuclear cytokine-activated IKKalpha controls prostate cancer metastasis by repressing Maspin. Nature 2007;446(7136):690–4.

72. Miller RE, Roudier M, Jones J, Armstrong A, Canon J, Dougall WC. RANK ligand inhibition plus docetaxel improves survival and reduces tumor burden in a murine model of prostate cancer bone metastasis. Mol Cancer Ther 2008;7(7):2160–9.

73. Dreicer R, Petrylak D, Agus D, Webb I, Roth B. Phase I/II study of bortezomib plus docetaxel in patients with advanced androgen-independent prostate cancer. Clin Cancer Res 2007;13(4):1208–15.

74. Cao W, Shiverick KT, Namiki K, et al. Docetaxel and bortezomib downregulate Bcl-2 and sensitize PC-3-Bcl-2 expressing prostate cancer cells to irradiation. World J Urol 2008;26(5):509–16.

75. Morris M, Beekman K, Kelly W, et al. Phase II study of bortezomib for castrate metastatic prostate cancer. Proc Am Soc Clin Oncol 2005;23:411S(abstract 4633).

76. Papandreou CN, Daliani DD, Nix D, et al. Phase I trial of the proteasome inhibitor bortezomib in patients with advanced solid tumors with observations in androgen-independent prostate cancer. J Clin Oncol 2004;22(11):2108–21.

77. Kaufman HL, Wang W, Manola J, et al. Phase II randomized study of vaccine treatment of advanced prostate cancer (E7897): a trial of the Eastern Cooperative Oncology Group. J Clin Oncol 2004;22(11):2122–32.

78. Kaufman H, Wang W, Manola J, et al. Phase II prime/boost vaccination using poxviruses expressing PSA in hormone dependent prostate cancer: follow up clinical results from ECOG 7897. Proc Am Soc Clin Oncol 2005;24:4501a.

79. Arlen PM, Gulley JL, Parker C, et al. A randomized phase II study of concurrent docetaxel plus vaccine versus vaccine alone in metastatic androgen-independent prostate cancer. Clin Cancer Res 2006;12(4):1260–9.

80. Garnett CT, Schlom J, Hodge JW. Combination of docetaxel and recombinant vaccine enhances T-cell responses and antitumor activity: effects of docetaxel on immune enhancement. Clin Cancer Res 2008;14(11):3536–44.

81. Roehl KA, Han M, Ramos CG, Antenor JA, Catalona WJ. Cancer progression and survival rates following anatomical radical retropubic prostatectomy in 3,478 consecutive patients: long-term results. J Urol 2004;172(3):910–4.

82. Pickles T, Morgan S, Morton G, Souhami L, Warde P, Lukka H. Adjuvant radiotherapy following radical prostatectomy: Genito-Urinary Radiation Oncologists of Canada Consensus Statement. Can Urol Assoc J (Journal de l'Association des urologues du Canada) 2008;2(2):95–9.

83. Sonpavde G, Chi KN, Powles T, et al. Neoadjuvant therapy followed by prostatectomy for clinically localized prostate cancer. Cancer 2007;110(12):2628–39.

84. Carson CC III, Zincke H, Utz DC, Cupps RE, Farrow GM. Radical prostatectomy after radiotherapy for prostatic cancer. J Urol 1980;124(2):237–9.

85. Garcia JA, Klein EA, Magi-Galluzzi C, Elson P, Triozzi P, Dreicer R. Clinical and biological effects of neoadjuvant sargramostim and thalidomide in patients with locally advanced prostate carcinoma. Clin Cancer Res 2008;14(10):3052–9.

86. Hussain M, Smith DC, El-Rayes BF, et al. Neoadjuvant docetaxel and estramustine chemotherapy in high-risk/locally-advanced prostate cancer. Urology 2003;61(4):774–80.

87. Dreicer R, Magi-Galluzzi C, Zhou M, et al. Phase II trial of neoadjuvant docetaxel before radical prostatectomy for locally advanced prostate cancer. Urology 2004;63(6):1138–42.

88. Febbo PG, Richie JP, George DJ, et al. Neoadjuvant docetaxel before radical prostatectomy in patients with high-risk localized prostate cancer. Clin Cancer Res 2005;11(14):5233–40.

89. Garzotto M, Myrthue A, Higano CS, Beer TM. Neoadjuvant mitoxantrone and docetaxel for high-risk localized prostate cancer. Urol Oncol 2006;24(3):254–9.

90. Friedman J, Dunn RL, Wood D, et al. Neoadjuvant docetaxel and capecitabine in patients with high risk prostate cancer. J Urol 2008;179(3):911–5; discussion 5–6.

91. Chi KN, Chin JL, Winquist E, Klotz L, Saad F, Gleave ME. Multicenter phase II study of combined neoadjuvant docetaxel and hormone therapy before radical prostatectomy for patients with high risk localized prostate cancer. J Urol 2008;180(2):565–70; discussion 70.

92. Eastham JA, Kelly WK, Grossfeld GD, Small EJ. Cancer and Leukemia Group B (CALGB) 90203: a randomized phase 3 study of radical prostatectomy alone versus estramustine and docetaxel before radical prostatectomy for patients with high-risk localized disease. Urology 2003;62(Suppl 1):55–62.

93. Eisenberger M, Kattan M, Kibel A, Sternberg C, Epstein J. Impact of central pathology review (CPR) of radical prostatectomy (RP) specimens for patient selection in the surgical adjuvant trial in prostate cancer (PCa) TAX-3501. J Clin Oncol 2008;26:abstr 5128.

94. Kibel AS, Rosenbaum E, Kattan MW, et al. Adjuvant weekly docetaxel for patients with high risk prostate cancer after radical prostatectomy: a multi-institutional pilot study. J Urol 2007;177(5):1777–81.

95. Montgomery B, Lavori P, Garzotto M, et al. Veterans Affairs Cooperative Studies Program Study 553: Chemotherapy after prostatectomy, a phase III randomized study of prostatectomy versus prostatectomy with adjuvant docetaxel for patients with high-risk, localized prostate cancer. Urology 2008;72(3):474–80.

96. Mason KA, Hunter NR, Milas M, Abbruzzese JL, Milas L. Docetaxel enhances tumor radioresponse in vivo. Clin Cancer Res 1997;3(12 Pt 1):2431–8.

97. Kumar P, Perrotti M, Weiss R, et al. Phase I trial of weekly docetaxel with concurrent three-dimensional conformal radiation therapy in the treatment of unfavorable localized adenocarcinoma of the prostate. J Clin Oncol 2004;22(10): 1909–15.

98. Perrotti M, Doyle T, Kumar P, et al. Phase I/II trial of docetaxel and concurrent radiation therapy in localized high risk prostate cancer (AGUSG 03-10). Urol Oncol 2008;26(3):276–80.

99. Ebrrahimi K, Ruckle H, Harper J, et al. Post prostatectomy multimodality adjuvant therapy for patients at high risk for prostate cancer relapse. In: American Urologic Association Annual Meeting, Orlando;2008.

100. Patel AR, Sandler HM, Pienta KJ. Radiation Therapy Oncology Group 0521: a phase III randomized trial of androgen suppression and radiation therapy versus androgen suppression and radiation therapy followed by chemotherapy with docetaxel/prednisone for localized, high-risk prostate cancer. Clinical Genitourin Cancer 2005;4(3):212–4.

Chapter 13
Beyond Docetaxel: Emerging Agents in the Treatment of Advanced Prostate Cancer

Jonathan Rosenberg

Abstract Increased understanding of the biology of advanced prostate cancer has yielded multiple targets that are worthy of evaluation. Multiple signaling pathways appear to play a role in the maintenance and progression of the malignant phenotype. These pathways, such as PI3 kinase/Akt pathway, the mTOR pathway, the Hsp90 pathway, and the insulin-like growth factor 1 pathway, are currently being investigated in clinical trials. Other fundamental processes such as histone deacetylation are also involved in prostate cancer progression. Testing agents targeting these pathways will provide crucial information regarding whether inhibition will yield clinical benefit for prostate cancer patients.

Keywords mTOR inhibition • Novel therapeutics • Histone deacetylation • Insulin-like growth factor 1 • HSP90

Introduction

Docetaxel chemotherapy is associated with improved overall survival in men with castration-resistant prostate cancer (CRPC). However, median survival of these patients remains under 2 years, and better options are needed. Several strategies to improve these outcomes have been pursued. Addition of novel agents to docetaxel represents one pathway forward. To date, adding another agent does not appear to add positively to docetaxel (e.g. DN101, GVAX, bevazicumab). Epidermal growth factor receptor (EGFR) pathway inhibition with erlotinib or gefitinib has been tested in phase II setting in CRPC, but does not seem to add substantial activity to docetaxel chemotherapy [1, 2]. Other investigational agents target pathways that appear important in prostate cancer pathogenesis, maintenance, and progression. These therapies target the PI3 kinase/Akt pathways, the mTOR pathway, the Hsp90 pathway, insulin-like growth factor 1 pathway, and histone deacetylation. Preclinical evidence supports the importance of these molecular pathways, although clinical testing of most of these agents remains immature. This chapter will review the available data and the current clinical status of agents targeting these pathways.

PI3 Kinase/Akt Pathways

The tumor suppressor gene encoding phosphatase and tensin homolog deleted on chromosome 10 (PTEN) is lost with high frequency in prostate cancer. This results in constitutive activation of the PI3 kinase/Akt pathway. The PI3 kinase is a complex heterodimeric molecule with multiple subcomponents which receives upstream signals from multiple receptor tyrosine kinases, including the insulin-like growth factor (IGF) receptor. These receptor tyrosine kinases activate the PI3 kinase, leading to Akt activation by PDK1 and 2. After phosphorylation by PDK1 and 2, Akt translocates to the nucleus, where it, in turn, phosphorylates many proteins to regulate diverse functions in the cell. While no activating point mutations of Akt have been identified in prostate cancer specimens, high Akt activity appears to be involved in prostate cancer growth and progression [3].

J. Rosenberg (✉)
Lank Center for Genitourinary Oncology,
Dana-Farber Cancer Institute, Boston, MA, USA
e-mail: jonathan_rosenberg@dfci.harvard.edu

W.D. Figg et al. (eds.), *Drug Management of Prostate Cancer*,
DOI 10.1007/978-1-60327-829-4_13, © Springer Science+Business Media, LLC 2010

Increased Akt activity has been demonstrated in more poorly differentiated prostate tumors and predicts biochemical recurrence [4, 5]. Furthermore, Akt activation has been implicated in the progression to castration resistance. In vitro studies with androgen-dependent LNCaP cells grown in the absence of androgens develop androgen-independent growth and high levels of Akt activation [6]. Akt activation was also increased in LNCaP xenografts grown in castrated mice, compared to the parental LNCaP cell line [7].

Akt and PI3 kinase inhibitors are currently under investigation in clinical trials in prostate cancer. Perifosine, an oral Akt inhibitor has been evaluated in a phase II study of patients with hormone-sensitive prostate cancer and rising PSA after definitive local therapy [8]. Twenty percent of patients treated had a reduction in PSA levels, but none had declines greater than 50%. PSA doubling time (compared to pretreatment doubling time) was not increased with perifosine treatment, and the median time to PSA progression was 6.6 months. This modest activity is insufficient to justify further single-agent testing of perifosine in prostate cancer, but combination studies with androgen deprivation therapy and chemotherapy are underway. Other Akt and PI3 kinase inhibitors are in early phase clinical trials and have not yet been specifically tested in prostate cancer.

mTOR Inhibition

The mammalian target of rapamycin (mTOR) lies downstream of PI3 kinase and Akt and is activated in PTEN-deleted tumors. mTOR is a serine/threonine kinase that receives signals from multiple upstream growth and nutrient sensing pathways and phosphorylates transcription factors that are critical for cell proliferation (S6K1 and 4E-BP1). mTOR inhibition using temsirolimus has demonstrated clinical benefit in patients with advanced renal cell carcinoma [9]. Preclinical testing suggests that Akt upregulation may be countered by mTOR inhibition. Transgenic mice expressing human Akt develop tumors in the ventral prostate; treatment with everolimus, an mTOR inhibitor, reverses the neoplastic phenotype [10]. Other preclinical works suggest that mTOR inhibition might restore chemotherapy sensitivity to a resistant prostate cancer cell line. PTEN-deficient PC-3 cells treated with rapamycin or temsirolimus were rendered sensitive to

doxorubicin, similar to PC-3 cells with normal PTEN expression both in vitro and in vivo [11].

Agents targeting mTOR have been tested in phase II studies in prostate cancer. A pharmacodynamic study of everolimus was conducted in patients with newly diagnosed prostate cancer about to undergo radical prostatectomy [12]. Preliminary results suggest that the pharmacodynamic effects of mTOR inhibition by everolimus can be detected in prostate tumor tissue, as measured by a reduced level of phospho-S6 kinase by immunohistochemistry. In a similar fashion, oral temsirolimus was tested in newly diagnosed prostate cancer patients who were about to undergo radical prostatectomy [13]. Decreases in mTOR activation as measured by S6 kinase phosphorylation were detected in patients treated with temsirolimus, although an associated increase in phospho-Akt and phospho-mTOR was seen. These results are consistent with other research works suggesting that upstream Akt activation is observed with mTOR inhibition, and may be a mechanism of resistance [14].

In CRPC, everolimus was tested in a phase II study [15]. Preliminary results from this study demonstrated a 2.5 month time to progression without any radiographic or PSA responses. Although these results were not encouraging, the majority of these patients were a chemotherapy refractory population. Everolimus was also tested in combination with docetaxel in a phase I study using FDG-PET imaging as a pharmacodynamic endpoint [16]. The combination was tolerable at doses of everolimus 10 mg daily with docetaxel 70 mg/m^2 every 3 weeks, with some evidence suggesting decreased FDG-avidity associated with PSA responses.

Hsp90 Pathway

Hsp90 is a highly expressed molecular chaperone that is significantly upregulated during cellular stress. It plays a role in the folding, translocation, and refolding of proteins in eukaryotic cells. Hsp90 has been demonstrated to play a role in the ability of cancer cells to evade normal regulatory pathways. In particular, Hsp90 has been shown to be critical for the proper folding and processing of the androgen receptor. The ability of Hsp90 to bind to target proteins is dependent on its ability to bind and hydrolyze ATP. Inhibitors of the ATP hydrolase activity prevent Hsp90 from associating with its target proteins. In vivo, treatment of prostate cancer cells with geldanamycin, an Hsp90 inhibitor, causes loss of AR activity and degradation of AR protein [17]. Based on the loss of AR activity, degradation of the AR protein, and provocative xenograft data demonstrating significant tumor regression, geldanamycin derivatives such as 17-AAG, which are less toxic, have been tested in prostate cancer. A phase II study of 17-AAG in CRPC patients previously treated with chemotherapy, unfortunately, did not result in any patients achieving a 50% decline in PSA, and the median time to progression was only 1.8 months [18]. Other Hsp90 inhibitors, such as 17-DMAG, are currently under investigation as single agents or in combination with other therapies for the treatment of prostate cancer.

Insulin-Like Growth Factor Pathway

Nonandrogen hormonal signaling appears to play an important role in the progression of CRPC. Of the cell membrane-associated receptor tyrosine kinases, the insulin-like growth factor 1 receptor (IGF1R) may play a key role. The IGF pathway regulates cell growth, protects cells from apoptosis, and promotes tumor cell invasion in a variety of human cancers. Clinical and epidemiological data suggest that elevated plasma IGF-1 levels are a risk factor for the development of prostate cancer and that IGF-1 increases the growth of prostate cancer cell cultures [19]. Elimination of IGF1R signaling suppresses growth and invasion in in vivo models of prostate cancer [20]. Furthermore, some androgen-dependent cell lines increase IGF1 and IGF1R expression when they develop androgen-independent growth [21, 22]. Therefore, targeting the IGF1 axis may play an important role in the future treatment of CRPC.

The IGF1 axis may be targeted in multiple ways. First, the available ligand to activate the pathway may be depleted. This may be accomplished by growth hormone pathway inhibition leading to decreased IGF1 secretion, increased binding of IGF1 to its binding proteins, or antibodies targeting the IGF molecule. Somatostatin analogues that lower IGF1 have been tested in CRPC and found to be associated with modest PSA response proportions. Lantreotide was associated with ≥50% PSA declines in 20% of CRPC patients [23]. Octreotide, in combination with dexamethasone, was associated with ≥50% PSA declines in 60% of

patients [24]. Further testing of somatostatin analogues is ongoing.

Second, receptor activation may be inhibited. Small-molecule tyrosine kinase inhibitors and receptor-binding antibodies may prove useful for this purpose. These are currently being tested in phase II clinical trials in prostate cancer. Meso-nordihydroguaiaretic acid (NDGA), derived from the creosote bush, inhibits the IGF1R tyrosine kinase and was observed to reduce androgen-dependent growth in in vitro studies. A phase I study with NDGA was completed in men with a rising PSA after definitive local therapy [25]. While transaminase elevations limited therapy, one of 11 patients experienced a ≥50% PSA decline, and several other patients had a prolongation of PSA doubling time. Further development of NDGA is ongoing.

Inhibition of the IGF1 receptor activation may also be achieved by binding and inactivating the receptor. The human monoclonal IgG1 antibody, IMC-A12, inhibits ligand-dependent receptor activation and is currently being tested in prostate cancer [26].

An expected toxicity associated with IGF1 inhibition would be cross-inhibition of the insulin receptor pathway and concomitant problems with hyperglycemia. The extent that this will be a concern with agents targeting this pathway remains an open question. These agents are currently being tested as single agents, and the potential for synergy with cytotoxic chemotherapy suggests that they will be tested in combinations in the future.

Histone Deacetylase Inhibitors

Transcription of genes depends on the interaction of transcription factors, DNA, and chromatin structural elements, such as histones. Regulation of transcription is affected by histone acetylation status. Histone deacetylation is carried out by histone deacetylases, of which there are three classes: class I, which is nuclear and associated with transcriptional repression; class II, which deacetylates larger proteins in both the cytoplasm and the nucleus; and HDAC6, which is specific for histones. Inhibition of histone deacetylation, resulting in hyperacetylation, leads to transcriptional activation of repressed genes. Preclinical evaluation of histone deacetylase inhibitors has suggested the presence of significant antiprostate cancer activity, although the mechanism of cancer cell death of these agents is not entirely elucidated. HDAC inhibitor-mediated cytotoxicity may result from several different mechanisms. One pathway that may be particularly important in prostate cancer is acetylation and disruption of heat shock protein client proteins, which shuttle the androgen receptor to the nucleus.

Romidepsin (FK228) inhibits class I HDAC's and Hsp90 function and has demonstrated preclinical evidence of efficacy in prostate cancer. Xenograft models of prostate cancer show reduced growth when treated with romidepsin, and this is potentiated in combination with docetaxel chemotherapy [27, 28]. Romidepsin was tested as a single agent in a phase II study of CRPC patients not previously treated with chemotherapy. One of 21 evaluable patients elicited a radiographically confirmed partial response, and the PSA response proportion was 7% [29]. Some patients experienced periods of disease stabilization, and this agent is being tested in combination with other agents in CRPC.

Vorinostat (SAHA) also has activity in preclinical models of prostate cancer [30]. Interestingly, there seems to be reduced activity of the compound in androgen receptor-negative prostate cancer cells, such as PC-3, and suppression of androgen signaling in the presence of the androgen receptor may sensitize prostate cancer cells to vorinostat [31]. A phase II study of vorinostat alone in patients previously treated with docetaxel chemotherapy did not demonstrate significant anticancer activity [32]. In that study of heavily pretreated patients, vorinostat was associated with a short time to progression and significant toxicity. Vorinostat is being tested in androgen-dependent prostate cancer in combination with androgen deprivation, based on the preclinical data suggesting that androgen deprivation may potentiate the actions of HDAC inhibition [33]. Other HDAC inhibitors, such as LBH589 and belinostat, are being evaluated in prostate cancer as well; no clinical data is available at this time.

Conclusion

Preclinical work has indicated that multiple biochemical pathways may play a role in the maintenance and progression of the malignant phenotype in prostate cancer, and many of these pathways may be targeted with novel agents. While none of the treatments referred to above have been proven to provide clinical benefit, further testing is ongoing.

References

1. Canil CM, Moore MJ, Winquist E, et al. Randomized phase II study of two doses of gefitinib in hormone-refractory prostate cancer: a trial of the National Cancer Institute of Canada-Clinical Trials Group. J Clin Oncol 2005;23(3): 455–60.
2. Gross M, Higano C, Pantuck A, et al. A phase II trial of docetaxel and erlotinib as first-line therapy for elderly patients with androgen-independent prostate cancer. BMC Cancer 2007;7:142.
3. Majumder PK, Sellers WR. Akt-regulated pathways in prostate cancer. Oncogene 2005;24(50):7465–74.
4. Malik SN, Brattain M, Ghosh PM, et al. Immunohistochemical demonstration of phospho-Akt in high Gleason grade prostate cancer. Clin Cancer Res 2002;8(4):1168–71.
5. Kreisberg JI, Malik SN, Prihoda TJ, et al. Phosphorylation of Akt (Ser473) is an excellent predictor of poor clinical outcome in prostate cancer. Cancer Res 2004;64(15):5232–6.
6. Murillo H, Huang H, Schmidt LJ, Smith DI, Tindall DJ. Role of PI3K signaling in survival and progression of LNCaP prostate cancer cells to the androgen refractory state. Endocrinology 2001;142(11):4795–805.
7. Graff JR, Konicek BW, McNulty AM, et al. Increased AKT activity contributes to prostate cancer progression by dramatically accelerating prostate tumor growth and diminishing p27Kip1 expression. J Biol Chem 2000;275(32):24500–5.
8. Chee KG, Longmate J, Quinn DI, et al. The AKT inhibitor perifosine in biochemically recurrent prostate cancer: a phase II California/Pittsburgh cancer consortium trial. Clin Genitourin Cancer 2007;5(7):433–7.
9. Hudes G, Carducci M, Tomczak P, et al. Temsirolimus, interferon alfa, or both for advanced renal-cell carcinoma. N Engl J Med 2007;356(22):2271–81.
10. Majumder PK, Febbo PG, Bikoff R, et al. mTOR inhibition reverses Akt-dependent prostate intraepithelial neoplasia through regulation of apoptotic and HIF-1-dependent pathways. Nat Med 2004;10(6):594–601.
11. Grunwald V, DeGraffenried L, Russel D, Friedrichs WE, Ray RB, Hidalgo M. Inhibitors of mTOR reverse doxorubicin resistance conferred by PTEN status in prostate cancer cells. Cancer Res 2002;62(21):6141–5.
12. Lerut E, Roskams T, Goossens E, et al. Molecular pharmacodynamic (MPD) evaluation of dose and schedule of RAD001 (everolimus) in patients with operable prostate carcinoma (PC). J Clin Oncol (Meeting Abstracts) 2005;23(16_suppl):3071.
13. Efstathiou E, Tsavachidou D, Wen S, Troncoso P, Mills GB, Logothetis CJ. Integrated quantative and spatial proteomic analysis of PI3kinase signaling in high grade prostate cancer (PCa) treated with Temsirolimus with or without androgen ablation. J Clin Oncol (Meeting Abstracts) 2008;26 (15_suppl):5071.
14. O'Reilly KE, Rojo F, She Q-B, et al. mTOR inhibition induces upstream receptor tyrosine kinase signaling and activates Akt. Cancer Res 2006;66(3):1500–8.
15. George DA, Armstrong AJ, Creel P, et al. A phase II study of RAD001 in men with hormone-refractory metastatic prostate cancer. Proceedings of the Genitourinary Cancers Symposium 2008: Abstract 181.

16. Ross RW, Manola J, Oh WK, et al. Phase I trial of RAD001 (R) and docetaxel (D) in castration resistant prostate cancer (CRPC) with FDG-PET assessment of RAD001 activity. J Clin Oncol (Meeting Abstracts) 2008;26(15_suppl):5069.

17. Smaletz O, Kelly WK, Horse-Grant D, et al. Epothilone B analogue (BMS-247550) with estramustine phosphate in patients with progressive castrate-metastatic prostate cancer. Proc Am Soc Clin Oncol 2002;21:732.

18. Heath EI, Hillman D, Vaishampayan U, et al. A phase II trial of 17-allylamino-17-demethoxygeldanamycin (17-AAG) in patients with hormone-refractory metastatic prostate cancer. J Clin Oncol (Meeting Abstracts) 2007;25(18_suppl): 15553.

19. Chan JM, Stampfer MJ, Giovannucci E, et al. Plasma insulin-like growth factor-I and prostate cancer risk: a prospective study. Science 1998;279(5350):563–6.

20. Wu JD, Odman A, Higgins LM, et al. In vivo effects of the human type I insulin-like growth factor receptor antibody A12 on androgen-dependent and androgen-independent xenograft human prostate tumors. Clin Cancer Res 2005;11(8):3065–74.

21. Krueckl SL, Sikes RA, Edlund NM, et al. increased insulin-like growth factor I receptor expression and signaling are components of androgen-independent progression in a lineage-derived prostate cancer progression model. Cancer Res 2004;64(23):8620–9.

22. Kiyama S, Morrison K, Zellweger T, et al. castration-induced increases in insulin-like growth factor-binding protein 2 promotes proliferation of androgen-independent human prostate LNCaP tumors. Cancer Res 2003;63(13):3575–84.

23. Maulard C, Richaud P, Droz JP, Jessueld D, Dufour-Esquerre F, Housset M. Phase I-II study of the somatostatin analogue lanreotide in hormone-refractory prostate cancer. Cancer Chemother Pharmacol 1995;36(3):259–62.

24. Koutsilieris M, Mitsiades CS, Bogdanos J, et al. Combination of somatostatin analog, dexamethasone, and standard androgen ablation therapy in stage D3 prostate cancer patients with bone metastases. Clin Cancer Res 2004;10(13):4398–405.

25. Ryan CJ, Harzstark AH, Rosenberg J, et al. A pilot dose-escalation study of the effects of nordihydroguareacetic acid on hormone and prostate specific antigen levels in patients with relapsed prostate cancer. BJU Int 2008;101(4):436–9.

26. Rowinsky EK, Youssoufian H, Tonra JR, Solomon P, Burtrum D, Ludwig DL. IMC-A12, a human IgG1 monoclonal antibody to the insulin-like growth factor I receptor. Clin Cancer Res 2007;13(18):5549s–55s.

27. Lai M-T, Yang C-C, Lin T-Y, Tsai F-J, Chen W-C. Depsipeptide (FK228) inhibits growth of human prostate cancer cells. Urologic Oncology: Seminars and Original Investigations 2008;26(2):182–9.

28. Zhang Z, Stanfield J, Frenkel E, Kabbani W, Hsieh J-T. Enhanced therapeutic effect on androgen-independent prostate cancer by depsipeptide (FK228), a histone deacetylase inhibitor, in combination with docetaxel. Urology 2007;70(2):396–401.

29. Parker C, Molife R, Karavasilis V, et al. Romidepsin (FK228), a histone deacetylase inhibitor: final results of a phase II study in metastatic hormone refractory prostate cancer (HRPC). J Clin Oncol (Meeting Abstracts) 2007;25 (18_suppl):15507.

30. Early clinical data and potential clinical utility of novel histone deacetylase inhibitors in prostate cancer. Clin Prostate Cancer 2005;4(2):83–5.

31. Marrocco DL, Tilley WD, Bianco-Miotto T, et al. Suberoylanilide hydroxamic acid (vorinostat) represses androgen receptor expression and acts synergistically with an androgen receptor antagonist to inhibit prostate cancer cell proliferation. Mol Cancer Ther 2007;6(1):51–60.

32. Bradley DA, Dunn R, Rathkopf D, et al. Vorinostat in hormone refractory prostate cancer (HRPC): trial results and IL-6 analysis. Proceedings of the Genitourinary Cancers Symposium 2008: Abstract 211.

33. Rokhlin OW, Glover RB, Guseva NV, Taghiyev AF, Kohlgraf KG, Cohen MB. Mechanisms of cell death induced by histone deacetylase inhibitors in androgen receptor-positive prostate cancer cells. Mol Cancer Res 2006;4(2):113–23.

Chapter 14
Platinum Agents in Prostate Cancer

Ashley Brick, Junyang Niu, Jiaoti Huang, and William K. Oh

Abstract The standard first-line treatment for metastatic castration-resistant prostate cancer (CRPC) is docetaxel chemotherapy. Platinum drugs, including cisplatin and carboplatin, when used as single agents and in combinations, have shown a moderate response in metastatic CRPC patients, as both first- and second-line treatment. Furthermore, the relationship between neuroendocrine differentiation and castration-resistant disease progression suggests that there may be a possible role for platinum agents. Newer platinum analogs, including picoplatin, oxaliplatin, and satraplatin have been recently studied in CRPC. Though a Phase III trial demonstrated a progression-free survival benefit favoring satraplatin plus prednisone versus prednisone alone, no overall survival benefit was demonstrated in the second-line setting. Further trials will be needed to demonstrate a clear role for platinum agents in CRPC.

Keywords Carboplatin • Neuroendocrine • Castration-resistant • Chemotherapy

Introduction

Docetaxel is currently the standard first-line chemotherapy for patients with metastatic castration-resistant prostate cancer (CRPC) [1, 2]. However, after progression on docetaxel chemotherapy, there is no uniformly accepted second-line chemotherapy [3]. Recent trials have suggested that treatment with platinum drugs alone or in combination with taxanes may have important clinical activity [4]. Although it was previously believed that platinum drugs had little activity in CRPC, these recent studies, which used palliation as well as PSA endpoints, have demonstrated clinical benefits. Also, newer and more potent platinum analogues, such as satraplatin and picoplatin, have shown activity in CRPC and have been studied in recent clinical trials [5–7].

Today it is not clear how prostate cancer (CaP) advances to a castration-resistant state. One mechanism proposes that neuroendocrine (NE) differentiation is a contributing factor to the progression towards CRPC [8]. Recent research has better elucidated the biology of NE differentiation in prostate cancer. Although several studies have focused on the relationship between NE differentiation and activity of platinum chemotherapy, it remains unclear if there is a "platinum-sensitive" subtype of CaP that can be biologically determined.

Neuroendocrine Differentiation in Prostate Cancer

NE differentiation is a consistent histologic feature of prostate cancer, making it a unique tumor among all epithelial malignancies [9]. However, the concept of NE differentiation has caused confusion among clinicians and basic researchers alike, which needs to be more clearly defined.

Epithelial components of the normal prostate include luminal secretory cells, basal cells, and a third

W.K. Oh (✉)
Division of Hematology and Medical Oncology, Dana-Farber Cancer Institute, New York, 10029 NY, USA
e-mail: william.oh@mssm.edu

W.D. Figg et al. (eds.), *Drug Management of Prostate Cancer*,
DOI 10.1007/978-1-60327-829-4_14, © Springer Science+Business Media, LLC 2010

minor component of NE cells. NE cells have neuron-like morphology ultrastructurally and endocrine function including the secretion of biogenic amines and neuropeptides. They are widely distributed in the normal prostate with only an occasional cell per gland or duct but cannot be easily distinguished from surrounding cell on H&E-stained sections under light microscopy. Immunohistochemical staining for NE markers such as chromogranin A, synaptophysin, and neuron-specific enolase (NSE) is a sensitive and specific method to identify such cells in formalin-fixed, paraffin-embedded tissue sections. The function of NE cells in normal prostate is unclear. NE cells are also present in prostate cancer. Very rarely, a prostate cancer is composed entirely of NE tumor cells. Depending on the morphologic features of tumor cells, the amount of necrosis, and the frequency of mitotic figures, such tumors may be classified as small cell carcinoma [10, 11], large cell neuroendocrine carcinoma [12], or carcinoid tumor [13–15]. Such pure neuroendocrine tumors are subtypes of prostatic epithelial malignancies and comprise no more than 1% of all tumors of the prostate. The vast majority of prostate cancers are adenocarcinomas with tumor cells showing luminal secretory cell features including the expression of androgen receptor (AR) and secretion of PSA. NE differentiation of prostate cancer commonly refers to the presence of rare individual NE cells or small nests of NE cells scattered among the more abundant luminal secretory-type cancer cells in conventional adenocarcinomas [16, 17]. By this definition, all adenocarcinomas of the prostate demonstrate some degree of NE differentiation [18].

NE tumor cells, unlike the non-NE secretory type tumor cells of CaP, do not express androgen receptor (AR) and are likely androgen-independent. It is therefore hypothesized that while hormonal therapy causes apoptosis of the AR-positive (androgen-dependent) secretory-type tumor cells, it will not affect NE tumor cells and may actually enrich the NE tumor cell population. The NE cells that survive hormonal therapy may, through secretion of their products, establish paracrine networks to stimulate androgen-independent proliferation of the secretory type tumor cells, leading to tumor recurrence. Therefore, the cellular heterogeneity of prostate cancer may explain the inability of hormonal therapy to eliminate all cancer cells and contribute to its eventual failure in most patients. Many studies suggest that ADT may induce NE differentiation and the latter contributes to the emergence of CRPC. For instance, NE differentiation is increased in high-grade and high-stage [19] localized tumors. Also, it has been shown that levels of circulating chromogranin A (CgA), a product of prostate NE cells, are higher in prostate cancer patients than in patients with benign prostatic conditions. In patients with CaP, serum levels of CgA correlate with both the clinical stage of disease, as well as with the degree to which the cancer has become hormone refractory [20]. Positive staining for CgA by immunohistochemistry of tumor tissue is an independent predictor of cancer progression in well and moderately differentiated prostate cancers [21]. In castration-resistant disease, elevated serum CgA is a significant predictor of poor prognosis, independent of serum PSA and other prognostic factors [22, 23]. Finally, in a gene expression profiling experiment of primary prostate cancers, Singh et al. showed that CgA is one of five genes that correlate strongly with the Gleason score and that this five gene expression model alone accurately predicts the outcome following radical prostatectomy [24].

The relationship of NE differentiation in prostate cancer with chemotherapy is not as well studied. Unlike the non-NE secretory type tumor cells that show proliferative activity, NE tumor cells are normally quiescent, and this may make them resistant to chemotherapeutic agents that target fast-proliferating tumor cells. Interestingly, it has been shown that higher chromogranin A level in patients with CRPC correlated with response to chemotherapy (paclitaxel and carboplatin or mitoxantrone), but not with overall survival [25]. Patients with a PSA response after chemotherapy more commonly had a CgA decrease of 25% or greater than those without a response [25].

The function of NE differentiation has been extensively studied in in vitro and in vivo assays. NE cells secrete biogenic amines, neuropeptides, and cytokines [26] and the non-NE tumor cells express receptors for many of NE cell products [27–33]. In vitro, some NE cell products stimulate proliferation of prostate cancer cells. For instance, interleukin-8 (IL-8), an angiogenic and mitogenic factor for many tumors including CaP, promotes proliferation of prostate cancer cells in the absence of androgen in an in vitro assay [34]. Tissue studies have similarly shown that NE cells in prostate cancer produce IL-8 and non-NE tumor cells express increased levels of the IL-8 receptor CXCR1 [35], suggesting that NE differentiation may be one of the factors contributing to the progression of CaP in a paracrine fashion [36–38]. Deeble et al. showed that LNCaP cells could be induced to show NE phenotype by constitutive expression of an activated form of the cyclic AMP-dependent protein kinase A catalytic subunit. Such NE-like cells could induce proliferation of LNCaP cells in vitro and xenograft tumors in vivo, particularly in castrated hosts [39]. In the CWR22 xenograft tumor model, there was a significant increase in the number of NE cells after castration that preceded the increase in tumor cell proliferation [40]. In the transgenic adenocarcinoma of the mouse prostate (TRAMP) tumor model and the PTEN knockout model, recurrent tumors after castration were also associated with increased NE differentiation [41, 42]. LNCaP xenograft tumors do not normally survive in castrated hosts, but an allograft mouse NE tumor (NE-10) implanted on the opposite flank could support LNCaP xenograft tumor in castrated mice, providing strong evidence for the function of NE differentiation in androgen-independent proliferation of prostate cancer [43]. In an uncastrated host, the same NE cells appear to enhance migration and invasion of LNCaP tumor cells [44].

As NE tumor cells likely represent the androgen-independent subpopulation of CaP cells and may be responsible for tumor recurrence, targeting NE cells in CRPC may thus provide a novel approach to treat this disease. It is known that platinum has activity against cancers with NE differentiation. Together with etoposide or irinotecan, it generates the highest response rates in small cell lung cancer and is the established first-line treatment option for this disease [45]. Pure small cell carcinoma of the prostate is a rare disease and is generally managed similarly to other extrapulmonary small cell carcinomas. Since most of these patients present with metastatic disease at diagnosis, treatment usually consists of cisplatin and etoposide. In those with more localized disease, treatment directed at the prostate with surgery or more commonly radiotherapy can be considered.

If the importance of NE differentiation of prostate cancer is confirmed over time, use of chemotherapies that specifically target NE cells may be a reasonable added option in the armamentarium of CaP treatment and it may provide a rationale for combining platinum drugs with others directed more specifically at the non-NE epithelial cancer cells.

First-Line Platinum Chemotherapy for Prostate Cancer

Single-Agent Cisplatin and Carboplatin

Platinum drugs were studied both as single therapies as well as in combination with taxane chemotherapy (Table 14.1). Cisplatin was the most common treatment in the time period before PSA evaluation. Twenty-five patients were treated with an every 3 weeks regimen of 50–75 mg/m^2 of single-agent cisplatin in 1979 by Yagoda et al. [46]. Twelve percent of patients achieved a partial response, and evaluation with the National Prostate Cancer Project criteria reported 24 patients with stable disease. A later study treated 18 patients with 50 mg/m^2 every 3 weeks with no patients achieving measurable response, leading investigators to conclude that the treatment course was not active [47]. In a 1993 review article, Yagoda and Petrylak reported an overall 12% partial response rate for 209 patients treated with cisplatin [48]. Further examination of both trials with cisplatin every 3 weeks indicated that treatment dose was low and activity level was a reflection of patient selection. This conclusion is based on other studies with higher treatment doses (1 mg/kg per week) for 6 weeks with responses visible in many sites including liver, lung, lymph nodes, and bone.

Carboplatin is a second-generation platinum chemotherapy with a different toxicity profile than cisplatin. The Eastern Cooperative Oncology Group (ECOG) treated 29 CPRC patients with 250–400 mg/m^2 carboplatin depending on renal function and previous radiation. Results show that one out of five (20%) patients with bidimensionally measurable disease achieved a partial response, 1 out of 24 patients with an abnormal bone scan had ≥50% regression in the number of sites with abnormal tracer uptake, and 3 out of 24 patients experienced clinical benefit [49]. Although investigators deemed carboplatin's activity insignificant, it is noted that compared with modern standards, the treatment dose was low and was not

Table 14.1 Single agent cisplatin and carboplatin in CRPC

Author, year	N	PSA response rate (%)	Measurable response rate (%)	Duration of response, median (months)
Cisplatin				
Merrin, 1978	21	–	43	5.8
Merrin, 1979	45	–	29	6
Merrin, 1979	54	–	31.4	7
Yagoda, 1979	25	–	12	2.5
Qazi, 1983	18	–	0	–
Moore, 1986	29	–	10	8
Carboplatin				
Trump, 1990	29	–	20	3
Canobbio, 1993	25	12	17	7
Miglietta, 1995	40	28	17	6.6
Jungi, 1998	27	8	6	NR
Castagneto, 2006	27	27	NR	NR

administered using the current area under the curve (AUC) method. Furthermore, the patient population included those with bone metastases, unlike prior cisplatin studies, and was therefore unable to be evaluated by standard, cross-sectional imaging techniques that were developed at that time.

In the post-PSA era, four clinical trials with weekly carboplatin all showed activity when evaluated by clinical benefit, measurable response, or PSA decline. Canobbio et al. calculated a 17% response rate when combining both measurable and evaluable disease (using PSA and prostatic acid phosphatase) [50]. Patients were treated with a weekly 150 mg/m^2 carboplatin dose, increasing dose intensity after treatments every 3 or 4 weeks. Miglietta et al. performed a second 35 patient study with an equal weekly treatment schedule. Ten patients (28%) had a PSA decline $\geq$50%, and the mean response duration was 6.6 months [51]. Another study by Jungi et al. treated 27 CRPC patients with 400 mg/m^2 carboplatin every 28 days. Thirteen out of 27 patients exhibited a decrease in pain, an improved performance status, and stabilization of metastases, resulting in a 48% clinical benefit response rate [52]. Moreover, 2 out of 24 evaluable patients (8%) showed a PSA response though investigators found no clear link between clinical benefit and PSA decline. At the 2006 Prostate Cancer Symposium, Castagneto et al. reported a study that evaluated 27 CRPC patients treated with 150 mg/m^2 weekly for 3 or 4 weeks. PSA decline $\geq$50% was achieved by 26.9% of patients after treatment [53]. These trials clearly suggest that carboplatin has defi-

nite though moderate activity in CRPC even with various weekly or monthly treatment schedules. No recent trials of carboplatin alone, using AUC dosing, have been reported.

Multiagent Regimens with Cisplatin and Carboplatin

Cisplatin in combination with other drugs is active in CRPC. A multiagent Phase II trial of cisplatin and doxorubicin reported clinical benefit in 24% of patients along with measurable improvement in prostatic acid phosphatase in 21% of patients [54]. Other trials evaluated cisplatin with the following agents: doxorubicin plus 5-flourouracil [55], strontium-89 [56], etopside plus pirarubicin [57], mitoxantrone [58], estramustine plus etoposide [59], and calcitriol plus dexamethasone [60].

Comparison between Strontium-89 (^{89}Sr) with and without cisplatin in a randomized Phase III trial showed mixed results. Seventy CRPC patients with painful bone metastases were evaluated with study endpoints of palliation of bone pain at 2 months, onset of new bone pain, progression of bone metastases, and survival. Cisplatin was infused three times in 11 days up to a total dose of 50 mg/m^2 before and after ^{89}Sr. Pain improvement at 2 months was reported to be 91% for combination therapy and 63% for ^{89}Sr alone. Bone metastases progression was 64% versus 27% favoring the single agent. There were no significant differences in the onset of new bone metastases or survival [61].

Table 14.2 Recent trials of estramustine, platinum, and taxane chemotherapy

Author, year	Phase	Regimen	Number of patients	PSA response rate	Measurable response rate
Kelly, 2001	II	Paclitaxel/estramustine/carboplatin	56	67	45
Urakami, 2002	II	Paclitaxel/estramustine/carboplatin	32	100	61
Solit, 2003	II	Paclitaxel/estramustine/carboplatin	30	60	65
Oh, 2004	II	Docetaxel/estramustine/carboplatin	40	68	52
Oh, 2005	I/II	Docetaxel/estramustine/carboplatin	30	63[a]	24[a]
Berry, 2006	II	Paclitaxel/estramustine/carboplatin	84	61	50[b]
Kikuno, 2006	II	Docetaxel/estramustine/carboplatin	40	95	
Breitz, 2008	II	Picoplatin/docetaxel	30	59	
Ross, 2008	II	Carboplatin/docetaxel	34	18	

[a]At the recommended Phase II dose, the PSA response rate was 75% in 12 patients and measurable responses were seen in two of five (40%) patients

[b]Reported as a pooled endpoint of measurable and/or PSA response

Docetaxel now serves as the standard upon which other agents are added. A number of clinical trials recently combined carboplatin with a taxane (docetaxel or paclitaxel) and estramustine and reported encouraging results (Table 14.2) [62–68]. Phase II trials reported PSA declines $\geq$50% in 60–100% of CRPC patients and objective response rates from 45 to 65% in the cohort of patients with measurable disease. The results further suggest that carboplatin may have success as a second-line therapy for some CRPC patients. However, it should be noted that patients were highly selected for these Phase II trials, and therefore, results may vary in a real world population.

New Platinum Drugs

Recently, various platinum analogs have been tested in the clinical trial setting with both CRPC as well as many other cancers, and a recent comprehensive summary of novel platinum compounds has been published. Oxaliplatin, a platinum analog with a favorable toxicity profile, has shown positive results in cisplatin-resistant cell lines. Droz et al. evaluated the activity of oxaliplatin with and without 5-fluorouracil in 54 CRPC patients in a randomized, multicenter Phase II study. PSA declines were reported in 11 and 19% of patients in each arm, even with more than 50% of the patient population already treated with chemotherapy (including cisplatin) [69].

Picoplatin is a new platinum therapy developed to overcome platinum resistance. A Phase I study conducted by Breitz et al. showed efficacy in CRPC patients treated with a combination of 120 mg/m^2 picoplatin and 75 mg/m^2 docetaxel with prednisone. Nineteen out of 32 evaluable patients (59%) reported a PSA response. At ASCO 2008, Breitz et al. presented a Phase II study which enrolled 30 CRPC on a treatment regimen of 120 mg/m^2 picoplatin and 75 mg/m^2 docetaxel every 3 weeks plus prednisone 5 mg PO bid. Current data report that 59% of evaluable patients achieved a PSA response of >50% decrease for at least 4 weeks indicating that platinum chemotherapy in combination with current therapy may have potential benefit for CRPC patients [6].

Platinum drugs have been tested in other cisplatin-resistant cancers including ovarian and lung cancer. Platinum compound ZD-0473 reported activity in both ovarian and lung cancer cell lines with moderate response rates achieved in both platinum-resistant cancers [69]. Additionally, lobaplatin has also been found to be of benefit in cisplatin-resistant cancer cell lines [70].

Although recent trials have targeted novel drugs in the hope of isolating a standard for second-line therapy, alternative approaches to improving platinum chemotherapy include improving the delivery of the drug to the cancer itself.

Platinum Drugs as Second-Line Therapy for CRPC

With no single standard of care for second-line therapy, patient participation in clinical trials remains a necessary priority [3]. Platinum drugs are currently in clinical development for treatment of CRPC for patients who progressed on docetaxel. Satraplatin and carboplatin represent two platinum analogs that have been tested recently in clinical trials.

In the randomized Phase III data from the SPARC (Satraplatin and Prednisone against Refractory Cancer) trial, 950 metastatic CRPC patients were enrolled to evaluate second-line satraplatin plus prednisone versus prednisone alone [73]. Patients were treated 2:1 to satraplatin 80 mg/m^2 days 1–5 for 5 weeks with 5 mg prednisone twice daily or to prednisone alone. Patients on satraplatin plus prednisone demonstrated a 42% improvement in progression-free survival (PFS) when compared to prednisone alone, as well as a prolonged time to pain progression and a higher PSA response rate. After 6 months, PFS was reported to be 30 and 17% for the satraplatin plus prednisone arm and the prednisone alone arm, respectively. At 12 months, satraplatin plus prednisone continued to show an increase in the percentage of PFS at 17% versus 7% in prednisone alone. These improvements, however, did not translate into a benefit in overall survival, and satraplatin did not receive approval by the Food and Drug Administration.

In a continued effort to expand the second-line therapy options in an environment of limited choices, Ross et al. enrolled 34 patients who progressed on docetaxel in a prospective, multicenter trial of docetaxel 60 mg/m^2 plus carboplatin AUC (4) every 3 weeks. Six out of 34 patients achieved a partial response according to PSA criteria (decrease in ≥50% in serum PSA), and ten patients had stable disease, with three out of ten remaining stable for ≥3 months [71]. Although not statistically significant, results showed that patients with a serum PSA drop ≥50% when treated initially with docetaxel alone were more likely to respond to the combination of docetaxel plus carboplatin. Of the CRPC patients with progressive disease during or shortly after initial treatment with single agent docetaxel, adding carboplatin resulted in PSA declines ≥50% in 18% of patients, and median PFS was 3 months with median response duration of 5.7 months. Further analysis included measurements of the circulating markers, chromagranin A (CgA) and neuron-specific enolase (NSE), from serum samples, showing a trend toward improved PSA response rate in patients with a lower CgA level at baseline; however, the data was not statistically significant.

In 2007, Nakabayashi et al. published a retrospective study evaluating docetaxel/carboplatin as first- and second-line chemotherapy for CRPC patients [72]. Study cohort included patients treated with first-line docetaxel/carboplatin plus estramustine as well as second-line docetaxel/carboplatin alone. The study evaluated 54 patients, and 24 out of them received first-line 140 mg estramustine three times daily plus carboplatin every 3–4 weeks and 20–70 mg/m^2 docetaxel. The remaining 30 patients received second-line 50–70 mg/m^2 docetaxel and carboplatin every 3–4 weeks. Results showed PSA declines of ≥50% in 88 and 20%, respectively, as well as a median overall survival of 17.7 and 14.9 months, respectively. Results suggest that adding carboplatin to traditional docetaxel treatment as second-line therapy positively influences activity in 20% of CRPC patients.

Conclusion

Platinum chemotherapy has been a part of treatment regimens for decades in many cancers including lung, ovarian, and testicular carcinomas. Unlike in these diseases, in which efficacy of platinum chemotherapy is clearly proven, its activity in prostate cancer remains less certain. Pre-PSA era trials evaluating cisplatin and carboplatin as single and as part of multiagent regimens did not demonstrate clear clinical benefit, though one can argue that the rules determining response in the 1980s and 1990s were ineffective. Carboplatin trials in the mid-1990s showed palliative benefit and PSA declines which led to further evaluation. In recent years, multiple trials have combined carboplatin with estramustine and a taxane and shown evidence of high PSA and measurable response rates. However, the question still remains as to the extent to which carboplatin influences PFS or overall survival in CRPC patients.

There is strong support for the consideration of platinum chemotherapy in the management of CRPC. Although docetaxel chemotherapy remains the standard of care for initial treatment of patients with metastatic prostate cancer, platinum chemotherapy alone or in combination with other drugs may have meaningful clinical benefit as second-line therapy for CRPC patients. The SPARC trial showed improvements in PFS˙ and pain response, though overall survival was not affected.

The possibility for specific subtypes of patients with CRPC achieving a greater response to platinum analogs than others requires continued efforts to define these distinct phenotypes.

References

1. Petrylak DP, Tangen CM, Hussain MH, et al. Docetaxel and estramustine compared with mitoxantrone and prednisone for advanced refractory prostate cancer. N Engl J Med 2004;351:1513–20.

2. Tannock IF, de Wit R, Berry WR, et al. Docetaxel plus prednisone or mitoxantrone plus prednisone for advanced prostate cancer. N Engl J Med 2004;351:1502–12.

3. Rosenberg JE, Oh WK. What is the current status of second-line chemotherapy for castration-resistant prostate cancer? Nat Clin Pract Urol 2008;5(12):650–1.

4. Oh WK, Tay M, Huang J. Is there a role for platinum chemotherapy in the treatment of patients with hormone-refractory prostate cancer? Cancer 2007;109(3):477–86.

5. Sternberg CN, Whelan P, Hetherington J, et al. Phase III trial of satraplatin, an oral platinum plus prednisone vs. prednisone alone in patients with hormone-refractory prostate cancer. Oncology 2005;68:2–9.

6. Breitz HB, Roman LA, Karlov PA, et al. A phase II study of picoplatin with docetaxel and prednisone in chemotherapy-naïve patients with metastatic hormone refractory prostate cancer (CRPC). J Clin Oncol 2008; 26 (May 20 Suppl; abstr 5153).

7. McKeage MJ. New-generation platinum drugs in the treatment of cisplatin-resistant cancers. Expert Opin Investig Drugs 2005;14:1033–46.

8. di Sant'Agnese PA. Neuroendocrine differentiation in human prostatic carcinoma. Hum Pathol 1992;23:287–96.

9. Huang J, diSant'Agnese PA. Neuroendocrine differentiation in prostate cancer: an overview. In: Lamberts S, editor. Advances in Oncology: The Expanding Role of Octreotide. Bristol: BioScientifica Ltd; 2002. p. 243–62.

10. Yao JL, Madeb R, Bourne P, et al. Small cell carcinoma of the prostate: an immunohistochemical study. Am J Surg Pathol 2006;30:705–12.

11. Wang W, Epstein JI. Small cell carcinoma of the prostate: a morphologic and immunohistochemical study of 95 cases. Am J Surg Pathol 2008;32:65–71.

12. Evans AJ, Humphrey PA, Belani J, van der Kwast TH, Srigley JR. Large cell neuroendocrine carcinoma of prostate: a clinicopathologic summary of 7 cases of a rare manifestation of advanced prostate cancer. Am J Surg Pathol 2006;30:684–93.

13. Lim KH, Huang MJ, Yang S, Hsieh RK, Lin J. Primary carcinoid tumor of prostate presenting with bone marrow metastases. Urology 2005;65:174.

14. Reyes A, Moran CA. Low-grade neuroendocrine carcinoma (carcinoid tumor) of the prostate. Arch Pathol Lab Med 2004;128:e166–8.

15. Ghannoum JE, DeLellis RA, Shin SJ. Primary carcinoid tumor of the prostate with concurrent adenocarcinoma: a case report. Int J Surg Pathol 2004;12:167–70.

16. Abrahamsson PA, Falkmer S, Falt K, Grimelius L. The course of neuroendocrine differentiation in prostatic carcinomas. An immunohistochemical study testing chromogranin A as an "endocrine marker". Pathol Res Pract 1989;185:373–80.

17. Abrahamsson PA, Wadstrom LB, Alumets J, Falkmer S, Grimelius L. Peptide-hormone- and serotonin-immunoreactive tumour cells in carcinoma of the prostate. Pathol Res Pract 1987;182:298–307.

18. Huang J, Yao JL, di Sant'agnese PA, Yang Q, Bourne PA, Na Y. Immunohistochemical characterization of neuroendocrine cells in prostate cancer. Prostate 2006;66:1399–406.

19. Puccetti L, Supuran CT, Fasolo PP, et al. Skewing towards neuroendocrine phenotype in high grade or high stage androgen-responsive primary prostate cancer. Eur Urol 2005;48:215–21; discussion 21–3.

20. Berruti A, Dogliotti L, Mosca A, et al. Circulating neuroendocrine markers in patients with prostate carcinoma. Cancer 2000;88:2590–7.

21. Theodoropoulos VE, Tsigka A, Mihalopoulou A, et al. Evaluation of neuroendocrine staining and androgen receptor expression in incidental prostatic adenocarcinoma: prognostic implications. Urology 2005;66:897–902.

22. Taplin ME, George DJ, Halabi S, et al. Prognostic significance of plasma chromogranin a levels in patients with hormone-refractory prostate cancer treated in Cancer and Leukemia Group B 9480 study. Urology 2005;66:386–91.

23. Berruti A, Mosca A, Tucci M, et al. Independent prognostic role of circulating chromogranin A in prostate cancer patients with hormone-refractory disease. Endocr Relat Cancer 2005;12:109–17.

24. Singh D, Febbo PG, Ross K, et al. Gene expression correlates of clinical prostate cancer behavior. Cancer Cell 2002;1:203–9.

25. Cabrespine A, Guy L, Gachon F, Cure H, Chollet P, Bay JO. Circulating chromogranin A and hormone refractory prostate cancer chemotherapy. J Urol 2006;175:1347–52.

26. Abdul M, Anezinis PE, Logothetis CJ, Hoosein NM. Growth inhibition of human prostatic carcinoma cell lines by serotonin antagonists. Anticancer Res 1994;14:1215–20.

27. Dizeyi N, Bjartell A, Nilsson E, et al. Expression of serotonin receptors and role of serotonin in human prostate cancer tissue and cell lines. Prostate 2004;59:328–36.

28. Aprikian AG, Han K, Chevalier S, Bazinet M, Viallet J. Bombesin specifically induces intracellular calcium mobilization via gastrin-releasing peptide receptors in human prostate cancer cells. J Mol Endocrinol 1996;16:297–306.

29. Reubi JC, Wenger S, Schmuckli-Maurer J, Schaer JC, Gugger M. Bombesin receptor subtypes in human cancers: detection with the universal radioligand (125)I-[D-TYR(6), beta-ALA(11), PHE(13), NLE(14)] bombesin(6–14). Clin Cancer Res 2002;8:1139–46.

30. Seethalakshmi L, Mitra SP, Dobner PR, Menon M, Carraway RE. Neurotensin receptor expression in prostate cancer cell line and growth effect of NT at physiological concentrations. Prostate 1997;31:183–92.

31. Magni P, Motta M. Expression of neuropeptide Y receptors in human prostate cancer cells. Ann Oncol 2001;12(Suppl 2): S27–9.

32. Wu G, Burzon DT, di Sant'Agnese PA, et al. Calcitonin receptor mRNA expression in the human prostate. Urology 1996;47:376–81.

33. van Leenders GJ, Aalders TW, Hulsbergen-van de Kaa CA, Ruiter DJ, Schalken JA. Expression of basal cell keratins in human prostate cancer metastases and cell lines. J Pathol 2001;195:563–70.

34. Lee LF, Louie MC, Desai SJ, et al. Interleukin-8 confers androgen-independent growth and migration of LNCaP: differential effects of tyrosine kinases Src and FAK. Oncogene 2004;23:2197–205.

35. Huang J, Yao JL, Zhang L, et al. Differential expression of interleukin-8 and its receptors in the neuroendocrine and non-neuroendocrine compartments of prostate cancer. Am J Pathol 2005;166:1807–15.

36. Vashchenko N, Abrahamsson PA. Neuroendocrine differentiation in prostate cancer: implications for new treatment modalities. Eur Urol 2005;47:147–55.

37. Evangelou AI, Winter SF, Huss WJ, Bok RA, Greenberg NM. Steroid hormones, polypeptide growth factors, hormone refractory prostate cancer, and the neuroendocrine phenotype. J Cell Biochem 2004;91:671–83.

38. Adam RM, Kim J, Lin J, et al. Heparin-binding epidermal growth factor-like growth factor stimulates androgen-independent prostate tumor growth and antagonizes androgen receptor function. Endocrinology 2002;143:4599–608.

39. Deeble PD, Cox ME, Frierson HF, Jr., et al. Androgen-independent growth and tumorigenesis of prostate cancer cells are enhanced by the presence of PKA-differentiated neuroendocrine cells. Cancer Res 2007;67:3663–72.

40. Huss WJ, Gregory CW, Smith GJ. Neuroendocrine cell differentiation in the CWR22 human prostate cancer xenograft: association with tumor cell proliferation prior to recurrence. Prostate 2004;60:91–7.

41. Kaplan-Lefko PJ, Chen TM, Ittmann MM, et al. Pathobiology of autochthonous prostate cancer in a pre-clinical transgenic mouse model. Prostate 2003;55:219–37.

42. Liao CP, Zhong C, Saribekyan G, et al. Mouse models of prostate adenocarcinoma with the capacity to monitor spontaneous carcinogenesis by bioluminescence or fluorescence. Cancer Res 2007;67:7525–33.

43. Jin RJ, Wang Y, Masumori N, et al. NE-10 neuroendocrine cancer promotes the LNCaP xenograft growth in castrated mice. Cancer Res 2004;64:5489–95.

44. Uchida K, Masumori N, Takahashi A, et al. Murine androgen-independent neuroendocrine carcinoma promotes metastasis of human prostate cancer cell line LNCaP. Prostate 2006;66(5):536–45.

45. Noda K, Nishiwaki Y, Kawahara M, et al. Irinotecan plus cisplatin compared with etoposide plus cisplatin for extensive small-cell lung cancer. N Engl J Med 2002; 346:85–91.

46. Yagoda A, Watson RC, Natale RB, et al. A critical analysis of response criteria in patients with prostatic cancer treated with cis-diamminedichloride platinum II. Cancer 1979;44:1553–62.

47. Qazi R, Khandekar J. Phase II study of cisplatin for metastatic prostatic carcinoma. An Eastern Cooperative Oncology Group study. Am J Clin Oncol 1983;6:203–5.

48. Yagoda A, Petrylak D. Cytotoxic chemotherapy for advanced hormone-resistant prostate cancer. Cancer 1993;71: 1098–109.

49. Trump DL, Marsh JC, Kvols LK, et al. A phase II trial of carboplatin (NSC 241240) in advanced prostate cancer, refractory to hormonal therapy. An Eastern Cooperative Oncology Group pilot study. Invest New Drugs 1990; 8(Suppl 1):S91–4.

50. Canobbio L, Guarneri D, Miglietta L, et al. Carboplatin in advanced hormone refractory prostatic cancer patients. Eur J Cancer 1993;29A:2094–6.

51. Miglietta L, Cannobbio L, Boccardo F. Assessment of response to carboplatin in patients with hormone-refractory prostate cancer: a critical analysis of drug activity. Anticancer Res 1995;15:2825–8.

52. Jungi WF, Bernhard J, Hurny C, et al. Effect of carboplatin on response and palliation in hormone-refractory prostate cancer. Swiss Group for Clinical Cancer Research (SAKK). Support Care Cancer 1998;6:462–8.

53. Castagneto B, Ferraris V, Perachino M, et al. Weekly administration of standardized low-dose carboplatin (CBDCA) in the treatment of advanced hormone refractory prostate cancer (CRPC): a phase II study. Proceedings GH Cancer Symposium 2006; abstract 243.

54. Citrin DL, Hogan TF. A phase II evaluation of adriamycin and cis-platinum in hormone resistant prostate cancer. Cancer 1982;50:201–6.

55. Droz JP, Fargeot P, Laplaige P, et al. Phase II trial of the association of doxorubicin, 5 FU and cis platinum in hormonally unresponsive metastatic carcinoma of the prostate. Prog Clin Biol Res 1987;243B:235–42.

56. Mertens WC, Porter AT, Reid RH, et al. Strontium-89 and low-dose infusion cisplatin for patients with hormone refractory prostate carcinoma metastatic to bone: a preliminary report. J Nucl Med 1992;33:1437–43.

57. Naito S, Ueda T, Kotoh S, et al. Treatment of advanced hormone-refractory prostate carcinoma with a combination of etoposide, pirarubicin and cisplatin. Cancer Chemother Pharmacol 1995;35:225–9.

58. Osborne CK, Blumenstein BA, Crawford ED, et al. Phase II study of platinum and mitoxantrone in metastatic prostate cancer: a Southwest Oncology Group Study. Eur J Cancer 1992;28:477–8.

59. Steineck G, Reuter V, Kelly WK, et al. Cytotoxic treatment of aggressive prostate tumors with or without neuroendocrine elements. Acta Oncol 2002;41:668–74.

60. Flaig TW, Barqawi A, Miller G, et al. A phase II trial of dexamethasone, vitamin D, and carboplatin in patients with hormone-refractory prostate cancer. Cancer 2006;107:266–74.

61. Tu SM, Millikan RE, Mengistu B, et al. Bone-targeted therapy for advanced androgen-independent carcinoma of the prostate: a randomised phase II trial. Lancet 2001; 357(9253):336–41.

62. Berry W, Friedland D, Fleagle J, et al. A phase II study of weekly paclitaxel/estramustine/carboplatin in hormone-refractory prostate cancer. Clin Genitourin Cancer 2006;5:131–7.

63. Kelly WK, Curley T, Slovin S, et al. Paclitaxel, estramustine phosphate, and carboplatin in patients with advanced prostate cancer. J Clin Oncol 2001;19:44–53.

64. Urakami S, Igawa M, Kikuno N, et al. Combination chemotherapy with paclitaxel, estramustine and carboplatin

for hormone refractory prostate cancer. J Urol 2002;168: 2444–50.

65. Solit DB, Morris M, Slovin S, et al. Clinical experience with intravenous estramustine phosphate, paclitaxel, and carboplatin in patients with castrate, metastatic prostate adenocarcinoma. Cancer 2003;98:1842–8.

66. Kikuno N, Urakami S, Nakamura S, et al. Phase-II study of docetaxel, estramustine phosphate, and carboplatin in patients with hormone-refractory prostate cancer. Eur Urol 2008;51(5):1252–8.

67. Oh WK, Halabi S, Kelly WK, et al. A phase II study of estramustine, docetaxel, and carboplatin with granulocyte-colony-stimulating factor support in patients with hormone-refractory prostate carcinoma: Cancer and Leukemia Group B 99813. Cancer 2003;98:2592–8.

68. Oh WK, Hagmann E, Manola J, et al. A phase I study of estramustine, weekly docetaxel, and carboplatin chemotherapy in patients with hormone-refractory prostate cancer. Clin Cancer Res 2005;11:284–9.

69. Hay MP. ZD-0473 AstraZeneca. Curr Opin Investig Drugs 2000;1:263–6.

70. McKeage MJ. Lobaplatin: a new antitumour platinum drug. Expert Opin Investig Drugs 2001;10:119–28.

71. Ross RW, Beer TM, Jacobus S, Bubley GJ, Taplin ME, Ryan CW, Huang J, Oh WK. A phase 2 study of carboplatin plus docetaxel in men with metastatic hormone-refractory prostate cancer who are refractory to docetaxel. Cancer 2008;112(3):521–6.

72. Nakabayashi M, Sartor O, Jacobus S, et al. Response to docetaxel (D)/carboplatin (C)-based chemotherapy as first- and second-line therapy in patients with metastatic hormone-refractory prostate cancer (CRPC). J Clin Oncol 2007 ASCO Annual Meeting Proceedings Part I. Vol 25, No. 18S (June 20 Supplement), 2007.

73. Sternberg CN, Petrylak DP, Sartor O, et al. Multinational, double-blind, phase III study of prednisone and either satraplatin or placebo in patients with castrate-refractory prostate cancer progressing after prior chemotherapy: the SPARC trial. J Clin Oncol 2009;27:5431–8.

Chapter 15
Clinical Pharmacology and Pharmacogenetics of Chemotherapy in Prostate Cancer

Tristan M. Sissung and William D. Figg

Abstract Cytotoxic chemotherapy using docetaxel, estramustine, and mitoxantrone is often employed to treat men with hormone-refractory prostate tumors. More recently, oral satraplatin has been studied as an alternative to docetaxel-based therapies. These cytotoxic agents have diverse mechanisms of action and disposition. Moreover, there is often wide inter-individual variation in the pharmacokinetics, toxicity, and clinical outcome following administration of these agents in patients with prostate cancer. This chapter summarizes what is known about the basic clinical pharmacology of these agents and discusses the mechanisms and implications of interindividual variation in treatment.

Keywords Docetaxel • Mitoxantrone • Estramustine • Satraplatin • Prostate cancer • Pharmacogenetics • Pharmacology

Introduction

In 2008, the National Cancer Institute documented 186,320 new cases and 28,660 deaths due to prostate cancer. The majority of deaths are expected to have occurred in men with metastatic castration-resistant prostate cancer (CRPC), and a large proportion of these men likely received cytotoxic chemotherapy prior to death. However, CRPC has only been effectively treated with cytotoxic agents as recently as 2004 with the approval of docetaxel as the standard of care in metastatic CRPC. Docetaxel-based therapy still only provides an approximate 2–3-month survival benefit over palliative care with mitoxantrone plus prednisone [1, 2]. Other chemotherapies, such as oral satraplatin, have been introduced in men with CRPC with limited success.

There is often great interindividual variation in the survival and palliative benefits of these chemotherapies despite their often-narrow therapeutic indices. Thus, treatment is more or less effective or toxic within certain subgroups based on differences in genetic, morphometric, physiological, and demographic parameters. Furthermore, there are notable differences in pharmacokinetics (PK) brought on by interindividual variation suggesting that individualized dosing could improve therapeutic outcome in some cases. The purpose of this chapter is to summarize what is currently known about the mechanism, clinical pharmacology, interindividual variability, and pharmacogenetics of the major cytotoxic agents that have been used in prostate cancer including docetaxel, estramustine, mitoxantrone, and satraplatin.

Docetaxel

Mechanism of Action

Docetaxel binds to β-tubulin and promotes the polymerization of microtubules while also inhibiting depolymerization. This disrupts the normal dynamics of microtubules that are required for formation of the cytoskeleton and the movement of the mitotic spindle, ultimately leading to cell cycle arrest in the G2/M phase and subsequent apoptosis. Docetaxel has other

W.D. Figg (✉)
Medical Oncology Branch, Center for Cancer Research
National Cancer Institute, National Institute of Health,
Bethesda, MD, USA
e-mail: wdfigg@helix.nih.gov

W.D. Figg et al. (eds.), *Drug Management of Prostate Cancer*,
DOI 10.1007/978-1-60327-829-4_15, © Springer Science+Business Media, LLC 2010

proapoptotic effects as well including inhibiting the antiapoptotic protein BCL2 overexpression, interactions with BCLxl, upregulation of p53, and antiangiogenic properties [3, 4].

Pharmacokinetics, Drug Distribution, and Pharmacodynamic Determinants

Docetaxel can be assayed in plasma with a detection range of 5–1,000 ng/mL by high performance liquid chromatography-mass spectrometry (HPLC-MS) [5–7]. Other methods have been developed to determine unbound docetaxel levels [8] as well as the concentration of its vehicle, polysorbate 80 [9], allowing for sophisticated PK determinations. Docetaxel is administered intravenously, and the distribution is generally accepted to be approximately 30–100 L/m^2 in most individuals. This rather large volume of distribution is consistent with ~98% of the drug being protein-bound. Polysorbate 80 in concentrations observed in patients treated with docetaxel is responsible for increasing the unbound fraction of docetaxel by 50% [10], resulting in greater exposure to docetaxel as well as greater likelihood of neutropenia [11, 12]. It has been proposed that polysorbate 80 is able to form micelar complexes with proteins, including serum albumin and α1-acid glycoprotein causing saturable binding of docetaxel that has also been observed with other drugs [13, 14], or by rapid degradation of polysorbate 80 by plasma esterases followed by oleic acid-mediated protein binding displacement of docetaxel [15]. Docetaxel is subjected to successive hydroxylation reactions by cytochrome P450 CYP3A4/5 at the C13 carbon on the *tert*-butyl sidechain resulting in hydroxy-docetaxel, two stereometric hydroxyoxazolidinones, and an oxazolidinone metabolite (called M1–M4, respectively), and approximately 75% of the drug is recovered in these relatively inactive metabolites [16] (Fig. 15.1). Docetaxel is primarily eliminated by excretion into the bile with approximately 5–10% being cleared by urinary excretion.

The importance of CYP3A enzymes on docetaxel metabolism was recently underscored in a study that found a sevenfold decrease in the clearance of docetaxel in mice lacking the *Cyp3a* gene cluster [17] and another study that found that individuals with certain high expression/function of *CYP3A* alleles had an approximate 64–75% increase in docetaxel clearance

[18, 19]. Both parent drug and docetaxel metabolites are transported across several biological barriers by the transporters ABCB1 [20], ABCC2 [21], and OATP1B3 [22] (see Fig. 15.1). The current literature suggests that docetaxel is taken into the liver by OATP1B3, inactivated by CYP3A4/5, eliminated through hepatobilliary secretion by ABCB1 and ABCC2, and undergoes enterohepatic recirculation that is mediated by ABCB1 [23]. Such metabolism and transport characteristics have also been noted in peripheral tissues including blood–brain and blood–nerve barriers [24–26], within hematopoietic cells [27, 28], and even within tumors themselves leading to multidrug resistance [29, 30]. Moreover, the genes encoding the above enzymes and transporters are all regulated by the pregnane X receptor (PXR; NR1I2), the constitutive androstane receptor (CAR; NR1I3) nuclear receptors that promiscuously bind to many different xenobiotic substrates and modulate gene expression [31, 32]. CYP1B1 also generates reactive estrogen species that may be responsible for docetaxel inefficacy by both interfering with docetaxel–microtubule interactions as well as covalently binding to docetaxel itself and reducing its potency [33, 34].

Nongenetic Sources of Variability in Docetaxel Pharmacology

Docetaxel variability is manifested in an approximate 10% difference in docetaxel clearance among individuals [35], an approximate 10–35% lower clearance in women than in men [18, 36, 37], wide variability in systemic exposure [38], alterations in toxicity determined by PK and/or drug distribution [39, 40], and ultimately alterations in progression and time to death [40, 41]. To date, variability in PK has been evaluated in a variety of populations with several different diseases, and it has been noted that hepatic function, gender dimorphism, age, and plasma protein levels (especially the α-acid glycoprotein, AAG) are important determinants of PK and pharmacodynamics (PD) [42]. It is expected that drug coadministration, comorbidity, diet, and myriad other factors also influence docetaxel PK/PD, although these remain poorly studied. Pharmacokinetic modeling in patients has revealed that the most important factors in determining interindividual variation in docetaxel clearance (L/h) are body surface area (BSA; m^2), age (years), AAG

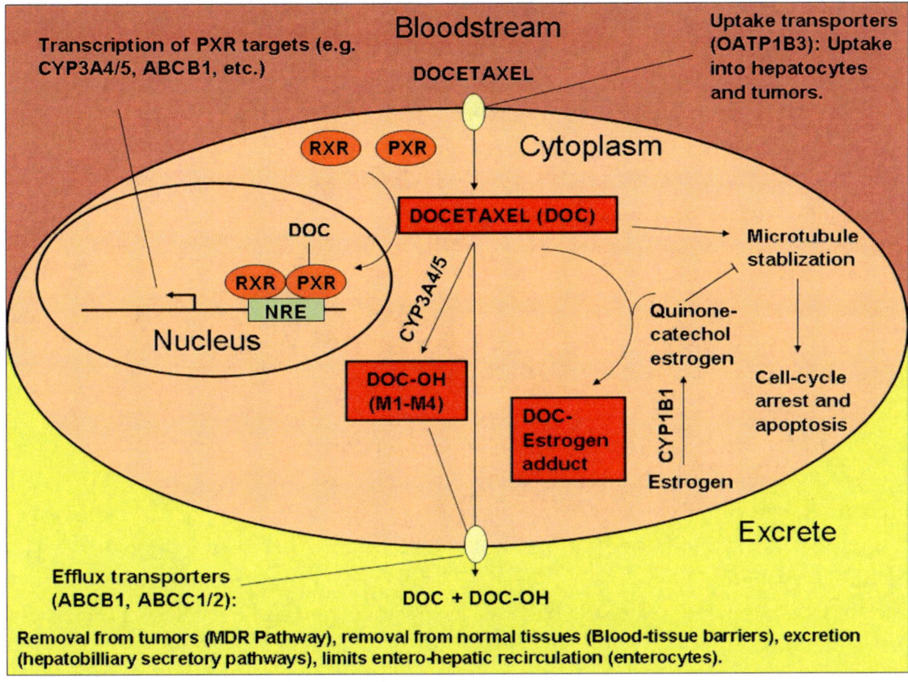

Fig. 15.1 Docetaxel metabolic and transport pathway. Docetaxel-related intracellular pathways, uptake, metabolism, and elimination

levels (g/L), albumin levels (g/L), and hepatic dysfunction affecting clearance of docetaxel (HEP12) as is shown in the following equation [43].

$$CL = BSA\,(22.1 - 3.55\,AAG - 0.095\,AGE + 0.2245\,ALB)\cdot(1 - 0.334\,HEP12)$$

As the aforementioned model suggests, the binding of docetaxel to serum proteins and liver function is especially important to determining variability in docetaxel pharmacology. Docetaxel binds to albumin, AAG, and lipoproteins in the serum, is primarily metabolized in the liver, and cleared through the hepatobiliary route.

Liver function abnormalities are associated with reduced docetaxel clearance that is highly variable as compared to patients with normal liver function, and much of this variability can be attributed to a reduced CYP3A activity phenotype – especially in patients with advanced liver dysfunction [11, 44]. However, liver metastases of prostate cancer are uncommon; therefore, liver impairment is not characteristic of this disease. Since AAG levels are highly variable in individuals with certain types of cancer as a result of proinflammatory pathways, AAG levels are also considered to be the very important determinants of variation in docetaxel plasma-protein binding properties [45]. Higher AAG levels are considered a surrogate for decreased unbound fraction available for elimination [46], an expected reduction in hematological toxicity [11], and a potential effect on nonhematological toxicity. Some have suggested that inflammation in the prostate may lead to prostate cancer, and that AAG can play a role in disease etiology [47, 48]. A strong, nonsignificant trend does indeed exist where men with metastatic prostate cancer have elevated AAG, while African American and Caucasian men also have higher levels of AAG than men of other races [49, 50]. However, it is unclear if AAG levels are clinically important covariates in docetaxel treatment of advanced prostate cancer, although this relationship has been demonstrated in non-small cell lung carcinoma – a disease with frequent liver involvement resulting in high AAG levels [51]. Finally, others have shown that castrate patients have a 50% higher clearance of docetaxel than noncastrate patients [52], resulting in increased likelihood of neutropenic events [53, 54]. Therefore, hormonal factors may change the metabolism of docetaxel in males.

Since albumin, AAG, and CYP3A are of liver origin, no changes are expected in most cases of advanced prostate cancer although AAG levels might be higher. It should also again be noted that since men have a rapid clearance of docetaxel than women, and that docetaxel clearance is even higher in men with metastatic prostate cancer than in noncastrate patients, liver function differences might be less important in prostate cancer than in other diseases. This may change only if the patient has massive liver involvement, which is very uncommon.

Renal function is also not expected to be an important determinant of docetaxel PK/PD given that so little docetaxel is cleared through the urine (~5–10%). Indeed, an individual with advanced renal disease receiving docetaxel at 65 mg/m^2 had similar pharmacokinetic parameters to patients without renal failure receiving the same treatment [55]. However, confirmation of these results in a larger patient cohort has not yet been published.

Several studies have related age to PK/PD parameters during docetaxel treatment. At the highest dose evaluated (75 mg/m^2), docetaxel PK were unchanged, although docetaxel-induced neutropenia was higher in the elderly cohort (16%) than in the younger cohort (0%) [56]. Another study found that docetaxel toxicity is also increased in elderly patients while pharamacokinetics remain unchanged [57]. However, the aforementioned studies evaluated few elderly patients ($n \leq 26$), and only a very small cohort of elderly patients with prostate cancer receiving single-agent docetaxel ($n \leq 6$) was evaluated. Furthermore, both of these studies were in contrast to a larger pharmacokinetic study, where clearance was modestly related to age (estimated at a 7% decrease in mean clearance for a 71-year-old patient) [58]. Other studies have evaluated elderly patients with non-small cell lung carcinoma and found that docetaxel at a dose of (30–60 mg/m^2) is well tolerated alone or in combination with cisplatin [59–61]. Thus, age might be associated with interindividual differences in docetaxel-related toxicity in a dose/schedule-dependant fashion, but age may only be modestly associated with PK.

Docetaxel Pharmacogenetics

Several pharmacogenetic studies have been completed studying genetic variation in docetaxel disposition genes including *ABCB1*, *ABCC2*, *ABCG2*, *CYP1B1*, *CYP3A4/5*, *NR1I2*, *NR1I3*, and *SLCO1B3* (encoding OATP1B3). The results from these studies will be summarized below in the following sections.

CYP3A4 and CYP3A5

Several have evaluated the *CYP3A4*1B* and *CYP3A5*3C* polymorphisms in relation to the PK of docetaxel. Most studies in this regard have been negative [62–68], although recent evidence suggests that these SNPs may be important when considered in the context of *CYP3A4/5* haplotype [18, 19]. Baker et al. found that carriers of a haplotype consisting of *CYP3A4*1B* (i.e., variant at rs2740574) and *CYP3A5*1A* alleles (i.e., wild type at *CYP3A5*3C*; rs776746) that was named *CYP3A4/5*2* had a 64% higher clearance of docetaxel and a 46% increase in clearance of another CYP3A4/5 substrate, midazolam. Those individuals ($n = 5$) carrying the *CYP3A4/5*2* haplotype may actually have a higher level of CYP3A expression in the liver due to increases in CYP3A4 expression brought on by the *CYP3A4*1B* allele [69], coupled with CYP3A5 expression in the liver in those patients not carrying the *CYP3A5*3* null allele. Another study in Caucasians had similar results with those individuals carrying *CYP3A4*1B* and *CYP3A5*1A* alleles having a 75% increase in docetaxel clearance, although this relationship depended on clearance data from only four patients [19].

It is important to note that the above findings cannot be extrapolated to other world populations as the haplotype is organized in a different fashion in non-Caucasians, and future investigations evaluating this haplotype must take interracial genetic variation into account. However, most investigations in the Caucasian population taking place prior to these studies did not evaluate the effect of *CYP3A4/5* haplotypes that might be better associated with clearance of substrate drugs, or outcome following treatment [62, 63, 65, 68]. Those studies in the Asian population suffered from very low power due to *CYP3A4/5* monomorphism [67], or low frequency of these SNPs in the Asian population [64, 66] and are thus inconclusive or difficult to interpret. African Americans also have a different haplotype organization, and no relationship has been found between *CYP3A4/5* SNPs and docetaxel PK/PD in this racial population [68]. In summary, the haplotype structure of *CYP3A4/5* is very likely an important determinant of pharmacogenetics relationships between these enzymes and docetaxel PK/PD in Caucasians, and *CYP3A4/5* haplotypes remain poorly studied in relation to docetaxel PK/PD in all world populations.

The ABCB1, ABCC2, ABCG2, and OATP1B3 Active Transporters of Docetaxel

Pharmacogenetics studies in active transporters in docetaxel treatment are quite complex as docetaxel transport seems to be responsible for drug distribution throughout the body including in and out of blood–brain/nerve barriers, hematopoeitic cells, enterocytes, and liver cells. For this reason, all of the aforementioned transporters might determine local drug levels in addition to overall PK of docetaxel; thus, genetic variation within this pathway might influence several tissues in a different fashion.

Earlier studies found that *ABCB1* polymorphisms were associated with clearance of docetaxel and midazolam [62, 64] and docetaxel toxicity [19]. Still other studies found no relationship between docetaxel PK and ABCB1 SNPs [19, 67]. Since Kimchi-Sarfaty et al. published rather convincing evidence that *ABCB1* haplotypes are related to protein folding and expression in a fashion that is more deterministic that any individual *ABCB1* SNP alone, two studies have investigated the combined effect of ABCB1 SNPs at the 1236C>T, 2677G>T/A, and 3435C>T loci.

Studies that investigated *ABCB1* 1236C>T, 2677G>T/A, 3435C>T SNPs alone and in diplotype combinations found that patients with castration-resistant prostate cancer (CRPC) receiving docetaxel alone and who carried 1236C-2677G-3435C linked alleles had improved overall survival, while patients carrying the 2677T-3435T diplotype had shorter median survival after treatment. Interestingly, patients with the 2677T-3435T haplotype also had higher on-study PSA that might be related to survival as those patients who had a higher disease burden. However, it may be that patients carrying certain *ABCB1* diplotypes had tumors that were more resistant to docetaxel therapy or alterations in clearance that were responsible for this relationship. However, no relationship with clearance was observed in a separate cohort of patients treated with docetaxel in this study, and other studies have found relationships with docetaxel outcomes that are independent of PK [19]. The present study also found that patients treated with docetaxel in combination with

thalidomide (not an ABCB1 substrate) had an increased likelihood to develop early onset neuropathy, while there was no relationship found in those treated with docetaxel alone. This is probably because thalidomide also causes neuropathies resulting in a higher neuropathy burden in the combination arm. Thus, small differences in efflux of docetaxel from nerve tissues due to *ABCB1* SNPs may contribute to onset of neuropathy in these patients. Finally, a trend toward increased neutropenia grade was also observed in patients homozygous for the 2677T-3435T haplotype. This study suggests that *ABCB1* SNPs contribute to survival and toxicity differences in men with CRPC and again demonstrates that haplotype analysis is important to determine associations with polymorphisms in docetaxel disposition genes and clinical outcome. A second study investigated variation in both individual genotypes and in the common haplotypes within *ABCB1* (1236C>T, 2677G>T/A, 3435C>T), *ABCC2* (−1019A>G, −24C>T, 1249G>A, IVS26 −34C>T, 3972C>T, 4544G>A), and *SLCO1B3* (334T>G, 439A>G, 699G>A, 767G>C, 1559A>C, 1679T>C) against docetaxel clearance data in Caucasian patients with various malignancies, including 24 patients with prostate cancer. None of the genotypes or haplotypes were related to docetaxel PK, as was consistent with the former study.

Other known docetaxel transporters have been less studied. The *ABCC2* rs12762549 SNP has been linked to docetaxel-induced neutropenia in the Asian population [67], although no associations between *ABCC2* polymorphisms, alone or in haplotype, have been found in relation to docetaxel PK [18]. Similar results were found for SNPs in *SLCO1B3*. Interestingly, the protein product of *SLCO1B3* (OATP1B3) is upregulated during prostate cancer progression [70, 71], although no study has linked *SLCO1B3* SNPs to docetaxel efficacy in this disease. Finally, the *ABCG2* Q141K polymorphism was associated with improved survival following treatment with combination docetaxel and vinorelbine or combination docetaxel and estramustine in men with CRPC [65]. The authors concluded that the increase in survival was related to inefficiency of the drug efflux pump leading to increased efficacy in some patients. However, since docetaxel is not an ABCG2 substrate [72], it is likely that ABCG2 effluxes another substrate that lowers docetaxel efficacy, or that decreases in ABCG2 pump efficiency brought on by the Q141K SNP [73] can alter the efflux of a substrate that is related to cancer progression (e.g., PhIP).

Other Docetaxel Pharmacogenetics Studies

Some studies have attempted to link docetaxel PK to polymorphisms in *PXR*, *CAR*, and *HNF4α* in the Asian population [66, 74]. The rationale for such studies is explained in Fig. 15.1 where nuclear receptors bind to docetaxel and increase the expression of genes related to docetaxel metabolism and transport. Such nuclear receptors are thus responsible for global regulation of genes involved in docetaxel disposition. While no such study has found a relationship with PK, a relationship between the Met49Val SNP in *HNF4α* and slower neutrophil recovery was observed [66]. This same study found that patients who were wild type for both *HNF4α* Met49Val and *CAR* Pro180Pro had an approximate 16% lower percentage neutrophil decrease from baseline. Thus, it seems that while *PXR* and *CAR* are polymorphic, the SNPs in these genes have not yet been found to be responsible for any detectible interindividual variation in relation to docetaxel. However, genetic variation in *HNF4α*, which regulates genes involved in cell growth and survival, might be responsible for the robustness of neutrophils when challenged by docetaxel treatment, and this might be related to variation in *PXR/CAR*. Further study is needed to both validate the above study and elucidate the molecular reasons behind these associations.

CYP1B1 has also been found to be related to docetaxel treatment. Early studies indicated that CYP1B1 might directly metabolize docetaxel [75], although a later study indicated rather convincingly that this was not true [76]. However, CYP1B1 was found to be highly expressed in the prostate tumors and seemed to be related to docetaxel treatment [34, 77]. Three studies have been published that have indicated that the *CYP1B1* L432V (*CYP1B1*3*) allele might be associated with docetaxel treatment efficacy in prostate cancer [33, 78, 79]. This relationship is likely due to more efficient metabolism of estrogen by individuals carrying the *CYP1B1*3* allele, resulting in increased levels of reactive estrogen metabolites that antagonize docetaxel by destablizing tubulin and directly adducting docetaxel itself. Indeed, higher levels of CYP1B1 estrogen metabolites have been observed in the urine of men with prostate cancer [80]. However, further studies are required to validate these data in the clinic and in the laboratory.

Mitoxantrone

Mechanism of Action

Anthracycline antibiotics, including mitoxantrone, are responsible for several different biological effects related to their role as anticancer agents. The main mechanism behind the antineoplastic effect of these agents is inhibition of topoisomerase II (TOPOII) resulting in inhibition of DNA repair [81]. Mitoxantrone also inhibits DNA replication and DNA-dependent RNA synthesis in its role as a DNA intercalating agent, DNA replication through inhibition of nuclear helicase, and can undergo reduction reactions resulting in the formation of quinone species that damage cellular components [82, 83]. However, mitoxantrone is significantly less reactive than other anthracyclines and thus does not form free radical intermediates as readily. For this reason, it is also less likely to cause cardiotoxicity, and higher dosages can be given without increasing the risk of cardiac failure [84]. Mitoxantrone has been observed bound to DNA, and it accumulates in the endoplasmic reticulum, cytosol, and in low-polarity environments consistent with cell membranes [85]. Unlike other cytotoxic agents, mitoxantrone cytotoxicity is cell cycle-independent, killing both proliferating and nonproliferating cells alike [86]. Mitxantrone plus steroidal therapy has been used for the treatment of CRPC for its palliative effects, but this therapy does not increase life expectancy [87–89].

Pharmacokinetics, Drug Distribution, and Pharmacodynamic Determinants

There is an approximate 13-fold interindividual variation in the area under the curve (AUC) exposure following mitoxantrone in patients with acute lymphoblastic leukemia (ALL) receiving 5 mg/m^2 every week for 3 weeks [90]. A population PK model demonstrated an approximately 46% interindividual variability in clearance [91]. For men suffering from CRPC, mitoxantrone is typically given at a dose level of 12 mg/m^2 every 3 weeks in combination with steroids such as prednisone. Mitoxantrone is distributed rapidly and extensively into the tissues while ~78% of the drug is protein bound. Two major mono- and dicarboxylic acid metabolites have been observed, although several metabolites are present. The primary routes of elimination of mitoxantrone include hepatobilliary (~25% over 5 days) and urinary excretion (6–11%; 65% of drug is unchanged).

Mitoxantrone is extruded from cells expressing the ATP-binding cassette transporters ABCB1 (MDR1, P-glycoprotein) [92], ABCC1 (MRP1) [93–95], ABCC2 (MRP2) [96], and ABCG2 (BCRP, MXR, ABCP) [97, 98], and it is also actively influxed into certain cells via an unknown mechanism [99]. Whereas these transporters are expressed in hepatic and renal cells, they could mediate mitoxantrone elimination pathways, and some of these transporters limit penetration of anthracyclines into certain tissues such as hematopoietic stem cells, thereby limiting toxicity [25]. Prostate tumors frequently upregulate ATP-binding cassette (ABC) transporters, such as ABCB1 and ABCG2 [100, 101], during the course of tumor progression. It is likely that resistance to mitoxantrone occurs due to multidrug resistance brought on by over-expression of active drug transporters. Overexpression of these transporters seems to be related to prolonged androgen deprivation [101, 102], acquired resistance to mitoxantrone [103], and the ability of normal and tumor stem cells to evade cytotoxicity [101, 104]. It is also possible that downregulation of an uncharacterized influx mechanism could also be responsible for mitoxantrone resistance, although this remains to be explored [99]. The pathways that regulate mitoxantrone metabolism have not yet been elucidated.

Nongenetic Sources of Variability in Pharmacology

Mitoxantrone clearance is reduced in patients with hepatic dysfunction, and patients with normal hepatic function with bilirubin >3.4 mg/dL have a threefold increase in AUC exposure following mitoxantrone. Thus, dose adjustments are required in patients with moderate to severe hepatic dysfunction. Advanced age does not appear to be related to mitoxantrone toxicity or outcome as the drug was well tolerated with similar response in patients with ALL >60 years of age at both high (80 mg/m^2; day 2) and low (12 mg/m^2; days 1–3) doses [105].

Pharmacogenetics

The common *ABCG2* 421C>A (Q141K) variant has been attributed to lowered expression of ABCG2 [106–110]. The Q141K polymorphism is responsible for an approximate two- to fivefold increase in drug sensitivity toward mitoxantrone in vitro as compared to the wild-type protein in four separate studies [73, 106, 111, 112]. The *ABCG2* 34G>A (V12M) allele has been linked to poor localization of ABCG2 resulting in a less functional protein [73], while a small proportion of the Japanese population (~2%) carries the *ABCG2* 376C>T (Q126stop) transition that results in protein truncation and a complete loss of ABCG2 function [106]. The V12M polymorphism was not associated with increased mitoxantrone sensitivity vs. the wild-type allele when expressed in PA137 and Flp-ln-293 cells [106, 112], but it abolished the effect of ABCG2 expression in LLC-PK1 cells treated with mitoxantrone [73]. Some speculate that the Q126stop truncation increases sensitivity through drastically lowering ABCG2 expression [106, 113], although no data have emerged to support this conclusion. Other alleles have been explored that are only found in small proportions of certain world populations or are only present in cancer cell lines [106, 112, 114, 115], but it is unclear if any of these are relevant to clinical treatment with mitoxantrone. Further, while ABC-transporter polymorphisms have been related to the PK of numerous anticancer drugs [116], ABCG2 and ABCB1 mRNA levels have been related to mitoxantrone treatment outcome in cancer [117], and ABCG2 was even initially discovered as a mediator of mitoxantrone resistance in cancer cell lines [97, 98], no clinical studies evaluating the relationship between transporter polymorphisms and mitoxantrone pharmacology have yet been published (based on a PubMed search of "transporter polymorphism mitoxantrone" revealing 22 articles; conducted December 19, 2008).

Estramustine

Mechanism of Action

Estramustine phosphate is a nor-nitrogen mustard-carbamate estradiol that is administered to men with prostate cancer. The initial design of estramustine targeted hormone-dependent cancers where estramustine was thought to bind hormone receptors and mediate DNA alkylation in the nucleus through the mustard-carbamate moiety [118]. Interestingly, the drug has little (if any) alykylating activity, and intact estramustine does not bind to hormone receptors. Estramustine does increase the levels of estradiol through hydrolysis of the nitrogen mustard moiety, thus increasing estradiol binding to the estrogen receptor [119]. Like mitoxantrone, estramustine has a range of biological effects that suppress cell growth in prostate tumors, and these include direct cytotoxicity, inhibition of mitosis, promotion of apoptosis, microtubule depolymerization, inhibition of DNA synthesis, TOPOII inhibition, blockade of tyrosine kinase, disruption of apoptotic regulators such as bcl-2, activation of death domain receptors (as reviewed by Ho et al. [120]), formation of oxygen radicals [121], and interaction with nuclear matrix proteins [122, 123].

Pharmacokinetics, Drug Distribution, and Pharmacodynamic Determinants

Estramustine phosphate is administered to men with prostate cancer orally at a dose level of approximately 300 mg twice daily. Most of the estramustine phosphate is retained within the body following drug administration. Estramustine phosphate is rapidly dephosphorylated to estramustine most likely through alkaline phosphatase found in nearly every tissue [124], and oral estramustine is subject to heavy first-pass metabolism through this mechanism. As such, the oral bioavailability of intact estramustine phosphate is low (~44–75%) with the majority of the drug being converted into other metabolites [121]. The dephosphorylated form (estramustine) is then oxidized to an estrone-bound mustard carbamate group (estromustine), and the carbamate–ester bond is subsequently hydrolyzed by carbaminidase forming estrone and a free carbamate mustard. All of these metabolic events, with the exception of the formation of estromustine, can take place in the prostate leading to an anticancer effect as previously explained. Following oral delivery, estromustine is the main metabolite found in plasma at an approximately 10- to 16-fold greater concentration than estramustine, while within tumors the estromustine:estramustine is approximately 2:1 [121],

and estramustine has more potent anticancer activity than estromustine [125]. Targeting to the prostate is perhaps due to the estramustine-binding protein (EMBP) being expressed within that tissue [126]. Following a single dose of estramustine phosphate (420 mg), the peak plasma concentration of estromustine (C_{max}) is achieved after approximately 2–3 h (~310–475 µg/mL in the plasma), and the plasma half-life of this metabolite is approximately 14 h [127]. Following carbaminidase metabolism, the liberated estrogen increases the levels of estradiol within a range similar to conventional estradiol therapy. Similar to endogenous estrogens, estramustine estrogen metabolites are cleared through the hepatobilliary and urinary routes, although at a slower rate due to the heavy tissue retention of the drug. Little is known as to the fate of the free mustard group [127]. Estramustine also increases the levels of sex-hormone-binding globulin (SHBG), elevation of plasma transcortin and cortisol, suppression of adrenocorticotropic hormone (ACTH) by the pituitary, and subsequent reduction in leutenizing hormone (as reviewed in [118]).

Nongenetic Sources of Variability in Pharmacology

The only well-studied source of variability in estramustine pharmacology has been in those individuals ingesting sources of calcium (e.g., milk and antacids) following an oral dose of estramustine. Absorption through the gastrointestinal tract is significantly inhibited by calcium, and the accumulation of estramustine and estromustine in tumors (glioma and astrocytoma) is significantly inhibited [121].

Pharmacogenetics

There have been few studies evaluating the pharmacogenetics of estramustine. Although a clinical trial was published demonstrating that ABCG2 Q141K was related to a more favorable clinical outcome following a combination of docetaxel and estramustine, it is unclear why this relationship exists [65]. The V158M polymorphism in catechol-*O*-methyltransferase (COMT) has been also been related to PSA-progression-free survival in men with prostate cancer, and the authors attribute this result to decreased formation of the microtubule-stabilizing agent 2-methoxyestradiol (2-ME) brought on by metabolism of estramustine-generated estrogens within prostate tumors [128]. It is also likely that this result is actually due to decreased conjugation of catechol estrogens within the prostate preventing their oxidation into procarcinogenic quinones and semiquinones [129, 130]. Finally, another study found that the risk of estramustine-induced peripheral edema and appetite loss was related to polymorphisms in the *type 7 17β-hydroxysteroid dehydrogenase* (*HSD17B7*) gene in men with prostate cancer [131]. Again, it is very difficult to understand why this might be as so little is known about HSD17B7 and its involvement in steroidogenesis or the formation of sex hormones.

Satraplatin

Mechanism of Action

Satraplatin, like other platinum-based chemotherapies (cisplatin, carboplatin, oxaloplatin), mediates its effects by binding to the DNA and forming inter- and intrastrand cross-links at adjacent purine bases, thus distorting the DNA template and preventing DNA replication. These compounds can also form mono-adducts to the DNA and bind to reactive thiols, amino, hydroxyl, or other groups on proteins and other cellular factors resulting in DNA–protein and other types of adducts (as reviewed in [132]). Such DNA binding often results in cell cycle arrest in the G2 phase and also activates several intracellular signaling pathways such those involved in DNA-damage repair, cell cycle arrest, and apoptosis [133–135]. The major active metabolite of satraplatin (JM118) is very similar to cisplatin except for a single cyclohexamine (instead of amine) moiety that contributes to its asymmetrical binding of the DNA. While JM118 still forms the aforementioned cross-links within DNA, chiral adducts can cause different DNA conformations and be processed differentially by intracellular machinery [136]. For example, satraplatin adducts evade the mismatch repair (MMR) pathway that is associated with resistance to cisplatin [137]. However, the X-ray crystal structure of the major satraplatin–DNA adduct has a remarkably similar structure

to that of *cis*- and oxaloplatin [138], and both adducts are efficiently repaired by the nucleotide excision repair (NER) pathway [139].

Pharmacokinetics, Drug Distribution, and Pharmacodynamic Determininants

Following oral administration, satraplatin is absorbed through the gastrointestinal mucosa and undergoes rapid deacetylation to form the major active satraplatin metabolite JM118 that accounts for ~20–40% of the administered platinum [140]. This deacetylation reaction is rather rapid as parent satraplatin has a half-life of only 6.3 min in whole blood in vitro to form JM118 and at least five other metabolites [141]. The majority of a dose of satraplatin becomes bound to red blood cells (~62%) while 38% is found in plasma. Of the plasma fraction, 71% of the platinum content is bound to proteins (especially albumin) and the remaining 29% is unbound [141].

Satraplatin was originally developed in the search for a platinum-based drug with significant oral bioavailability with a similar toxicity profile to carboplatin (i.e., dose-limiting toxicities including myelosuppression) instead of the more toxic cisplatin (i.e., dose-limiting toxicities are nephro- and GI toxicity) [142]. As such it has rather higher bioavailability than other platinum drugs (i.e., cisplatin, carboplatin, and oxaloplatin). Satraplatin was also developed with the aim to find platinum species that can overcome cisplatin resistance mechanisms, and satraplatin evades certain pathways that confer resistance in human cell lines [142]. First, satraplatin demonstrates activity in cells that do not express the copper-ion uptake transporter CRT1, although forced expression of the copper efflux transporters ATP7A and ATP7B conferred resistance to JM118 [143]. As was previously mentioned, JM118 also evades the MMR pathway and thus confers partial resistance in tumor cell lines that upregulate repair pathways to overcome cisplatin cytotoxicity, as was noted by Kelland et al. [144]. However, since JM118 and cisplatin are removed with similar kinetics by the NER pathway [139], and JM-118 lesions are repairable when bound to certain genes [134], it appears that the partial resistance to JM118 noted by Kelland et al. was only due to MMR evasion [142]. Resistance to satraplatin or

JM118 appears to be mediated by increased levels of glutathione [133] and increased intracellular detoxification mechanisms [145].

Unlike other platinum compounds. JM118 demonstrates activity in prostate cancer cells with a IC_{50} of approximately 0.5–1.0 µM, although oxaliplatin has a slightly higher activity toward cytotoxicity in cells with a functional androgen receptor (LNCaP), and the activity of JM118 is similar to cisplatin in androgen-independent cell lines (PC3 and DU145) [146]. Yet, cisplatin and other platinum-based therapies have typically not demonstrated clinically significant therapeutic outcome in men with CRPC [147]. This may explain the recent findings of the SPARC (Satraplatin and Prednisone Against Refractory Cancer) trial where satraplatin was found to only have a palliative effect as overall survival in CRPC was not different between patients treated with satraplatin plus prednisone, or prednisone alone [150]. However, satraplatin has been shown to confer sensitivity to taxane treatment [145] and shows synergistic activity with docetaxel in vivo [148]. Moreover, satraplatin is able to evade docetaxel mechanisms of resistance such as the upregulation of multidrug resistance transporters (e.g., ABCB1, ABCC1/2) that remove docetaxel, but not satraplatin, from prostate cancer cells [146]. Although there are currently trials treating patients with the combination docetaxel plus satraplatin, it remains to be seen if the combination docetaxel plus satraplatin shows clinical benefit despite the undesirable results of satraplatin as monotherapy in hormone-resistant prostate cancer.

Nongenetic Sources of Variability in Pharmacology

Satraplatin inhibits several cytochrome P450 enzymes such as CYP1A1, CYP1A2, CYP2A6, CYP2C8, CYP2D6, CYP2E1, and CYP3A4 [149]. This inhibition was noncompetitive and occurred with low IC50 values (~1.0 µM for metabolite formation of testosterone and paclitaxel, respectively). However, the potential drug–drug and gene–drug interactions have not been well studied in the literature. It is expected that since satraplatin inhibits so many drug-metabolizing enzymes, cotreatment with other medications will be complicated by such interactions.

Conclusion

Prostate cancer has been treated using several different classes of drugs with diverse mechanisms of action, although only docetaxel alone, or docetaxel in combination with estramustine has offered an established survival benefit in CRPC thus far. Given that cytotoxic drugs have such a narrow therapeutic window (i.e., maximum efficacy and minimum toxicity) within the population suffering from advanced prostate cancer, interindividual variation as it applies to both PK and clinical outcome must be better explored to identify optimal dosing and individuals who are more likely to benefit from treatment with these agents. It is hoped that the information gleaned from such studies will be utilized to improve therapy with cytotoxic agents and eventually lead to the design of superior therapeutic options.

References

1. Petrylak DP, Tangen CM, Hussain MH, et al. Docetaxel and estramustine compared with mitoxantrone and prednisone for advanced refractory prostate cancer. N Engl J Med 2004;351: 1513–20.
2. Tannock IF, de Wit R, Berry WR, et al. Docetaxel plus prednisone or mitoxantrone plus prednisone for advanced prostate cancer. N Engl J Med 2004;351: 1502–12.
3. Kraus LA, Samuel SK, Schmid SM, Dykes DJ, Waud WR, Bissery MC. The mechanism of action of docetaxel (Taxotere) in xenograft models is not limited to bcl-2 phosphorylation. Invest New Drugs 2003;21: 259–68.
4. Pienta KJ. Preclinical mechanisms of action of docetaxel and docetaxel combinations in prostate cancer. Semin Oncol 2001;28: 3–7.
5. Kuppens IE, van Maanen MJ, Rosing H, Schellens JH, Beijnen JH. Quantitative analysis of docetaxel in human plasma using liquid chromatography coupled with tandem mass spectrometry. Biomed Chromatogr 2005;19: 355–61.
6. Parise RA, Ramanathan RK, Zamboni WC, Egorin MJ. Sensitive liquid chromatography-mass spectrometry assay for quantitation of docetaxel and paclitaxel in human plasma. J Chromatogr B Analyt Technol Biomed Life Sci 2003;783: 231–6.
7. Wang LZ, Goh BC, Grigg ME, Lee SC, Khoo YM, Lee HS. A rapid and sensitive liquid chromatography/tandem mass spectrometry method for determination of docetaxel in human plasma. Rapid Commun Mass Spectrom 2003;17: 1548–52.
8. Mortier KA, Lambert WE. Determination of unbound docetaxel and paclitaxel in plasma by ultrafiltration and liquid chromatography-tandem mass spectrometry. J Chromatogr B Analyt Technol Biomed Life Sci 2006;1108: 195–201.

9. Sparreboom A, Zhao M, Brahmer JR, Verweij J, Baker SD. Determination of the docetaxel vehicle, polysorbate 80, in patient samples by liquid chromatography-tandem mass spectrometry. J Chromatogr B Analyt Technol Biomed Life Sci 2002;773: 183–90.

10. Loos WJ, Baker SD, Verweij J, Boonstra JG, Sparreboom A. Clinical pharmacokinetics of unbound docetaxel: role of polysorbate 80 and serum proteins. Clin Pharmacol Ther 2003;74: 364–71.

11. Baker SD, Li J, ten Tije AJ, et al. Relationship of systemic exposure to unbound docetaxel and neutropenia. Clin Pharmacol Ther 2005;77: 43–53.

12. Minami H, Kawada K, Sasaki Y, et al. Pharmacokinetics and pharmacodynamics of protein-unbound docetaxel in cancer patients. Cancer Sci 2006;97: 235–41.

13. Guentert TW, Oie S, Paalzow L, et al. Interaction of mixed micelles formed from glycocholic acid and lecithin with the protein binding of various drugs. Br J Clin Pharmacol 1987;23: 569–77.

14. Reynolds JA. The role of micelles in protein–detergent interactions. Methods Enzymol 1979;61: 58–62.

15. Petitpas I, Grune T, Bhattacharya AA, Curry S. Crystal structures of human serum albumin complexed with mono-unsaturated and polyunsaturated fatty acids. J Mol Biol 2001;314: 955–60.

16. Shou M, Martinet M, Korzekwa KR, Krausz KW, Gonzalez FJ, Gelboin HV. Role of human cytochrome P450 3A4 and 3A5 in the metabolism of taxotere and its derivatives: enzyme specificity, interindividual distribution and metabolic contribution in human liver. Pharmacogenetics 1998;8: 391–401.

17. van Herwaarden AE, Wagenaar E, van der Kruijssen CM, et al. Knockout of cytochrome P450 3A yields new mouse models for understanding xenobiotic metabolism. J Clin Invest 2007;117: 3583–92.

18. Baker S, Verweij J, Cusatis G, et al. Pharmacogenetic pathway analysis of docetaxel elimination. Clin Pharmacol Ther 2008;85(2): 155–63.

19. Tran A, Jullien V, Alexandre J, et al. Pharmacokinetics and toxicity of docetaxel: role of CYP3A, MDR1, and GST polymorphisms. Clin Pharmacol Ther 2006;79: 570–80.

20. Bardelmeijer HA, Ouwehand M, Buckle T, et al. Low systemic exposure of oral docetaxel in mice resulting from extensive first-pass metabolism is boosted by ritonavir. Cancer Res 2002;62: 6158–64.

21. Huisman MT, Chhatta AA, van Tellingen O, Beijnen JH, Schinkel AH. MRP2 (ABCC2) transports taxanes and confers paclitaxel resistance and both processes are stimulated by probenecid. Int J Cancer 2005;116: 824–9.

22. Smith NF, Acharya MR, Desai N, Figg WD, Sparreboom A. Identification of OATP1B3 as a high-affinity hepatocellular transporter of paclitaxel. Cancer Biol Ther 2005;4: 815–8.

23. van Zuylen L, Verweij J, Nooter K, Brouwer E, Stoter G, Sparreboom A. Role of intestinal P-glycoprotein in the plasma and fecal disposition of docetaxel in humans. Clin Cancer Res 2000;6: 2598–603.

24. Cordon-Cardo C, O'Brien JP, Casals D, et al. Multidrug-resistance gene (P-glycoprotein) is expressed by endothelial cells at blood-brain barrier sites. Proc Natl Acad Sci U S A 1989;86: 695–8.

25. Saito T, Zhang ZJ, Ohtsubo T, et al. Homozygous disruption of the mdrla P-glycoprotein gene affects blood-nerve barrier function in mice administered with neurotoxic drugs. Acta Otolaryngol 2001;121: 735–42.

26. Saito T, Zhang ZJ, Shibamori Y, et al. P-glycoprotein expression in capillary endothelial cells of the 7th and 8th nerves of guinea pig in relation to blood-nerve barrier sites. Neurosci Lett 1997;232: 41–4.

27. Drach D, Zhao S, Drach J, et al. Subpopulations of normal peripheral blood and bone marrow cells express a functional multidrug resistant phenotype. Blood 1992;80: 2729–34.

28. Fruehauf S, Wermann K, Buss EC, et al. Protection of hematopoietic stem cells from chemotherapy-induced toxicity by multidrug-resistance 1 gene transfer. Recent Results Cancer Res 1998;144: 93–115.

29. Gottesman MM, Fojo T, Bates SE. Multidrug resistance in cancer: role of ATP-dependent transporters. Nat Rev Cancer 2002;2: 48–58.

30. Ieiri I, Takane H, Otsubo K. The MDR1 (ABCB1) gene polymorphism and its clinical implications. Clin Pharmacokinet 2004;43: 553–76.

31. Burk O, Koch I, Raucy J, et al. The induction of cytochrome P450 3A5 (CYP3A5) in the human liver and intestine is mediated by the xenobiotic sensors pregnane X receptor (PXR) and constitutively activated receptor (CAR). J Biol Chem 2004;279: 38379–85.

32. Lehmann JM, McKee DD, Watson MA, Willson TM, Moore JT, Kliewer SA. The human orphan nuclear receptor PXR is activated by compounds that regulate CYP3A4 gene expression and cause drug interactions. J Clin Invest 1998;102: 1016–23.

33. Sissung TM, Danesi R, Price DK, et al. Association of the CYP1B1*3 allele with survival in patients with prostate cancer receiving docetaxel. Mol Cancer Ther 2008;7: 19–26.

34. Sissung TM, Price DK, Sparreboom A, Figg WD. Pharmacogenetics and regulation of human cytochrome P450 1B1: implications in hormone-mediated tumor metabolism and a novel target for therapeutic intervention. Mol Cancer Res 2006;4: 135–50.

35. Baker SD, Sparreboom A, Verweij J. Clinical pharmacokinetics of docetaxel: recent developments. Clin Pharmacokinet 2006;45: 235–52.

36. Kloft C, Wallin J, Henningsson A, Chatelut E, Karlsson MO. Population pharmacokinetic-pharmacodynamic model for neutropenia with patient subgroup identification: comparison across anticancer drugs. Clin Cancer Res 2006;12: 5481–90.

37. Rudek MA, Sparreboom A, Garrett-Mayer ES, et al. Factors affecting pharmacokinetic variability following doxorubicin and docetaxel-based therapy. Eur J Cancer 2004;40: 1170–8.

38. Bruno R, Olivares R, Berille J, et al. Alpha-1-acid glycoprotein as an independent predictor for treatment effects and a prognostic factor of survival in patients with non-small cell lung cancer treated with docetaxel. Clin Cancer Res 2003;9: 1077–82.

39. Bruno R, Hille D, Riva A, et al. Population pharmacokinetics/pharmacodynamics of docetaxel in phase II studies in patients with cancer. J Clin Oncol 1998;16: 187–96.

40. Sissung TM, Baum CE, Deeken J, et al. ABCB1 genetic variation influences the toxicity and clinical outcome of patients with androgen-independent prostate cancer treated with docetaxel. Clin Cancer Res 2008;14: 4543–9.

41. Veyrat-Follet C, Bruno R, Olivares R, Rhodes GR, Chaikin P. Clinical trial simulation of docetaxel in patients with cancer as a tool for dosage optimization. Clin Pharmacol Ther 2000;68: 677–87.

42. Strother RM, Sweeney C. Lessons learned from development of docetaxel. Expert Opin Drug Metab Toxicol 2008;4: 1007–19.

43. Clarke SJ, Rivory LP. Clinical pharmacokinetics of docetaxel. Clin Pharmacokinet 1999;36: 99–114.

44. Hooker AC, Ten Tije AJ, Carducci MA, et al. Population pharmacokinetic model for docetaxel in patients with varying degrees of liver function: incorporating cytochrome P4503A activity measurements. Clin Pharmacol Ther 2008;84: 111–8.

45. Urien S, Barre J, Morin C, Paccaly A, Montay G, Tillement JP. Docetaxel serum protein binding with high affinity to alpha 1-acid glycoprotein. Invest New Drugs 1996;14: 147–51.

46. Puisset F, Chatelut E, Sparreboom A, et al. Dexamethasone as a probe for CYP3A4 metabolism: evidence of gender effect. Cancer Chemother Pharmacol 2007;60: 305–8.

47. De Marzo AM, Marchi VL, Epstein JI, Nelson WG. Proliferative inflammatory atrophy of the prostate: implications for prostatic carcinogenesis. Am J Pathol 1999;155: 1985–92.

48. Lucia MS, Torkko KC. Inflammation as a target for prostate cancer chemoprevention: pathological and laboratory rationale. J Urol 2004;171: S30–4; discussion S5.

49. Kuvibidila S, Rayford W. Correlation between serum prostate-specific antigen and alpha-1-antitrypsin in men without and with prostate cancer. J Lab Clin Med 2006;147: 174–81.

50. Ward AM, Cooper EH, Houghton AL. Acute phase reactant proteins in prostatic cancer. Br J Urol 1977;49: 411–8.

51. Puisset F, Alexandre J, Treluyer JM, et al. Clinical pharmacodynamic factors in docetaxel toxicity. Br J Cancer 2007;97: 290–6.

52. Baker SD, Scher HI, Li J, et al. Effect of androgen-ablation and hormonal cycling on docetaxel clearance in patients with metastatic prostate cancer. Proc ASCO (abst 4608) 2005.

53. Rathkopf D, Carducci MA, Morris MJ, et al. Phase II trial of docetaxel with rapid androgen cycling for progressive non-castrate prostate cancer. J Clin Oncol 2008;26: 2959–65.

54. Sinibaldi VJ, Elza-Brown K, Schmidt J, et al. Phase II evaluation of docetaxel plus exisulind in patients with androgen independent prostate carcinoma. Am J Clin Oncol 2006;29: 395–8.

55. Hochegger K, Lhotta K, Mayer G, Czejka M, Hilbe W. Pharmacokinetic analysis of docetaxel during haemodialysis in a patient with locally advanced non-small cell lung cancer. Nephrol Dial Transplant 2007;22: 289–90.

56. ten Tije AJ, Verweij J, Carducci MA, et al. Prospective evaluation of the pharmacokinetics and toxicity profile of docetaxel in the elderly. J Clin Oncol 2005;23: 1070–7.

57. Hurria A, Fleming MT, Baker SD, et al. Pharmacokinetics and toxicity of weekly docetaxel in older patients. Clin Cancer Res 2006;12: 6100–5.

58. Bruno R, Vivier N, Veyrat-Follet C, Montay G, Rhodes GR. Population pharmacokinetics and pharmacokinetic-pharmacodynamic relationships for docetaxel. Invest New Drugs 2001;19: 163–9.

59. Kaira K, Tsuchiya S, Sunaga N, et al. A phase I dose escalation study of weekly docetaxel and carboplatin in elderly patients with nonsmall cell lung cancer. Am J Clin Oncol 2007;30: 51–6.

60. LeCaer H, Barlesi F, Robinet G, et al. An open multicenter phase II trial of weekly docetaxel for advanced-stage non-small-cell lung cancer in elderly patients with significant comorbidity and/or poor performance status: The GFPC 02-02b study. Lung Cancer 2007;57: 72–8.

61. Takigawa N, Segawa Y, Kishino D, et al. Clinical and pharmacokinetic study of docetaxel in elderly non-small-cell lung cancer patients. Cancer Chemother Pharmacol 2004;54: 230–6.

62. Bosch TM, Huitema AD, Doodeman VD, et al. Pharmacogenetic screening of CYP3A and ABCB1 in relation to population pharmacokinetics of docetaxel. Clin Cancer Res 2006;12: 5786–93.

63. Engels FK, Loos WJ, Mathot RA, van Schaik RH, Verweij J. Influence of ketoconazole on the fecal and urinary disposition of docetaxel. Cancer Chemother Pharmacol 2007;60: 569–79.

64. Goh BC, Lee SC, Wang LZ, et al. Explaining interindividual variability of docetaxel pharmacokinetics and pharmacodynamics in Asians through phenotyping and genotyping strategies. J Clin Oncol 2002;20: 3683–90.

65. Hahn NM, Marsh S, Fisher W, et al. Hoosier Oncology Group randomized phase II study of docetaxel, vinorelbine, and estramustine in combination in hormone-refractory prostate cancer with pharmacogenetic survival analysis. Clin Cancer Res 2006;12: 6094–9.

66. Hor SY, Lee SC, Wong CI, et al. PXR, CAR and HNF4alpha genotypes and their association with pharmacokinetics and pharmacodynamics of docetaxel and doxorubicin in Asian patients. Pharmacogenomics J 2008;8: 139–46.

67. Kiyotani K, Mushiroda T, Kubo M, Zembutsu H, Sugiyama Y, Nakamura Y. Association of genetic polymorphisms in SLCO1B3 and ABCC2 with docetaxel-induced leukopenia. Cancer Sci 2008;99: 967–72.

68. Lewis LD, Miller AA, Rosner GL, et al. A comparison of the pharmacokinetics and pharmacodynamics of docetaxel between African-American and Caucasian cancer patients: CALGB 9871. Clin Cancer Res 2007;13: 3302–11.

69. Daly AK. Significance of the minor cytochrome P450 3A isoforms. Clin Pharmacokinet 2006;45: 13–31.

70. Hamada A, Sissung T, Price DK, et al. Effect of SLCO1B3 haplotype on testosterone transport and clinical outcome in caucasian patients with androgen-independent prostatic cancer. Clin Cancer Res 2008;14: 3312–8.

71. Sharifi N, Hamada A, Sissung T, et al. A polymorphism in a transporter of testosterone is a determinant of androgen independence in prostate cancer. BJU Int 2008;102: 617–21.

72. Bessho Y, Oguri T, Achiwa H, et al. Role of ABCG2 as a biomarker for predicting resistance to CPT-11/SN-38 in lung cancer. Cancer Sci 2006;97: 192–8.

73. Mizuarai S, Aozasa N, Kotani H. Single nucleotide polymorphisms result in impaired membrane localization and reduced atpase activity in multidrug transporter ABCG2. Int J Cancer 2004;109: 238–46.

74. Tham LS, Holford NH, Hor SY, et al. Lack of association of single-nucleotide polymorphisms in pregnane X receptor, hepatic nuclear factor 4alpha, and constitutive androstane receptor with docetaxel pharmacokinetics. Clin Cancer Res 2007;13: 7126–32.

75. Rochat B, Morsman JM, Murray GI, Figg WD, McLeod HL. Human CYP1B1 and anticancer agent metabolism: mechanism for tumor-specific drug inactivation? J Pharmacol Exp Ther 2001;296: 537–41.

76. Bournique B, Lemarie A. Docetaxel (Taxotere) is not metabolized by recombinant human CYP1B1 in vitro, but acts as an effector of this isozyme. Drug Metab Dispos 2002;30: 1149–52.

77. Carnell DM, Smith RE, Daley FM, et al. Target validation of cytochrome P450 CYP1B1 in prostate carcinoma with protein expression in associated hyperplastic and premalignant tissue. Int J Radiat Oncol Biol Phys 2004;58: 500–9.

78. Brandi G, de Rosa F, Danesi R, Montini GC, Biasco G. Durable complete response to frontline docetaxel in an advanced prostate cancer patient with favourable CYP1B1 isoforms: suggestion for changing paradigms? Eur Urol 2008;54(4):938–41.

79. Figg WD, Li H, Sissung T, et al. Pre-clinical and clinical evaluation of estramustine, docetaxel and thalidomide combination in androgen-independent prostate cancer. BJU Int 2007;99: 1047–55.

80. Markushin Y, Gaikwad N, Zhang H, et al. Potential biomarker for early risk assessment of prostate cancer. Prostate 2006;66: 1565–71.

81. Tewey KM, Rowe TC, Yang L, Halligan BD, Liu LF. Adriamycin-induced DNA damage mediated by mammalian DNA topoisomerase II. Science 1984;226: 466–8.

82. Bachur NR, Yu F, Johnson R, Hickey R, Wu Y, Malkas L. Helicase inhibition by anthracycline anticancer agents. Mol Pharmacol 1992;41: 993–8.

83. Myers CE, McGuire WP, Liss RH, Ifrim I, Grotzinger K, Young RC. Adriamycin: the role of lipid peroxidation in cardiac toxicity and tumor response. Science 1977;197: 165–7.

84. Hande KR. Clinical applications of anticancer drugs targeted to topoisomerase II. Biochim Biophys Acta 1998;1400: 173–84.

85. Vibet S, Maheo K, Gore J, Dubois P, Bougnoux P, Chourpa I. Differential subcellular distribution of mitoxantrone in relation to chemosensitization in two human breast cancer cell lines. Drug Metab Dispos 2007;35: 822–8.

86. Levine S, Gherson J. Morphologic effects of mitoxantrone and a related anthracenedione on lymphoid tissues. Int J Immunopharmacol 1986;8: 999–1007.

87. Berry W, Dakhil S, Modiano M, Gregurich M, Asmar L. Phase III study of mitoxantrone plus low dose prednisone versus low dose prednisone alone in patients with asymptomatic hormone refractory prostate cancer. J Urol 2002;168: 2439–43.

88. Kantoff PW, Halabi S, Conaway M, et al. Hydrocortisone with or without mitoxantrone in men with hormone-refractory prostate cancer: results of the cancer and leukemia group B 9182 study. J Clin Oncol 1999;17: 2506–13.

89. Tannock IF, Osoba D, Stockler MR, et al. Chemotherapy with mitoxantrone plus prednisone or prednisone alone for symptomatic hormone-resistant prostate cancer: a Canadian randomized trial with palliative end points. J Clin Oncol 1996;14: 1756–64.

90. Schleyer E, Kamischke A, Kaufmann CC, Unterhalt M, Hiddemann W. New aspects on the pharmacokinetics of mitoxantrone and its two major metabolites. Leukemia 1994;8: 435–40.

91. Launay MC, Iliadis A, Richard B. Population pharmacokinetics of mitoxantrone performed by a NONMEM method. J Pharm Sci 1989;78: 877–80.

92. Schurr E, Raymond M, Bell JC, Gros P. Characterization of the multidrug resistance protein expressed in cell clones stably transfected with the mouse mdr1 cDNA. Cancer Res 1989;49: 2729–33.

93. Morrow CS, Smitherman PK, Diah SK, Schneider E, Townsend AJ. Coordinated action of glutathione S-transferases (GSTs) and multidrug resistance protein 1 (MRP1) in antineoplastic drug detoxification. Mechanism of GST A1-1- and MRP1-associated resistance to chlorambucil in MCF7 breast carcinoma cells. J Biol Chem 1998;273: 20114–20.

94. Schneider E, Horton JK, Yang CH, Nakagawa M, Cowan KH. Multidrug resistance-associated protein gene overexpression and reduced drug sensitivity of topoisomerase II in a human breast carcinoma MCF7 cell line selected for etoposide resistance. Cancer Res 1994;54: 152–8.

95. Morrow CS, Peklak-Scott C, Bishwokarma B, Kute TE, Smitherman PK, Townsend AJ. Multidrug resistance protein 1 (MRP1, ABCC1) mediates resistance to mitoxantrone via glutathione-dependent drug efflux. Mol Pharmacol 2006;69: 1499–505.

96. Hooijberg JH, Broxterman HJ, Kool M, et al. Antifolate resistance mediated by the multidrug resistance proteins MRP1 and MRP2. Cancer Res 1999;59: 2532–5.

97. Doyle LA, Yang W, Abruzzo LV, et al. A multidrug resistance transporter from human MCF-7 breast cancer cells. Proc Natl Acad Sci U S A 1998;95: 15665–70.

98. Miyake K, Mickley L, Litman T, et al. Molecular cloning of cDNAs which are highly overexpressed in mitoxantrone-resistant cells: demonstration of homology to ABC transport genes. Cancer Res 1999;59: 8–13.

99. Pan G, Elmquist WF. Mitoxantrone permeability in MDCKII cells is influenced by active influx transport. Mol Pharm 2007;4: 475–83.

100. Bhangal G, Halford S, Wang J, Roylance R, Shah R, Waxman J. Expression of the multidrug resistance gene in human prostate cancer. Urol Oncol 2000;5: 118–21.

101. Huss WJ, Gray DR, Greenberg NM, Mohler JL, Smith GJ. Breast cancer resistance protein-mediated efflux of androgen in putative benign and malignant prostate stem cells. Cancer Res 2005;65: 6640–50.

102. Fedoruk MN, Gimenez-Bonafe P, Guns ES, Mayer LD, Nelson CC. P-glycoprotein increases the efflux of the androgen dihydrotestosterone and reduces androgen responsive gene activity in prostate tumor cells. Prostate 2004;59: 77–90.

103. Allen JD, Schinkel AH. Multidrug resistance and pharmacological protection mediated by the breast cancer resistance protein (BCRP/ABCG2). Mol Cancer Ther 2002;1: 427–34.

104. Hirschmann-Jax C, Foster AE, Wulf GG, et al. A distinct "side population" of cells with high drug efflux capacity in human tumor cells. Proc Natl Acad Sci U S A 2004;101: 14228–33.

105. Feldman EJ, Seiter K, Damon L, et al. A randomized trial of high- vs standard-dose mitoxantrone with cytarabine in elderly patients with acute myeloid leukemia. Leukemia 1997;11: 485–9.

106. Imai Y, Nakane M, Kage K, et al. C421A polymorphism in the human breast cancer resistance protein gene is associated with low expression of Q141K protein and low-level drug resistance. Mol Cancer Ther 2002;1: 611–6.

107. Kobayashi D, Ieiri I, Hirota T, et al. Functional assessment of ABCG2 (BCRP) gene polymorphisms to protein expression in human placenta. Drug Metab Dispos 2005;33: 94–101.

108. Kolwankar D, Glover DD, Ware JA, Tracy TS. Expression and function of ABCB1 and ABCG2 in human placental tissue. Drug Metab Dispos 2005;33: 524–9.

109. Kondo C, Suzuki H, Itoda M, et al. Functional analysis of SNPs variants of BCRP/ABCG2. Pharm Res 2004;21: 1895–903.

110. Sparreboom A, Gelderblom H, Marsh S, et al. Diflomotecan pharmacokinetics in relation to ABCG2 421C>A genotype. Clin Pharmacol Ther 2004;76: 38–44.

111. Morisaki K, Robey RW, Ozvegy-Laczka C, et al. Single nucleotide polymorphisms modify the transporter activity of ABCG2. Cancer Chemother Pharmacol 2005;56: 161–72.

112. Tamura A, Wakabayashi K, Onishi Y, et al. Re-evaluation and functional classification of non-synonymous single nucleotide polymorphisms of the human ATP-binding cassette transporter ABCG2. Cancer Sci 2007;98: 231–9.

113. Sugimoto Y, Tsukahara S, Ishikawa E, Mitsuhashi J. Breast cancer resistance protein: molecular target for anticancer drug resistance and pharmacokinetics/pharmacodynamics. Cancer Sci 2005;96: 457–65.

114. Honjo Y, Hrycyna CA, Yan QW, et al. Acquired mutations in the MXR/BCRP/ABCP gene alter substrate specificity in MXR/BCRP/ABCP-overexpressing cells. Cancer Res 2001;61: 6635–9.

115. Polgar O, Deeken JF, Ediriwickrema LS, et al. The 315-316 deletion determines the BXP-21 antibody epitope but has no effect on the function of wild type ABCG2 or the Q141K variant. Mol Cell Biochem 2008;322(1–2): 63–71.

116. Sissung TM, Gardner ER, Gao R, Figg WD. Pharmacogenetics of membrane transporters: a review of current approaches. Methods Mol Biol 2008;448: 41–62.

117. Benderra Z, Faussat AM, Sayada L, et al. Breast cancer resistance protein and P-glycoprotein in 149 adult acute myeloid leukemias. Clin Cancer Res 2004;10: 7896–902.

118. Sandberg AA. Metabolic aspects and actions unique to Estracyt. Semin Oncol 1983;10: 3–15.

119. Muechler EK, Kohler D. Interaction of the cytotoxic agent estramustine phosphate (Estracyt) with the estrogen receptor of the human uterus. Gynecol Oncol 1979;8: 330–8.

120. Ho SM. Estrogens and anti-estrogens: key mediators of prostate carcinogenesis and new therapeutic candidates. J Cell Biochem 2004;91: 491–503.

121. Bergenheim AT, Henriksson R. Pharmacokinetics and pharmacodynamics of estramustine phosphate. Clin Pharmacokinet 1998;34: 163–72.

122. Hartley-Asp B, Kruse E. Nuclear protein matrix as a target for estramustine-induced cell death. Prostate 1986;9: 387–95.

123. Pienta KJ, Lehr JE. Inhibition of prostate cancer growth by estramustine and etoposide: evidence for interaction at the nuclear matrix. J Urol 1993;149: 1622–5.

124. Tritsch GL, Shukla SK, Mittelman A, Murphy GP. Estracyt (NSC 89199) as a substrate for phosphatases in human serum. Invest Urol 1974;12: 38–9.

125. Kreis W, Budman DR, Calabro A. Unique synergism or antagonism of combinations of chemotherapeutic and hormonal agents in human prostate cancer cell lines. Br J Urol 1997;79: 196–202.

126. Forsgren B, Bjork P, Carlstrom K, Gustafsson JA, Pousette A, Hogberg B. Purification and distribution of a major protein in rat prostate that binds estramustine, a nitrogen mustard derivative of estradiol-17 beta. Proc Natl Acad Sci U S A 1979;76: 3149–53.

127. Gunnarsson PO, Forshell GP. Clinical pharmacokinetics of estramustine phosphate. Urology 1984;23: 22–7.

128. Suzuki M, Mamun MR, Hara K, et al. The Val158Met polymorphism of the catechol-O-methyltransferase gene is associated with the PSA-progression-free survival in prostate cancer patients treated with estramustine phosphate. Eur Urol 2005;48: 752–9.

129. Lu F, Zahid M, Saeed M, Cavalieri EL, Rogan EG. Estrogen metabolism and formation of estrogen-DNA adducts in estradiol-treated MCF-10F cells. The effects of 2,3,7,8-tetrachlorodibenzo-p-dioxin induction and catechol-O-methyltransferase inhibition. J Steroid Biochem Mol Biol 2007;105: 150–8.

130. Zahid M, Saeed M, Lu F, Gaikwad N, Rogan E, Cavalieri E. Inhibition of catechol-O-methyltransferase increases estrogen-DNA adduct formation. Free Radic Biol Med 2007;43: 1534–40.

131. Suzuki M, Muto S, Hara K, et al. Single-nucleotide polymorphisms in the 17beta-hydroxysteroid dehydrogenase genes might predict the risk of side-effects of estramustine phosphate sodium in prostate cancer patients. Int J Urol 2005;12: 166–72.

132. Boulikas T, Vougiouka M. Cisplatin and platinum drugs at the molecular level. (Review). Oncol Rep 2003;10: 1663–82.

133. Mellish KJ, Barnard CF, Murrer BA, Kelland LR. DNA-binding properties of novel cis- and trans platinum-based anticancer agents in 2 human ovarian carcinoma cell lines. Int J Cancer 1995;62: 717–23.

134. O'Neill CF, Koberle B, Masters JR, Kelland LR. Gene-specific repair of Pt/DNA lesions and induction of apoptosis by the oral platinum drug JM216 in three human ovarian carcinoma cell lines sensitive and resistant to cisplatin. Br J Cancer 1999;81: 1294–303.

135. Siddik ZH. Cisplatin: mode of cytotoxic action and molecular basis of resistance. Oncogene 2003;22: 7265–79.

136. Benedetti M, Malina J, Kasparkova J, Brabec V, Natile G. Chiral discrimination in platinum anticancer drugs. Environ Health Perspect 2002;110 Suppl 5: 779–82.

137. Fink D, Nebel S, Aebi S, et al. The role of DNA mismatch repair in platinum drug resistance. Cancer Res 1996;56: 4881–6.

138. Silverman AP, Bu W, Cohen SM, Lippard SJ. 2.4-A crystal structure of the asymmetric platinum complex [Pt(ammine)(cyclohexylamine)]2+ bound to a dodecamer DNA duplex. J Biol Chem 2002;277: 49743–9.

139. Reardon JT, Vaisman A, Chaney SG, Sancar A. Efficient nucleotide excision repair of cisplatin, oxaliplatin, and Bis-aceto-ammine-dichloro-cyclohexylamine-platinum(IV) (JM216) platinum intrastrand DNA diadducts. Cancer Res 1999;59: 3968–71.

140. Raynaud FI, Mistry P, Donaghue A, et al. Biotransformation of the platinum drug JM216 following oral administration to cancer patients. Cancer Chemother Pharmacol 1996;38: 155–62.

141. Carr JL, Tingle MD, McKeage MJ. Rapid biotransformation of satraplatin by human red blood cells in vitro. Cancer Chemother Pharmacol 2002;50: 9–15.

142. Kelland L. Broadening the clinical use of platinum drug-based chemotherapy with new analogues. Satraplatin and picoplatin. Expert Opin Investig Drugs 2007;16: 1009–21.

143. Samimi G, Howell SB. Modulation of the cellular pharmacology of JM118, the major metabolite of satraplatin, by copper influx and efflux transporters. Cancer Chemother Pharmacol 2006;57: 781–8.

144. Kelland LR, Abel G, McKeage MJ, et al. Preclinical antitumor evaluation of bis-acetato-ammine-dichloro-cyclohexylamine platinum(IV): an orally active platinum drug. Cancer Res 1993;53: 2581–6.

145. Samimi G, Kishimoto S, Manorek G, Breaux JK, Howell SB. Novel mechanisms of platinum drug resistance identified in cells selected for resistance to JM118 the active metabolite of satraplatin. Cancer Chemother Pharmacol 2007;59: 301–12.

146. Wosikowski K, Lamphere L, Unteregger G, et al. Preclinical antitumor activity of the oral platinum analog satraplatin. Cancer Chemother Pharmacol 2007;60: 589–600.

147. Yagoda A, Petrylak D. Cytotoxic chemotherapy for advanced hormone-resistant prostate cancer. Cancer 1993;71: 1098–109.

148. Lamphere L, Wang S, Casazza AM. Synergistic antitumor activity of the combination of satraplatin (S) and docetaxel (D) in H460 human non-small cell lung carcinoma (NSCLC) xenografted in nude mice. Proc Am Assoc Cancer Res 2006;47: Abstract no. 563.

149. Ando Y, Shimizu T, Nakamura K, et al. Potent and non-specific inhibition of cytochrome P450 by JM216, a new oral platinum agent. Br J Cancer 1998;78: 1170–4.

150. Sternberg CN, Petrylak DP, Sartor O, et al. Multinational, double-blind, phase III study of prednisone and either satraplatin or placebo in patients with castrate-refractory prostate cancer progressing after prior chemotherapy: the SPARC trial. J Clin Oncol 2009;27: 5431–8.

Chapter 16
Microtubule Targeting Agents

Antonio Tito Fojo and David E. Adelberg

Abstract Microtubules are intracellular filamentous structures that comprise the cytoskeleton of all eukaryotic cells. They play a critical role in various cellular processes such as mitosis and have become an essential target for the chemotherapeutic approach to a wide spectrum of malignancies. It is thus crucial to understand the basic biology of the microtubule and be familiar with the various microtubule targeting agents used clinically. This chapter provides an overview of microtubule physiology and the novel microtubule-targeting chemotherapeutic agents that are currently being evaluated for the treatment of taxane-refractory, castration-resistant prostate cancer.

Keywords Cytoskeleton • Microtubule • Tubulin • Chemotherapy • Prostate cancer

Introduction

Because of its crucial roles in cellular physiology, it is not surprising that the microtubule cytoskeleton has emerged as one of the most effective targets for cancer therapeutics. Interest in this validated target has led to the identification of an increasing number of structurally diverse compounds that interact with soluble tubulin and the microtubule cytoskeleton. Compounds that interact with tubulin and/or the microtubules can be divided into two major classes: By preferentially binding to the alpha/beta-tubulin heterodimer, agents comprising

A.T. Fojo (✉)
Experimental Therapeutics Section, Medical Oncology Branch, Center for Cancer Research, National Cancer Institute, Bethesda, MD, USA
e-mail: fojot@mail.nih.gov

the first class (depolymerizing or destabilizing agents) inhibit microtubule polymerization. In contrast, agents with a binding site on the microtubule polymer act principally by stabilizing microtubules (polymerizing or stabilizing agents). Depolymerizing agents include vinblastine (Velbe®), vincristine (Oncovin®), vinorelbine (Navelbine®), vindesine (Eldisine®), vinflunine, cryptophycins, halichondrins, dolastatins, estramustine, 2-methoxyestradiol (2-ME), colchicine, and combretastatins [1–3]. Microtubule-stabilizing agents include paclitaxel (Taxol®, the first identified in this class), docetaxel (Taxotere®), the epothilones, including the recently approved epothilone B analog, ixabepilone (Ixempra®), and other mechanistically similar but structurally unrelated natural products such as discodermolide, the eleutherobins, sarcodictyins, laulimalide, rhazinilam, and certain steroids and polyisoprenyl benzophenones [2, 4].

The Microtubule Cytoskeleton: Structure, Function, and the Importance of Microtubule Dynamics

Agents targeting tubulin and the microtubule have emerged as active chemotherapeutic agents because of the essential function microtubules perform in eukaryotes. These diverse cellular functions include important roles in mitosis, meiosis, motility, maintenance of cell shape, and intracellular trafficking of macromolecules and organelles [5–7]. As the name implies, microtubules are hollow cylindrical tubes and these are formed by the self-association of alpha/beta-tubulin heterodimers into polymers. The tubulin heterodimers associate in a head-to-tail fashion to form linear filaments, referred to as protofilaments, and 12–13 of these in turn associate

W.D. Figg et al. (eds.), *Drug Management of Prostate Cancer*,
DOI 10.1007/978-1-60327-829-4_16, © Springer Science+Business Media, LLC 2010

in a lateral manner to form hollow microtubules. On cross section, one sees the protofilaments assembled in a circle lining the outside of a hollow tubule. The arrangement of the protofilaments imparts polarity to the structure. The alpha subunits of the tubulin dimer are exposed at the "minus end" while the beta subunits are found at the "plus end" of the polymer. In cells, the minus end of a microtubule associates with the microtubule-organizing center (MTOC or centrosome) near the nucleus. From this anchored position, the microtubules radiate outward with their plus ends near the periphery of the cell. Gamma-tubulin (γ-tubulin) is localized at the MTOC and plays an important role in the process of microtubule nucleation by interacting with alpha-tubulin [6]. Gamma-tubulin combines with several proteins to form a circular structure known as the γ-tubulin ring complex (γ-TuRC). This complex acts as a scaffold for α/β-tubulin dimers to begin polymerization – the process of enucleation. It also acts as a cap for the minus end that associates with it, thus directing microtubule growth toward the (+) direction.

During polymerization, α- and β-subunits bound together as tubulin dimers are added to the growing ends of microtubules. GTP binding and hydrolysis at the exchangeable or *E-site* of beta-tubulin is crucial for assembly and for dynamic instability (GTP also binds to alpha-tubulin, but at the nonexchangeable or *N-site*). Microtubule assembly requires that GTP be bound to beta-tubulin, and this is hydrolyzed shortly after assembly. After hydrolysis, the guanine nucleotide becomes nonexchangeable, and so microtubules are mostly composed of (GTP:alpha-tubulin/GDP:beta-tubulin). The kinetics of GDP-tubulin is different from that of GTP-tubulin. Whereas GTP tubulin is stable, GDP-tubulin is prone to depolymerization. If a GDP-bound tubulin is present at the tip of a microtubule it is likely to fall off, and consequently the growing end is usually "capped" with GTP (or GDP·Pi):beta-tubulin. This GTP-cap allows microtubules, which are inherently unstable, to be stabilized by GTP (or GDP·Pi)-tubulin at the growing ends. However, when hydrolysis catches up to the tip of the microtubule and the GTP cap is lost, it begins a rapid depolymerization and shrinkage phase with the protofilaments peeling outward. This switch from growth to shrinking is called a *catastrophe*. GTP-bound tubulin can begin adding to the tip of the microtubule again, providing a new cap and protecting the microtubule from shrinking. This is referred to as *rescue*. This nonequilibrium behavior, termed *dynamic instability*, makes microtubules highly dynamic structures able to undergo rapid transitions between growth and shrinkage.

Dynamic instability of microtubules in vivo is regulated by interaction with other proteins. For example, during prophase of mitosis, microtubules grow out from the centrosome. If the plus end of a microtubule makes contact with a chromosome, it becomes stabilized. Otherwise rapid disassembly at the plus end ensues, and the tubulin dimers are available for growth of another microtubule.

There are numerous proteins that can interact with free tubulin dimers and/or microtubules and in so doing influence microtubule dynamics. Proteins, such as stathmin bind exclusively to tubulin dimers, thereby increasing the catastrophe rate and promoting depolymerization. By comparison, the microtubule-associated proteins (MAPs) associate with and stabilize microtubules by decreasing the frequency and duration of catastrophes and/or increasing the frequency and duration of rescues. The activities of many of these microtubule-destabilizing and microtubule-stabilizing proteins can be regulated in a cell cycle-dependent manner by phosphorylation and dephosphorylation.

Finally we should note here that while we commonly divide microtubule-targeting agents into two classes, depolymerizing/destabilzing and polymerizing/stabilizing, these properties refer to their effect at high drug concentrations and high tubulin concentrations. But we also know that in addition to these effects on the mass of tubulin, both classes of agents also suppress dynamic instability. This ability to quiet dynamics is central to the anticancer mechanisms of such drugs.

Microtubule-Depolymerizing Agents

Microtubule-depolymerizing agents are defined by their ability to decrease the polymer mass when present at equal concentrations compared with tubulin – although as noted they impact microtubule dynamics and do this at concentrations far lower than those needed to affect the polymer mass. Three classes of microtubule-depolymerizing agents have been distinguished based on binding analysis with purified tubulin: (1) agents that competitively inhibit the binding of vinca to microtubules (the vinca alkaloids), (2) agents that competitively inhibit colchicine-binding to tubulin (the colchicine class), and (3) agents that inhibit the binding of vinca alkaloids to tubulin, but do so in a noncompetitive manner and contain a peptide-based core structure – peptides and depsipeptides [8].

The Vinca Alkaloids

The vinca alkaloids, a group of compounds originally derived from the common periwinkle plant include vinblastine, vincristine, vindesine, and vinorelbine. The interactions of the vinca alkaloids with both tubulin and with microtubules have been extensively characterized [2, 9–11]. They bind to the β-tubulin subunit at a distinct region known as the vinca domain [12, 13]. At high concentrations, vinblastine inhibits microtubule polymerization by binding to both soluble tubulin and directly to tubulin in microtubules. The evidence is clear in demonstrating that vinblastine can bind to soluble tubulin – a binding that is rapid, reversible, and relatively weak ($K_A \sim 2 \times 104$ M^{-1}) [11, 14, 15]. This binding to soluble tubulin induces a conformational change, which leads to both self-association of tubulin and increases in the affinity of vinblastine for tubulin [9, 11, 16]. While it has not been possible to resolve whether free vinblastine or vinblastine–tubulin aggregates bind to microtubule ends, it is clear that vinblastine binds to microtubule ends with high affinity at some 16–17 high-affinity binding sites (k_d, 1–2 μM) present at the ends of an individual microtubule that as noted above is composed of 12–14 microfilaments [14]. Interestingly, at high concentrations, vinblastine also binds stoichiometrically with markedly reduced affinity (k_d, 0.3 mM) to tubulin along the length of the microtubule [17, 18].

The inhibition of microtubule polymerization by high concentrations of vinblastine – the property that characterizes the vinca alkaloids as depolymerizing agents – occurs through several mechanisms. Perhaps the most important is the inhibition of polymerization that results from preventing further tubulin addition consequent to the binding of vinblastine or vinblastine–tubulin aggregates to microtubule plus ends. In addition, at vinblastine levels that are far substoichiometric to the tubulin concentration drug binding to soluble tubulin induces rather than polymerization into microtubules.

Finally, at high concentrations, vinblastine can bind the low-affinity sites along the microtubule surface, leading to depolymerization as tubulin dimers are "peeled away" from the microtubule ends [17]. In contrast to its effect on microtubule polymerization, high-affinity binding to the microtubule ends at the 16–17 high-affinity binding sites noted above mediates its effects on microtubule dynamics. Because this binding occurs at low vinblastine concentrations, it does not appreciably decrease the polymer mass, instead suppressing dynamic instability and treadmilling. Because of vinblastine's high affinity for the plus ends of microtubules, concentrations as low as 0.14 μM suppress the rate of microtubule treadmilling, a measure of dynamicity, by 50% when only 1–2 vinblastine molecules are bound to the microtubule [14]. Treadmilling is a phenomenon that occurs when one end of a microfilament grows in length while the other end shrinks resulting in a section of filament seemingly "moving" across a microfilament. This is due to the constant removal of the tubulin dimers from one end of the microfilaments while dimers are constantly added at the other end. In addition to its effect on treadmilling, vinblastine suppresses growth and shortening and increases the percentage of time microtubules spend in an attenuated or paused state, neither growing nor shortening. These effects of vinblastine on dynamic instability are produced exclusively at the plus ends and are thought to be mediated by an increase in the stability of the GTP cap [19]. It has been proposed that this strengthening of the microtubule cap is brought about by a conformational change induced by the binding of even a few vinblastine molecules to the plus end of a microtubule that strengthens the affinity of the tubulin to which vinblastine is bound for adjacent tubulin subunits near the end. Interestingly, vinblastine reduces the quantity of stably bound GDP-Pi at microtubule ends [20]. Thus, the increase in cap stability may be brought about by a change in the chemical nature of the cap.

The Colchicine Class

The interaction of colchicine with tubulin and microtubules presents another variation in the mechanisms by which microtubule-targeted drugs inhibit microtubule function. Considerable evidence has indicated that the binding of colchicine to tubulin is an unusually slow process involving a conformational change in the tubulin that locks the colchicine into a site in the form of a final-state tubulin–colchicine complex from which the colchicine very poorly dissociates [9, 21].

As with the vinca alkaloids, high colchicine concentrations depolymerize microtubules, a property that assigns them to the microtubule-depolymerizing class of agents. Colchicine inhibits microtubule polymerization by binding primarily to microtubule ends rather than to the pool of soluble tubulin dimers, although it does not appear to directly bind the microtubule ends. Rather, as is thought to occur with vinblastine, colchicine first forms a poorly reversible complex with tubulin, which in turn copolymerizes together with other free tubulin dimers into the microtubule at both ends [9, 22–25]. However, unlike vinblastine that selectively binds the plus ends of the microtubule, colchicine can bind at both the plus and the minus ends of the microtubule [24] but does not bind along the length of the microtubule [26].

While the incorporation of colchicine into microtubule ends can lead to microtubule depolymerization, the ends remain competent to grow and shorten. However, as with vinblastine, the ability of the ends to both grow and shorten is compromised, affecting microtubule dynamics. As with the vinca alkaloids, low substoichiometric colchicine concentrations well below the concentration of tubulin free in solution suppress microtubule dynamics [9]. Indeed, suppression of treadmilling occurs even when relatively few colchicine–tubulin complexes have been incorporated at the plus ends of microtubule [25]. Like vinblastine, the inhibition of treadmilling by colchicines occurs at steady state without affecting the mass of assembled microtubules [25, 27]. Also like vinblastine, colchicine-binding to the plus ends of microtubules increases the fraction of time microtubules spend in an attenuated state, neither growing nor shortening, thus suppressing the rate and extent of microtubule growth and shortening [28].

Colchicine-Like Compounds

Colchicine is a highly soluble alkaloid that was first isolated from the meadow saffron *Colchicum autumnale* and has been widely used for the treatment of gout [29]. However, because its toxicity profile prevented colchicine's widespread use investigators from numerous disciplines have searched for simplified, less toxic analogs. The search has led to the identification of numerous compounds that are either structurally similar or that bind to the colchicine-binding site and are considered functionally similar. One such compound is combretastatin A-4, originally isolated from the African willow tree *Combretum caffrum* and structurally related to colchicines. In vitro studies have shown that combretastatin A-4 and several related analogs inhibit tubulin polymerization and interact with tubulin at or near the colchicine-binding site [30]. The combretastatins contain two phenyl rings linked by a two-carbon bridge, with several methoxy substitutions on the ring system [31]. Because of its limited water solubility the clinical development of combretastatin A-4 was not possible, and this led to the synthesis of combretastatin A-4 phosphate (CA-4-P), a prodrug that rapidly dephosphorylates in vivo to the active compound combretastatin A-4 [32]. In animal models, CA-4-P leads to rapid and selective disruption of the tumor vasculature resulting in hemorrhagic necrosis of tumors [33]. The mechanism of this disruption of the tumor vasculature has been debated, with some investigators advocating apoptosis of proliferating endothelial cells as the cause and others suggesting that by inhibiting endothelial cell migration CA-4-P inhibits angiogenesis [33, 34].

Another antimitotic compound that binds to the colchicine site of tubulin is 2-ME, a naturally occurring metabolite of estradiol, which is normally excreted in the urine [35]. 2-ME competitively binds to the colchicine-binding site of β-tubulin, and depending on the reaction conditions it either inhibits tubulin polymerization or results in the formation of a polymer with altered stability [36]. While its principal mode of toxicity is likely inhibition of tubulin polymerization with impaired microtubule trafficking and mitotic arrest, the thought that 2-ME could inhibit angiogenesis was a principal catalyst for its clinical development not as a microtubule-targeting agent but as an "antiangiogenic" agent [35, 37].

A final member of this class that has undergone clinical development is mivobulin isethionate (CI-980), a synthetic water-soluble compound that competitively binds tubulin at the colchicine-binding site and inhibits tubulin polymerization [38]. Interest in this compound was heightened by its broad spectrum of activity in murine and human tumor models that were cross-resistant to a wide range of chemotherapeutics [39].

Peptides and Depsipeptides

The dolastatin peptides, originally isolated from the small Indian Ocean sea hare Dollabella auricularia are small linear peptide molecules that interfere with tubulin by binding at the vinca/peptide region. Interestingly, speculation that the dolastatins were microbial products and not actually produced by D. auricularia has been confirmed. The assortment of amino acids in the peptides comprising the dolastatins pointed to a probable cyanobacterial (blue-green "algae") origin now identified as a marine cyanobacteria known to be grazed by *D. auricularia.*

Although vinblastine and dolastatin have similar quantitative effects on assembly reactions, dolastatin 10 has been shown to accumulate to higher levels and remain in cells longer – an observation ascribed to differences in the interactions of the two drugs with tubulin, with dolastatin having much higher affinity [40]. Thus, if one is to preserve drug-induced structures by HPLC, vinblastine but not dolastatin must be present in the column equilibration buffer [41, 42]. Furthermore, underscoring dolastatin's affinity for tubulin, an unbound dolastatin 10 peak can only be detected when the drug:tubulin ratio is greater than one. Moreover, the apparent Ka value for dolastatin 10 ($3.8 \times 10^7\,M^{-1}$) [42] is 21-fold higher than that obtained for vinblastine ($1.8 \times 10^6\,M^{-1}$) [43]. At the cellular level, these differences result in markedly higher retention of dolastatin 10 as compared with vinblastine.

Dolastatin 10, a four amino acid peptide (dolavaline, valine, dolaisoleuine, dolaproine) linked to a complex primary amine (dolaphenine), is cytotoxic at subnanomolar concentrations [12]. Studies have shown that the dolaisoleuine amino acid residue is critical for the inhibition of tubulin polymerization but that the dolaproine or dolavaline amino acids can be modified without inhibiting tubulin polymerization [44, 45]. For example, auristatin PE (TZT-1027), a structurally modified dolastatin 10 analog, has a phenylalanine in place of the terminal dolaphenine [46].

Dolastatin 10 inhibits microtubule assembly and polymerization of tubulin [44]. Because dolastatin 10 noncompetitively inhibits vinblastine-binding, it was originally thought to bind at the vinca alkaloid site; however, it was subsequently shown to inhibit binding of rhizoxin and phomopsin A to tubulin, indicating that it binds to the rhizoxin/maytansine region on tubulin [47]. Studies of auristatin PE have shown that it inhibits tubulin polymerization similar to dolastatin 10 [48, 49].

The Mechanism of Action of Paclitaxel and Other Microtubule-Stabilizing Compounds

In 1967, Monroe Wall working with extracts from the bark of the yew tree (*Taxus brevifolia*) named a compound "taxol" based on its source and because it was an alcohol. Now known by the generic name paclitaxel and the trade name Taxol®, it was first described in a landmark study by Wall, Mansukh Wani, and their colleagues that began the era of microtubule-stabilizing agents – an era that only became apparent when studies conducted by Horwitz and her colleagues in 1979 showed it was able to increase the rate and extent of microtubule assembly in vitro and to stabilize microtubules in vitro and in cells [50–52]. The first experiments demonstrated that paclitaxel at nanomolar concentrations inhibited the replication of HeLa cells by blocking cells in metaphase. Previously studied drugs such as colchicine and the vinca alkaloids were known to block cells in mitosis, but unlike those agents, paclitaxel treatment resulted in microtubules' reorganization with the appearance of distinct microtubule bundles.

The formation of *stable microtubule bundles*, now recognized as diagnostic of microtubule stabilization, suggested that paclitaxel enhanced microtubule assembly and stabilized existing microtubules. These hypotheses were confirmed by several experiments including early studies showing paclitaxel-stabilized microtubules against cold-induced depolymerization and augmented assembly of microtubules at steady state by promoting the elongation of existing microtubules as well as spontaneous nucleation of new microtubules [53]. In the absence of paclitaxel, polymerization occurred after a lag period of 3–4 min while in the presence of paclitaxel, the lag period was eliminated, indicating that paclitaxel enhanced the initiation phase of microtubule polymerization [51]. Furthermore, paclitaxel polymerized tubulin even at cold temperatures and in the absence of MAPs and GTP. The microtubules that formed in the presence of paclitaxel were resistant to cold (4°C) and Ca^{2+}-induced depolymerization.

Paclitaxel also affects microtubule structure, reducing the number of microfilaments from a normal average of 13 to an average of 12 [54].

Sedimentation assays to assess the binding of [³H] paclitaxel to microtubule protein [55] found that although both podophyllotoxin and vinblastine were able to inhibit the binding of [³H]paclitaxel to microtubule protein unlike unlabeled paclitaxel, which competitively displaced [³H]paclitaxel from microtubules, podophyllotoxin and vinblastine did not. Although the latter two drugs reduced the mass of paclitaxel-stabilized microtubules, the specific activity of bound [³H]paclitaxel remained constant. This data was consistent with competition between paclitaxel and either podophyllotoxin or vinblastine for different forms of tubulin (the dimeric or soluble form and the polymeric or microtubule form) and not competition for a single binding site. Finally the observation that preassembled microtubules bound [³H]paclitaxel with the same stoichiometry as microtubules assembled in the presence of [³H]paclitaxel led to the conclusion that paclitaxel bound specifically and reversibly to the polymerized form of tubulin with a stoichiometry approaching unity [56]. Subsequent studies identified the paclitaxel-binding site in the β-tubulin subunit of intact microtubules, a conclusion that is now widely accepted after having been confirmed by electron crystallography [57]. There is no evidence that paclitaxel binds to soluble tubulin dimer.

In contrast to cells exposed to microtubule-destabilizing agents, cells exposed to high concentrations of paclitaxel present with an increase in the mass of microtubule polymer and microtubule bundle formation in interphase cells. Bundle formation has become a hallmark of paclitaxel-binding and is now recognized as a property of microtubule stabilization [52]. However, as with the microtubule-destabilizing agents an effect on the polymer mass occurs only above a threshold concentration of the drug. At paclitaxel concentrations below 10 nM, there is no obvious effect on polymer mass and only a fraction of the paclitaxel-binding sites on the microtubule is occupied; instead the principal drug effect is suppression of microtubule dynamics [58, 59]. Because this effect at low paclitaxel concentrations is similar to that observed with low concentrations of vinblastine and other microtubule-destabilizing agents it has been suggested that both drug classes block mitosis by decreasing the dynamics of spindle microtubules. However, the two drug classes exhibit different mitotic effects at low concentrations [60]. Microtubule-stabilizing drugs, including paclitaxel and the epothilones, induce multipolar spindles but cannot sustain a mitotic block resulting in aneuploidy as cells exit from an aberrant mitosis [60, 61]. In contrast, destabilizing drugs such as the vinca alkaloids do not lead to aneuploidy at low concentrations [61].

The Interaction of Paclitaxel and Microtubules

Early studies employing photoaffinity labeling with initial [³H]-paclitaxel demonstrated that paclitaxel binds specifically to the beta-subunit of tubulin [56, 62–66]. A more detailed definition of the contact sites between beta-tubulin and paclitaxel became possible when paclitaxel analogs bearing photoreactive groups became available. These studies led to the isolation of photolabeled beta-tubulin peptides containing amino-acid residues 1–31 [62], 217–233 [63], and Arg282 [65]. Eventually, excellent agreement was found between the binding site predicted using the various photoaffinity analogs and that determined by electron crystallography [67].

Nontaxane Microtubule-Stabilizing Drugs

The clinical success of paclitaxel first and then docetaxel (Taxotere®) in the treatment of cancer patients catalyzed an extensive search for additional microtubule-stabilizing compounds. Different approaches led to the identification of several natural products unrelated to the taxanes that were found to stabilize microtubules [68–70]. The first and most extensively characterized were epothilones A and B, two novel polyketide natural products isolated from the fermentation broth of a soil Myxobacterium, *Sorangium cellulosum* strain 90. As with taxol, the epothilones were found to polymerize tubulin, form microtubule bundles, and arrest cells in mitosis [68]. Compared with paclitaxel, both epothilones were reported to be more potent in promoting microtubule assembly in vitro. The identification of the epothilones suggested that additional agents with microtubule stabilizing properties likely existed, an expectation that was affirmed by the isolation of discodermolide from *Discodermia dissolute,* a Caribbean sponge. Like the epothilones, discodermolide was shown to induce microtubule assembly in vitro, microtubule bundling, and mitotic arrest [69, 71, 72]. Subsequent studies led to the isolation of eleutherobin, a diterpene glycoside, from an *Eleutherobia* species of soft, red-colored coral found near Western Australian, the closely related sarcodictyins and finally the laulimalides, complex macrolide compounds isolated from the marine sponge *Cacospongia mycofijiensis* [73–75]. With the exception of laulimalide, these agents can stabilize and competitively inhibit the binding of [^{3}H]-paclitaxel to microtubules [72, 76]. This has been explained by proposing that all drugs except laulimalide interact at the same or an overlapping binding domain as paclitaxel on beta-tubulin, with laulimalide possibly binding to α-tubulin [77]. However, emerging evidence from electron crystallographic studies might challenge the extent to which the binding sites overlap. While all of these agents can stabilize mammalian microtubules, this property might be too crude or imprecise to discriminate binding sites. Identifying/characterizing the binding site on the microtubule may eventually be of value in the design of analogs or even synthetic compounds targeting microtubules.

The Role of Microtubule Stability and Dynamics in Drug Sensitivity

Selection of cell lines resistant to microtubule targeting agents has provided insight into drug action and intrinsic drug sensitivity. Early selections employed microtubule-destabilizing agents since these had been discovered first and approved for clinical use. These selections led to the isolation of resistant cells harboring mutations in tubulin, manifested by alterations in protein migration or cells with reduced intracellular drug concentrations mediated by the multidrug transporter, P-glycoprotein [78, 79]. The advent of paclitaxel, and its clinical success, followed by the realization of its limitations and the occurrence of resistance then led to widespread interest and the isolation of cells resistant to paclitaxel and then to other microtubule-stabilizing agents. The expectation was that given the drug's specificity for its target, tubulin, mutations would emerge that would

impair rug binding and identify the binding site. However, in the majority of resistant cell lines, mutations mapping to putative drug binding sites that would interfere with drug binding were not found [80–82]. Instead the mutations or adaptations found were such that they affected microtubule stability and dynamics, and in turn, drug sensitivity. While unexpected, this outcome might be explained by considering the fact that because tubulin is an essential cellular protein the mutations it can "tolerate" might be constrained. Specifically, mutations that arise in drug-resistant cells must both confer resistance to the selecting drug while not interfering with areas essential for the function of tubulin, since cellular survival would not be possible. The high degree of sequence conservation across species is an evidence that a large portion of the protein is essential, and thus possibly "off limits" to the emergence of a mutation.

In this context, two models have been proposed to help us understand the relationship between resistance to microtubule-targeting agents and the importance of microtubule stability and dynamics. The first hypothesis posits that under normal circumstances microtubule stability or polymerization is maintained within a limited range. According to this model, the *intrinsic sensitivity* to a microtubule-targeting agent depends on the basal level of microtubule stability/polymerization [83–85]. Thus, in a cell with a higher basal level of polymerized tubulin (microtubules) it is easier for a microtubule-stabilizing agent to achieve its goal, and such a cell is more sensitive to a microtubule-stabilizing agent. One should note that since a drug such as paclitaxel preferentially (exclusively) binds microtubules (polymerized tubulin) – not tubulin dimers – a cell with a more stable polymer presents more sites for drug binding and would be more sensitive to paclitaxel. Conversely, cells with less stable or polymerized tubulin (i.e., microtubules) should be resistant to drugs such as paclitaxel, but have greater sensitivity to depolymerizing agents such as vinblastine whose goal is to destabilize microtubules and whose target is tubulin dimers. The model also offers a potential explanation for why low paclitaxel concentrations are required by some paclitaxel-resistant cell lines for normal growth – the cells require low concentrations of paclitaxel to stabilize a microtubule that is otherwise too unstable. Remembering that in these "drug-dependent cells", the acquired mutation emerged while cells were kept in a medium containing paclitaxel, one can posit that the mutation (in a site other than the paclitaxel-binding site) perturbed polymer stability to such an extent – actually the polymer is so hypostable – that normal microtubule function is only possible in the presence of some "stabilizing drug".

A second model evolved from the observation that at low concentrations both microtubule-stabilizing and -destabilizing agents impact microtubule *dynamics* without affecting the microtubule polymer mass [58, 86, 87]. In a manner analogous to the model that implicates tubulin stability (in the form of microtubules) as crucial for drug sensitivity, microtubule dynamics is also crucial for drug sensitivity: increased dynamics confers resistance to microtubule-stabilizing agents while reduced dynamics underlies insensitivity to destabilizing compounds. Therefore, in paclitaxel-resistant cell lines, the equilibrium is shifted in favor of highly dynamic microtubules antagonizing the effects of paclitaxel [59, 86–88]. An increase in microtubule dynamics also provides a survival advantage to a cell challenged with a microtubule-stabilizing drug such as paclitaxel.

Resistance to Microtubule-Stabilizing Agents

A full discussion of resistance mechanisms is beyond the scope of this chapter and the reader is referred to other reviews [89]. To date, the evidence accumulated has been obtained principally with paclitaxel, and to a lesser extent with the epothilones, and colchicines as well as other destabilizing agents. However, it is likely that these changes/mechanisms apply to varying extents to all microtubule-stabilizing agents. The following mechanisms have been identified or proposed: (1) changes in the absolute or relative expression levels of tubulin isotypes; (2) tubulin mutations that impact longitudinal/lateral interactions and can alter microtubule dynamics; (3) ubulin mutations that affect either binding of regulatory proteins or GTP; (4) posttranslational modifications that affect the binding of regulatory protein; (5) altered expression and posttranslational modifications of proteins that regulate the dynamics/stability of the microtubules; (6) altered drug binding to the microtubule often secondary to acquired mutations; and (7) alterations in signaling pathways.

Role of Microtubule Targeting Agents in the Treatment of Castration-Resistant Prostate Cancer

Castration-resistant prostate cancer (CRPC) is defined as a rising serum prostate-specific antigen (PSA) despite castrate levels of testosterone. CRPC is an incurable condition projected to cause almost 27,360 deaths in America alone in 2009 [90]. The microtubule-stabilizing agent docetaxel with prednisone is the current first-line, standard of care for advanced prostate cancer resistant to androgen-ablative therapy [91, 92]. This is based on two landmark phase III trials published in the New England Journal of Medicine in 2004 in which docetaxel-based chemotherapy was shown to provide both a survival and palliative advantage for patients with CRPC when compared with mitoxantrone and prednisone [91, 92]. While a detailed discussion of the role of taxanes for CRPC is presented elsewhere in this publication, it is important to note that the survival advantage of docetaxel over mitoxantrone is only 2–3 months [91, 92], and a significant proportion of patients with castration-resistant prostate cancer become refractory to taxane-based treatments [93]. The efficacy of taxane-based therapies for CRPC is limited by the development of drug resistance. Taxane resistance is mediated predominantly, but not exclusively, by overexpression of the transmembrane transporter P-glycoprotein, leading to the multidrug resistance phenotype [94]. Thus, novel microtubule-targeted agents are needed that can be used in the setting of taxane-refractory, castration-resistant prostate cancer. Such agents include the epothilone class of drugs as well as the semisynthetic taxoid compound XRP6258 (cabazitaxel, Jevtana®, Sanofi-Aventis). The subsequent sections of this chapter focus on the clinical development of these agents.

Epothilones in Castration-Resistant Prostate Cancer

Epothilones are macrolides that were isolated from the myxobacterium *Sorangium cellulosum* [94]. These nontaxane microtubule-stabilizing agents in clinical development include epothilone B (patupilone;

EPO906, Novartis), ixabepilone (azaepothilone B; BMS-247550, Bristol-Myers Squibb), BMS-310705 (a water-soluble epothilone B derivative, Bristol-Myers Squibb), ZK-EPO (ZK-219477, a third-generation epothilone B derivative, Schering AG), and KOS-862 (epothilone D; desoxyepothilone B, Kosan Biosciences) [94]. Similar to the taxanes, the epothilones promote microtubule stabilization and lead to mitotic arrest at the G2/M phase of the cell cycle, ultimately inducing apoptosis [94]. However, it has been shown that the epothilones differ from the taxanes with respect to the binding site on β-tubulin and thus, the epothilones represent a distinct class of antimicrotubule agents [96].

Preclinical Data

The epothilones have demonstrated potent antitumor activity in vitro as well as in experimental animal models of prostate cancer [93]. In cell culture assays utilizing human prostate cancer cell lines DU145 and PC-3M, epothilone B (patupilone; EPO906) and aza-epothilone B (ixabepilone®; BMS-247550) have demonstrated more potent cytotoxicity than paclitaxel (Taxol®) [97]. In athymic murine xenograft models of castrate-resistant prostate cancer using these same two human prostate cancer cell lines, administration of epothilone B (patupilone) was associated with the inhibition of tumor growth, followed by sustained regression [98].

Preclinical studies have shown that epothilones have cytotoxic activity against taxane-resistant tumor models and thus lack cross-resistance with the taxanes [93]. Possible explanations for this include the minimal effect on epothilone cytotoxicity generated by

either P-glycoprotein overexpression or mutations in β-tubulin, both of which are known to mediate taxane resistance [99–101].

Phase I Clinical Trials of the Epothilones

Multiple dosing schedules of patupilone and its semisynthetic derivative ixabepilone (BMS – 247550) have been studied in phase I trials. The toxicity profiles of the epothilones are diverse and depend on the particular agent and administration schedule [94] Table 16.1.

Patupilone has been evaluated as a single agent in several regimens, including dosing once every 3 weeks [102] with a maximum tolerated dosage (MTD) of 8 mg/m^2, and a weekly schedule [103] with an MTD of 2.5 mg/m^2. The most common dose-limiting toxicities for both schedules of patupilone were diarrhea and fatigue [93, 94]. Multiple phase I studies of ixabepilone (BMS-247550) have been reported in the literature and two of them will be discussed here. An accelerated titration phase I trial of BMS-247550 in 17 patients was reported in 2005 [104]. BMS-247550 was administered as a 1-h infusion every 3 weeks; all patients received prophylaxis for hypersensitivity reactions with steroids and histamine antagonists. The MTD of every 3-week administration of BMS-247550 in this study was 40 mg/m^2 with neutropenia being the dose-limiting toxicity [104]. A subsequent accelerated dose-escalation phase I trial of ixabepilone was reported in 2007 in which BMS-247550 was given as a 1-h infusion every 3 weeks to patients with advanced solid tumors or relapsed/refractory non-Hodgkin's lymphoma. Sixty-one patients were enrolled and the most common dose-limiting toxicities were neutropenia,

Table 16.1 Epothilones in clinical development

Epothilones	Other names	Characteristics	Clinical phase of development	Manufacturer
Ixabepilone	BMS247550	Aza-epothilone B	FDA approval for breast cancer	Bristol-Myers Squibb
Patupilone	EPO906	Epothilone B (natural epothilone)	Phase III	Novartis
BMS-310705	NA	Water-soluble, semisynthetic analog of epothilone B	Phase I (terminated)	Bristol-Myers Squibb
KOS-862	NA	Epothilone D (deoxyepothilone B)	Phase II (terminated)	Bristol-Myers Squibb
KOS-1584	NA	9,10-didehydroepothilone D	Phase I	Roche and Bristol-Myers Squibb
ZK-EPO	NA	Synthetic epothilone	Phase II	Schering

Adapted with permission from Macmillan Publishers Ltd [97]. Copyright 2009
NA not available

stomatitis/pharyngitis, myalgia, and arthralgia. The MTD of ixabepilone in this study was determined to be 50 mg/m^2 when given as a 1-h infusion every 3 weeks [105]. A 3-h infusion time is recommended, because a higher risk for neurotoxicity was observed with the shorter infusion time [96, 104]. The current FDA-approved dose and schedule for ixabepilone in phase II trials is 40 mg/m^2 I.V. over 3 h, given once every 3 weeks [96]. The most common grade 3 or 4 toxicity associated with single-agent ixabepilone at 40-mg/m^2 dose every 3 weeks is neutropenia [96], although it should be noted that grade 3 peripheral sensory neuropathy was also commonly encountered. Phase I clinical trials have shown that single-agent patupilone and ixabepilone have activity against castration-resistant prostate cancer, and this finding has led to subsequent phase II evaluations of these two drugs.

Phase II Clinical Trials of the Epothilones for CRPC

To date, ixabepilone and patupilone have provided the most convincing data regarding clinical activity in patients with castration-resistant prostate cancer [93]. The phase II SWOG0111 clinical trial [106] evaluated ixabepilone (at 40 mg/m^2 over 3 h once every 3 weeks) in 42 patients [median age, 73 years; median prostate specific antigen (PSA) level 111 ng/mL] with chemotherapy-naïve, metastatic castration-resistant prostate cancer [106]. The primary objective was to assess the proportion of patients achieving a ≥50% reduction in PSA levels in response to ixabepilone. Of the 42 patients treated with ixabepilone, 14 patients (33%) had a confirmed PSA response; the majority of these patients (72%) had PSA declines of greater than 80%, and two patients achieved undetectable PSA (<0.2 ng/mL) [106]. Among the 20 patients with measurable disease, one patient had an unconfirmed complete response and two patients had unconfirmed partial responses [106]. There were no confirmed objective complete responses. The estimated progression-free survival was 6 months (95% CI, 4–8 months), and the median survival was 18 months (95% CI, 13–24 months). All grade 4 toxicities were neutropenia or leukopenia. The most frequent grade 3 adverse events were neuropathy, hematologic toxicity, flu-like symptoms, and infection. The SWOG0111 trial has thus demonstrated that single-agent ixabepilone has activity in chemotherapy-naive metastatic CRPC (Table 16.2).

Combination studies have been undertaken to determine if there is a synergistic clinical effect when ixabepilone is added to estramustine phosphate (EMP) therapy for the treatment of castration-resistant prostate cancer. Smaletz et al. [112] performed a dose-escalation study of BMS-247550 and determined that 35 mg/m^2 given over 3 h on day 1 of a 21-day cycle was the MTD when

Table 16.2 Phase II clinical trials of epothilones in patients with metastatic castration-resistant prostate cancer

Agents	References	Clinical setting of CRPC	Number of patients	Response rate (%) PSA decline 50%	Tumor shrinkage
Ixabepilone (40 mg/m^2 Q3 weeks)	Hussain et al. [106]	Chemotherapy-naive	42	33	ND
Ixabepilone (35 mg/m^2 Q3 weeks)	Galsky et al. [107]	Chemotherapy-naive	45	48	32
Ixabepilone (35 mg/m^2 Q3 weeks) with estramustine (280 mg TID on D1-5)	Galsky et al. [107]	Chemotherapy-naive	47	69	48
Ixabepilone (35 mg/m^2 Q3 weeks) or mitoxantrone (14 mg/m^2 Q3 weeks) with prednisone	Rosenberg et al. [108]	Taxane-refractory	41	17	4
Ixabepilone (20 mg/m^2 weekly for 3/4 weeks)	Wilding et al. [109]	Chemo-naïve	31	32.3	20.8
Ixabepilone (20 mg/m^2 weekly for 3/4 weeks)	Wilding et al. [109]	Taxane-refractory	36	22.2	7.1
Patupilone (10 mg/m^2 Q3 weeks)	Chi et al. [110]	Taxane-refractory	19	42	0
Patupilone (2.5 mg/m^2 weekly for 3/4 weeks)	Hussain et al. [111]	First-line or second-line	45	13	0

Adapted with permission from Macmillan Publishers Ltd [97]. Copyright 2009

CRPC castration-resistant prostate cancer, *ND* not determined, *PSA* prostate-specific antigen administered in combination with EMP (280 mg three times daily on days 1–5 of the 21-day cycle) for the treatment of chemotherapy-naïve patients with metastatic CRPC. Neutropenia was the dose-limiting toxicity that established the MTD. A subsequent multicenter, randomized noncomparative phase II trial [107] was undertaken to test the safety and clinical efficacy of ixabepilone (BMS-247550; 35 mg/m^2 every 3 weeks) with and without EMP (280 mg three times daily on days 1–5 of a 21-day cycle) in chemotherapy-naïve patients with metastatic CRPC. The primary endpoint was the proportion of patients achieving a ≥50% post-therapy reduction in PSA [107]. Forty-five patients were randomized to receive ixabepilone alone and 47 patients received the combination. Posttherapy PSA declines of at least 50% occurred more frequently in the combination group than in the monotherapy group; 31 of 45 patients (69%; 95% CI, 55–82%) in the combination cohort compared to 21 of 44 patients (48%; 95% CI, 33–64%) in the ixabepilone only group [107]. In patients with measurable disease, the objective response rate as assessed by RECIST criteria was also higher in the combination group than in the monotherapy group. Partial responses were observed in 11 of 23 (48%; 95% CI, 27–68%) patients in the combination cohort compared to 8 of 25 patients (32%; 95% CI, 14–50%) in the monotherapy group [107]. The most common toxic effects were neutropenia and neuropathy; treatment was discontinued due to neuropathy in eight patients (18%) in the combination cohort compared to 13 patients (28%) in the monotherapy group [107].

Rosenberg et al. [108] performed a multicenter, noncomparative, crossover phase II trial in which patients with castrate-resistant, taxane-refractory metastatic prostate cancer were randomized to receive either ixabepilone (35 mg/m^2 once every 3 weeks) or mitoxantrone (14 mg/m^2 once every 3 weeks plus daily oral prednisone). The primary objective was to determine if a ≥50% reduction in serum PSA would occur in at least 25% of these highly pretreated patients. Forty-one patients were accrued to each arm of the study. PSA declines of ≥50% were observed in 17% of ixabepilone-treated patients (95% CI, 7–32) and in 20% of mitoxantrone/prednisone treated patients (95% CI, 9–35) [108]. In those patients with evaluable measurable disease, partial responses were observed in 1 of 24 ixabepilone-treated and 2 of 21 mitoxantrone/prednisone-treated patients. Median overall survival was 10.4 months for those receiving ixabepilone and

9.8 months with mitoxantrone [108]. Assessment of survival by treatment cohort is confounded by the fact that 16 of 41 patients (39%) on second-line ixabepilone crossed over to MP treatment and 30 of 41 patients (73%) on second-line mitoxantrone/prednisone crossed over to ixabepilone therapy. The most common grade three and four toxicity associated with second-line treatment was neutropenia (54% in the ixabepilone cohort and 63% in the mitoxantrone cohort) [108]. These results indicate that single-agent ixabepilone has modest activity as second line chemotherapy in this population of taxane-refractory CRPC patients [93].

Wilding et al. [109] have published in abstract form updated results of a phase II trial examining the toxicity and antitumor activity of ixabepilone when administered on a weekly basis to both chemotherapy-naïve and taxane-refractory patients with castration-resistant prostate cancer. Ixabepilone was administered at a dose of 20 mg/m^2 weekly for three out of a total 4 week cycle. Patients were stratified to one of three arms, either chemotherapy-naïve, prior taxane-only treatment or a third arm which had received two prior chemotherapy regimens. The primary objective was a ≥50% reduction in serum PSA by Consensus Criteria in at least 50% of the chemotherapy-naïve patients and in at least 30% of the patients in each of the other two cohorts [109]. Rates of PSA response were higher in the chemotherapy-naïve group (10 of 31 patients, 32.3%) than in the group who had received prior taxane-only therapy (8 of 36 patients, 22.2%) [109]. For those patients with measurable disease, 20.8% in the chemotherapy-naïve group and 7.1% in the taxane-only group had evidence of partial objective responses by RECIST criteria [109]. The most common toxicities seen were neutropenia, sensory neuropathy, and fatigue. The toxicity profile for the weekly administration of ixabepilone compared favorably to the every-3-week schedule, with a decreased rate of myelosuppression in those patients who were chemotherapy-naïve.

Epothilone B (patupilone) has been evaluated in two separate phase II trials. Chi et al. published results in abstract form [110] of a phase II trial of patupilone (10 mg/m^2 IV every 3 weeks) for taxane-refractory, metastatic CRPC. PSA reduction of at least 50% was the primary endpoint with progression-free and overall survival, along with measurable disease response as secondary endpoints. At the time of abstract publication, 19 of 33 enrolled patients had data available and 8/19 patients (42%) had a reduction in serum PSA of at least 50%. No patients with measurable disease at that time had an objective response by RECIST criteria [110]. The most common grade 3 or 4 adverse events were diarrhea and fatigue with no hematologic adverse events [110].

Hussain et al. [111] report on a single arm phase II trial, the purpose of which was to establish the safety and efficacy of this agent in patients with castration-resistant prostate cancer. Forty-five patients with CRPC (median age 69 years; documented metastatic disease not required) were administered patupilone at a dose of 2.5 mg/m^2 weekly for 3 weeks of a 4-week cycle. 64% of patients had prior chemotherapy (55% having received previous taxane therapy). Six of 45 patients (13%) had a $\geq$50% decline in PSA; three of these patients had received prior taxane therapy. No patient with measurable disease had an objective response by RECIST criteria. Median overall survival was 13.4 months. The most common adverse events were grade 3 diarrhea and fatigue with no patients experiencing neutropenia or thrombocytopenia [111].

Beer et al. [113] have reported results of a phase II study evaluating the potential role of KOS-862 (epothilone D) in patients with docetaxel-refractory, castration-resistant prostate cancer. Epothilone D was administered at a dose of 100 mg/m^2 weekly for three out of a 4 week cycle. Because of excess toxicity and limited clinical efficacy of KOS-862, further investigational studies are not planned [95].

Phase II trials of the epothilones patupilone and ixabepilone for the treatment of patients with CRPC have demonstrated single-agent antitumor activity as well as incomplete cross-resistance with the taxanes [94]. Phase III trials are now needed to confirm the activity of the epothilones and better define their role in the treatment algorithm for castration-resistant prostate cancer [93].

Cabazitaxel, a Novel Taxane for the Treatment of Advanced CRPC

Cabazitaxel is a semisynthetic novel taxoid compound [114]. Preclinical in vitro studies have shown that cabazitaxel not only promotes tubulin polymerization and stabilizes microtubules as potently as docetaxel, but it also demonstrates greater cytotoxicity than docetaxel in a broad array of cancer cell lines with P-glycoprotein overexpression. Cabazitaxel displays decreased affinity for the P-glycoprotein 1 drug efflux pump. Additional preclinical studies with cabazitaxel have shown antitumor activity in mice bearing human DU-145 prostatic adenocarcinoma xenografts [114].

Phase I and II trials demonstrated antitumor activity in solid tumors including docetaxel-refractory mCRPC and that neutropenia was the primary dose-limiting toxicity [115, 116]. In June 2010, cabazitaxel (Jevtana, XRP6258) received US Food and Drug Administration approval for second-line use in combination with prednisone for the treatment of patients with metastatic CRPC previously treated with a docetaxel-containing treatment regimen. It was reviewed under the agency's priority review program, an expedited 6-month review for drugs that offer an advance in treatment or provide a treatment where none exists. The approval was based on data from the international Phase III TROPIC trial conducted in 755 patients with mCRPC who all had been previously treated with docetaxel [117]. They were randomized to receive either cabazitaxel (25 mg/m^2) or mitoxantrone (12 mg/m^2), both administered intravenously every three weeks in combination with prednisone (CP vs. MP). The median overall survival was 15.1 months with cabazitaxel and 12.7 months with mitoxantrone (HR= 0.70; 95% CI, 0.59-0.83; p< 0.0001). Investigator-assessed tumor response rates using RECIST criteria were 14.4% for CP vs 4.4% for MP (p=0.0005), although no complete responses were observed on either treatment arm. The most common ($\geq$5%) grade 3/4 adverse reactions were neutropenia, leukopenia, anemia, febrile neutropenia, diarrhea, fatigue and asthenia. The most common fatal adverse reactions in cabazitaxel-treated patients were infections and renal failure. The most frequent grade 3/4 toxicity was neutropenia (CP=81.7%; MP=58.0%) and rates of febrile neutropenia were 7.5% and 1.3%, respectively. Granulocyte colony-stimulating factor (G-CSF) may be administered to reduce the risks of neutropenic complications associated with cabazitaxel use and primary prophylaxis with G-CSF should be considered in patients with high-risk clinical features.

With the approval of cabazitaxel, there is now a new treatment option for patients with the most advanced stage of prostate cancer and for whom there have been few options available. Cabazitaxel in combination with prednisone is the first and only FDA approved regimen to provide significant survival benefit in patients previously treated with a docetaxel-based regimen.

Conclusion

Microtubules are polymers composed of α,β-tubulin heterodimers. These filamentous structures associate to form the cytoskeleton of all eukaryotic cells. They also play critical roles in normal cellular physiology such as mitosis. There is a dynamic interplay between the intracellular pool of tubulin, and the mature microtubule. Many chemotherapeutic agents have been developed that shift the balance of this dynamic relationship in favor of either soluble or polymerized tubulin and these microtubule-targeting agents play a critical role in many different types of malignancies, including castration-resistant prostate cancer.

References

1. Hamel E, Covell DG. Antimitotic peptides and depsipeptides. Curr Med Chem Anticancer Agents 2002;2:19–53.
2. Jordan MA. Mechanism of action of antitumor drugs that interact with microtubules and tubulin. Curr Med Chem Anticancer Agents 2002;2:1–17.
3. Jordan MA, Wilson L. Microtubules as a target for anticancer drugs. Nat Rev Cancer 2004;4:253–65.
4. Jimenez-Barbero J, Amat-Guerri F, Snyder JP. The solid state, solution and tubulin-bound conformations of agents that promote microtubule stabilization. Curr Med Chem Anticancer Agents 2002;2(1):91–122.
5. Desai A, Mitchison TJ. Microtubule polymerization dynamics. Annu Rev Cell Dev Biol 1997;13:83–117.
6. Oakley BR. An abundance of tubulins. Trends Cell Biol 2000;10:537–42.
7. Sharp DJ, Rogers GC, Scholey JM. Microtubule motors in mitosis. Nature 2000;407:41–7.
8. Calvert PM, O'Neill V, Twelves C, et al. A phase I clinical and pharmacokinetic study of EPO906 (Epothilone B), given every three weeks, in patients with advanced solid tumors. Proc Am Soc Clin Oncol 2001;20:A429.
9. Wilson L, Jordan MA. Pharmacological probes of microtubule function. In: Hyams J, Lloyd C, editors. Microtubules. New York: Wiley; 1994. p. 59–84.
10. Jordan MA, Wilson L. The use of drugs to study the role of microtubule assembly dynamics in living cells, Molecular motors and the cytoskeleton. Methods Enzymol, vol. 298. 1998. p. 252–76.
11. Lobert S, Correia J. Energetics of vinca alkaloid interactions with tubulin. Methods Enzymol 2000;323:77–103.
12. Bai RB, Pettit GR, Hamel E. Dolastatin 10. a powerful cytostatic peptide derived from a marine animal. Inhibition of tubulin polymerization mediated through the vinca alkaloid binding domain. Biochem Pharmacol 1990;39:1941–9.
13. Bai RB, Pettit GR, Hamel E. Binding of dolastatin 10 to tubulin at a distinct site for peptide antimitotic agents near the exchangeable nucleotide and vinca alkaloid sites. J Biol Chem 1990;265:17141–9.
14. Wilson L, Jordan MA, Morse A, Margolis RL. Interaction of vinblastine with steady-state microtubules in vitro. J Mol Biol 1982;159:129–49.
15. Correia JJ, Lobert S. Physiochemical aspects of tubulin-interacting antimitotic drugs. Curr Pharm Des 2001;7(13):1213–28.
16. Na GC, Timasheff SN. Thermodynamic linkage between tubulin self-association and the binding of vinblastine. Biochemistry 1980;19(7):1347–54.
17. Jordan MA, Margolis RL, Himes RH, Wilson L. Identification of a distinct class of vinblastine binding sites on microtubules. J Mol Biol 1986;187:61–73.
18. Singer WD, Jordan MA, Wilson L, Himes RH. Binding of vinblastine to stabilized microtubules. Mol Pharmacol 1989;36(3):366–70.
19. Panda D, Jordan MA, Chin K, Wilson L. Differential effects of vinblastine on polymerization and dynamics at opposite microtubule ends. J Biol Chem 1996;271:29807–12.
20. Panda D, Miller H, Wilson L. Determination of the size and chemical nature of the stabilizing cap at microtubule ends using modulators of polymerization dynamics. Biochemistry 2002;41:1609–17.
21. Hastie SB. Interactions of colchicine with tubulin. Pharmacol Ther 1991;512:377–401.
22. Sternlicht H, Ringel I. Colchicine inhibition of microtubule assembly via copolymer formations. J Biol Chem 1979;254:10540–50.
23. Sternlicht H, Ringel I, Szasz J. Theory for modelling the copolymerization of tubulin and tubulin-colchicine complex. Biophys J 1983;42:255–67.
24. Farrell KW, Wilson L. The differential kinetic stabilization of opposite microtubule ends by tubulin–colchicine complexes. Biochemistry 1984;23:3741–8.
25. Skoufias D, Wilson L. Mechanism of inhibition of microtubule polymerization by colchicine: inhibitory potencies of unliganded colchicine and tubulin–colchicine complexes. Biochemistry 1992;31:738–46.
26. Margolis RL, Rauch CT, Wilson L. Mechanism of colchicine dimer addition to microtubule ends: implications for the microtubule polymerization mechanism. Biochemistry 1980;19:5550–7.
27. Wilson L, Farrell KW. Kinetics and steady-state dynamics of tubulin addition and loss at opposite microtubule ends: the mechanism of action of colchicine. Ann N Y Acad Sci 1986;466:690–708.
28. Panda D, Goode BL, Feinstein SC, Wilson L. Kinetic stabilization of microtubule dynamics at steady state by tau and microtubule-binding domains of tau. Biochemistry 1995;34:11117–27.
29. Jordan A, Hadfield JA, Lawrence NJ, et al. Tubulin as a target for anticancer drugs: agents which interact with the mitotic spindle. Med Res Rev 1998;18:259–96.
30. Pettit GR, Cragg GM, Singh SB. Antineoplastic agents, 122. Constituents of *Combretum caffrum*. J Nat Prod 1987;50:386–91.
31. Tozer GM, Kanthou C, Parkins CS, et al. The biology of the combretastatins as tumour vascular targeting agents. Int J Exp Pathol 2002;83:21–38.
32. Pettit GR, Temple Jr C, Narayanan VL, et al. Antineoplastic agents 322. Synthesis of combretastatin A-4 prodrugs. Anticancer Drug Des 1995;10:299–309.

33. Dark GG, Hill SA, Prise VE, et al. Combretastatin A-4, an agent that displays potent and selective toxicity toward tumor vasculature. Cancer Res 1997;57:1829–34.

34. Ahmed B, Van Eijk LI, Bouma-Ter Steege JC, et al. Vascular targeting effect of combretastatin A-4 phosphate dominates the inherent angiogenesis inhibitory activity. Int J Cancer 2003;105:20–5.

35. Schumacher G, Neuhaus P. The physiological estrogen metabolite 2-methoxyestradiol reduces tumor growth and induces apoptosis in human solid tumors. J Cancer Res Clin Oncol 2001;127:405–10.

36. D'Amato RJ, Lin CM, Flynn E, et al. 2-Methoxyestradiol, an endogenous mammalian metabolite, inhibits tubulin polymerization by interacting at the colchicine site. Proc Natl Acad Sci U S A 1994;91:3964–8.

37. Fotsis T, Zhang Y, Pepper MS, et al. The endogenous oestrogen metabolite 2-methoxyoestradiol inhibits angiogenesis and suppresses tumour growth. Nature 1994;368:237–9.

38. de Ines C, Leynadier D, Barasoain I, et al. Inhibition of microtubules and cell cycle arrest by a new 1-deaza-7, 8-dihydropteridine antitumor drug, CI 980, and by its chiral isomer, NSC 613863. Cancer Res 1994;54:75–84.

39. Waud WR, Leopold WR, Elliott WL, et al. Antitumor activity of ethyl 5-amino-1,2-dihydro-2-methyl-3-phenyl-pyrido [3,4-b]pyrazin-7-ylcarbamate, 2-hydroxyethanesulfonate, hydrate (NSC 370147) against selected tumor systems in culture and in mice. Cancer Res 1990;50:3239–44.

40. Verdier-Pinard P, Kepler JA, Pettit GR, Hamel E. Sustained intracellular retention of dolastatin 10 causes its potent antimitotic activity. Mol Pharmacol 2000;57:180–7.

41. Singer WD, Hersh RT, Himes RH. Effect of solution variables on the binding of vinblastine to tubulin. Biochem Pharmacol 1988;37:2691–6.

42. Bai R, Taylor GF, Schmidt JM, Williams MD, Kepler JA, Pettit GR, et al. Interaction of dolastatin 10 with tubulin: Induction of aggregation and binding and dissociation reactions. Mol Pharmacol 1995;47:965–76.

43. Safa AR, Hamel E, Felsted RL. Photoaffinity labeling of tubulin subunits with a photoactive analogue of vinblastine. Biochemistry 1987;26:97–102.

44. Bai RL, Pettit GR, Hamel E. Structure-activity studies with chiral isomers and with segments of the antimitotic marine peptide dolastatin 10. Biochem Pharmacol 1990;40: 1859–64.

45. Bai R, Roach MC, Jayaram SK, et al. Differential effects of active isomers, segments, and analogs of dolastatin 10 on ligand interactions with tubulin. Correlation with cytotoxicity. Biochem Pharmacol 1993;45:1503–15.

46. Pettit GR, Srirangam JK, Barkoczy J, et al. Antineoplastic agents 337. Synthesis of dolastatin 10 structural modifications. Anticancer Drug Des 1995;10:529–44.

47. Li Y, Kobayashi H, Hashimoto Y, et al. Interaction of marine toxin dolastatin 10 with porcine brain tubulin: competitive inhibition of rhizoxin and phomopsin A binding. Chem Biol Interact 1994;93:175–83.

48. Otani M, Natsume T, Watanabe JI, et al. TZT-1027, an antimicrotubule agent, attacks tumor vasculature and induces tumor cell death. Jpn J Cancer Res 2000;91:837–44.

49. Natsume T, Watanabe J, Tamaoki S, et al. Characterization of the interaction of TZT-1027, a potent antitumor agent, with tubulin. Jpn J Cancer Res 2000;91:737–47.

50. Wani MC, Taylor HL, Wall ME, Coggan P, McPhail AT. Plant antitumor agents. VI. The isolation and structure of taxol, a novel antileukemic and antitumor agent from *Taxus brevifolia*. J Am Chem Soc 1971;93:2325–7.

51. Schiff PB, Fant J, Horwitz SB. Promotion of microtubule assembly in vitro by taxol. Nature 1979;277:665–7.

52. Schiff PB, Horwitz SB. Taxol stabilizes microtubules in mouse fibroblast cells. Proc Natl Acad Sci U S A 1980;77: 1561–5.

53. Schiff PB, Horwitz SB. Taxol assembles tubulin in the absence of exogenous guanosine 5′-triphosphate or microtubule-associated proteins. Biochemistry 1981;20:3247–52.

54. Diaz JF, Valpuesta JM, Chacon P, Diakun G, Andreu JM. Changes in microtubule protofilament number induced by Taxol binding to an easily accessible site. Internal microtubule dynamics. J Biol Chem 1998;273:33803–10.

55. Parness J, Horwitz SB. Taxol binds to polymerized tubulin in vitro. J Cell Biol 1981;91:479–87.

56. Rao S, Horwitz SB, Ringel I. Direct photoaffinity labeling of tubulin with taxol. J Natl Cancer Inst 1992;84:785–8.

57. Lowe J, Li H, Downing KH, Nogales E. Refined structure of alpha beta-tubulin at 3.5 Å resolution. J Mol Biol 2001;313: 1045–57.

58. Jordan MA, Toso RJ, Thrower D, Wilson L. Mechanism of mitotic block and inhibition of cell proliferation by taxol at low concentrations. Proc Natl Acad Sci U S A 1993;90: 9552–6.

59. Derry WB, Wilson L, Jordan MA. Substoichiometric binding of taxol suppresses microtubule dynamics. Biochemistry 1995;34:2203–11.

60. Chen JG, Horwitz SB. Differential mitotic responses to microtubule-stabilizing and -destabilizing drugs. Cancer Res 2002;62:1935–8.

61. Torres K, Horwitz SB. Mechanisms of taxol-induced cell death are concentration dependent. Cancer Res 1998;58: 3620–6.

62. Rao S, Krauss NE, Heerding JM, Swindell CS, Ringel I, Orr GA, et al. 3′-(p-azidobenzamido)taxol photolabels the N-terminal 31 amino acids of beta-tubulin. J Biol Chem 1994;269:3132–4.

63. Rao S, Orr GA, Chaudhary AG, Kingston DG, Horwitz SB. Characterization of the taxol binding site on the microtubule. 2-(m-Azidobenzoyl)taxol photolabels a peptide (amino acids 217-231) of beta-tubulin. J Biol Chem 1995;270: 20235–8.

64. Orr GA, Rao S, Swindell CS, Kingston DG, Horwitz SB. Photoaffinity labeling approach to map the taxol-binding site on the microtubule. Methods Enzymol 1998;298: 238–52.

65. Rao S, He L, Chakravarty S, Ojima I, Orr GA, Horwitz SB. Characterization of the taxol binding site on the microtubule. Identification of Arg(282) in beta-tubulin as the site of photoincorporation of a 7-benzophenone analogue of taxol. J Biol Chem 1999;274:37990–4.

66. Rao S, Aberg F, Nieves E, Horwitz SB, Orr GA. Identification by mass spectrometry of a new alpha-tubulin isotype expressed in human breast and lung carcinoma cell lines. Biochemistry 2001;40:2096–103.

67. Nogales E, Wolf SG, Downing KH. Structure of the alpha beta tubulin dimer by electron crystallography. Nature 1998;391:199–203. erratum in: Nature 393:191.

68. Bollag DM, McQueney PA, Zhu J, Hensens O, Koupal L, Liesch J, et al. Epothilones, a new class of microtubule-stabilizing agents with a taxol-like mechanism of action. Cancer Res 1995;55:2325–33.

69. ter Haar E, Kowalski RJ, Hamel E, Lin CM, Longley RE, Gunasekera SP, et al. Discodermolide, a cytotoxic marine agent that stabilizes microtubules more potently than taxol. Biochemistry 1996;35:243–50.

70. He L, Orr GA, Horwitz SB. Novel molecules that interact with microtubules and have functional activity similar to taxol. Drug Discov Today 2001;6:1153–64.

71. Hung DT, Chen J, Schreiber SL. (+)-Discodermolide binds to microtubules in stoichiometric ratio to tubulin dimers, blocks taxol binding and results in mitotic arrest. Chem Biol 1996;3:287–93.

72. Kowalski RJ, Giannakakou P, Gunasekera SP, Longley RE, Day BW, Hamel E. The microtubule-stabilizing agent discodermolide competitively inhibits the binding of paclitaxel (Taxol) to tubulin polymers, enhances tubulin nucleation reactions more potently than paclitaxel, and inhibits the growth of paclitaxel-resistant cells. Mol Pharmacol 1997; 52:613–22.

73. Long BH, Carboni JM, Wasserman AJ, Cornell LA, Casazza AM, Jensen PR, et al. Eleutherobin, a novel cytotoxic agent that induces tubulin polymerization, is similar to paclitaxel (taxol). Cancer Res 1998;58:1111–5.

74. Hamel E, Sackett DL, Vourloumis D, Nicolaou KC. The coral-derived natural products eleutherobin and sarcodictyins A and B: effects on the assembly of purified tubulin with and without microtubule-associated proteins and binding at the polymer taxoid site. Biochemistry 1999;38:5490–8.

75. Mooberry SL, Tien G, Hernandez AH, Plubrukarn A, Davison BS. Laulimalide and isolaulimalide, new paclitaxel-like microtubule-stabilizing agents. Cancer Res 1999;59: 653–60.

76. Pryor DE, O'Brate A, Bilcer G, Diaz JF, Wang Y, Kabaki M, et al. The microtubule stabilizing agent laulimalide does not bind in the taxoid site, kills cells resistant to paclitaxel and epothilones, and may not require its epoxide moiety for activity. Biochemistry 2002;41:9109–15.

77. Pineda O, Farras J, Maccari L, Manetti F, Botta M, Vilarrasa J. Computational comparison of microtubule-stabilising agents laulimalide and peloruside with taxol and colchicine. Bioorg Med Chem Lett 2004;14:4825–9.

78. Fojo AT, Whang-Peng J, Gottesman MM, Pastan I. Amplification of DNA sequences in human multidrug-resistant KB carcinoma cells. Proc Natl Acad Sci U S A 1985;82:7661–5.

79. Hari M, Wang Y, Veeraraghavan S, Cabral F. Mutations in alpha- and beta-tubulin that stabilize microtubules and confer resistance to colcemid and vinblastine. Mol Cancer Ther 2003;2:597–605.

80. Giannakakou P, Sackett DL, Kang YK, Zhan Z, Buters JT, Fojo T, et al. Paclitaxel-resistant human ovarian cancer cells have mutant beta-tubulins that exhibit impaired paclitaxel-driven polymerization. J Biol Chem 1997;272: 17118–25.

81. Giannakakou P, Sackett DL, Ward Y, Webster KR, Blagosklonny MV, Fojo T. p53 is associated with cellular microtubules and is transported to the nucleus by dynein. Nat Cell Biol 2000;2:709–17.

82. Hari M, Loganzo F, Annable T, Tan X, Musto S, Morilla DB, et al. Paclitaxel-resistant cells have a mutation in the paclitaxel-binding region of beta-tubulin (Asp26Glu) and less stable microtubules. Mol Cancer Ther 2006;5:270–8.

83. Cabral FR, Brady RC, Schibler MJ. A mechanism of cellular resistance to drugs that interfere with microtubule assembly. Ann N Y Acad Sci 1986;466:745–56.

84. Cabral F, Barlow SB. Mechanisms by which mammalian cells acquire resistance to drugs that affect microtubule assembly. FASEB J 1989;3:1593–9.

85. Minotti AM, Barlow SB, Cabral F. Resistance to antimitotic drugs in Chinese hamster ovary cells correlates with changes in the level of polymerized tubulin. J Biol Chem 1991;266: 3987–94.

86. Wilson L, Jordan MA. Microtubule dynamics: taking aim at a moving target. Chem Biol 1995;2:569–73.

87. Jordan MA, Wilson L. Microtubules and actin filaments: dynamic targets for cancer chemotherapy. Curr Opin Cell Biol 1998;10:123–30.

88. Goncalves A, Braguer D, Kamath K, Martello L, Briand C, Horwitz S, et al. Resistance to taxol in lung cancer cells associated with increased microtubule dynamics. Proc Natl Acad Sci U S A 2001;98:11737–42.

89. Fojo AT, Menefee M. Microtubule targeting agents: basic mechanisms of multidrug resistance (MDR). Semin Oncol 2005;32:S3–8.

90. Jemal A, Siegel R, Ward E, et al. Cancer Statistics, CA Cancer. J Clin 2009;59:225–49.

91. Tannock IF, de Wit R, Berry W, et al. Docetaxel plus prednisone or mitoxantrone plus prednisone for advanced prostate cancer. N Engl J Med 2004;351:1502–12.

92. Petrylak DP, Tangen CM, Hussain M, et al. Docetaxel and estramustine compared with mitoxantrone and prednisone for advanced refractory prostate cancer. N Engl J Med 2004;351:1513–20.

93. Dawson N. Epothilones in prostate cancer: review of clinical experience. Ann Oncol 2007;18 Suppl 5:v22–7.

94. Lee JJ, Kelly WK. Epothilones: tubulin polymerization as a novel target for prostate cancer therapy. Nat Clin Pract Oncol 2009;6(2):85–92.

95. Beardsley EK, Chi KN. Systemic therapy after first-line docetaxel in metastatic castration-resistant prostate cancer. Curr Opin Support Palliat Care 2008;2:161–6.

96. Rivera E, Lee J, Davies A. Clinical development of ixabepilone and other epothilones in patients with advanced solid tumors. Oncologist 2008;13:1207–23.

97. Sepp-Lorenzino L, Balog A, Su DS, et al. The microtubule-stabilizing agents epothilones A and B and their desoxy-derivatives induce mitotic arrest and apoptosis in human prostate cancer cells. Prostate Cancer Prostatic Dis 1999;2: 41–52.

98. O'Reilly T, McSheehy PM, Wenger F, et al. Patupilone (epothilone B, EPO906) inhibits growth and metastasis of experimental prostate tumors in vivo. Prostate 2005;65: 231–40.

99. Altmann KH. Recent developments in the chemical biology of epothilones. Curr Pharm Des 2005;11:1595–613.

100. Kowalski RJ, Giannakakou P, Hamel E. Activities of the microtubule-stabilizing agents epothilones A and B with purified tubulin and in cells resistant to paclitaxel (Taxol®). J Biol Chem 1997;272:2534–41.

101. Wartmann M, Altmann KH. The biology and medicinal chemistry of epothilones. Curr Med Chem Anticancer Agents 2002;2:123–48.

102. Calvert PM, O'Neill V, Twelves C, et al. A phase I clinical and pharmacokinetic study of EPO906 (Epothilone B), given every three weeks, in patients with advanced solid tumors. Proc Am Soc Clin Oncol 2001;20:A429.

103. Rubin EH, Rothermel J, Fisseha T, et al. Phase I dose-finding study of weekly single-agent patupilone in patients with advanced solid tumors. J Clin Oncol 2005;23:9120–9.

104. Gadgeel SM, Wozniak A, Boinpally RR, et al. Phase I clinical trial of BMS-247550, a derivative of epothilone B, using accelerated titration 2B design. Clin Cancer Res 2005;11:6233–9.

105. Aghajanian C, Burris HA, Jones S, et al. Phase I study of the novel epothilone analog Ixabepilone (BMS-247550) in patients with advanced solid tumors and lymphomas. J Clin Oncol 2007;25:1082–8.

106. Hussain M, Tangen CM, Lara Jr PN, et al. Ixabepilone (epothilone B analogue BMS-247550) is active in chemotherapy-naïve patients with hormone-refractory prostate cancer: a Southwest Oncology Group trial S0111. J Clin Oncol 2005;23:8724–9.

107. Galsky MD, Small EJ, Oh WK, et al. Multi-institutional randomized phase II trial of the epothilone B analog ixabepilone (BMS-247550) with or without estramustine phosphate in patients with progressive castrate metastatic prostate cancer. J Clin Oncol 2005;23:1439–46.

108. Rosenberg JE, Weinberg VK, Kelly WK, et al. Activity of second-line chemotherapy in docetaxel-refractory hormone refractory prostate cancer patients. Randomized phase 2 study of ixabepilone or mitoxantrone and prednisone. Cancer 2007;110(3):556–63.

109. Wilding G, Chen Y, DiPaola RP, et al. E3803: updated results on phase II study of a weekly schedule of BMS-247550 for patients with castrate refractory prostate cancer (CRPC). J Clin Oncol 2008;26(Suppl):A5070.

110. Chi KN, Beardsley EK, Venner PM, et al. A phase II study of patupilone in patients with metastatic hormone refractory prostate cancer (HRPC) who have progressed after docetaxel. J Clin Oncol 2008;26(15S) May 20 Suppl:516.

111. Hussain A, DiPaola RS, Baron AD, et al. Phase II trial of weekly patupilone in patients with castration-resistant prostate cancer. Ann Oncol 2009;20:492–7.

112. Smaletz O, Galsky M, Scher HI, et al. Pilot study of epothilone B analog (BMS-247550) and estramustine phosphate in patients with progressive metastatic prostate cancer following castration. Ann Oncol 2003;14:1518–24.

113. Beer TM, Higano CS, Saleh M, et al. Phase II study of KOS-862 in patients with metastatic androgen independent prostate cancer previously treated with docetaxel. Invest New Drugs 2007;25:565–70.

114. Sanofi-aventis. XRP6258 investigator's brochure. Antony (France): Sanofi-aventis; 2000.

115. Mita AC, Denis LJ, Rowinsky EK, et al. Phase I and pharmacokinetic study of XRP6258 (RPR 116258A), a novel taxane administered as a 10 hour infusion every 3 weeks in patients with advanced solid tumors. Clin Cancer Res 2009;15(2):723–30.

116. Pivot X, Koralewski P, Hidalgo JL, et al. A multicenter phase II study of XRP6528 administered as a 1-h i.v. infusion every 3 weeks in taxane-resistant metastatic breast cancer patients. Ann Oncol 2008;19(9):1547–52.

117. De Bono JS, Oudard S, Ozguroglu M, et al. Cabazitaxel or mitosantrone with presdnisone in patients with metastatic castration-resistant prostate cancer (mCRPC) previously treated with docetaxel: Final results of a multinational phase III trial (TROPIC). ASCO Annual Meeting Proceedings. J Clin Oncol 2010;28:4508.

Part III
Angiogenesis

Chapter 17
Principles of Antiangiogenic Therapy

Cindy H. Chau and William D. Figg

Abstract Angiogenesis is a critical process to both tumor growth and metastasis in prostate cancer. The markers of angiogenesis in prostate cancer have been identified and could potentially provide prognostic information in addition to clinicopathological data and patient outcome. Promising preclinical studies have led to the initiation of phase I/II studies of antiangiogenic therapy in combination with docetaxel-based chemotherapy in patients with castration-resistant prostate cancer. This chapter describes the mechanisms of the angiogenic process, establishes its role in prostate cancer, and discusses the markers of angiogenesis in prostate cancer, in an attempt to provide an overall understanding of the basic principles of antiangiogenic therapy.

Keywords Angiogenesis • Angiogenic switch • Angiogenesis inhibitor • Microvessel density • Antiangiogenic therapy

Introduction

Cancer metastasis occurs when cancer cells break away from the primary tumor and penetrate into lymphatic and blood vessels, circulating through the bloodstream to invade and grow in the normal tissues elsewhere. Understanding the metastatic process requires characterizing the growth and invasion of solid tumors and identifying the environmental cues that trigger and/or govern this event. Early cancer researchers investigating the conditions necessary for cancer metastasis observed that one of the critical events required for tumor growth is an increased vascularization and the formation of a new network of blood vessels called *angiogenesis*. Over 70 years ago, the existence of tumor-derived factors responsible for promoting new vessel growth was postulated [1], and it was found that tumor growth is essentially dependent on vascular induction and the development of a neovascular supply [2]. By the late 1960s, Dr. Judah Folkman and colleagues had begun the search for a tumor angiogenesis factor [3]. In his landmark report, Folkman proposed that inhibition of angiogenesis by means of holding tumors in a nonvascularized dormant state would be an effective strategy to treat human cancer, and hence laid the groundwork for the concept behind the development of "antiangiogenic" drugs [4]. This fostered the search for angiogenic factors, regulators of angiogenesis, and antiangiogenic molecules over the next three decades and shed light on angiogenesis as an important therapeutic target for the treatment of cancer and other diseases.

Successful development and clinical translation of antiangiogenic agents depends on understanding the biology of angiogenesis in tumor progression and the regulatory proteins that govern this angiogenic process. This chapter provides an overview of the principles of antiangiogenic therapy by presenting the mechanisms behind the angiogenic process followed by a discussion of the markers of angiogenesis in prostate cancer. The next chapters in this section cover the investigational antiangiogenic agents used in the treatment of metastatic castration-resistant prostate cancer (CRPC) as well as the pharmacogenetics of angiogenesis.

C.H. Chau (✉)
Medical Oncology Branch, Center for Cancer Research, National Cancer Institute/NIH, 9000 Rockville Pike, Bethesda, MD 20892, USA
e-mail: chauc@mail.nih.gov

W.D. Figg et al. (eds.), *Drug Management of Prostate Cancer*,
DOI 10.1007/978-1-60327-829-4_17, © Springer Science+Business Media, LLC 2010

Mechanisms of the Angiogenic Process

Angiogenic Switch and Regulatory Proteins

Tumor development and progression depends on angiogenesis. Recruitment of new blood vessels to the tumor site is required for delivery of nutrients and oxygen to the cancerous growths and removal of waste products [5]. Cancer cells promote angiogenesis at an early stage of tumorigenesis beginning with the release of molecules that send signals to the surrounding normal host tissue and stimulating the migration of microvascular endothelial cells (ECs) in the direction of the angiogenic stimulus. These angiogenic factors not only mediate EC migration but also EC proliferation and microvessel formation in tumors undergoing the switch to the angiogenic phenotype [6].

Experimental evidence for this "angiogenic switch" was observed when hyperplastic islets in transgenic mice (RIP-Tag model) switch from small (<1 mm), white microscopic dormant tumors to red, rapidly growing tumors [6]. Dormant tumors have been discovered during autopsies of individuals who died of causes other than cancer [7]. These autopsy studies suggest that the vast majority of microscopic, in situ cancers never switch to the angiogenic phenotype during a normal lifetime. Such incipient tumors are usually not neovascularized and can remain harmless to the host for long periods of time as microscopic lesions that are in a state of dormancy [8, 9]. These nonangiogenic tumors cannot expand beyond the initial microscopic size and become clinically detectable, lethal tumors until they have switched to the angiogenic phenotype [10–12] through neovascularization and/or blood vessel co-option [13]. Depending on the tumor type and the environment, this switch can occur at different stages of the tumor progression pathway and ultimately depends on a net balance of positive and negative regulators. Thus, the angiogenic phenotype may result from the production of growth factors by tumor cells and/or the downregulation of negative modulators.

Changes in this angiogenic balance affecting the levels of activator and inhibitor molecules dictate whether an EC will be in a quiescent or an angiogenic state. Normally, the inhibitors predominate, thereby blocking growth. Should a need for new blood vessels arise, the balance will shift in favor of the angiogenic state with an increase in the amount of activators and a decrease in inhibitors. This prompts the activation, growth, and division of vascular ECs, resulting in the formation of new blood vessels. The activated ECs produce and release matrix metalloproteinases (MMPs) into the surrounding tissue. These degradative enzymes breakdown the extracellular matrix to allow the ECs to migrate into the surrounding tissues and organize themselves into hollow tubes that eventually evolve into a mature network of blood vessels.

Proangiogenic factors or positive regulators of angiogenesis include vascular endothelial growth factor (VEGF), basic fibroblast growth factor, (bFGF), platelet-derived growth factor (PDGF), placental growth factor (PlGF), transforming growth factor-β, pleiotrophins, and others [14]. VEGF (also known as vascular permeability factor) is a potent proangiogenic growth factor and its expression is upregulated by most cancer-cell types. It stimulates endothelial-cell proliferation, migration, and survival as well as induces increased vascular permeability. The different forms of VEGF bind to transmembrane tyrosine kinase receptors (RTKs) on ECs: VEGFR1 (Flt-1), VEGFR2 (KDR/Flk-1), or VEGFR3 (Flt-4) [15]. This results in receptor dimerization, activation, and autophosphorylation of the tyrosine kinase domain, thereby triggering downstream signaling pathways. bFGF is present in basement membranes and in the subendothelial extracellular matrix of blood vessels. When activated, it can mediate the formation of new blood vessels. Other signaling molecules that may represent attractive therapeutic targets include PDGF and angiopoietin-2 (Ang-2). PDGF-B/PDGF receptor-β plays an important role in the recruitment of pericytes and maturation of the microvasculature [16]. Ang-2 (which binds the Tie-2 receptor) is mostly expressed in tumor-induced neovasculature, whereby its selective inhibition results in reduced EC proliferation [17].

Activation of the hypoxia-inducible factor-1α (HIF-1α) via tumor-associated hypoxic conditions is also involved in the upregulation of several angiogenic factors [18]. The angiogenic switch can downregulate angiogenesis suppressor proteins that include endostatin, angiostatin, thrombospondin, and others (reviewed in ref. [19, 20]). Most notable is the link between many oncogenes and angiogenesis and the significant role oncogenes play in driving the angiogenic switch. These proangiogenic oncogenes not only induce the expression of stimulators but may also downregulate inhibitors of angiogenesis (reviewed in ref. [21]).

Endogenous Inhibitors of Angiogenesis

The first angiogenesis inhibitor was reported in 1980 and involved low-dose administration of interferon-alpha [22–24]. Over the next decade, several compounds were discovered to have potent antiangiogenic activity and included protamine and platelet-factor 4 [25], trahydrocortisol [26], and the fumagillin analogue TNP-470 [27]. Additionally, at least 28 endogenous angiogenesis inhibitors have been identified to date [19, 20].

The infrequency of microscopic in situ tumors that actually undergo the angiogenic switch (<1%) suggests that naturally occurring endogenous inhibitors exist in the body to defend against the angiogenic switch in pathological conditions and limit physiological angiogenesis [8]. These circulating endogenous inhibitors could also prevent microscopic metastases from growing into visible tumors. The discovery of angiostatin, an internal fragment of plasminogen, first revealed that an angiogenesis inhibitory peptide could be enzymatically released from a parent protein that lacked this inhibitory property [28]. Soon thereafter endostatin, an internal fragment of collagen XVIII, demonstrated for the first time that a basement-membrane collagen contained an antiangiogenic peptide [29]. Endostatin is the most well-studied endogenous angiogenesis inhibitor (reviewed in ref. [30]). Other potent endogenous angiogenesis inhibitors include thrombospondin-1 (TSP-1) [31] and tumstatin, a 232-amino acid antiangiogenic peptide in the alpha3 chain of collagen type IV [32]. The discovery that these endogenous angiogenesis inhibitors can suppress the growth of primary tumors raises the possibility that such inhibitors might also be able to slow tumor metastasis. Indeed inhibition of angiogenesis by angiostatin significantly reduced the rate of metastatic spread.

Perhaps the most compelling genetic evidence that endogenous inhibitors suppress pathologic angiogenesis was observed in studies using mice deficient in tumstatin, endostatin, or TSP-1 [33]. These experiments demonstrate that normal physiological levels of the inhibitors can retard the tumor growth, and that

their absence leads to enhanced angiogenesis and increased tumor growth by two- to threefold. Tumors grow twofold faster in the tumstatin/TSP-1 double-knockout mice compared with either the tumstatin- or the TSP-1-deficient mice. Additionally, tumor growth in transgenic mice overexpressing endostatin specifically in the ECs (a 1.6-fold increase in the circulating levels) is threefold slower than the tumor growth in wild-type mice. Collectively, these results strongly suggest that endogenous inhibitors of angiogenesis can act as endothelium-specific tumor suppressors.

The connection between a tumor suppressor protein and angiogenesis is best illustrated by the classic tumor suppressor p53. p53 is known to link the biology of the cell cycle to tumorigenesis and for its role in regulating tumor cell proliferation. However, p53 can also inhibit angiogenesis by increasing the expression of TSP-1 [34], by repressing VEGF [35] and bFGF binding protein [36], and by degrading HIF-1 [37], which blocks downstream induction of VEGF expression. Furthermore, a recent study revealed that p53-mediated inhibition of angiogenesis occurs in part via the antiangiogenic activity of endostatin and tumstatin [38]. This landmark finding clearly demonstrates that p53 not only controls cell proliferation but can also repress tumor angiogenesis through enzymatic mobilization of these endogenous angiogenesis inhibitor proteins to prevent ECs from being recruited into the dormant, microscopic tumors and thereby preventing the switch to the angiogenic phenotype [39]. It remains to be established whether other angiogenesis inhibitors are regulated by p53 or by other tumor suppressor genes.

Angiogenesis and Prostate Cancer

The significance of angiogenesis in prostate cancer is well established with the identification of several markers of angiogenesis in CaP, with microvessel density (MVD) and VEGF being two of the most commonly measured (Table 17.1). In general, many studies have demonstrated the direct correlation of angiogenesis with Gleason score, pathological stage, progression, metastasis, and survival [40, 41]. Weidner et al. determined that patients with metastatic prostate cancer have a higher mean MVD than those without metastasis [42]. VEGF expression is significantly

Table 17.1 Markers of angiogenesis in prostate cancer

Markers of angiogenesis	References
MVD (factor VIII; CD34)	[40, 41, 43, 52, 53, 55, 59]
VEGF	[43, 44, 47, 48, 53, 59]
Serum VEGF	[45, 84]
Matrix metalloproteinases (MMP-2, MMP-9)	[44]
bFGF	[47]
Serum bFGF	[46, 84]
IL-8	[50]
Serum IL-8	[49]
Endoglin	[51]
p53	[52]
Tumor-associated macrophages	[52, 54, 55]
Tissue factor	[56]
Hypoxia-inducible factor 1	[57, 58]

increased in prostate tumors (relative to normal tissue), which directly correlates with MVD, tumor stage and grade, and disease-specific survival in patients with CaP [43]. A strong expression of VEGF is detected in neuroendocrine-differentiated tumor cells [43], and the coexpression of VEGF with MMP-2 and MMP-9 further increases the malignant potential of prostate tumors [44]. Serum VEGF levels are significantly higher in patients with metastatic prostate cancer than in patients with localized disease [45].

Several additional growth factors are thought to enhance angiogenesis in prostate cancer. Although bFGF is a known endothelial mitogen, the prognostic role of bFGF and its receptor (FGFR1) in prostate cancer has been controversial. Previous studies have shown that serum bFGF levels are elevated in most men with CaP and had a relatively high sensitivity (83%) in detecting carcinoma in patients with serum prostate-specific antigen (PSA) levels below 4.0 ng/mL as well as in differentiating between patients with local and advanced disease [46]. Others have reported that while serum bFGF and VEGF were not helpful in differentiating between patients with benign and malignant prostatic disease [47], together they are correlated with poor prostate cancer survival [48]. Serum levels of interleukin-8 (IL-8) are significantly elevated in men with prostate cancer and bone metastases compared with patients with localized disease [49], and the expression of IL-8 correlates directly with Gleason score, tumor stage, and MVD [50]. Endoglin, a receptor for TGF-β that is expressed on proliferating ECs, has direct association with MVD, Gleason score, tumor stage and CaP metastasis and is a prognostic marker

for survival in a subgroup of patients with Gleason score 5, 6, and 7 tumors [51]. While mutations in the *p53* gene have been associated with increased MVD and higher stage and grade of CaP [52], the regulation of VEGF in CaP appears to be independent of p53 expression [53]. Other markers that have shown a positive association with angiogenesis in prostate cancer include tumor-associated macrophages [54, 55] and tissue factor [56].

The role of HIF in prostate cancer development and its transition to a metastatic and castrate-resistant state remain to be elucidated. HIF, a key mediator of VEGF expression, is upregulated in the majority of prostate tumor tissues, compared with normal and benign prostate tissues, and its expression is induced in prostate cancer in situ [57]. Immunohistochemical studies of HIF-1α in clinical specimens of high-grade prostate intraepithelial neoplasia lesions, considered the precursor of a majority of invasive prostate adenocarcinoma, show an increase in HIF-1α relative to the respective normal epithelium, stromal cells, and benign prostatic hyperplasia [58]. These findings suggest that upregulation of HIF-1α is an early event in prostate carcinogenesis. Additionally, studies have shown that complete androgen blockade downregulates VEGF expression possibly via inhibition of HIF-1 with concomitant upregulation of thrombospondin and induction of EC apoptosis [59, 60]. Moreover, androgens can activate HIF-1, driving VEGF expression in androgen-sensitive LNCaP cells. This regulation is mediated through an autocrine loop involving epidermal growth factor/phosphatidylinositol 3'-kinase/protein kinase B, which in turn activate HIF-1α and HIF-1-regulated gene expression [61]. In prostate cancer cells, the androgen receptor (AR) has been shown to enhance HIF-1-mediated gene expression and that HIF-1 interacts with the AR on the *PSA* gene promoter, thereby activating its expression [62]. Thus, HIF-1 might be involved in AR-mediated gene expression in prostate cancer and implicated in tumor growth and progression. Furthermore, single nucleotide polymorphisms (SNPs) in the oxygen-dependent degradation domain of the HIF-1α gene, which enhance HIF-1α activity and hence increase transcription of downstream angiogenesis-related genes, have been identified in prostate cancer cell lines and clinical samples [63]. One of the SNPs (P582S) is associated with an increased risk of prostate cancer [64, 65]. Taken together, these findings indicate the importance of HIF-1-mediated VEGF and

AR regulation in prostate tumorigenesis and identify HIF-1 as a possible prime target for prostate cancer therapy.

Antiangiogenic Therapy: Rationale and Classification

Rationale

Antiangiogenic therapy stems from the fundamental concept that tumor growth, invasion, and metastatsis are angiogenesis-dependent. The microvascular EC recruited by a tumor has become an important second target in cancer therapy. Unlike the cancer cell (the primary target of cytotoxic chemotherapy) that is genetically unstable with unpredictable mutations, the genetic stability of ECs may make them less susceptible to acquired drug resistance [66]. Moreover, ECs in the microvascular bed of a tumor may support 50–100 tumor cells. Coupling this amplification potential together with the lower toxicity of most angiogenesis inhibitors results in the use of antiangiogenic therapy that should be significantly less toxic than conventional chemotherapy. Therefore, treating both the cancer cell and the EC in a tumor may be more effective than treating the cancer cell alone.

Classification of Antiangiogenic Agents

The proof of concept that targeting angiogenesis is an effective strategy for treating cancer came with the approval of the first angiogenesis inhibitor, bevacizumab, by the US Food and Drug Admistration (FDA) following a phase III study showing a survival benefit. Since then, several antiangiogenesis agents have received FDA approval for cancer treatment and numerous investigational angiogenesis inhibitors currently are being tested in clinical trials of prostate cancer. The reader is referred to [67] for a general overview of the current state of drug development of angiogenesis inhibitors.

The inhibitors being investigated fall into several different categories, depending on their mechanism of action. Some inhibit ECs directly, while others inhibit the angiogenesis signaling cascade or block the ability of ECs to break down the extracellular matrix. Some antiangiogenic agents either target VEGF directly through neutralizing the protein, block the tumor expression of the angiogenic factor, or block the receptor for the angiogenic factor on the ECs. Finally, these inhibitors may also be characterized by the degree of their blocking potential: drugs that block one main angiogenic protein, drugs that block two or three main angiogenic proteins, or drugs that have a broad spectrum effect, blocking a range of angiogenic regulators [67]. These broad spectrum inhibitors may target the angiogenic regulators and/or signaling pathways in both the tumor and ECs.

There are two general classes of angiogenesis inhibitors. A *direct angiogenesis inhibitor* blocks vascular ECs from proliferating, migrating, or increasing their survival in response to proangiogenic proteins. Direct angiogenesis inhibitors are less likely to induce acquired drug resistance because they target the genetically stable ECs. Examples in this category include angiostatin and TSP-1. Other drugs, which interact with the integrin protein, also can promote the destruction of proliferating ECs. Integrins are cell surface adhesion molecules that play an essential role in cell–cell and cell–matrix adhesion. They are responsible for transmitting signals important for cell migration, invasion, proliferation, and survival. One member of the integrin family, $\alpha 5\beta 3$-integrin, is expressed on tumor and ECs. The involvement of integrin in tumor angiogenesis was demonstrated in studies that show the $\beta 4$ subunit of integrin promoting endothelial migration and invasion [68].

Indirect angiogenesis inhibitors decrease or block the expression of a tumor cell product, neutralize the tumor product itself, or block its receptor on ECs. Examples of drugs that interfere with the angiogenesis signaling pathway include bevacizumab, sorafenib, and sunitinab. These drugs target the major signaling pathways in tumor angiogenesis: VEGF, PDGF, and their respective receptors as well as other growth factors and/or signaling pathways. As such, most indirect angiogenesis inhibitors are designed to target these signaling pathways and can block the activity of one, two, or a broad spectrum of proangiogenic proteins and/or their receptors. The limitation to indirect inhibitors is that over time tumor cells may acquire mutations that lead to increased expression of other proangiogenic proteins not blocked by the indirect inhibitor.

This may give the appearance of drug resistance and warrants the addition of a second antiangiogenic agent, one that would target the expression of these upregulated proangiogenic proteins.

Angiogenesis inhibitors may also be referred to as either being *exclusive* or *inclusive*. Drugs that are *exclusively* antiangiogenic only have one known function, which is to exhibit antiangiogenic activity. Examples of these drugs include bevacizumab, VEGF-Trap, etc. For other angiogenesis inhibitors, the antiangiogenic activity is *included* with other functions of the drug. Among them are certain cancer agents that exhibit dual roles. In many cases, the antiangiogenic activity is discovered as a secondary function after the drug has received FDA approval for a different primary function. For example, bortezomib is a proteasome inhibitor that is approved for multiple myeloma and later found to possess antiangiogenic acitivity via inhibiting VEGF. Certain orally available small molecule drugs display their antiangiogenic activity through inducing the expression of endogenous angiogenesis inhibitors such as celecoxib, a cox-2 inhibitor, which inhibits angiogenesis by increasing levels of endostatin [30]. Both bortezomib and celecoxib are under clinical investigation as potential angiogenesis inhibitors in prostate cancer clinical trials.

Combination Therapies

Tumor angiogenesis is a highly complex process involving multiple growth factors and their receptor signaling pathways. Based on current evidence, with a few exceptions, effective therapy will probably rely on a combinatorial approach that involves targeting multiple pathways simultaneously. A number of studies have shown that antiangiogenic agents in combination with chemotherapy or radiotherapy result in additive or synergistic effects. Several models have been proposed to explain the mechanism responsible for this potentiation, keying in on the chemosensitizing effects of antiangiogenic therapy [69]. One hypothesis is that antiangiogenic therapy may normalize the tumor vasculature, thus resulting in improved oxygenation, better blood perfusion and, consequently, improved delivery of chemotherapeutic drugs [70]. A second model suggests that chemotherapy delivered at low doses and at close, regular intervals with no extended

drug-free break periods preferentially damages ECs in the tumor neovasculature [71, 72] and suppresses circulating endothelial progenitor cells [73, 74]. This regimen, also called metronomic chemotherapy, sustains antiangiogenic activity and reduces acute toxicity [75]. Thus, the efficacy of metronomic chemotherapy may increase when administered in combination with specific antiangiogenic drugs. Finally, the third model addresses the use of antiangiogenic drugs to slow down tumor cell repopulation between successive cycles of cytotoxic chemotherapy [76]. This model underscores the importance of timing and sequence in achieving the maximal therapeutic benefit from combination therapies. Nevertheless, it remains a challenge to establish the most effective timing and combination of antiangiogenic agents, other targeted therapies, and conventional therapies to improve clinical outcomes, particularly in patients with CRPC who become refractory to docetaxel chemotherapy.

Surrogate Markers of Antiangiogenic Therapy

Antiangiogenesis therapy has created a need to develop effective biomarkers to assess the activity of these inhibitors. Surrogate markers of tumor angiogenesis activity are important to guide clinical development of these agents and to select patients most likely to benefit from this approach. Several avenues are currently being investigated and include tumor biopsy analysis, MVD, noninvasive vascular imaging (positron emission tomography, MRI) and measuring circulating biomarkers (levels of angiogenic factors in serum, plasma, urine, or circulating ECs) [77]. Thus, reliable surrogate markers of activity are desparately needed to monitor and evaluate the clinical efficacy of these new drugs.

Resistance to Antiangiogenic Therapy

Resistance to VEGF inhibitors may be observed in late stage tumors when tumors re-grow during treatment, after an initial period of growth suppression from these antiangiogenic agents. This resistance to VEGF inhibitors involves reactivation of tumor angiogenesis and increased expression of other proangiogenic factors. As the disease progresses, it is possible that redundant pathways might be implicated, with VEGF being replaced by other angiogenic pathways, warranting the addition of a second antiangiogenesis agent that would target these secondary growth factors and/or their activated receptor pathways. Perhaps the administration of angiogenic drugs at earlier stages of the disease may be a more effective and beneficial approach. In addition, tumor cells bearing genetic alterations of the *p53* gene may display a lower apoptosis rate under hypoxic conditions, which might reduce their reliance on vascular supply and thereby their responsiveness to antiangiogenic therapy [78]. Therefore, the selection and overgrowth of tumor-variant cells that are hypoxia resistant and thus less dependent [78] on angiogenesis and vasculature remodeling resulting in vessel stabilization [79] could also explain the resistance to antiangiogenic drugs. Finally, among the possible mechanisms for acquired resistance to antiangiogenic drugs [80, 81] perhaps the most intriguing finding is that although ECs are assumed to be genetically stable, they may under some circumstances harbor genetic abnormalities and thus acquire resistance as well [82, 83].

Conclusion

Antiangiogenic therapy has been established as a fourth modality in cancer treatment validating that angiogenesis as an important target for cancer. The role of angiogenesis in prostate cancer is well established, and the inhibition of this process has been shown to suppress tumor growth and metastasis in both preclinical prostate cancer models and in current clinical studies. Angiogenesis inhibition is likely to be a part of standard treatment strategy for CaP in the near future. Hence, current research efforts are needed to develop better surrogate markers of tumor angiogenesis and selection markers, determine the optimal dosing strategy, define the target patient population, and identify the most effective combination therapy to ensure that patients will fully benefit from these new agents as well as determine the tumor types and stages that will benefit most from antiangiogenic therapy. Much progress is needed in understanding the emergence of targeted therapy resistance and assessing the potential cumulative toxicities that arise from combination therapies of multiple antiangiogenic regimens. Nonetheless, while chemotherapy will remain a mainstay of cancer treatment for years to come, antiangiogenic therapy represents a promising add-on strategy for the treatment of prostate cancer for patients with CRPC.

References

1. Ide AG, Baker NH, Warren SL. Vascularization of the Brown Pearce rabbit epithelioma transplant as seen in the transparent ear chamger. Am J Roentgenol 1939;42:891–9.
2. Algire GH, Chalkley HW, Legallais FY, Park HD. Vascular reactions of normal and malignant tissues in vivo. I. Vascular reactions of mice to wounds and to normal and neoplastic transplants. J Natl Cancer Inst 1945;6:73–85.
3. Folkman J, Merler E, Abernathy C, Williams G. Isolation of a tumor factor responsible for angiogenesis. J Exp Med 1971;133:275–88.
4. Folkman J. Tumor angiogenesis: therapeutic implications. N Engl J Med 1971;285:1182–6.
5. Papetti M, Herman IM. Mechanisms of normal and tumor-derived angiogenesis. Am J Physiol Cell Physiol 2002;282:C947–70.
6. Hanahan D, Folkman J. Patterns and emerging mechanisms of the angiogenic switch during tumorigenesis. Cell 1996;86:353–64.
7. Black WC, Welch HG. Advances in diagnostic imaging and overestimations of disease prevalence and the benefits of therapy. N Engl J Med 1993;328:1237–43.
8. Folkman J, Kalluri R. Cancer without disease. Nature 2004;427:787.
9. Weidner N, Semple JP, Welch WR, Folkman J. Tumor angiogenesis and metastasis – correlation in invasive breast carcinoma. N Engl J Med 1991;324:1–8.
10. Udagawa T, Fernandez A, Achilles EG, Folkman J, D'Amato RJ. Persistence of microscopic human cancers in mice: alterations in the angiogenic balance accompanies loss of tumor dormancy. FASEB J 2002;16:1361–70.
11. Naumov GN, Bender E, Zurakowski D, et al. A model of human tumor dormancy: an angiogenic switch from the nonangiogenic phenotype. J Natl Cancer Inst 2006;98:316–25.
12. Holmgren L, O'Reilly MS, Folkman J. Dormancy of micrometastases: balanced proliferation and apoptosis in the presence of angiogenesis suppression. Nat Med 1995;1:149–53.
13. Holash J, Maisonpierrc PC, Compton D, et al. Vessel cooption, regression, and growth in tumors mediated by angiopoietins and VEGF. Science 1999;284:1994–8.
14. Relf M, LeJeune S, Scott PA, et al. Expression of the angiogenic factors vascular endothelial cell growth factor, acidic and basic fibroblast growth factor, tumor growth factor beta-1, platelet-derived endothelial cell growth factor, placenta growth factor, and pleiotrophin in human primary breast cancer and its relation to angiogenesis. Cancer Res 1997;57:963–9.

15. Ferrara N, Gerber HP, LeCouter J. The biology of VEGF and its receptors. Nat Med 2003;9:669–76.
16. Lindahl P, Johansson BR, Leveen P, Betsholtz C. Pericyte loss and microaneurysm formation in PDGF-B-deficient mice. Science 1997;277:242–5.
17. Oliner J, Min H, Leal J, et al. Suppression of angiogenesis and tumor growth by selective inhibition of angiopoietin-2. Cancer Cell 2004;6:507–16.
18. Carmeliet P, Dor Y, Herbert JM, et al. Role of HIF-1alpha in hypoxia-mediated apoptosis, cell proliferation and tumour angiogenesis. Nature 1998;394:485–90.
19. Folkman J. Endogenous angiogenesis inhibitors. APMIS 2004;112:496–507.
20. Nyberg P, Xie L, Kalluri R. Endogenous inhibitors of angiogenesis. Cancer Res 2005;65:3967–79.
21. Rak J, Yu JL, Klement G, Kerbel RS. Oncogenes and angiogenesis: signaling three-dimensional tumor growth. J Investig Dermatol Symp Proc 2000;5:24–33.
22. Brouty-Boye D, Zetter BR. Inhibition of cell motility by interferon. Science 1980;208:516–8.
23. Dvorak HF, Gresser I. Microvascular injury in pathogenesis of interferon-induced necrosis of subcutaneous tumors in mice. J Natl Cancer Inst 1989;81:497–502.
24. Sidky YA, Borden EC. Inhibition of angiogenesis by interferons: effects on tumor- and lymphocyte-induced vascular responses. Cancer Res 1987;47:5155–61.
25. Taylor S, Folkman J. Protamine is an inhibitor of angiogenesis. Nature 1982;297:307–12.
26. Crum R, Szabo S, Folkman J. A new class of steroids inhibits angiogenesis in the presence of heparin or a heparin fragment. Science 1985;230:1375–8.
27. Ingber D, Fujita T, Kishimoto S, et al. Synthetic analogues of fumagillin that inhibit angiogenesis and suppress tumour growth. Nature 1990;348:555–7.
28. O'Reilly MS, Holmgren L, Shing Y, et al. Angiostatin: a novel angiogenesis inhibitor that mediates the suppression of metastases by a Lewis lung carcinoma. Cell 1994;79:315–28.
29. O'Reilly MS, Boehm T, Shing Y, et al. Endostatin: an endogenous inhibitor of angiogenesis and tumor growth. Cell 1997;88:277–85.
30. Folkman J. Antiangiogenesis in cancer therapy – endostatin and its mechanisms of action. Exp Cell Res 2006;312:594–607.
31. Lawler J. Thrombospondin-1 as an endogenous inhibitor of angiogenesis and tumor growth. J Cell Mol Med 2002;6:1–12.
32. Maeshima Y, Manfredi M, Reimer C, et al. Identification of the anti-angiogenic site within vascular basement membrane-derived tumstatin. J Biol Chem 2001;276:15240–8.
33. Sund M, Hamano Y, Sugimoto H, et al. Function of endogenous inhibitors of angiogenesis as endothelium-specific tumor suppressors. Proc Natl Acad Sci U S A 2005;102:2934–9.
34. Dameron KM, Volpert OV, Tainsky MA, Bouck N. Control of angiogenesis in fibroblasts by p53 regulation of thrombospondin-1. Science 1994;265:1582–4.
35. Zhang L, Yu D, Hu M, et al. Wild-type p53 suppresses angiogenesis in human leiomyosarcoma and synovial sarcoma by transcriptional suppression of vascular endothelial growth factor expression. Cancer Res 2000;60:3655–61.
36. Sherif ZA, Nakai S, Pirollo KF, Rait A, Chang EH. Down-modulation of bFGF-binding protein expression following restoration of p53 function. Cancer Gene Ther 2001;8:771–82.
37. Ravi R, Mookerjee B, Bhujwalla ZM, et al. Regulation of tumor angiogenesis by p53-induced degradation of hypoxia-inducible factor 1alpha. Genes Dev 2000;14:34–44.
38. Teodoro JG, Parker AE, Zhu X, Green MR. p53-mediated inhibition of angiogenesis through up-regulation of a collagen prolyl hydroxylase. Science 2006;313:968–71.
39. Folkman J. Tumor suppression by p53 is mediated in part by the antiangiogenic activity of endostatin and tumstatin. Sci STKE 2006;2006:pe35.
40. Bono AV, Celato N, Cova V, Salvadore M, Chinetti S, Novario R. Microvessel density in prostate carcinoma. Prostate Cancer Prostatic Dis 2002;5:123–7.
41. Borre M, Offersen BV, Nerstrom B, Overgaard J. Microvessel density predicts survival in prostate cancer patients subjected to watchful waiting. Br J Cancer 1998;78:940–4.
42. Weidner N, Carroll PR, Flax J, Blumenfeld W, Folkman J. Tumor angiogenesis correlates with metastasis in invasive prostate carcinoma. Am J Pathol 1993;143:401–9.
43. Borre M, Nerstrom B, Overgaard J. Association between immunohistochemical expression of vascular endothelial growth factor (VEGF), VEGF-expressing neuroendocrine-differentiated tumor cells, and outcome in prostate cancer patients subjected to watchful waiting. Clin Cancer Res 2000;6:1882–90.
44. Kuniyasu H, Troncoso P, Johnston D, et al. Relative expression of type IV collagenase, E-cadherin, and vascular endothelial growth factor/vascular permeability factor in prostatectomy specimens distinguishes organ-confined from pathologically advanced prostate cancers. Clin Cancer Res 2000;6:2295–308.
45. Duque JL, Loughlin KR, Adam RM, Kantoff PW, Zurakowski D, Freeman MR. Plasma levels of vascular endothelial growth factor are increased in patients with metastatic prostate cancer. Urology 1999;54:523–7.
46. Meyer GE, Yu E, Siegal JA, Petteway JC, Blumenstein BA, Brawer MK. Serum basic fibroblast growth factor in men with and without prostate carcinoma. Cancer 1995;76:2304–11.
47. Trojan L, Thomas D, Knoll T, Grobholz R, Alken P, Michel MS. Expression of pro-angiogenic growth factors VEGF, EGF and bFGF and their topographical relation to neovascularisation in prostate cancer. Urol Res 2004;32:97–103.
48. West AF, O'Donnell M, Charlton RG, Neal DE, Leung HY. Correlation of vascular endothelial growth factor expression with fibroblast growth factor-8 expression and clinico-pathologic parameters in human prostate cancer. Br J Cancer 2001;85:576–83.
49. Lehrer S, Diamond EJ, Mamkine B, Stone NN, Stock RG. Serum interleukin-8 is elevated in men with prostate cancer and bone metastases. Technol Cancer Res Treat 2004;3:411.
50. Murphy C, McGurk M, Pettigrew J, et al. Nonapical and cytoplasmic expression of interleukin-8, CXCR1, and CXCR2 correlates with cell proliferation and microvessel density in prostate cancer. Clin Cancer Res 2005;11:4117–27.
51. Wikstrom P, Lissbrant IF, Stattin P, Egevad L, Bergh A. Endoglin (CD105) is expressed on immature blood vessels

and is a marker for survival in prostate cancer. Prostate 2002;51:268–75.

52. Mehta R, Kyshtoobayeva A, Kurosaki T, et al. Independent association of angiogenesis index with outcome in prostate cancer. Clin Cancer Res 2001;7:81–8.

53. Strohmeyer D, Rossing C, Bauerfeind A, et al. Vascular endothelial growth factor and its correlation with angiogenesis and p53 expression in prostate cancer. Prostate 2000;45:216–24.

54. Lissbrant IF, Stattin P, Wikstrom P, Damber JE, Egevad L, Bergh A. Tumor associated macrophages in human prostate cancer: relation to clinicopathological variables and survival. Int J Oncol 2000;17:445–51.

55. Sivridis E, Giatromanolaki A, Papadopoulos I, Gatter KC, Harris AL, Koukourakis MI. Thymidine phosphorylase expression in normal, hyperplastic and neoplastic prostates: correlation with tumour associated macrophages, infiltrating lymphocytes, and angiogenesis. Br J Cancer 2002;86: 1465–71.

56. Abdulkadir SA, Carvalhal GF, Kaleem Z, et al. Tissue factor expression and angiogenesis in human prostate carcinoma. Hum Pathol 2000;31:443–7.

57. Du Z, Fujiyama C, Chen Y, Masaki Z. Expression of hypoxia-inducible factor 1alpha in human normal, benign, and malignant prostate tissue. Chin Med J (Engl) 2003; 116:1936–9.

58. Zhong H, Semenza GL, Simons JW, De Marzo AM. Up-regulation of hypoxia-inducible factor 1alpha is an early event in prostate carcinogenesis. Cancer Detect Prev 2004;28:88–93.

59. Mazzucchelli R, Montironi R, Santinelli A, Lucarini G, Pugnaloni A, Biagini G. Vascular endothelial growth factor expression and capillary architecture in high-grade PIN and prostate cancer in untreated and androgen-ablated patients. Prostate 2000;45:72–9.

60. Quinn DI, Henshall SM, Sutherland RL. Molecular markers of prostate cancer outcome. Eur J Cancer 2005;41:858–7.

61. Mabjeesh NJ, Willard MT, Frederickson CE, Zhong H, Simons JW. Androgens stimulate hypoxia-inducible factor 1 activation via autocrine loop of tyrosine kinase receptor/ phosphatidylinositol 3′-kinase/protein kinase B in prostate cancer cells. Clin Cancer Res 2003;9:2416–25.

62. Horii K, Suzuki Y, Kondo Y, et al. Androgen-dependent gene expression of prostate-specific antigen is enhanced synergistically by hypoxia in human prostate cancer cells. Mol Cancer Res 2007;5:383–91.

63. Fu XS, Choi E, Bubley GJ, Balk SP. Identification of hypoxia-inducible factor-1alpha (HIF-1alpha) polymorphism as a mutation in prostate cancer that prevents normoxia-induced degradation. Prostate 2005;63:215–21.

64. Chau CH, Permenter MG, Steinberg SM, et al. Polymorphism in the hypoxia-inducible factor 1alpha gene may confer susceptibility to androgen-independent prostate cancer. Cancer Biol Ther 2005;4:1222–5.

65. Orr-Urtreger A, Bar-Shira A, Matzkin H, Mabjeesh NJ. The homozygous P582S mutation in the oxygen-dependent degradation domain of HIF-1 alpha is associated with increased risk for prostate cancer. Prostate 2007;67:8–13.

66. Kerbel RS. Inhibition of tumor angiogenesis as a strategy to circumvent acquired resistance to anti-cancer therapeutic agents. Bioessays 1991;13:31–6.

67. Folkman J. Angiogenesis: an organizing principle for drug discovery? Nat Rev Drug Discov 2007;6:273–86.

68. Nikolopoulos SN, Blaikie P, Yoshioka T, Guo W, Giancotti FG. Integrin beta4 signaling promotes tumor angiogenesis. Cancer Cell 2004;6:471–83.

69. Kerbel RS. Antiangiogenic therapy: a universal chemosensitization strategy for cancer? Science 2006;312:1171–5.

70. Jain RK. Normalization of tumor vasculature: an emerging concept in antiangiogenic therapy. Science 2005;307: 58–62.

71. Browder T, Butterfield CE, Kraling BM, et al. Antiangiogenic scheduling of chemotherapy improves efficacy against experimental drug-resistant cancer. Cancer Res 2000;60: 1878–86.

72. Klement G, Baruchel S, Rak J, et al. Continuous low-dose therapy with vinblastine and VEGF receptor-2 antibody induces sustained tumor regression without overt toxicity. J Clin Invest 2000;105:R15–24.

73. Bertolini F, Paul S, Mancuso P, et al. Maximum tolerable dose and low-dose metronomic chemotherapy have opposite effects on the mobilization and viability of circulating endothelial progenitor cells. Cancer Res 2003;63:4342–6.

74. Mancuso P, Colleoni M, Calleri A, et al. Circulating endothelial-cell kinetics and viability predict survival in breast cancer patients receiving metronomic chemotherapy. Blood 2006;108:452–9.

75. Kerbel RS, Kamen BA. The anti-angiogenic basis of metronomic chemotherapy. Nat Rev Cancer 2004;4:423–36.

76. Hudis CA. Clinical implications of antiangiogenic therapies. Oncology (Williston Park) 2005;19:26–31.

77. Davis DW, McConkey DJ, Abbruzzese JL, Herbst RS. Surrogate markers in antiangiogenesis clinical trials. Br J Cancer 2003;89:8–14.

78. Yu JL, Rak JW, Coomber BL, Hicklin DJ, Kerbel RS. Effect of p53 status on tumor response to antiangiogenic therapy. Science 2002;295:1526–8.

79. Glade Bender J, Cooney EM, Kandel JJ, Yamashiro DJ. Vascular remodeling and clinical resistance to antiangiogenic cancer therapy. Drug Resist Updat 2004;7: 289–300.

80. Sweeney CJ, Miller KD, Sledge GW, Jr. Resistance in the anti-angiogenic era: nay-saying or a word of caution? Trends Mol Med 2003;9:24–9.

81. Kerbel RS, Yu J, Tran J, et al. Possible mechanisms of acquired resistance to anti-angiogenic drugs: implications for the use of combination therapy approaches. Cancer Metastasis Rev 2001;20:79–86.

82. Streubel B, Chott A, Huber D, et al. Lymphoma-specific genetic aberrations in microvascular endothelial cells in B-cell lymphomas. N Engl J Med 2004;351:250–9.

83. Hida K, Hida Y, Amin DN, et al. Tumor-associated endothelial cells with cytogenetic abnormalities. Cancer Res 2004; 64:8249–55.

84. Walsh K, Sherwood RA, Dew TK, Mulvin D. Angiogenic peptides in prostatic disease. BJU Int 1999;84:1081–3.

Chapter 18
Bevacizumab in Advanced Prostate Cancer

Aymen A. Elfiky and William Kevin Kelly

Abstract Prostate cancer is the leading non-cutaneous malignancy in American men. Only the combination of docetaxel and prednisone has been shown to improve survival in patients with metastatic castration-resistant prostate cancer. Typically responses to docetaxel in patients with castrate-resistant disease are modest and additional therapies are needed. Angiogenesis has been shown to be a prerequisite event for tumor growth and metastasis in prostate cancer. Several strategies have been used to target angiogenesis in prostate cancer, which include blocking of pro-angiogenic factors via monoclonal antibodies or small-molecule inhibitors that target downstream signaling pathways for angiogenesis, direct inhibition of endothelial cells, or targeting other receptors involved in cell adhesion, proliferation, and survival. The following sections will discuss further the rationale for targeting the angiogenesis pathway in prostate cancer and the emergence of bevacizumab as a promising agent for the treatment of prostate cancer.

Keywords Angiogenesis • Prostate cancer • Drugs • Bevacizumab

Mechanism of Angiogenesis

For survival, tumor cells must obtain a steady supply of oxygen and nutrients needed to support metabolic activity. A tumor that relies on existing vasculature can reach a size of only about 2 mm. In tumor cells, increased production of pro-angiogenic factors occurs as the result of a phenomenon known as the "angiogenic switch." Pathological angiogenesis results from disruption of the regulatory processes that normally maintain the stability of the vascular system. Although usually confined to a localized area, the growth of new blood vessels during pathological angiogenesis is excessive and it often involves the intrusion of these vessels into an area where their presence is harmful. Growth factors generated as a result of the "angiogenic switch" enable a tumor to increase its supply of nutrients via tumor angiogenesis. Tumor angiogenesis begins when vascular endothelial growth factor (VEGF) and other growth factors diffuse away from the tumor and come into contact with established blood vessels of surrounding tissues. These factors activate endothelial cells that line the walls of existing vessels, trigger the angiogenic cascade, and lead to the sprouting of new capillaries [1].

VEGF plays a central role in the regulation of angiogenesis. Many environmental factors stimulate VEGF expression, including hypoxia, low pH, hormones (e.g., progesterone, estrogen), growth factors (e.g., epidermal growth factor [EGF], TGF-β[beta], bFGF, PDGF, insulin-like growth factor [IGF]-1), and cytokines (e.g., IL-1α[alpha], IL-6). Tumorigenic mutations involving p53, p73, src, ras, vHL, and Bcr-Abl can also stimulate VEGF expression. VEGF binds and activates its receptor (VEGFR), resulting in stimulation of downstream signaling cascades such as phospholipase C, protein kinase C, the cytoplasmic tyrosine kinase src, $\alpha v\beta 5$ integrins, phosphatidylinositol-3-kinase, ras, and MAP kinase. These downstream signaling pathways in endothelial cells lead to inhibition of apoptosis, stimulation of mitosis, and cytoskeletal changes associated with motility [1].

W.K. Kelly (✉)
Solid Tumor Oncology, Department of Medical Oncology, Associate Director of Translation Research, Jefferson Kimmel Cancer Center, Thomas Jefferson University, Suite 314, Philadelphia, PA 19107, USA
e-mails: wm.kevin.kelly@jefferson.edu; wm.kevin.kelly@yale.edu

W.D. Figg et al. (eds.), *Drug Management of Prostate Cancer*,
DOI 10.1007/978-1-60327-829-4_18, © Springer Science+Business Media, LLC 2010

VEGF (also known as VEGF-A) is part of a family of related proteins with similar structural motifs, including placenta growth factor (PlGF), VEGF-B, VEGF-C, VEGF-D, and VEGF-E (viral VEGF homolog), identified in the parapoxvirus Orf virus (Fig. 18.1). The family of VEGF proteins binds to several different VEGFRs with distinct binding and signaling properties. VEGFR1 (Flt-1), VEGFR2 (Flk-1, KDR), and VEGFR3 (Flt-4) have similar structural features and form homodimers upon ligand binding. Alternative splicing leads to the production of a soluble form of VEGFR-1, which does not bind to the membrane and functions as a negative regulator of VEGF signaling. The neuropilins, a distinct family of receptors, also interact with members of the VEGF family. Neuropilin-1 may function as co-receptor, enhancing VEGF interactions with VEGFR2. VEGFR1 interacts with PlGF, VEGF-B, and VEGF-A. The function of VEGFR1 remains to be elucidated. VEGFR1 signaling is only weakly activated by VEGF. VEGFR1 may function as a decoy receptor, much like soluble VEGFR1. VEGFR2 interacts with VEGF-C and D in

addition to VEGF. This receptor is the major mediator of the mitogenic and angiogenic effects of VEGF. VEGFR-3 only interacts with VEGF-C and D and is involved in lymphangiogenesis [1].

Because tumors require new blood vessel development in order to grow and metastasize, tumor vasculature provides a useful target for anticancer therapy. In preclinical models, therapies that inhibit the activity of the VEGF pathway have been shown to slow tumor progression. Therapies that inhibit the VEGF pathway in combination with chemotherapy or radiation therapy has been shown to be synergistic in preclinical models. VEGF is over-expressed in many types of human tumors, and its over-expression is frequently associated with malignant progression. Inhibiting VEGF represents a promising anticancer approach, as it targets the key regulator of angiogenesis. A mouse monoclonal antibody that neutralizes the activity of human VEGF (A.4.6.1) is the precursor antibody to Bevacizumab [Avastin™ (BV)]. BV is a recombinant humanized monoclonal antibody that binds to VEGF with high specificity and affinity, resulting in potent

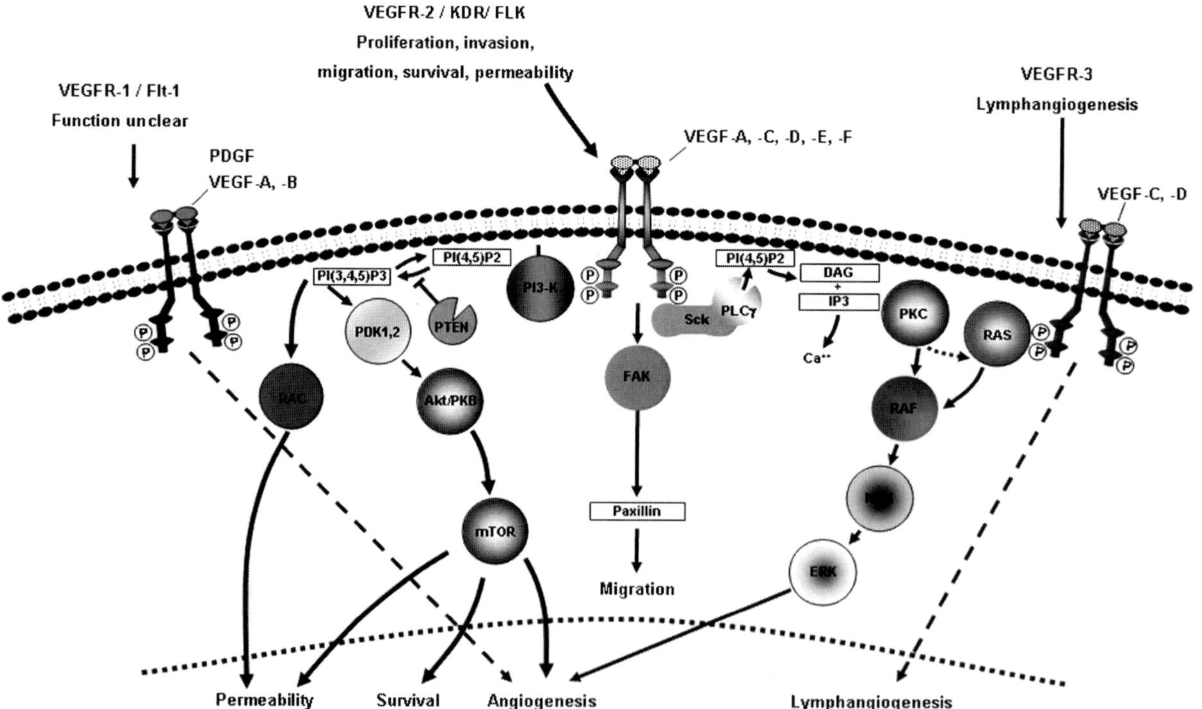

Fig. 18.1 VEGF family pathways

VEGF-neutralizing activity. Once bound, BV prevents VEGF interactions with VEGFR-1 (Flt-1) and VEGFR-2 (KDR) on the surface of endothelial cells, inhibiting VEGF-stimulated downstream signaling events. The estimated half-life of Bevacizumab is about 20 days (with a range of 11–50 days) [2].

Rationale for Targeting the Angiogenesis Pathway in Prostate Cancer

Inhibition of angiogenesis prevents the growth of tumor cells at the primary site and can prevent the emergence of metastasis [3]. Efforts to inhibit angiogenesis as a means of controlling the growth and spread of cancer cells began more than 30 years ago when it was demonstrated that progressive tumor growth is contingent upon formation of new vessels that support proliferation [4–6]. With the implication of tumor angiogenesis in the pathological progression of a number of tumor models, numerous angiogenic growth factors, many of which may be targeted with modern drugs, have been identified. These include VEGF, platelet-derived endothelial cell growth factor (PD-ECGF), basic fibroblast growth factor (bFGF), platelet-derived growth factor (PDGF), IGFs, angiogenin, thrombospondin, angiopoeitins, and integrins [7]. Additionally, early studies importantly demonstrated that higher microvessel density counts, a measure of angiogenesis, was associated with metastasis in solid tumors such as breast, lung, and bladder cancer [8–11], and was considered a negative prognostic indicator for several solid tumors, including prostate cancer [12]. Weidner et al. reported on 74 radical prostatectomy specimens that were stained for endothelial cells using factor VIII-related antigen and in which microvessel density was counted per 200 fields [12]. After a median follow-up of between 30 and 50 months, 29 of the 74 patients were found to have metastases. The mean number of microvessels counted for the patients with metastatic disease was 76.8 microvessels per 200 field (median, 66; SD, 44.6), a much higher count compared with the 39.2 microvessels per 200 field (median, 36; SD, 18.6) ($P < 0.0001$) found in the 45 patients who did not develop metastasis during the length of the follow-up period. This suggests that microvessel density appears to be a predictor of tumor metastasis in prostate cancer. Furthermore, this increase

in microvessel density was limited to invasive cancer areas and was notably different from surrounding benign areas of prostate tissue within the same patient [13]. Such observations have supported an increased focus on angiogenesis as a therapeutic target in prostate cancer.

VEGF Targeted Inhibition

The use of angiogenesis inhibitors is rapidly emerging as a promising treatment strategy in a variety of solid tumors, currently including prostate cancer [14]. Importantly, the inevitable emergence of drug resistance that is seen with the use of cytotoxic chemotherapy alone may be overcome by targeting endothelial cells that possess little or no inherent mutation [15]. In addition, there is evidence suggesting enhanced efficacy of cytotoxic chemotherapy when it is combined with specific angiogenesis inhibitors as a result of vessel normalization and improvement in intratumoral or interstitial fluid pressure, allowing for better delivery of chemotherapy to areas of tumor [16, 17].

Specific strategies, which have been used to target angiogenesis in prostate cancer, include blocking of pro-angiogenic factors such as VEGF via monoclonal antibodies such as bevacizumab or other small molecule inhibitors targeting downstream signaling pathways for angiogenesis, direct inhibition of endothelial cells, or targeting other receptors involved in cell adhesion, proliferation, and survival [18].

The Clinical Role of Bevacizumab in Prostate Cancer

Preclinical Data

VEGF plays a role in the pathogenesis and progression of human prostate cancer [19, 20]. Flk-1/KDR receptors are expressed in human prostate cancer, and their presence correlates with higher grade lesions [21]. VEGF is present in both localized and metastatic prostate tumors as well as the plasma of patients with metastatic disease, and increasing expression correlates with disease progression [22–24]. In patients with castrate-resistant disease, both plasma and urine VEGF levels are independent predictors of survival [25, 26]. In vivo and in situ molecular analysis demonstrated that castration leads to tumor regression and concomitant decrease in VEGF expression [27, 28]. Subsequently, replacement of androgens to long term castrated rats stimulated eightfold increase rise in VEGF content. In studies with the Shionogi murine tumor (an androgen-dependent mammary tumor), castration leads to tumor regression with a marked decrease in VEGF within 1 week. Once these tumors relapse in the absence of androgens, the dominant angiogenic factor is VEGF.

Antibodies to VEGF have caused tumor regression in preclinical prostate tumor models [29–31]. In human prostate cancer xenograft, an oral inhibitor of VEGF (ZD6474) produced greater inhibition of tumor growth than orchiectomy but increased tumor necrosis was observed when ZD6474 was combined with orchiectomy. In studies that evaluated, androgen-independent AT-1 prostate cancer cells that were grown inside the ventral prostate of adult non-castrated rats, ZD6474 decreased tumor vascular density, increased tumor hypoxia and apoptosis, and decreased tumor growth [32]. Similar effects were seen with castration that suggested castration and inhibition of VEGF may work through similar mechanisms. In these studies, the combination of ZD6474 and castration had synergistic effects on the tumor growth.

These studies suggests that VEGF pathway specifically plays a critical role in development and progression of prostate cancer, and that inhibitors of the VEGF signaling in combination with other standard treatments may improve the outcomes of patients with prostate cancer.

Success of Bevacizumab in Cancer

Bevacizumab has been approved by the FDA for first- and second-line therapy of metastatic colorectal cancer (CRC), first-line therapy of non-small cell lung cancer (NSCLC), and more recently metastatic HER2-negative breast cancer. In patients with CRC, bevacizumab was shown to extend patients' lives by about 5 months when given intravenously as a combination treatment along with the standard regimen of ironotecan, 5-fluorouracil (5FU), and leucovorin [33]. In the second-line setting, an absolute 17% improvement in

overall survival (OS) and a 26% relative reduction in risk of death has been shown in patients receiving the combination of bevacizumab plus FOLFOX-4 compared with those receiving FOLFOX-4 alone [34]. This study is noteworthy as it was the first Phase III study to demonstrate the ability of bevacizumab to enhance the efficacy of an oxaliplatin-based regimen.

The recommendation for the initial systemic treatment of patients with unresectable, locally advanced, recurrent, or metastatic, nonsquamous, NSCLC is based on the demonstration of a statistically significant improvement in OS in patients receiving bevacizumab with carboplatin and paclitaxel compared with those receiving carboplatin and paclitaxel alone [35].

The recent approval in breast cancer was based on the demonstration of an improvement in progression-free survival (PFS) in patients receiving bevacizumab with paclitaxel compared with those receiving paclitaxel alone as a first-line treatment for metastatic breast cancer [36].

Most of the data elucidating the toxicities associated with bevacizumab have come from trials in CRC. Specific adverse effects, which have been attributed to bevacizumab, include hemorrhage (2–9.3%), thromboembolism (0–19%), proteinuria (1–28%), hypertension (7–25%), and perforation (0–3.3%).

Clinical Trials in Castration-Resistant Prostate Cancer

Bevacizumab is a humanized monoclonal antibody that was developed from a murine antihuman VEGF monoclonal antibody that functions as an inhibitor of all major isoforms of VEGF-A [37]. A series of phase II and III clinical trials are being conducted to evaluate response to single-agent therapy as well as response to therapy in combination with other agents, which have demonstrated effect on prostate cancer and offered the potential of a synergistic effect when administered with bevacizumab (Table 18.1). Bevacizumab as a single agent in castration-resistant prostate cancer has shown modest clinical activity. In a phase II study, 15 patients with castration-resistant disease were treated with 10 mg/kg rhuMAb VEGF every 14 days for six infusions followed by additional treatment for selected patients exhibiting a response or stable disease. After 12 weeks of therapy, none of the 15 patients evaluable

Table 18.1 Selected clinical trials of bevacizumab in prostate cancer

Clinical trials	Study designation	Disease designation	Agents
CALGB 9006	Phase II	HRPC	Bevacizumab, docetaxel, and estramustine
NCI-04-C-0257	Phase II	HRPC	Bevacizumab, thalidomide, and docetaxel
CALGB 90401	Phase III	HRPC	Docetaxel and prednisone with or without bevacizumab
WSU-2006-064	Phase II	HRPC	Bevacizumab
NCT00321646	Phase II	High-risk, localized PC	Neoadjuvant Bevacizumab plus Docetaxel before surgery
BRIVMRC-3031500	Phase II	High-risk, locally advanced PC	Bevacizumab plus ADT and RT
NCT00574769	Phase I/II	HRPC	Bevacizumab plus Docetaxel and RAD001 (mTOR inhibitor)
TORI GU-01	Phase II	High-risk, localized PC	Adjuvant Bevacizumab plus erlotinib following surgery
NCT00658697	Phase II	Rising PSA after local therapy	Bevacizumab, Docetaxel, and ADT followed by continued Bevacizumab and ADT

for tumor response had an objective complete or partial response. Three possible mixed responses were observed. No patient achieved a >50% decrease in serum PSA, although four patients (27%) had a PSA decline of <50%. The median time to objective progression was 3.9 months, and the median time to PSA progression was 2 months. Toxicity was generally mild with asthenia present in 6/15 (40%). Two patients developed severe hyponatremia, although the association with rhuMAb VEGF was unclear. The conclusion was that single-agent rhuMAb VEGF in this dose and schedule did not produce significant objective responses in this population. It was recommended that further development of this agent in prostate cancer should include its evaluation in combination with other therapies [38].

Because of the encouraging safety profile in prostate cancer and data from other malignancies showing enhanced clinical activity and benefit when combined with a cytotoxic agent, several combinational studies have been done. The investigators from the Cancer and Leukemia Group B (CALGB) performed a phase II trial investigating the role of bevacizumab with estramustine and docetaxel in patients with progressive castrate metastatic prostate cancer (CALGB 90006) [39]. Seventy-nine patients were treated with this combination (EMP-280 mg po TID days 1–5; Docetaxel 70 mg/m² – day 2; Bevacizumab 15 mg/kg over 30 min-day 2). Typical premedication for Docetaxel was given, and daily 2 mg of coumadin was administered to help prevent any thromboembolic disease related to the estramustine. Patients tolerated the therapy well. There was one death due to mesenteric vein thrombosis, one unrelated death due to a perforated sigmoid colon diverticulum, two patients with a CNS bleed, and two patients each with pulmonary embolism and deep venous thrombosis. Although these thromboembolic events were of concern, the overall incidence was not dramatically higher than what has been observed with estramustine and docetaxel without bevacizumab. An increase in neutropenia without neutropenic fever was observed. Additionally, an increased number of infections were also seen. The other toxicities were similar to what were published studies from Savarese and colleagues with estramustine, docetaxel, and hydrocortisone [40]. Perhaps, most importantly, the results observed with this combination compared favorably with other concurrent combinations tested by the CALGB. Compared with another CALGB triplet trial in which carboplatin was added to estramustine and docetaxel (CALGB 99813) [41], the use of bevacizumab resulted in a post-therapy PSA decline in 58 out of 72 (81%) patients compared with 68% of the patients treated with the carboplatin regimen, median time to objective disease progression of 9.7 months compared with 8.1, median time to PSA failure of 9.9 vs. 9 months, and OS of 21 months compared with 18 months. DiLorenzo et al. also evaluated the combination of docetaxel (60 mg/m²) and bevacizumab (10 mg/kg) every 3 weeks in patients with castrate-resistant disease, who had been treated with up to two prior chemotherapy regimens with one being docetaxel. Twenty heavily pretreated patients were enrolled, 11 (55%) of the patients had major PSA declines posttherapy and one third of the evaluable patients achieved a partial response [42]. Of interest, four patients who had no response to docetaxel previously had significant post-therapy PSA decline with the combination. This would suggest that bevacizumab may reverse docetaxel resistance in some patients either by improving drug delivery or by another mechanism that still needs to be elucidated.

Colleagues at the National Cancer Institute (NCI) conducted a trial using the combination of bevacizumab (15 mg/kg) with docetaxel (75 mg/m^2) every 3 weeks, prednisone 5 mg twice daily, and thalidomide 200 mg every night, with thromboprophylaxis. Sixty evaluable patients with unfavorable characteristics evidenced by a high Gleason score and a short PSA doubling time were enrolled. Ninety percent of patients receiving the combination therapy had PSA declines of $\geq$ 50%, and 88% achieved a PSA decline of $\geq$ 30% within the first 3 months of treatment. The median time to progression was 18.3 months, and the median overall survival was 28.2 months [43]. Significant toxicities reported were febrile neutropenia, syncope, GI perforation or fistula, thrombosis, and grade 3 bleeding.

These encouraging data have lead to a randomized phase III double-blinded study comparing Docetaxel and prednisone with bevacizumab or placebo (CALGB 90401) [44] (Fig. 18.2). Preliminary results of the study have been reported. In an intent to treat analysis there was no significant difference in the median survival between the two arms (22.6 for the Docetaxel, prednisone and bevacizumab vs. 21.6 months for Docetaxel and prednisone alone, p = 0.181; Hazard ratio (HR) = 0.91). The median progression free survival favored patients treated on the bevacizumab arm (9.9 months verses 7.5 months, p< 0.0001; HR = 0.77). Secondary endpoints of $\geq$ 50% post-therapy PSA declines (69.5% vs. 53.2%, p = .0002) and objective response proportions (57.9 % vs. 53.2%, p = .0113) significantly favored the bevacizumab treated patients. Overall summary for maximum hematologic and non-hematologic adverse events showed that there was an increase in morbidity and mortality associated with docetaxel, prednisone and bevacizumab in this elderly population. This study showed that the addition of bevacizumab to docetaxel and prednisone did increase progression free survival; objective and PSA response along with the toxicity, but not the overall survival. The lack of survival benefit may have been related to the heterogeneity of the study population as well as impact of secondary chemotherapies on the primary outcome of the study. Further randomized studies are needed to define the role of anti-angiogenic therapy in this metastatic castrate resistant prostate cancer. (Kelly, WK et al. Jouranl of Clinical Oncology Proceeding 2010 ASCO, LBA 4511, Chicago, Ill June 4-8, 2010).

Bevacizumab in Castrate-Sensitive Prostate Cancer

Preclinical data demonstrate a strong association between castration and VEGF expression as well as a synergy between androgen deprivation and blockage of the VEGF pathway. This would suggest that castration and VEGF inhibition may lead to increased prostate cell death and prolong the effects of castration. Moreover, it is foreseeable that bringing bevacizumab to the forefront in treating patients with castrate-sensitive disease could potentially improve androgen deprivation therapy (ADT) clinical activity.

However, as we introduce biologic agents such as bevacizumab to earlier disease populations that have longer OSs, investigators need to ensure that these agents are not increasing other morbidities such as cardiovascular disease. Men with prostate cancer have a higher rate of non-cancer mortality than men in the general population with some of this excess mortality related to treatment. Keating and collogues, in an observational study of 73,196 patients with prostate cancer from the SEER database, showed that the use of GnRH agonists was associated with increased risk of incident of diabetes, coronary heart disease, myocardial infarction, and sudden cardiac arrest [45]. An increased risk of diabetes and coronary heart disease was evident even with 1–4 months of initiating GnRH analog therapy. Thus, the addition of any agent to ADT must consider the impact on non-cancer morbidity and mortality. Ultimately, to bring such a combination of bevacizumab plus ADT therapy forward into an asymptomatic population will require establishing the safety of this combination along with understanding the biological and clinical effects of these therapies

CALGB 90401 SCHEMA

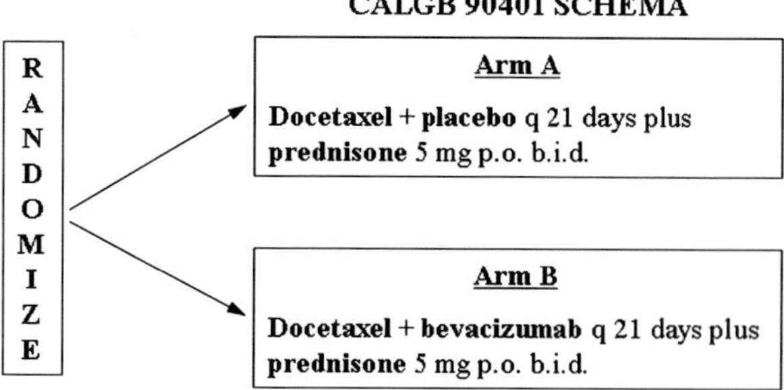

Fig. 18.2 CALGB 90401 clinical trial treatment schema

combined in androgen-dependent patients. Several trials are currently ongoing to further explore the safety and clinical activity of anti-angiogenesis agents in combination with ADT.

Future Directions

The search for better angiogenic inhibitors in terms of potency, tolerability, safety, and efficacy is a burgeoning field in all aspects of cancer research. It holds true promise with remarkable objective tumor response in synergism with conventional cytotoxic chemotherapy. Bevacizumab has a significant potential to augment the impact of other cytotoxic agents when given in combination. However, a significant limitation for bevacizumab as well as other agents working along related pathways is the concerns over debilitating toxicities in some patients. In this context, studies investigating the optimal dosing regimen and duration of treatment with bevacizumab combination therapies are needed to help circumvent a number of the toxicities. As in other malignancies, biomarkers and prognostic models that select patients for angiogenesis therapy are desperately needed. These data to date remain encouraging, and the ongoing trials will help determine the role of bevacizumab in patients with prostate cancer.

References

1. Ferrara N, Gerber HP, LeCouter J. The biology of VEGF and its receptors. Nat Med 2003;9:669–76.
2. Kim KJ, Li B, Winer J, et al. Inhibition of vascular endothelial growth factor-induced angiogenesis suppresses tumour growth in vivo. Nature 1993;362:841–4.
3. Fidler IJ, Ellis LM. The implications of angiogenesis for the biology and therapy of cancer metastasis. Cell 1994;79: 185–8.
4. Folkman J. Tumor angiogenesis: therapeutic implications. N Engl J Med 1971;285:1182–6.
5. Folkman J. Anti-angiogenesis: new concept for therapy of solid tumors. Ann Surg 1972;175:409–16.
6. Folkman J. Tumor angiogenesis: a possible control point in tumor growth. Ann Intern Med 1975;82:96–100.
7. Wray CJ, Rilo HL, Ahmad SA. Colon cancer angiogenesis and antiangiogenic therapy. Expert Opin Investig Drugs 2004;13:631–41.
8. Jaeger TM, Weidner N, Chew K, et al. Tumor angiogenesis correlates with lymph node metastases in invasive bladder cancer. J Urol 1995;154:69–71.
9. Macchiarini P, Fontanini G, Hardin MJ, Squartini F, Angeletti CA. Relation of neovascularisation to metastasis of non-small-cell lung cancer. Lancet 1992;340:145–6.
10. Weidner N, Folkman J, Pozza F, et al. Tumor angiogenesis: a new significant and independent prognostic indicator in early-stage breast carcinoma. J Natl Cancer Inst 1992;84:1875–87.
11. Weidner N, Semple JP, Welch WR, Folkman J. Tumor angiogenesis and metastasis – correlation in invasive breast carcinoma. N Engl J Med 1991;324:1–8.
12. Weidner N, Carroll PR, Flax J, et al. Tumor angiogenesis correlates with metastasis in invasive prostate carcinoma. Am J Pathol 1993;143:401–9.
13. Siegal JA, Yu E, Brawer MK. Topography of neovascularity in human prostate carcinoma. Cancer 1995;75:2545–51.
14. Folkman J, Browder T, Palmblad J. Angiogenesis research: guidelines for translation to clinical application. Thromb Haemost 2001;86:23–33.
15. Kerbel RS. Inhibition of tumor angiogenesis as a strategy to circumvent acquired resistance to anti-cancer therapeutic agents. Bioessays 1991; 13:31–6.
16. Gerber HP, Ferrara N. Pharmacology and pharmacodynamics of bevacizumab as monotherapy or in combination with cytotoxic therapy in preclinical studies. Cancer Res 2005; 65:671–80.
17. Jain RK. Normalization of tumor vasculature: an emerging concept in antiangiogenic therapy. Science 2005;307:58–62.
18. Epstein RJ. VEGF signaling inhibitors: more pro-apoptotic than antiangiogenic. Cancer Metastasis Rev 2007;26: 443–52.
19. Ferrara N. Role of vascular endothelial growth factor in regulation of angiogenesis. Kidney Int 1999;56:794–814.
20. Ferrara N and Davis-Smyth T. The biology of vascular endothelial growth factor. Endrocrinology 1997;18:1–22.
21. Ferrer FA, Miller LJ, et al. Expression of vascular endothelial receptors inhuman prostate cancer. Urology 1999;43:567–72.
22. Ferrer FA, Miller LJ, et al. Vascular endothelial growth factor (VEGF) expression in human prostate cancer: in situ and in vitro expression of FEGG by human prostate cancer cells. J Urol 1997;157:2329–33.
23. Duque J, Loughlin K, et al. Plasma levels of vascular endothelial growth factor are increased in patients with metastatic prostate cancer. Urology 1999;45:523–27.
24. Duque JL, Loughlin KR, et al. Measurement of plasma levels of vascular endothelial growth factor in prostate cancer patients: relationship with clinical stage, Gleason score, prostate volume, and serum prostate-specific antigen. Clinics 2006;61(5):401–8.
25. Bok R, Halabi S, et al. VEGF and bFGF urine levels as predictors of outcome in hormone refractory prostate cancer patients: a CALGB study. Cancer Res 2001;61:2533–6.
26. George D, Halabi S, et al. Prognostic significance of plasma vascular endothelial growth factor (VEGF) levels in patients with hormone refractory prostate cancer: a CALGB study. Clin Cancer Res 2001;7:1932–6.
27. Joseph IBJK, Nelson JB, et al. Androgens regulate vascular endothelial growth factor content in normal and malignant prostate tissues. Clin Cancer Res 1997;3:2507–11.
28. Jain A, Safabakhsh N, et al. Endothelial cell death, angiogenesis, and microvascular function after castration in an androgen-dependent tumor: role of vascular endothelial growth factor. Proc Natl Acad Sci U S A 1998;95:10820–25.

29. Kirschenbaum A, Wang J, et al. Inhibition of vascular endothelial cell growth factor suppresses the in vitro growth of human prostate cancer tumors. Urol Oncol 1997;3:3–10.

30. Borgstrom P, Bourdon M, et al. Neutralizing anti-vascular endothelial growth factor antibody completely inhibits angiogenesis and growth of human prostate carcinoma micro-tumors in vivo. Prostate 1998;35:1–10.

31. Melynk O, Simmerman M, et al. Neutralizing anti-vascular endothelial growth factor antibody inhibits further growth of established prostate cancer and metastases in pre-clinical model. J Urol 1999;161:960–63.

32. Hammarsten P, Halin S, et al. Inhibitory effects of castration in an orthotopic model of androgen-independent prostate cancer can be mimicked and enhanced by angiogenesis inhibition. Clin Cancer Res 2006;12(24):7431–6.

33. Hurwitz H, Fehrenbacher L, Novotny W, Cartwright T, Hainsworth J, et al. Bevacizumab plus irinotecan, fluorouracil, and leucovorin for metastatic colorectal cancer. N Engl J Med 2004;350:2335–42.

34. Giantonio BJ, Catalano PJ, Meropol NJ, O'Dwyer PJ, Mitchell EP, Alberts SR, Schwartz MA, Benson AB. High-dose bevacizumab improves survival when combined with FOLFOX4 in previously treated advanced colorectal cancer: results from the Eastern Cooperative Oncology Group (ECOG) study E3200. ASCO 2005 (abstract 2).

35. Sandler A, Gray R, Perry MC, et al. Paclitaxel-carboplatin alone or with bevacizumab for non-small-cell lung cancer. N Engl J Med 2006;355(24):2542–50.

36. Miller K, Wang M, Gralow J, et al. A randomized phase III trial of paclitaxel versus paclitaxel plus bevacizumab as first-line therapy for locally recurrent or metastatic breast cancer: a trial coordinated by the Eastern Cooperative Oncology Group (E2100). Breast Cancer Res Treat 2005;94 (suppl 1):S6 (abstract 3).

37. Presta LG, Chen H, O'Connor SJ, et al. Humanization of an antivascular endothelial growth factor monoclonal antibody for the therapy of solid tumors and other disorders. Cancer Res 1997;57:4593–99.

38. Reese DM, Fratesi P, Corry M, et al. A phase II trial of humanized anti-vascular endothelial growth factor antibody for the treatment of androgen-independent prostate cancer. Prostate 2001;3:65–70.

39. Picus J, Halabi S, Rini B, et al. The use of bevacizumab with docetaxel and estramustine in hormone refractory prostate cancer: initial results of CALGB 90006. Proc Am Soc Clin Oncol 2003;22:1578.

40. Savarese DM, Halabi S, Hars V, et al. Phase II study of docetaxel, estramustine, and low-dose hydrocortisone in men with hormone-refractory prostate cancer: a final report of CALGB 9780. J Clin Oncol 2001;19(9):2509–16.

41. Oh WK, Halabi S, Kelly WK, et al. A phase II study of estramustine, docetaxel, and carboplatin with granulocyte-colony-stimulating factor support in patients with hormone-refractory prostate carcinoma: cancer and Leukemia Group B 99813. Cancer 2003;98(12):2592–8.

42. Di Lorenzo G, Figg WD, Fossa SD, et al. Combination of bevacizumab and docetaxel in docetaxel-pretreated hormone-refractory prostate cancer: a phase 2 study. Eur Urol 2008;54(5):1089–94.

43. Ning YM, Gulley JL, Arlen PM, et al. A phase II trial of bevacizumab, thalidomide, docetaxel, and prednisone in patients with metastatic castration-resistant prostate cancer. J Clin Oncol 2010;28:2070–6.

44. Kelly WK, Halabi S, Carducci MA, et al. A randomized, double-blind, placebo-controlled phase III trial comparing docetaxel, prednisone, and placebo with docetaxel, prednisone, and bevacizumab in men with metastatic castration-resistant prostate cancer (mCRPC): Survival results of CALGB 90401. ASCO Annual Meeting Proceedings J Clin Oncol 2010;28:LBA4511.

45. Keating NL, O'Malley AJ, et al. Diabetes and cardiovascular disease during androgen deprivation therapy for prostate cancer. J Clin Oncol 2006;24(27):4448–56.

Chapter 19
Thalidomide and Analogs

Erin R. Gardner, Giuseppe Di Lorenzo, and William D. Figg

Abstract Thalidomide (Thalomid®), originally marketed as a sedative in Europe in the 1950s but withdrawn after teratogenicity was observed, has experienced a resurgence of interest due to its apparent anti-angiogenic and immunomodulatory properties. Thalidomide is currently in clinical testing for the treatment of prostate cancer. Numerous studies that have been completed, or are currently ongoing, have demonstrated promising activity. Thalidomide has been tested as a single agent and in combination with both targeted agents, such as bevacizumab, and traditional cytotoxic drugs, such as paclitaxel and docetaxel, in the majority of the studies. A range of thalidomide analogs have been generated in an effort to improve the clinical activity while reducing the side effect profile. Lenalidomide (Revlimid™), an immunomodulatory analog of thalidomide, has entered clinical trials in prostate cancer and is being tested in many of the same combinations. This chapter reviews the clinical trials of thalidomide and lenalidomide initiated or completed to date, including dosing, clinical response, and toxicity.

Keywords Thalidomide•Lenalidomide•Angiogenesis • Prostate cancer • Immunomodulatory

Introduction

Thalidomide was originally developed by the German company Chemie Gruenthal in the 1950s as an oral sedative and was widely prescribed outside of the US for off-label usage as an antiemetic. It was withdrawn from the market in 1961 after thalidomide was found to be teratogenic, causing phocomelia in over 10,000 babies, whose mothers had taken the drug during their first trimester of pregnancy [1].

Over 30 years later, a resurgence of interest in thalidomide occurred when D'Amato et al. reported that it was an inhibitor of angiogenesis [2]. They postulated that the observed limb defects were directly caused by inhibition of blood vessel growth in the developing fetal limb bud and demonstrated that thalidomide inhibits blood vessel growth in the chicken chorioallantoic membrane assay and inhibits bFGF-stimulated corneal neovascularization in treated rabbits. Interestingly, thalidomide is believed to exert its anti-angiogenic effects only when metabolized, as reported by several groups, though the exact mechanism of action has not been elucidated [2, 3]. In addition to its anti-angiogenic activity, thalidomide has also been shown to inhibit COX-2 and have immunomodulatory and anti-inflammatory activity [4].

The observed anti-angiogenic activity of thalidomide is of particular interest for the treatment of prostate cancer and other solid tumors. Numerous studies have shown that tumor angiogenesis correlates with both early hormone-dependent prostate growth and development of metastatic tumors [5–7].

In late 1997, thalidomide (marketed as Thalomid®, by Celgene Corp.) was granted the US Food and Drug Administration (FDA) approval for the treatment of erythema nodosum leprosum, a serious skin

W.D. Figg (✉)
Medical Oncology Branch, National Cancer Institute, NIH, Bethesda, MD, USA
e-mail: wdfigg@helix.nih.gov

W.D. Figg et al. (eds.), *Drug Management of Prostate Cancer*,
DOI 10.1007/978-1-60327-829-4_19, © Springer Science+Business Media, LLC 2010

complication of leprosy. In 2006, thalidomide was granted the accelerated FDA approval for the treatment of multiple myeloma, in combination with dexamethasone.

Because of the severe teratogenicity of thalidomide, all distribution is heavily restricted and monitored, under Celgene's S.T.E.P.S. program (System for Thalidomide Education and Prescribing Safety) [8]. This program was designed to minimize the chance of fetal exposure, and requires prescribers and pharmacists to register with the program. For male patients, the program involves extensive counseling about the risks and benefits, along with requirements for taking the drug. Additionally, male patients are instructed to use a latex condom during sexual intercourse, regardless of vasectomy, because of the presence of thalidomide in semen.

Thalidomide as a Single Agent

On the basis of the anti-angiogenic activity of thalidomide reported by D'Amato et al., and the numerous publications linking angiogenesis with prostate cancer progression, an open-label, randomized Phase II study of thalidomide was initiated at the National Cancer Institute [9]. This study enrolled a total of 63 men with castration-resistant prostate cancer (CRPC), 50 of which received 200 mg/day (the low-dose arm) and 13 of which received 1,200 mg/day (the high-dose arm). The high-dose arm was poorly tolerated, and many patients could not be escalated above 200 mg/day owing to the side effects, primarily sedation and fatigue. This arm was terminated early, as none of the 13 patients had a >50% decline in prostate-specific antigen (PSA). However, a total of 28% of patients had a >40% decline in PSA. Four patients maintained a >50% decline in PSA for more than 150 days. This is of note considering that thalidomide has been shown to upregulate the expression of PSA in prostate cancer cells [10]. However, by computed tomography (CT) or bone scan criteria, there were no partial responses (PR). Microvessel count and the expression of angiogenic markers (vascular endothelial growth factor, VEGF, and basic fibroblast growth factor, bFGF) were also evaluated in biopsy samples, although a correlation with response was not observed. Conversely, circulating bFGF did appear to decrease in patients who received the drug for more than 4 months. Figg et al. reported that constipation, dizziness, edema, fatigue, mood changes were the most prevalent toxicities observed [9]. Molloy et al. published detailed information about the development of thalidomide-induced neuropathy in this trial [11]. Of the eight patients remaining on study at 6 months, three patients had clinical and electrophysiologic evidence of sensory neuropathy. The three patients who remained on study after 9 months of treatment had all developed symptoms of peripheral neuropathy since the previous examination [11].

A second open-label Phase II study of thalidomide as a single agent was subsequently reported by Drake et al. [12]. Twenty men with CRPC received 100 mg/day thalidomide for up to 6 months. A >50% decline in PSA was observed in three (15%) of the treated men. A correlation between PSA and serum bFGF and VEGF was observed, with 5 of the 6 men whose PSA declined also exhibiting a decrease in circulating bFGF and VEGF. Similar to the initial study published by Figg et al., the most commonly observed adverse effects were constipation, fatigue ("sedation hangover"), and dizziness. Although these side effects were generally mild, all seven of the men who completed 6 months of thalidomide therapy exhibited subclinical peripheral neuropathy.

Both the Figg and Drake studies enrolled patients with CRPC, a population that has typically been heavily pretreated and has significant tumor burden. However, as angiogenesis inhibitors are anticipated to be cytostatic, halting tumor progression rather than resulting in regression, it has been hypothesized that treatment earlier in the course of the disease process would be more beneficial. Recently, a double-blind randomized crossover Phase III study of thalidomide vs. placebo control in patients with stage D0 androgen-dependent prostate cancer following limited hormonal ablation was completed [13]. The study enrolled 159 patients and after 6 months of intermittent GnRH agonist treatment (with leuprolide or goserelin), therapy with thalidomide (200 mg/day) or placebo was initiated. The median time to PSA progression for the thalidomide group was 17.1 months vs. 6.6 months on placebo ($p=0.0002$). Despite thalidomide having no effect on testosterone normalization, there was a clear effect on PSA progression. Neuropathy was evident with prolonged use of thalidomide.

Much interest is focused on the role of the tumor microenvironment and how interruption of the interaction between the tumor and its surrounding normal stroma may result in inhibition of tumor progression. Efstathiou et al. evaluated the effect of thalidomide on the tumor microenvironment by treating 18 men with 200–600 mg/day for 12 weeks immediately prior to radical prostatectomy [14]. All patients were started at a dosage of 200 mg/day and the dose was then escalated to 600 mg/day in the absence of grade 3 or 4 toxicity. Serum PSA levels declined in 17 of the 18 men enrolled, with a median reduction of 42% after 12 weeks of treatment. Similar to previous studies, the most frequent toxicities observed were low-grade somnolence, fatigue, neurotoxicity, and constipation. Following radical prostatectomy, thalidomide-treated prostate tissue was compared with untreated match-control prostate tissue using microarrays. VEGF and interleukin-6 (IL-6), both of which are involved in prostate cancer angiogenesis, were significantly lower in the thalidomide treated group, in both the tumor epithelium and the stroma. Significantly decreased expression of Smoothened (Smo), a key component of the sonic hedgehog signaling pathway was observed, as was a decrease in the matrix metalloproteinases (MMPs), MMP-2 and MMP-9 expression, in thalidomide-treated tissue when compared with control. These observations suggest that thalidomide is affecting the tumor microenvironment in a manner that may result in a decrease in the invasiveness of the tumor phenotype [14]. Table 19.1 provides a summary of single agent thalidomide trials in men with prostate cancer.

Thalidomide in Combination Therapy

In 2004, docetaxel (Taxotere®), a traditional cytotoxic agent, was approved in combination with prednisone for advanced CRPC, based on the improved overall survival when compared with mitoxantrone plus prednisone [15]. Docetaxel had previously been shown to have activity in CRPC both as a single agent and in combination with estramustine [16–18]. In 1999, a randomized Phase II clinical study compared thalidomide plus weekly docetaxel with weekly docetaxel alone as first-line treatment in men with CRPC [19]. Twenty-five men were randomized to receive 30 mg/m^2 docetaxel intravenously each week for 3 out of 4 weeks. Fifty men were randomized to the same regimen with the addition of 200 mg daily oral thalidomide. At a median follow-up time of 26.4 months, the proportion of patients with >50% decline in PSA was higher in the combination group (53% in the docetaxel/thalidomide group compared with 37% for docetaxel alone). In addition, overall survival at 18 months was greater in the combination treatment arm when compared with docetaxel alone (68.2% vs. 42.9%). Median progression-free survival (PFS) was also longer in the docetaxel/thalidomide cohort (5.9 months when compared with 3.7 months). However, none of these findings were statistically significant. The majority of observed toxicities were expected based on earlier studies of these two agents. However, of serious concern was the observation that 12 of the first 43 patients in the docetaxel/thalidomide cohort experienced thromboembolic events, either venous thrombosis, transient ischemic

Table 19.1 Summary of single agent thalidomide trials in prostate cancer

Investigator	Patients enrolled	Dose	Clinical results	Major toxicities
Figg et al. [9]	63 men with CRPC (50 low-dose and 13 high-dose)	200 mg/day (low-dose) or 1,200 mg/day (high-dose)	28% of patients >40% PSA decline	Sedation, fatigue, constipation, dizziness, edema, mood changes, neuropathy
Drake et al. [12]	20 men with CRPC	100 mg/day	15% of patients >50% PSA decline	Constipation, fatigue, dizziness, peripheral neuropathy
Figg et al. [13]	159 men with stage D0 androgen-dependent disease (randomized crossover)	200 mg/day	Median time to PSA progression 17.1 months vs. 6.6 with placebo	Standard toxicities, neuropathy
Efstathiou et al. [14]	18 men with prostate cancer, prior to radical prostatectomy	200–600 mg/day	PSA decline in 17/18 mean enrolled (median of 42% decline after 12 weeks of treatment)	Somnolence, fatigue, neurotoxicity, and constipation

CRPC castration-resistant prostate cancer; *PSA* prostate-specific antigen attack, or stroke. Conversely, none of the patients receiving docetaxel alone experienced thromboembolic events. The addition of low-molecular-weight heparin (LMWH) to the combination regimen prevented any further events from occurring [19].

Numerous subsequent studies continued to combine thalidomide with traditional cytotoxic chemotherapy. One study added estramustine to the combination of docetaxel and thalidomide described earlier, based on the synergistic activity of estramustine with docetaxel and promising preclinical activity of this triple combination [20]. A total of 20 patients with metastatic CRPC were enrolled into this phase II clinical trial. PFS was 7.2 months and 18 of the patients had a >50% decline in PSA. Two of the 10 patients with soft-tissue lesions had a partial response based on CT scan. The majority of patients (17/20) required a dose reduction of at least one of the three agents, and 65% of patients experienced grade 3 or 4 toxicities. On the basis of the incidence of thromboembolic events in the initial docetaxel-thalidomide trial, LMWH was administered to all patients. Despite this prophylactic treatment, two patients experienced thromboembolic events [19]. Based on the results of this trial, a larger, randomized study is required to confirm that the addition of thalidomide to the combination of docetaxel and estramustine is warranted.

The same regimen was also tested in a community-based study of elderly men, using 100–200 mg/day thalidomide [21]. Ten of 17 patients (59%) experienced a PSA decline of >50%, with one PR and seven stable disease (SD) by RECIST criteria. Following 6 months of treatment, those responding or with SD switched over to maintenance thalidomide only. Overall, three patients experienced life threatening deep vein thrombosis (despite warfarin prophylaxis), and more than half of the patients receiving 200 mg/day thalidomide required dose reductions. The authors concluded that in elderly men with CRPC, this combination did not represent an improvement over the previously reported efficacy of docetaxel or estramustine, especially in light of the apparent toxicity [21].

A similar study was performed by Mathew et al. that combined thalidomide and estramustine with another taxane, paclitaxel [22]. The trial was designed as a Phase I/II, to establish the maximum tolerated dose (MTD) of thalidomide, when used in this combination. The MTD was established at 600 mg/day, in combination with 100 mg/m^2 paclitaxel (days 3 and 10) and 140 mg estramustine (three times daily on days

1–5 and 8–12). However, the majority of patients could not be escalated beyond 400 mg/day thalidomide, because of the somnolence or fatigue. Regardless, 76% of evaluable patients experienced >50% decline in PSA, with 5 of 18 patients with measurable disease exhibiting an objective response. Interestingly, 64% of the patients with disease refractory to previous taxane therapy had >50% decline in PSA. The overall median time to progression was 3 months and median survival duration was 13.6 months. Grade 3/4 toxicities included neutropenia, fatigue, dyspnea, and thromboembolic events (despite prophylactic low-dose warfarin and aspirin). Because of the early and cumulative toxicity observed with thalidomide, Mathew et al. recommended future dosing of thalidomide in this combination not to exceed 200 mg/day.

The use of low-dose thalidomide in combination therapy was also confirmed in a small Phase I study evaluating thalidomide and paclitaxel in combination with doxorubicin in men with CRPC [23]. The thalidomide dose was escalated from 200 to 400 mg/day, and the MTD was determined to be 300 mg/day. This regimen also proved to be efficacious in this heavily pretreated population. All nine patients evaluable for response experienced at least SD, with 5 of the 9 having PSA declines of >50%. Neutropenia was the most common grade 3/4 toxicity, occurring in 9 of the 12 patients across all dose levels [23]. A Phase II study at the University of Pittsburgh is currently underway, evaluating thalidomide and doxorubicin, without paclitaxel, in men with CRPC [24].

Romero et al. recently investigated the oral combination of dexamethasone and thalidomide in patients with CRPC, who had progressed after chemotherapy [25]. Steroid-only treatments (prednisone, hydrocortisone, or dexamethasone) had previously exhibited some activity in CRPC [26–31]. In this study of 39 men, median PFS was 84 days. Ten individuals (26%) had at least a 50% decline in PSA with no radiological or clinical progression. An additional 14 individuals exhibited a decline in PSA, but had other progression by 12 weeks. In addition to poor efficacy, this regimen resulted in five thromboembolic events and significant neuropathy [25].

A phase I study by Di Lorenzo et al. evaluated the combination of thalidomide and cyclophosphamide in 16 highly pretreated men with CRPC [32]. The MTD of thalidomide was found to be 100 mg/day, because of one incident each of grade 3 peripheral neuropathy and venous thrombosis in the 200 mg/day cohort. This low MTD is perhaps unsurprising considering that it has previously been reported that cyclophosphamide alters the pharmacokinetics of thalidomide, prolonging the half-life and increasing drug exposure [33]. In this heavily pretreated population, only 2 of 13 evaluable patients had a decline in PSA >50% [32].

The combination of thalidomide and granulocyte stimulating factor (GM-CSF) was initially evaluated in 22 men with CRPC, based on the observed single agent activity of these two therapies [34]. Patients received GM-CSF three times weekly, and oral thalidomide dose was escalated up to 200 mg/day. All patients experienced a decline in PSA, with five patients (23%) exhibiting a decrease of >50%. Furthermore, two patients achieved an objective reduction in measurable soft tissue disease [34]. This relatively well-tolerated regimen was subsequently evaluated in a Phase II study enrolling patients with hormone-naïve disease [35]. Thalidomide was initially administered at 100 mg/day, and escalated up to 400 mg/day based on individual tolerance. Of 20 evaluable patients, 18 experienced a decline in PSA (median of 59%, range 26–89%). The median duration of response was 11 months [35]. A subsequent study was initiated by the same investigators, adding docetaxel to the thalidomide and GM-CSF regimen in patients with

hormone-naïve prostate cancer, but has since been terminated [36].

Laber et al. reported the results of a Phase I study of thalidomide, capecitabine, and temozolomide that included two patients with advanced prostate cancer [37]. Thalidomide was administered at 100 mg/day. Both of the men with prostate cancer experienced a partial response, suggesting that this regimen may warrant further study.

Finally, a promising phase II trial combining thalidomide with bevacizumab (to block multiple antiangiogenic pathways) along with docetaxel and prednisone is currently underway [38]. Thalidomide (200 mg) and prednisone (10 mg) are being administered daily, with docetaxel (75 mg/m^2) and bevacizumab (15 mg/kg) given every 3 weeks. A total of 60 patients with metastatic mCRPC have been enrolled. Ninety percent of patients receiving the combination therapy had PSA declines of $\geq$ 50%, and 88% achieved a PSA decline of $\geq$ 30% within the first 3 months of treatment. The median time to progression was 18.3 months with a median overall survival of 28.2 months [38]. The addition of bevacizumab and thalidomide to docetaxel is an active combination with manageable toxicities and future studies are warranted in this patient population. Table 19.2 summarizes the completed clinical trials of thalidomide combinations in prostate cancer.

Table 19.2 Summary of completed thalidomide combination trials in prostate cancer

Investigator	Patients enrolled	Thalidomide dose	Combination agents	Clinical Results	Major toxicities
Dahut et al. [19]	75 men with CRPC (50 randomized to combination, 25 to docetaxel alone)	200 mg/day	30 mg/m^2 docetaxel weekly	No statistically significant findings. Overall survival at 18 months: 68.2% vs. 42.9% for docetaxel alone. Median PFS: 5.9 months vs. 3.7 months for docetaxel alone	Fatigue, edema, constipation, sensory neuropathy. High incidence of thromboembolic events led to addition of prophylactic LMWH
Figg et al. [20]	20 men with metastatic CRPC	200 mg/day	30 mg/m^2 docetaxel weekly on days 1, 8 and 15, plus estramustine (3×/day on days 1–3, 8–10, and 15–17 of each 28-day cycle)	PFS of 7.2 months. PSA decline of >50% in 18/20 patients. Two PR in patients with soft tissue lesions	17/20 patients required dose reductions in 1 or more drug. Nausea, sedation, constipation, alopecia, sensory neuropathy. 2 thrombotic events, despite prophylactic anticoagulation
Frank et al. [21]	17 elderly men with CRPC	100–200 mg/day	25 mg/m^2 docetaxel weekly on days 1, 8, and 15, plus 140 mg estramustine 3×/day, 3× per week	PSA decline of >50% in 10/17 patients. 1 PR, 7 SD. Median survival of 17 months	Major grade 3/4 toxicities included: DVT, asthenia, edema and dyspnea. More than half of the patients required dose reductions of thalidomide from 200 mg

Table 19.2 (continued)

Investigator	Patients enrolled	Thalidomide dose	Combination agents	Clinical Results	Major toxicities
Mathew et al. [22]	40 men with CRPC (10 Phase I + 30 Phase II)	200–600 mg/day (600 established as thalidomide MTD)	100 mg/m² paclitaxel on days 3 and 10, 140 mg estramustine 3×/day on days 1–5 and 8–12 of 21-day cycle	PSA decline of >50% in 29/38 patients. Objective response in 5/18 patients with measurable disease	Major grade 3/4 toxicities included: neutropenia, fatigue, dyspnea and thromboembolic events
Amato and Sarao [23]	12 men with CRPC	200–400 mg/day (300 established as thalidomide MTD)	100 mg/m² paclitaxel and 20 mg/m² doxorubicin weekly for 3 weeks of each 5 week cycle	PSA decline of >50% in 5/9 evaluable patients	Major grade 3/4 toxicities included: neutropenia, fatigue, constipation and leukopenia
Romero et al. [25]	39 men with CRPC, following one or more cytotoxic treatment	100–400 mg/day	0.75 mg dexamethasone twice daily	PSA decline of >50% in 10/39 patients. Median PFS: 84 days	Major grade 3/4 toxicities included: neuropathy, thrombotic events and fatigue
Di Lorenzo et al. [32]	16 men with CRPC	100–200 mg/day (100 established as MTD)	50 mg/day oral cyclophosphamide	PSA decline of >50% in 2/16 patients	Grade 3/4 toxicities included neutropenia, anemia, constipation, peripheral neuropathy and venous thrombosis
Dreicer et al. [34]	22 men with CRPC	100–200 mg/day	250 µg GM-CSF three times weekly	PSA decline of >50% in 5/22 patients	Grade 3/4 toxicities included neutropenia, fatigue, venous thrombosis and hyperglycemia

CRPC castration-resistant prostate cancer; *DVT* deep vein thrombosis; *LMWH* low molecular weight heparin; *MTD* maximum tolerated dose; *PFS* progression free survival; *PSA* prostate-specific antigen

Thalidomide Analogs

Numerous thalidomide analogs have been synthesized to optimize the antiangiogenic and anti-tumor properties of thalidomide, while reducing the side effects [39]. This includes efforts to reduce teratogenticity, improve TNF-alpha inhibitory activity, or eliminate the need for metabolism. Of the thalidomide analogs currently in development, two agents in a class termed immunomodulatory drugs (IMiDs) have entered clinical testing. Lenalidomide (Revlimid®, CC-5013) and CC-4047 (Actimid®) act similarly to thalidomide, but have improved TNF-alpha inhibitory activity [39]. Initial in vitro and in vivo testing has suggested that lenalidomide possesses anti-migratory and anti-angiogenic activity [40]. It was shown to inhibit vascularization in a dose-dependent manner in the rat mesenteric window assay. Furthermore, endothelial cell migration was inhibited by lenalidomide in vitro [40]. In 2006, Lenalidomide was approved for use in combination with dexamethasone in patients with multiple myeloma by the US FDA.

Lenalidomide as a Single Agent

A Phase I study of oral lenalidomide was initiated in 2002 by Dahut et al. [41]. Although open to any patient with a refractory solid tumor or lymphoma, 35 of the 45 patients accrued presented with prostate cancer. Lenalidomide was initially administered orally once per day continuously from 5 to 20 mg. This was subsequently modified, with patients receiving lenalidomide for the first 21 days of each 28-day cycle, starting at 15 mg/day and dose escalating to 40 mg/day. The most frequent grade 1 and 2 toxicities included fatigue, nausea, pruritus/rash, neutropenia, and neuropathy.

Neutropenia was the most commonly observed grade 3/4 toxicity. SD was observed in a total of 12 patients, 9 of whom had prostate cancer. However, no durable PSA responses were noted [41].

In 2006, a randomized, double-blinded clinical study was initiated, enrolling patients with evidence of biochemical relapse following surgery or radiation [42]. Patients were randomized to receive either 5 or 25 mg/day of lenalidomide. An open-label phase II clinical trial was started in early 2008 to assess the toxicity and efficacy of lenalidomide in chemotherapy-naïve CRPC patients [43]. The drug is being administered orally at a dose of 25 mg/day for 21 days of each 28-day cycle. As of September 2008, both studies are continuing patient recruitment.

Lenalidomide in Combination Therapy

Several combination studies with lenalidomide have been initiated, many of which are designed based on completed thalidomide trials, using lenalidomide in place of thalidomide. Lenalidomide is currently being evaluated in combination with ketoconazole, based on the hypothesis that the immune stimulatory activity might augment the activity of ketoconazole against prostate cancer in chemotherapy-naïve men with castrate-resistant disease [44]. Patients receive 25 mg/day oral lenalidomide on a 21 out of 28 day schedule, along with 400 mg ketoconazole three times daily continuously. As of May 2008, the study was still open to accrual. Toxicity has been reasonable, with fatigue commonly observed. Ten (56%) of the 18 evaluable patients had PSA declines of >50%. Of the four individuals with measurable disease, three have achieved a partial response and the fourth has SD with tumor volume reduction [44].

A Phase I dose-finding study of lenalidomide in combination with docetaxel (based on the activity observed with thalidomide plus docetaxel) was initiated by Moss et al. [45]. As of early 2007, dosing has been escalated to 75 mg/m^2 docetaxel every 3 weeks, with an oral daily dose of lenalidomide up to 20 mg/day on days 1–14. No dose limiting toxicities had been observed and the MTD was not reached. Nine (47.4%) of the 19 evaluable patients experienced a PSA decline of >50%. Of the 13 patients with measurable disease, 12 experienced a partial response or SD [45].

A combination study in men with metastatic CRPC who had previously received taxane therapy employed a 28-day lead-in of 10 mg lenalidomide (daily, 21/28 days) followed by the addition of weekly paclitaxel at 100 mg/m^2 [46]. Subsequent deescalation of the lenalidomide dose to 5 mg was necessary. In addition, five of the ten total patients enrolled discontinued therapy due to toxicity. Only one of the nine evaluable patients had a minor PSA decline during the lenalidomide lead-in. Overall, weekly paclitaxel combined with even low-dose lenalidomide was very poorly tolerated in this patient population [46].

Following on from the promising results of combining GM-CSF with thalidomide, a Phase I/II clinical trial was started with GM-CSF and lenalidomide in patients with CRPC [47]. Lenalidomide was administered daily at 25 mg/day on days 1–21 of each 28-day cycle. At an interim analysis, four of 17 evaluable patients had experienced a PSA decline of >50%. Fatigue and diarrhea were the most common side effects observed [47].

Finally, a Phase II study of lenalidomide, ketoconazole, and hydrocortisone was opened in 2007 and is continuing to accrue men with CRPC [48].

Summary

Overall, thalidomide has demonstrated potentially promising activity against prostate cancer, especially in combination with cytotoxic or antiangiogenic agents. Activity has been observed both in earlier stage disease and in heavily pretreated populations of men with metastatic CRPC. Thalidomide appears to be altering the tumor microenvironment and may be working via several different mechanisms. However, it is apparent from the completed studies that the dose must be carefully determined in each regimen to minimize the toxicity. None of the published clinical studies of thalidomide have shown a benefit of doses of higher than 200 mg/day, and several have utilized 100 mg/day. Of particular concern is the occurrence of thromboembolic events, even with the administration of prophylactic anticoagulation, and the development of sensory neuropathy.

Initial results with lenalidomide are suggestive of activity in prostate cancer. To date, the most efficacious regimen appears to be the combination of lenalidomide with ketoconazole. In vitro and preclinical testing differs greatly between thalidomide and lenalidomide, and the two agents are likely working via different mechanisms of action. As such, different combinations may be required to achieve the best activity with each agent.

References

1. Giving Thalidomide a Second Chance. 1997. (Accessed August 18, 2008, at http://www.fda.gov/fdac/features/1997/697_thal.html).
2. D'Amato RJ, Loughnan MS, Flynn E, Folkman J. Thalidomide is an inhibitor of angiogenesis. Proc Natl Acad Sci USA 1994;91:4082–5.
3. Bauer KS, Dixon SC, Figg WD. Inhibition of angiogenesis by thalidomide requires metabolic activation, which is species-dependent. Biochem Pharmacol 1998;55:1827–34.
4. Lepper ER, Smith NF, Cox MC, Scripture CD, Figg WD. Thalidomide metabolism and hydrolysis: mechanisms and implications. Curr Drug Metab 2006;7:677–85.
5. Lissbrant IF, Lissbrant E, Damber JE, Bergh A. Blood vessels are regulators of growth, diagnostic markers and therapeutic targets in prostate cancer. Scand J Urol Nephrol 2001;35:437–52.
6. Siegal JA, Yu E, Brawer MK. Topography of neovascularity in human prostate carcinoma. Cancer 1995;75:2545–51.
7. Weidner N, Carroll PR, Flax J, Blumenfeld W, Folkman J. Tumor angiogenesis correlates with metastasis in invasive prostate carcinoma. Am J Pathol 1993;143:401–9.
8. S.T.E.P.S. System for Thalidomide Education and Prescribing Safety. (Accessed August 18, 2008, at http://www.thalomid.com/steps_program.aspx).
9. Figg WD, Dahut W, Duray P, et al. A randomized phase II trial of thalidomide, an angiogenesis inhibitor, in patients with androgen-independent prostate cancer. Clin Cancer Res 2001;7:1888–93.
10. Dixon SC, Kruger EA, Bauer KS, Figg WD. Thalidomide up-regulates prostate-specific antigen secretion from LNCaP cells. Cancer Chemother Pharmacol 1999;43 Suppl:S78–84.
11. Molloy FM, Floeter MK, Syed NA, et al. Thalidomide neuropathy in patients treated for metastatic prostate cancer. Muscle Nerve 2001;24:1050–7.
12. Drake MJ, Robson W, Mehta P, Schofield I, Neal DE, Leung HY. An open-label phase II study of low-dose thalidomide in androgen-independent prostate cancer. Br J Cancer 2003;88:822–7.
13. Figg WD, Hussain MH, Gulley JL, et al. A double blind randomized crossover study of oral thalidomide versus placebo in patients with androgen dependent prostate cancer treated by intermittent androgen ablation. J Urol 2009;181(3):1104–13.
14. Efstathiou E, Troncoso P, Wen S, et al. Initial modulation of the tumor microenvironment accounts for thalidomide activity in prostate cancer. Clin Cancer Res 2007;13:1224–31.
15. Tannock IF, de Wit R, Berry WR, et al. Docetaxel plus prednisone or mitoxantrone plus prednisone for advanced prostate cancer. N Engl J Med 2004;351:1502–12.
16. Petrylak DP, Macarthur RB, O'Connor J, et al. Phase I trial of docetaxel with estramustine in androgen-independent prostate cancer. J Clin Oncol 1999;17:958–67.
17. Petrylak DP, Tangen CM, Hussain MH, et al. Docetaxel and estramustine compared with mitoxantrone and prednisone for advanced refractory prostate cancer. N Engl J Med 2004;351:1513–20.
18. Picus J, Schultz M. Docetaxel (Taxotere) as monotherapy in the treatment of hormone-refractory prostate cancer: preliminary results. Semin Oncol 1999;26:14–8.
19. Dahut WL, Gulley JL, Arlen PM, et al. Randomized phase II trial of docetaxel plus thalidomide in androgen-independent prostate cancer. J Clin Oncol 2004;22:2532–9.
20. Figg WD, Li H, Sissung T, et al. Pre-clinical and clinical evaluation of estramustine, docetaxel and thalidomide combination in androgen-independent prostate cancer. BJU Int 2007;99:1047–55.
21. Frank R, Versea L, Cohen N, Long J, Nair K. Low-dose docetaxel, estramustine and thalidomide followed by maintenance thalidomide in androgen-independent prostate cancer (AIPC): final results of a phase II community based study in elderly men. J Clin Oncol 2007;25:15609.
22. Mathew P, Logothetis CJ, Dieringer PY, et al. Thalidomide/estramustine/paclitaxel in metastatic androgen-independent prostate cancer. Clin Genitourin Cancer 2006;5:144–9.
23. Amato RJ, Sarao H. A phase I study of paclitaxel/doxorubicin/thalidomide in patients with androgen- independent prostate cancer. Clin Genitourin Cancer 2006;4:281–6.
24. Thalidomide and Doxil in Patients with Androgen Independent Prostate Cancer (AIPC). 2008. (Accessed August 25, 2008, at http://www.clinicaltrials.gov).
25. Romero S, Stanton G, DeFelice J, Schreiber F, Rago R, Fishman M. Phase II trial of thalidomide and daily oral dexamethasone for treatment of hormone refractory prostate cancer progressing after chemotherapy. Urol Oncol 2007;25:284–90.
26. Akakura K, Suzuki H, Ueda T, et al. Possible mechanism of dexamethasone therapy for prostate cancer: suppression of circulating level of interleukin-6. Prostate 2003;56:106–9.
27. Berry W, Dakhil S, Modiano M, Gregurich M, Asmar L. Phase III study of mitoxantrone plus low dose prednisone versus low dose prednisone alone in patients with asymptomatic hormone refractory prostate cancer. J Urol 2002;168:2439–43.
28. Kantoff PW, Halabi S, Conaway M, et al. Hydrocortisone with or without mitoxantrone in men with hormone-refractory prostate cancer: results of the cancer and leukemia group B 9182 study. J Clin Oncol 1999;17:2506–13.
29. Saika T, Kusaka N, Tsushima T, et al. Treatment of androgen-independent prostate cancer with dexamethasone: a prospective study in stage D2 patients. Int J Urol 2001;8:290–4.
30. Storlie JA, Buckner JC, Wiseman GA, Burch PA, Hartmann LC, Richardson RL. Prostate specific antigen levels and clinical response to low dose dexamethasone for hormone-refractory metastatic prostate carcinoma. Cancer 1995;76:96–100.
31. Tannock IF, Osoba D, Stockler MR, et al. Chemotherapy with mitoxantrone plus prednisone or prednisone alone for symptomatic hormone-resistant prostate cancer: a Canadian randomized trial with palliative end points. J Clin Oncol 1996;14:1756–64.

32. Di Lorenzo G, Autorino R, De Laurentiis M, et al. Thalidomide in combination with oral daily cyclophosphamide in patients with pretreated hormone refractory prostate cancer: a phase I clinical trial. Cancer Biol Ther 2007;6:313–7.

33. Chung F, Wang LC, Kestell P, Baguley BC, Ching LM. Modulation of thalidomide pharmacokinetics by cyclophosphamide or 5,6-dimethylxanthenone-4-acetic acid (DMXAA) in mice: the role of tumour necrosis factor. Cancer Chemother Pharmacol 2004;53:377–83.

34. Dreicer R, Klein EA, Elson P, Peereboom D, Byzova T, Plow EF. Phase II trial of GM-CSF + thalidomide in patients with androgen-independent metastatic prostate cancer. Urol Oncol 2005;23:82–6.

35. Amato RJ, Hernandez-McClain J, Henary H. Phase 2 study of granulocyte-macrophage colony-stimulating factor plus thalidomide in patients with hormone-naive adenocarcinoma of the prostate. Urol Oncol 2009;27(1):8–13.

36. Safety and Efficacy Study of GM-CSF, Thalidomide Plus Docetaxel in Prostate Cancer. (Accessed August 25, 2008, at http://clinicaltrials.gov/ct2/show/NCT00450008).

37. Laber DA, Khan MI, Kloecker GH, Schonard C, Taft BS, Salvador C. A phase I study of thalidomide, capecitabine and temozolomide in advanced cancer. Cancer Biol Ther 2007;6:840–5.

38. Ning YM, Gulley JL, Arlen PM, et al. A phase II trial of bevacizumab, thalidomide, docetaxel, and prednisone in patients with metastatic castration-resistant prostate cancer. J Clin Oncol 2010;28:2070–6.

39. Aragon-Ching JB, Li H, Gardner ER, Figg WD. Thalidomide analogues as anticancer drugs. Recent Patents Anticancer Drug Discov 2007;2:167–74.

40. Dredge K, Horsfall R, Robinson SP, et al. Orally administered lenalidomide (CC-5013) is anti-angiogenic in vivo and inhibits endothelial cell migration and Akt phosphorylation in vitro. Microvasc Res 2005;69:56–63.

41. Dahut W, Tohnya T, Aragon-Ching J, et al. Phase I study of oral lenalidomide in patients with refractory metastatic cancer. J Clin Pharmacol 2009;49(6):650–60.

42. Study of 2 Different Doses of Revlimid in Biochemically Relapse Prostate Cancer. (Accessed August 26, 2008, at http://clinicaltrials.gov/ct2/show/NCT00348595).

43. Phase II Study Evaluating Toxicity and Efficacy of Lenalidomide (Revlimid) in Chemotherapy-Naive Androgen Independent Prostate Cancer Patients. (Accessed 26 August, 2008, at http://clinicaltrials.gov/ct2/show/NCT00654186).

44. Garcia J, Triozzi P, Elson P, et al. Clinical activity of ketoconazole and lenalidomide in castrate progressive prostate carcinoma (CPPCA): Preliminary results of a phase II trial. J Clin Oncol 2008;26:abstr 5143.

45. Moss R, Mohile S, Shelton G, Melia J, Petrylak D. A phase I open-label study using lenalidomide and docetaxel in androgen independent prostate cancer (AIPC). In: 2007 Prostate Cancer Symposium; 2007; Orlando, FL, Abstract 89.

46. Pagliaro L, Tannir N, Tu S, et al. A modular phase I study of lenalidomide and paclitaxel in metastatic castration-resistant prostate cancer with prior taxane therapy. J Clin Oncol 2008;26:Abstract 13545.

47. Dreicer R, Garcia J, Smith S, et al. Phase I/II trial of GM-CSF and lenalidomide in patients with hormone refractory prostate cancer (HRPC). J Clin Oncol 2007;25:Abstract 15515.

48. Ketoconazole, Hydrocortisone, and Lenalidomide in Treating Patients with Prostate Cancer That Did Not Respond to Hormone Therapy. (Accessed August 26, 2008, at http://clinicaltrials.gov/ct2/show/NCT00460031).

Chapter 20
Investigational Angiogenesis Inhibitors

Jeanny B. Aragon-Ching and William Dahut

Abstract Targeting angiogenesis is an evolving field of cancer research. Tumor angiogenesis is considered as an important step in the progression and metastasis of prostate cancer. Several pathways that converge toward promotion of growth, proliferation, and survival of prostate cancer cells have been targeted, including modulation of proangiogenic factors such as vascular endothelial growth factor (VEGF), tyrosine kinases, cytokines, and the extracellular matrix. Accurately measuring antitumor activity remains a challenge with the use of investigational angiogenesis inhibitors in prostate cancer.

Keywords Antiangiogenesis • Clinical trials • Prostate cancer • Tyrosine kinases

Introduction

Angiogenesis has rapidly emerged as a target for anticancer therapy in the last decade. Since the discovery by Dr. Judah Folkman that tumors require blood supply in order to proliferate [1], the strategy of inhibiting angiogenesis has become one of the most promising fields in cancer research. Almost all neoplasms exhibit neovascularization properties either within the tumor itself or its surrounding stroma by altering homeostatic mechanisms [2]. Tumor neovascularization is a multistep process that involves a complex interaction between proangiogenic stimuli, basement membrane disruption, endothelial cell migration to the extracellular matrix, endothelial cell proliferation, reorganization, and organization into new blood vessels [3]. Targeting angiogenesis involves blocking several different pathways in the angiogenesis cascade. This occurs either directly by targeting endothelial cells or indirectly by decreasing or blocking proangiogenic factors or its endothelial cell receptors, and may vary also by the ability to block one, two, or several factors [4]. At the forefront of investigational angiogenesis inhibitors is the lead agent bevacizumab, a monoclonal antibody to vascular endothelial growth factor (VEGF). Bevacizumab in combination with chemotherapy is approved by the Food and Drug Administration (FDA) for the treatment of metastatic colon, lung, and breast cancer [5]. Although limited activity has been shown using single agent bevacizumab [6, 7], increased activity is seen when combined with chemotherapy [8–10], possibly due to normalization of the tumor vasculature [11], allowing for better delivery of chemotherapeutic drugs. Metastatic prostate cancer has also been shown to exhibit increased angiogenic activity [12]. As such, there is significant interest in targeting angiogenesis in prostate cancer.

Evidence for the Role of Angiogenesis in Prostate Cancer

Tumor angiogenesis is a highly complex process with distinct yet overlapping mechanisms. Early studies showed that aberrant blood formation as well as increasing microvessel density (MVD) count, which was a measure of angiogenesis, were associated with

J.B. Aragon-Ching (✉)
Department of Medicine, George Washington University, Washington, DC, USA
e-mail: jaragonching@mfa.gwu.edu

W.D. Figg et al. (eds.), *Drug Management of Prostate Cancer*,
DOI 10.1007/978-1-60327-829-4_20, © Springer Science+Business Media, LLC 2010

recurrence or metastasis in malignancies including melanoma [13, 14], breast [15, 16], lung [17], and bladder cancer [18]. Elevated circulating VEGF and other soluble growth factors have been associated with poorer prognosis in prostate cancer [19, 20]. Numerous studies have looked at the role of angiogenesis in prostate cancer and attempted to correlate the extent of angiogenesis with the risk for progression. One study examined the microvessel density using immunoperoxidase technique of staining endothelial cells for Factor VIII-related antigen [12] in radical prostatectomy specimens of 74 patients with invasive prostate cancers, of whom 29 eventually developed metastasis. Patients with metastatic disease had a higher mean MVD compared to those without metastasis. In another study using immunostaining against the von Willebrand factor to stain endothelial cells, 64 consecutive radical prostatectomy specimens were quantified for mean and maximal MVD [21]. Maximal MVD was found to be an important independent prognostic variable for survival in men with prostate cancer. Several other studies have reported the utility of microvessel density as a predictor of disease specific survival in prostate cancer, either alone [22, 23] or in combination with standard prognostic factors for prediction of extraprostatic disease extension [24].

Prostate cancer cells also express and/or are regulated by a variety of cytokines or proteins that are involved in angiogenesis, basement membrane degradation, VEGF interaction, or endothelial cell activation [25].

For instance, VEGF mRNA and protein were found to be overexpressed in the highly metastatic LNCaP prostate cancer cell line variant LNCaP-LN3 compared to the less metastatic potential variant LNCaP-Pro5 [26]. Although basic fibroblast growth factor (bFGF) was not found to be overexpressed in this study, other in vitro studies have found augmented response to bFGF either alone or in addition to VEGF [27, 28]. Other factors found to be upregulated in prostate cancer include the hypoxia-inducible factor-1 (HIF-1) [29–32], cyclooxygenase-2 (COX-2) [33], urokinase-type plasminogen activator [34, 35], matrix metalloproteinases [36–38], and cytokines such as interleukin-8 [39] and tumor necrosis factor (TNF) [40, 41]. Several other dysregulated pathways that are involved in the angiogenic signaling cascade have been described, including the Ras/Raf/Mek/Erk pathway [42–44] and phosphatidylinositol-3 kinase/protein kinase B (PI3/AKT) [31, 45] signaling pathway via inactivation of phosphatase and tensin homologue (PTEN) [46], all contributing toward tumor angiogenesis and proliferation.

Investigational Angiogenesis Inhibitors

The emergence of different pathways and molecular targets for angiogenesis inhibition has resulted in a robust field of research investigation in prostate cancer (see Table 20.1). This section describes the clinical

Table 20.1 Selected antiangiogenic agents in clinical development for prostate cancer

Mechanisms and drugs	Cellular targets	Clinical phase of development	References
Anti-VEGF agents			
Bevacizumab	VEGF-A	Phase II in combination with docetaxel and thalidomide	[57]
		Phase III in combination with docetaxel and estramustine	[54, 55]
VEGF Trap	VEGF, PlGF	Phase I in combination with docetaxel	[61]
		Phase III in combination with docetaxel	[62]
Small-molecule tyrosine kinase inhibitors			
AZD2171	VEGFR1, VEGFR2, VEGFR-3, PDGFR, c-Kit	Phase I single agent	[76]
		Phase II single agent	[77]
Sorafenib	VEGFR, PDGFR, c-Kit, Raf kinase	Phase II single agent	[68–70]
		Phase II in combination with docetaxel	[71]
Tandutinib (MLN518/CT53518)	FLT3, PDGFR, c-Kit	Phase II single agent	[78]
Agents that target extracellular matrix, cytokines, or cell-matrix adhesion			
Thalidomide	Unknown, immunomodulatory	Phase II in combination with docetaxel and bevacizumab	[57]
Cilengitide (EMD-121974)	Alpha-5 beta-3 integrin	Phase II single agent	[90]

FLT3 FMS-like tyrosine kinase 3; *PDGFR* platelet-derived growth factor receptor; *PlGF* platelet growth factor; *VEGF* vascular endothelial growth factor

trials investigating agents that inhibit various targets, including the VEGF ligands and its receptors, receptor tyrosine kinases involved in angiogenic signaling, and the epithelial-stromal interactions including proteinases and cytokines that support the surrounding microenvironment.

Targeting VEGF and VEGF-Receptor (VEGF-R) Family

The VEGF family of ligands and receptors constitute a diverse yet distinct pathway of activating signals that result ultimately in proliferation, endothelial cell migration, and survival of newly formed vasculature [47, 48]. At least seven members of this family have been described [49–51]. VEGF-A isoform is the most widely studied mediator of tumor angiogenesis [52] and binds to major VEGF receptors 1 and 2 (VEGFR1 and VEGFR2), leading to receptor dimerization and a cascade of signaling pathways. The lead angiogenesis inhibitor bevacizumab was a humanized IgG monoclonal antibody against all isoforms of VEGF-A [53]. An early clinical trial using single-agent bevacizumab in prostate cancer used a dose of 10 mg/kg every 2 weeks for six infusions. Results showed no objective or partial responses by day 70 in the eight patients who had measurable disease and no significant PSA declines, although there were PSA declines of <50% in 4 of 15 patients [7]. Although single-agent bevacizumab lacked significant activity in prostate cancer, the encouraging results from other clinical trials using combined bevacizumab and chemotherapy led to a Cancer and Leukemia Group B (CALGB) trial 90006 that combined bevacizumab with docetaxel and estramustine [54]. The CALGB 90006 trial enrolled 79 patients, and a 77% PSA response rate was observed (defined as PSA decline of >50% in 58 of 75 patients with sufficient PSA data) [55]. Forty-four percent (15 out of 34 patients who had measurable disease) achieved a partial response (PR), and 32% achieved stable disease (SD) for at least 6 weeks. In another study, the CALGB 90401 trial had the primary objective of comparing overall survival between men with chemotherapy-naïve metastatic castration-resistant prostate cancer (CRPC) treated with docetaxel and prednisone and those treated with docetaxel, prednisone, and bevacizumab [56]. Preliminary results demonstrate that

despite an improvement in PFS, measurable disease response and post-therapy PSA decline, the addition of bevacizumab to docetaxel and prednisone did not improve OS in men with mCRPC, and was associated with greater morbidity and mortality. A trial at the National Cancer Institute (NCI) utilized a combination of bevacizumab given at 15 mg/kg every 3 weeks, which constituted one cycle, in combination with docetaxel 75 mg/m^2 every 3 weeks, thalidomide 200 mg daily, prednisone 10 mg daily, with appropriate thromboprophylaxis. This phase II trial accrued 60 patients with metastatic CRPC, with a median of 66 years (range 44–79), median Gleason score of 8, on-study PSA of 99 ng/mL (range: 6.0–4,399), and prestudy PSA doubling time of 1.6 months (0.3–18.2, 81% <3 months) [57]. Ninety percent of patients receiving the combination therapy had PSA declines of ≥ 50%, with a median time to progression of 18.3 months and a median OS of 28.2 months. The four drug regimen was generally tolerable with manageable toxicities [57]. Thus, despite the negative findings in the CALGB 90401 study, there still may be a role for antiangiogenic agents in advanced prostate cancer. Future studies are needed to address treatment combinations and to clarify the role of angiogenesis as a target in mCRPC (see Chap. 18, Bevacizumab in Advanced Prostate Cancer).

Another strategy for targeting VEGF is through blocking the VEGF receptors. One of the most potent VEGF-R inhibitors is a decoy receptor fusion protein, which comprises the extracellular domains of VEGFR1 and VEGFR2, fused to the constant region (Fc portion) of human IgG1 [58]. Earlier studies using truncated soluble VEGFR1 inhibitors, while effective at inhibiting VEGF bioactivity and angiogenesis, also exhibited poor pharmacokinetic profile and had to be administered more frequently and at high concentrations [59, 60]. Engineering of the parental VEGF Trap (aflibercept) by switching the Ig domains resulted in a fusion protein that interacts minimally with the extracellular matrix, thus improving its pharmacokinetic profile while maintaining in vivo tumor growth suppression [58]. A phase I dose escalation study using aflibercept in combination with docetaxel 75 mg/m^2 every 3 weeks has been preliminarily reported [61]. The recommended dosing of aflibercept at 6 mg/kg with docetaxel did not show any exacerbation of docetaxel-related side effects. In prostate cancer, a phase III trial using aflibercept with docetaxel and prednisone is currently ongoing, with the primary objective of determining improvement in overall survival for metastatic CRPC [62].

While these agents targeting VEGF are very promising, patterns of resistance against antiangiogenic agents given in combination with chemotherapy, are slowly emerging [52].

Targeting Receptor Tyrosine Kinases Involved in Angiogenesis

Tyrosine kinases are key enzymes that play a major role in regulating various cellular processes that modulate signaling for tumor growth, proliferation, and survival [63]. Binding of VEGF to VEGFR2 triggers intracellular signaling cascade via autophosphorylation and activation of the tyrosine kinase domains [64, 65], thus promoting and sustaining angiogenesis. As such, small-molecule inhibitors that target these receptor tyrosine kinases have been investigated in prostate cancer.

Sorafenib is a multikinase inhibitor that targets Raf kinase and the tyrosine kinases including VEGF-R, platelet derived growth factor receptor (PDGF-R), stem cell factor receptor c-kit, and c-Ret [66]. Preclinical tumor models have shown apoptosis in response to sorafenib inhibition [67]. Dysregulation of the Ras/Raf/Mitogen activated protein (Map) kinase was also associated with prostate cancer progression [43, 44], providing the rationale for the use of sorafenib in prostate cancer. There have been several studies utilizing sorafenib for metastatic CRPC [68–70]. Modest response has been observed using this agent, with apparent lack of reliability in using PSA as a measure of response. One trial enrolled an initial 22 out of 46 patients [68]. No PSA declines >50% were noted. However, discordance between increasing PSA values and improvement in bone lesions by bone scan was observed in two patients, and accrual to the full 46 patients continued. A search for alternative biomarkers using phosphorylated extracellular signal regulated kinase (Erk) also showed no consistent correlation with response. Another trial enrolled 57 patients with metastatic CRPC and had a primary end point of PFS of ≥ 12 weeks based on PSA progression [70]. Of the eight patients with measurable disease, four patients were categorized with SD. Of the 47 patients evaluable for PSA response, 11 patients achieved SD according

to PSA-based criteria, with two additional patients who had PSA declines > 50%. These trials also showed immediate posttreatment PSA declines without administration of any further therapy, suggesting possible modulation of PSA secretion by sorafenib [68]. Combinations using sorafenib and docetaxel are currently underway for metastatic CRPC patients [71].

Sunitinib is another small-molecule inhibitor targeting VEGFR1 and VEGFR2, along with PDGF-R, c-kit, and *RET* kinases [72]. It has exhibited antitumor properties in preclinical models, especially in combination with docetaxel [73]. As such, a phase 1 and 2 dose escalating trial using docetaxel and sunitinib in chemotherapy-naïve patients with metastatic CRPC is currently being investigated [74].

A promising, highly potent, ATP-competitive small-molecule that inhibits all VEGF receptors has also shown activity in prostate cancer. AZD2171 (cediranib) has been studied in patients with advanced solid malignancies with hypertension as the most frequently observed dose limiting toxicity (DLT) [75]. A phase I dose escalation study utilizing AZD2171 in patients with prostate cancer has been completed [76]. Similar to sorafenib, posttreatment PSA declines were noted in four patients within 30 days following drug discontinuation. There was also one objective response noted. A phase II clinical trial using AZD2171 as second line therapy for patients with metastatic CRPC who have failed prior docetaxel is currently ongoing at the NCI [77]. The primary endpoint was a 30% 6 month probability of progression-free survival using clinical and radiographic criteria. Of the 18 patients currently enrolled, significant decreases in lymph node as well as other sites of metastases, including the lung, liver, and bone lesions have been documented despite discordant effect on PSA levels. Of the 11 patients who had measurable disease, two patients had PR. Correlative dynamic contrast enhanced-magnetic resonance imaging (DCE-MRI) showed circulatory and vascular changes which correlated with clinical response to AZD2171 in some patients.

Tandutinib is another small-molecule compound that inhibits the autophosphorylation of FLT3 (FMS-Like Tyrosine kinase-3), c-KIT, and PDGF receptor tyrosine kinases, thereby inhibiting cellular proliferation and inducing apoptosis. Tandutinib has also been reported to have activity in metastatic CRPC patients who have progressed on taxanes [78]. This phase II trial used oral tandutinib at 500 mg twice daily dosage given every 28 days with the primary endpoint of measuring freedom from disease progression in 8 weeks. Two (13%) out of 15 evaluable patients were free from symptomatic or radiological progression beyond 8 weeks (35, 50 weeks), and PSA declines of 50% and 40%, respectively were seen in these two patients. Unlike sorafenib and AZD2171, no PSA declines were noted following drug discontinuation.

Targeting the Extracellular Matrix, Cytokines, and Cell–Matrix Adhesion

It is increasingly being recognized that different cytokines such as FGF, transforming growth factor (TGF), endothelial cell-activating factors, stromal fibroblasts, and components of the tumor microenvironment, all help to sustain angiogenesis [79, 80]. To this end, thalidomide and its analogues have been widely studied for its antiangiogenic and immunomodulatory effects in prostate cancer [81–83], with encouraging results (see Chap. 19, Thalidomide and Analogs). The thalidomide analogue lenalidomide has also been studied in solid tumors [84], and in combination with docetaxel in prostate cancer [85]. This open-label phase I trial utilized docetaxel at two dose levels every 3 weeks at 60 mg/m^2 and 75 mg/m^2, prednisone 5 mg twice a day, and lenalidomide at doses of 10 mg, 15 mg, 20 mg, or 25 mg. Of the 13 patients with measurable disease, five patients achieved PR (38.5%) and seven patients (53.9%) had SD. Another phase I trial combining lenalidomide with docetaxel [86] in patients with solid tumors showed that of the nine patients with prostate cancer, SD was seen in five patients and PSA declines of 32–95% were observed.

5,6-Dimethylxanthenone acetic acid (DMXAA) is an agent that disrupts the tumor vasculature by directly causing apoptosis and necrosis as well as tumor necrosis factor (TNF) induction [87]. A randomized phase II trial in metastatic prostate cancer utilizing docetaxel 75 mg/m^2 every 3 weeks, with or without DMXAA at 1,200 mg/m^2 every 21 days has been completed. Sixty-two and a half percent of patients in the DMXAA treatment arm had at least a 30% reduction in PSA during the first 3 months, compared with 47.4% patients in the control arm, who received docetaxel alone [88], with tolerable safety profiles.

An integral component in the maintenance of the basal membrane is the integrins, which are heterodimer transmembrane receptors composed of an alpha and beta subunit in the extracellular matrix, of which the heterodimers α(alpha)Vβ(beta)3 and α(alpha)Vβ(beta)5 were the earliest known integrin targets for inhibiting endothelial cell-cell interactions, endothelial cell-matrix interactions, and tumor angiogenesis [89]. Integrins recognize several ligands via their arginine-glycine-aspartic acid (RGD) sequence, including, but not limited to, laminin, fibrinogen, fibronectin, thrombospondin, matrix metalloproteinase-2 (MMP-2), and FGF-2. Several approaches in blocking integrins are in development, including monoclonal antibodies against integrins and synthetic peptides or peptidomimetics that contain the RGD sequence. One of the synthetic peptides in development which has been studied in a phase II clinical trial for chemotherapy-naïve asymptomatic metastatic CRPC patients is cilengitide (EMD 121974) [90]. The primary endpoint was a 6-month objective progression-free rate, excluding PSA as a criterion. Using a Simon two-stage design, patients were randomized to cilengitide 500 mg or 2,000 mg intravenously twice a week in 6-week cycles. SD was documented as the best objective response in 27% of patients on the 500 mg arm and 36% on 2,000 mg arm. No significant trends in biologic markers such as *N*-telopeptides were noted. Based on this activity, accrual to the second stage was halted.

The potential role of MMPs in prostate cancer progression has also been investigated [91]. Several agents that modulate angiogenesis partly via MMP inhibition include endostatin [92], TNP-470 [93], and perhaps 2-methoxyestradiol [94]. Although these agents have been studied in prostate cancer, significant meaningful clinical responses have not been seen.

Conclusions

Targeting angiogenesis is a burgeoning field of cancer research. Early investigations have established the improved utility of combining these targeted agents with cytotoxic chemotherapy without undue additional toxicity. Specific challenges include defining outcome measures, especially since PSA is proving to be an unreliable surrogate marker for response or progression.

The search for appropriate biomarkers as surrogates for response is ongoing and must be clinically validated, including circulating levels of proangiogenic factors, circulating tumor cells or endothelial cells, and assessment of functional imaging, such as DCE-MRI. In addition, patterns of resistance against these antiangiogenic agents, are slowly emerging [52]. It had been an initially held belief that endothelial cells were genetically stable and thus might not develop resistance. However, some harbor cytogenetic abnormalities would render them with acquired resistance [95]. Increasing recognition of varying mechanisms of resistance would be valuable in developing strategies for circumventing this resistance patterns. One possible approach is to use combinational therapies, whether with additional cytotoxic chemotherapy or another antiangiogenic agent that utilizes a different activating pathway. The optimal dosing schedule as well as potential long-term safety antiangiogenic agents alone or in combination must also be addressed.

References

1. Folkman J. Tumor angiogenesis: therapeutic implications. N Engl J Med 1971;285:1182–6.
2. Fidler IJ. Modulation of the organ microenvironment for treatment of cancer metastasis. J Natl Cancer Inst 1995;87:1588–92.
3. Folkman J, Watson K, Ingber D, et al. Induction of angiogenesis during the transition from hyperplasia to neoplasia. Nature 1989;339:58–61.
4. Folkman J. Angiogenesis: an organizing principle for drug discovery? Nat Rev Drug Discov 2007;6:273–86.
5. FDA Approval for Bevacizumab-National Cancer Institute. (Accessed May 20, 2008, at http://www.cancer.gov/cancer-topics/druginfo/fda-bevacizumab)
6. Cohen MH, Gootenberg J, Keegan P, et al. FDA drug approval summary: bevacizumab plus FOLFOX4 as second-line treatment of colorectal cancer. Oncologist 2007;12:356–61.
7. Reese DM, Fratesi P, Corry M, et al. A Phase II trial of humanized anti-vascular endothelial growth factor antibody for the treatment of androgen-independent prostate cancer. Prostate 2001;3:65–70.
8. Hurwitz H, Fehrenbacher L, Novotny W, et al. Bevacizumab plus irinotecan, fluorouracil, and leucovorin for metastatic colorectal cancer. N Engl J Med 2004;350:2335–42.
9. Hurwitz HI, Fehrenbacher L, Hainsworth JD, et al. Bevacizumab in combination with fluorouracil and leucovorin: an active regimen for first-line metastatic colorectal cancer. J Clin Oncol 2005;23:3502–8.
10. Sandler A, Gray R, Perry MC, et al. Paclitaxel-carboplatin alone or with bevacizumab for non-small-cell lung cancer. N Engl J Med 2006;355:2542–50.
11. Jain, RK. Normalization of tumor vasculature: an emerging concept in antiangiogenic therapy. Science 2005;307:58–62.
12. Weidner N, Carroll PR, Flax J, et al. Tumor angiogenesis correlates with metastasis in invasive prostate carcinoma. Am J Pathol 1993;143:401–9.
13. Srivastava A, Laidler P, Hughes LE, et al. Neovascularization in human cutaneous melanoma: a quantitative morphological and Doppler ultrasound study. Eur J Cancer Clin Oncol 1986;22:1205–9.
14. Srivastava A, Laidler P, Davies RP, et al. The prognostic significance of tumor vascularity in intermediate-thickness (0.76–4.0 mm thick) skin melanoma. A quantitative histologic study. Am J Pathol 1988;133:419–23.
15. Weidner N, Folkman J, Pozza F, et al. Tumor angiogenesis: a new significant and independent prognostic indicator in early-stage breast carcinoma. J Natl Cancer Inst 1992;84:1875–87.
16. Weidner N, Semple JP, Welch WR, Folkman, J. Tumor angiogenesis and metastasis – correlation in invasive breast carcinoma. N Engl J Med 1991;324:1–8.
17. Macchiarini P, Fontanini G, Hardin MJ, et al. Relation of neovascularisation to metastasis of non-small-cell lung cancer. Lancet 1992;340:145–6.
18. Jaeger TM, Weidner N, Chew K, et al. Tumor angiogenesis correlates with lymph node metastases in invasive bladder cancer. J Urol 1995;154:69–71.
19. Borre M, Nerstrom B, Overgaard J. Association between immunohistochemical expression of vascular endothelial growth factor (VEGF), VEGF-expressing neuroendocrine-differentiated tumor cells, and outcome in prostate cancer patients subjected to watchful waiting. Clin Cancer Res 2000;6:1882–90.
20. Shariat SF, Anwuri VA, Lamb DJ, et al. Association of preoperative plasma levels of vascular endothelial growth factor and soluble vascular cell adhesion molecule-1 with lymph node status and biochemical progression after radical prostatectomy. J Clin Oncol 2004;22:1655–63.
21. Offersen BV, Borre M, Overgaard, J. (1998) Immunohistochemical determination of tumor angiogenesis measured by the maximal microvessel density in human prostate cancer. APMIS 1998;106:463–9.
22. Borre M, Offersen BV, Nerstrom B, Overgaard J. Microvessel density predicts survival in prostate cancer patients subjected to watchful waiting. Br J Cancer 1998;78:940–4.
23. Borre M, Bentzen SM, Nerstrom B, Overgaard J. Tumor cell proliferation and survival in patients with prostate cancer followed expectantly. J Urol 1998;159:1609–14.
24. Bostwick DG, Wheeler TM, Blute M, et al. Optimized microvessel density analysis improves prediction of cancer stage from prostate needle biopsies. Urology 1996;48:47–57.
25. Nicholson B, Theodorescu D. Angiogenesis and prostate cancer tumor growth. J Cell Biochem 2004;91:125–50.
26. Balbay MD, Pettaway CA, Kuniyasu H, et al. Highly metastatic human prostate cancer growing within the prostate of athymic mice overexpresses vascular endothelial growth factor. Clin Cancer Res 1999;5:783–9.
27. Gaudric A, N'Guyen T, Moenner M, et al. Quantification of angiogenesis due to basic fibroblast growth factor in a modified rabbit corneal model. Ophthalmic Res 1992;24:181–8.
28. Pepper MS, Ferrara N, Orci L, Montesano R. Potent synergism between vascular endothelial growth factor and basic

fibroblast growth factor in the induction of angiogenesis in vitro. Biochem Biophys Res Commun 1992;189:824–31.

29. Zhong H, Agani F, Baccala AA, et al. Increased expression of hypoxia inducible factor-1alpha in rat and human prostate cancer. Cancer Res 1998;58:5280–4.

30. Zhong H, DeMarzo AM, Laughner E, et al. Overexpression of hypoxia-inducible factor 1alpha in common human cancers and their metastases. Cancer Res 1999;59:5830–5.

31. Zhong H, Chiles K, Feldser D, et al. Modulation of hypoxia-inducible factor 1alpha expression by the epidermal growth factor/phosphatidylinositol 3-kinase/PTEN/AKT/FRAP pathway in human prostate cancer cells: implications for tumor angiogenesis and therapeutics. Cancer Res 2000;60:1541–5.

32. Kimbro KS, Simons JW. Hypoxia-inducible factor-1 in human breast and prostate cancer. Endocr Relat Cancer 2006;13:739–49.

33. Liu XH, Kirschenbaum A, Yao S, et al. Upregulation of vascular endothelial growth factor by cobalt chloride-simulated hypoxia is mediated by persistent induction of cyclooxygenase-2 in a metastatic human prostate cancer cell line. Clin Exp Metastasis 1999;17:687–94.

34. Hoosein NM, Boyd DD, Hollas WJ, et al. Involvement of urokinase and its receptor in the invasiveness of human prostatic carcinoma cell lines. Cancer Commun 1991;3:255–64.

35. Hollas W, Hoosein N, Chung LW, et al. Expression of urokinase and its receptor in invasive and non-invasive prostate cancer cell lines. Thromb Haemost 1992;68:662–6.

36. Nagakawa O, Murakami K, Yamaura T, et al. Expression of membrane-type 1 matrix metalloproteinase (MT1-MMP) on prostate cancer cell lines. Cancer Lett 2000;155:173–9.

37. Trudel D, Fradet Y, Meyer F, et al. Membrane-type-1 matrix metalloproteinase, matrix metalloproteinase 2, and tissue inhibitor of matrix proteinase 2 in prostate cancer: identification of patients with poor prognosis by immunohistochemistry. Hum Pathol 2008;39:731–9.

38. Trudel D, Fradet Y, Meyer F, et al. Significance of MMP-2 expression in prostate cancer: an immunohistochemical study. Cancer Res 2003;63:8511–5.

39. Inoue K, Slaton JW, Eve BY, et al. Interleukin 8 expression regulates tumorigenicity and metastases in androgen-independent prostate cancer. Clin Cancer Res 2000;6:2104–19.

40. Ferrer FA, Miller LJ, Andrawis RI, et al. Vascular endothelial growth factor (VEGF) expression in human prostate cancer: in situ and in vitro expression of VEGF by human prostate cancer cells. J Urol 1997;157:2329–33.

41. Ferrer FA, Miller LJ, Andrawis RI, et al. Angiogenesis and prostate cancer: in vivo and in vitro expression of angiogenesis factors by prostate cancer cells. Urology 1998;51:161–7.

42. Erlich S, Tal-Or P, Liebling R, et al. Ras inhibition results in growth arrest and death of androgen-dependent and androgen-independent prostate cancer cells. Biochem Pharmacol 2006;72:427–36.

43. Gioeli D, Mandell JW, Petroni GR, et al. Activation of mitogen-activated protein kinase associated with prostate cancer progression. Cancer Res 1999;59:279–84.

44. Gioeli D. Signal transduction in prostate cancer progression. Clin Sci (Lond) 2005;108:293–308.

45. Malik SN, Brattain M, Ghosh PM, et al. Immunohistochemical demonstration of phospho-Akt in high Gleason grade prostate cancer. Clin Cancer Res 2002;8:1168–71.

46. Giri D, Ittmann M. Inactivation of the PTEN tumor suppressor gene is associated with increased angiogenesis in clinically localized prostate carcinoma. Hum Pathol 1999;30:419–24.

47. Hicklin DJ, Ellis LM. Role of the vascular endothelial growth factor pathway in tumor growth and angiogenesis. J Clin Oncol 2005;23:1011–27.

48. Ferrara N. VEGF and the quest for tumor angiogenesis factors. Nat Rev Cancer 2002;2:795–803.

49. Yamazaki Y, Morita T. Molecular and functional diversity of vascular endothelial growth factors. Mol Divers 2006;10:515–27.

50. Epstein RJ. (2007) VEGF signaling inhibitors: More pro-apoptotic than anti-angiogenic. Cancer Metastasis Rev 2007;26:443–52.

51. Neufeld G, Cohen T, Gengrinovitch S, Poltorak Z. Vascular endothelial growth factor (VEGF) and its receptors. FASEB J 1999;13:9–22.

52. Kerbel RS. Tumor angiogenesis. N Engl J Med 2008;358:2039–49.

53. Presta LG, Chen H, O'Connor SJ, et al. Humanization of an anti-vascular endothelial growth factor monoclonal antibody for the therapy of solid tumors and other disorders. Cancer Res 1997;57:4593–9.

54. Picus J, Halabi S, Rini B, et al. The use of bevacizumab with docetaxel and estramustine in hormone refractory prostate cancer: Initial results of CALGB 90006 [abstract]. Proc Am Soc Clin Oncol 2003;22:No. 1578.

55. Picus J. Docetaxel/bevacizumab (Avastin) in prostate cancer [abstract]. Cancer Invest 2004;22:60:No. 46.

56. Kelly WK, Halabi S, Carducci MA, et al. A randomized, double-blind, placebo-controlled phase III trial comparing docetaxel, prednisone, and placebo with docetaxel, prednisone, and bevacizumab in men with metastatic castration-resistant prostate cancer (mCRPC): Survival results of CALGB 90401. ASCO Annual Meeting Proceedings J Clin Oncol 2010;28:LBA4511.

57. Ning YM, Gulley JL, Arlen PM, et al. A phase II trial of bevacizumab, thalidomide, docetaxel, and prednisone in patients with metastatic castration-resistant prostate cancer. J Clin Oncol 2010;28:2070–6.

58. Holash J, Davis S, Papadopoulos N, et al. VEGF-Trap: a VEGF blocker with potent antitumor effects. Proc Natl Acad Sci USA 2002;99:11393–8.

59. Ferrara N, Chen H, Davis-Smyth T, et al. Vascular endothelial growth factor is essential for corpus luteum angiogenesis. Nat Med 1998;4:336–40.

60. Gerber HP, Vu TH, Ryan AM, et al. VEGF couples hypertrophic cartilage remodeling, ossification and angiogenesis during endochondral bone formation. Nat Med 1999;5:623–8.

61. Isambert N, Freyer G, Zanetta S, et al. A phase I dose escalation and pharmacokinetic (PK) study of intravenous aflibercept (VEGF trap) plus docetaxel (D) in patients (pts) with advanced solid tumors: Preliminary results [abstract]. J Clin Oncol 2008:No. 3599.

62. NCT00519285. Aflibercept in combination with docetaxel in metastatic androgen independent prostate cancer (VENICE). (Accessed April 15, 2008 at http://clinicaltrials.gov/ct2/show/NCT00519285)

63. Arora A, Scholar EM. Role of tyrosine kinase inhibitors in cancer therapy. J Pharmacol Exp Ther 2005;315:971–9.

64. Bergsland EK. Vascular endothelial growth factor as a therapeutic target in cancer. Am J Health Syst Pharm 2004;61:S4–11.

65. Parikh AA, Ellis LM. The vascular endothelial growth factor family and its receptors. Hematol Oncol Clin North Am 2004;18:951–71,vii.

66. Wilhelm S, Carter C, Lynch M, et al. Discovery and development of sorafenib: a multikinase inhibitor for treating cancer. Nat Rev Drug Discov 2006;5:835–44.

67. Yu C, Bruzek LM, Meng XW, et al. The role of Mcl-1 down-regulation in the proapoptotic activity of the multikinase inhibitor BAY 43-9006. Oncogene 2005;24:6861–9.

68. Dahut WL, Scripture C, Posadas E, et al. A phase II clinical trial of sorafenib in androgen-independent prostate cancer. Clin Cancer Res 2008;14:209–14.

69. Chi KN, Ellard SL, Hotte SJ, et al. A phase II study of sorafenib in patients with chemo-naive castration-resistant prostate cancer. Ann Oncol 2008;19:746–51.

70. Steinbild S, Mross K, Frost A, et al. A clinical phase II study with sorafenib in patients with progressive hormone-refractory prostate cancer: a study of the CESAR Central European Society for Anticancer Drug Research-EWIV. Br J Cancer 2007;97:1480–5.

71. NCT00414388. Sorafenib to overcome resistance to systemic chemotherapy in androgen-independent prostate cancer. (Accessed September 22, 2007 at http://clinicaltrials.gov/show/NCT00414388)

72. Chow LQ, Eckhardt SG. Sunitinib: from rational design to clinical efficacy. J Clin Oncol 2007;25:884–96.

73. Guerin O, Formento P, Lo Nigro C, et al. Supra-additive antitumor effect of sunitinib malate (SU11248, Sutent) combined with docetaxel. A new therapeutic perspective in hormone refractory prostate cancer. J Cancer Res Clin Oncol 2008;134:51–7.

74. NCT00137436. Study of SU11248 in combination with docetaxel and prednisone in patients with prostate cancer. (Accessed September 22, 2007 at http://clinicaltrials.gov/show/NCT00137436)

75. Drevs J, Siegert P, Medinger M, et al. Phase I clinical study of AZD2171, an oral vascular endothelial growth factor signaling inhibitor, in patients with advanced solid tumors. J Clin Oncol 2007;25:3045–54.

76. Ryan CJ, Stadler WM, Roth B, et al. Phase I dose escalation and pharmacokinetic study of AZD2171, an inhibitor of the vascular endothelial growth factor receptor tyrosine kinase, in patients with hormone refractory prostate cancer (HRPC). Invest New Drugs 2007;25:445–51.

77. Karakunnel JJ, Gulley J, Arlen P, et al. Phase II trial of cediranib (AZD2171) in docetaxel-resistant, castrate-resistant prostate cancer (CRPC) [abstract]. J Clin Oncol 2008;26:(May 20 suppl), No. 189.

78. Mathew P, Pagliaro LC, Tannir NM, et al. Single-agent platelet-derived growth factor (PDGF) receptor inhibitor therapy for castration-resistant prostate cancer with bone metastases [abstract]. J Clin Oncol 2008:No.5164.

79. Janvier R, Sourla A, Koutsilieris M, Doillon C. Stromal fibroblasts are required for PC-3 human prostate cancer cells to produce capillary-like formation of endothelial cells in a three-dimensional co-culture system. Anticancer Res 1997;17:1551–7.

80. Hepburn PJ, Griffiths K, Harper ME. Angiogenic factors expressed by human prostatic cell lines: effect on endothelial cell growth in vitro. Prostate 1997;33:123–32.

81. Dahut WL, Gulley JL, Arlen PM, et al. Randomized phase II trial of docetaxel plus thalidomide in androgen-independent prostate cancer. J Clin Oncol 2004;22:2532–9.

82. Figg WD, Arlen P, Gulley J, et al. A randomized phase II trial of docetaxel (taxotere) plus thalidomide in androgen-independent prostate cancer. Semin Oncol 2001;28:62–6.

83. Franks ME, Macpherson GR, Figg WD. Thalidomide. Lancet 2004;363:1802–11.

84. Tohnya TM, Ng SS, Dahut WL, et al. A phase I study of oral CC-5013 (lenalidomide, Revlimid), a thalidomide derivative, in patients with refractory metastatic cancer. Clin Prostate Cancer 2004;2:241–3.

85. Moss R, Mohile S, Shelton G, et al. A phase I open-label study using lenalidomide and docetaxel in androgen-independent prostate cancer (AIPC) [abstract]. In ASCO Prostate Cancer Symposium: Orlando, FL, February 22–24, 2007, No. 89.

86. Sanborn SL, Cooney M, Gibbons J, et al. Phase I trial of daily lenalidomide and docetaxel given every three weeks in patients with advanced solid tumors. In ASCO Genitourinary Symposium: San Francisco, CA February 25–28, 2008, Abstract #183.

87. Rustin GJ, Bradley C, Galbraith S, et al. 5,6-Dimethylxanthenone-4-acetic acid (DMXAA), a novel anti-vascular agent: phase I clinical and pharmacokinetic study. Br J Cancer 2003;88:1160–7.

88. Pili R, Rosenthal M, and AS1404-203 study group investigators. Addition of DMXAA (ASA404) to docetaxel in patients with hormone-refractory metastatic prostate cancer (HRMPC): update from a randomized, phase II study. J Clin Oncol 2008;26(May 20 suppl), No. 5007.

89. Stupp R, Ruegg C. Integrin inhibitors reaching the clinic. J Clin Oncol 2007;25:1637–8.

90. Bradley DA, Daignault S, Ryan C, et al. Cilengitide in asymptomatic metastatic androgen independent prostate cancer (AIPC) patients (pts): A randomized phase II trial [abstract]. J Clin Oncol 2008;26(May 20 suppl), No. 5144.

91. Madigan MC, Kingsley EA, Cozzi PJ, et al. The role of extracellular matrix metalloproteinase inducer protein in prostate cancer progression. Cancer Immunol Immunother 2008;57:1367–79.

92. Kim YM, Jang JW, Lee OH, et al. Endostatin inhibits endothelial and tumor cellular invasion by blocking the activation and catalytic activity of matrix metalloproteinase. Cancer Res 2000;60:5410–3.

93. Logothetis CJ, Wu KK, Finn LD, et al. Phase I trial of the angiogenesis inhibitor TNP-470 for progressive androgen-independent prostate cancer. Clin Cancer Res 2001;7:1198–203.

94. Dahut WL, Lakhani NJ, Gulley JL, et al. Phase I clinical trial of oral 2-methoxyestradiol, an antiangiogenic and apoptotic agent, in patients with solid tumors. Cancer Biol Ther 2006;5:22–7.

95. Hida K, Hida Y, Amin DN, et al. Tumor-associated endothelial cells with cytogenetic abnormalities. Cancer Res 2004;64:8249–55.

Chapter 21
Pharmacogenetics of Angiogenesis

Guido Bocci, Giuseppe Pasqualetti, Antonello Di Paolo, Francesco Crea, Mario Del Tacca, and Romano Danesi

Abstract Angiogenesis is a complex cascade of events involving extensive interplay between cells, soluble factors, and extracellular matrix components. Soluble factors including cytokines and growth factors have multifaceted stimulatory or inhibitory roles, thereby finely tuning the process. The angiogenic potential of tumors was initially demonstrated in animal models, and it is now recognized that angiogenesis not only precedes tumor growth but is also necessary for metastasis. Vascular endothelial growth factor (VEGF) plays a central role in prostate angiogenesis. Genetic variability of VEGF involves mainly the untranslated region of the gene and may be associated with increased VEGF transcription and protein expression. Indeed, the -1154G>A polymorphism increases VEGF transcription and has been associated with significantly increased risk of prostate cancer. Hypoxia inducible factor-1α (HIF-1α) is a transcription factor overexpressed in early stage prostate cancer; through its binding to hypoxic responsive elements, it activates the transcription of a wide variety of genes as a part of the cellular response to hypoxia, including VEGF, and potentially plays a key role in prostate cancer development and response to antiangiogenic drugs. Therefore, angiogenesis-related genes seem to have an important role in prostate cancer risk and aggressiveness, thus influencing the outcome of antiangiogenic treatments and survival of patients.

Keywords Antiangiogenic therapy • Cancer risk • HIF • MMP • Single nucleotide polymorphisms • TNF • VEGF

R. Danesi (✉)
Division of Pharmacology and Chemotherapy,
Department of Internal Medicine, University of Pisa, Pisa, Italy
e-mail: r.danesi@med.unipi.it

Introduction

The increasing incidence of prostate cancer and the pivotal role that tumor-driven angiogenesis has in the aggressive behavior of this malignancy [1] have led to the evaluation of several antiangiogenic drugs in prostate cancer clinical trials [2]. As a matter of fact, the inhibition of endothelial cell proliferation and normalization of blood vessels may circumvent several mechanisms of chemoresistance, allowing the achievement of a better clinical response. During the last years, the therapeutic scenario has been significantly changed because of the introduction in clinical trials of newer drugs acting at different levels along the angiogenic pathway. However, the most interesting targets are represented by the vascular endothelial growth factor-A (VEGF-A) and/or its receptors, against which monoclonal antibodies, "small molecules" inhibitors of the tyrosine kinase domain or immunomodulatory agents have been tested.

Bevacizumab is a monoclonal antibody targeting the VEGF-A isoform, to prevent the binding of the growth factor to its receptors, hence inhibiting the angiogenesis process. While bevacizumab did not show meaningful activity as a single agent in prostate cancer patients [3], when it was combined with other drugs (i.e., docetaxel and thalidomide), it was effective in reducing the levels of PSA [4]. Thalidomide, whose antiangiogenic activity has been demonstrated in several in vitro and in vivo animal models, although its exact molecular mechanism remains to be fully elucidated, it seems to be effective in castration-resistant prostate cancer (CRPC) patients [5], because in several studies, performed in CRPC subjects, thalidomide alone or in combination with other agents (i.e., docetaxel and bevacizumab) was able to increase the response rate

W.D. Figg et al. (eds.), *Drug Management of Prostate Cancer*,
DOI 10.1007/978-1-60327-829-4_21, © Springer Science+Business Media, LLC 2010

observed with docetaxel alone and measured as decline of PSA >50% [6, 7]. These encouraging results are prompting to the evaluation of the thalidomide analog lenalidomide [8], which shows an improved tolerability and similar effectiveness with respect to thalidomide in clinical trials in patients affected by multiple myeloma [9].

VEGF and endothelial growth factor (EGF) stimulation of prostate cancer cells occurs via the activation of the tyrosine-kinase (TK) domain within the cytoplasmic portion of the VEGF receptor (VEGFR) and EGF receptor (EGFR) (Fig. 21.1). Because this step is crucial for signal transduction, several TK inhibitors have been developed and some of them are now in clinical evaluation for the treatment of prostate cancer. Among the newer drugs, sorafenib (BAY 43-9006), an inhibitor of B-raf and C-raf isoforms, is able to reduce signal transduction through VEGFR2, VEGFR3, and the platelet-derived growth factor receptor (PDGF)-β [10]. In castration-resistant prostate cancer patients, the drug has been demonstrated to be effective as single agent when responses were assessed by PSA levels and RECIST criteria [11], despite other studies showed some discordances between PSA and objective responses [12, 13]. Other inhibitors of VEGF TK

activity are under clinical evaluation in prostate cancer patients. AZD2171, a pan-VEGFR inhibitor [14] and sunitinib (SU011248) seem to have a promising role in prostate cancer treatment. Finally, integrin signaling (cilengitide, EMD 121974) as well as mammalian target of rapamycin (RAD001) are being evaluated as potential target of angiogenesis in prostate cancer [3]. Figure 21.2 shows the multiple advantages of optimal antiangiogenic therapy and its potential for combination with conventional treatments.

Genetic Variants of VEGF Gene and Prostate Cancer

Polymorphisms are naturally occurring DNA sequence variations, which differ from mutations in that they occur in the healthy population and have a frequency of at least 1%. Approximately, 90% of DNA polymorphisms are single nucleotide polymorphisms (SNPs) due to single base substitutions [15]. Others include insertion/deletion polymorphisms, minisatellite polymorphisms, and microsatellite polymorphisms. Although most polymorphisms are functionally neutral (i.e.,

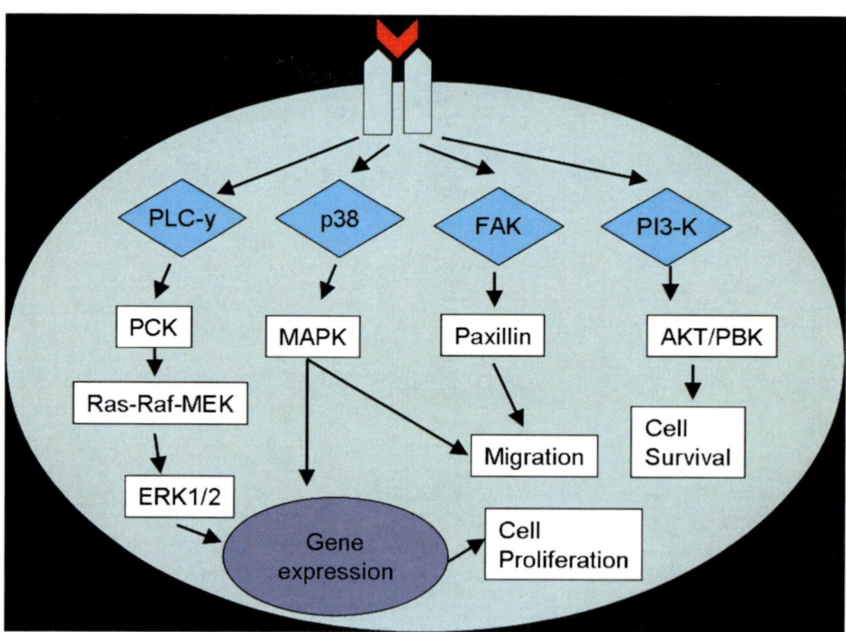

Fig. 21.1 VEFG intracellular signaling via VEGFR-2. The binding of VEGF to VEGFR-2 produces a number of intracellular reactions that promote endothelial cells survival, migration, and proliferation. *PLC-α* phospholipase C-α; *PCK* protein kinase C; *ERK* extracellular regulated kinase; *MAPK* mitogen activate protein kinase; *FAK* focal adhesion kinase; *PI3-K* phosphatidyl inositol 3′ kinase; *Akt/PBK* protein kinase B

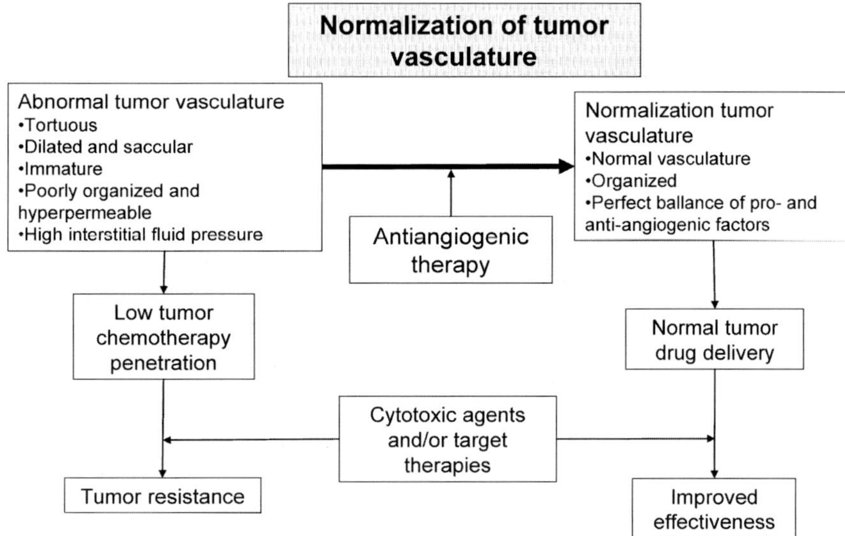

Fig. 21.2 Normalization of tumor vasculature after treatment with antiangiogenic agents might improve the effectiveness of chemotherapy

intronic and exonic synonymous SNPs), some have effects on regulation of gene expression or on the function of the coded protein [15]. These functional polymorphisms, despite having low penetrance, could contribute to the differences between individuals in susceptibility to and severity of disease as well as to responsiveness to drug treatment. Certain polymorphisms alone, in combination or by interaction with environmental factors may affect the angiogenic pathway and thereby susceptibility to the development of selected cancers [15]. Identification of the role of angiogenic gene polymorphisms that influence cancer susceptibility and/or severity may improve the understanding of tumor angiogenesis and may influence risk stratification and detection, use of new treatment strategies, and definition of prognosis of the disease [15].

Studies specifically addressing the involvement of genetic variants of angiogenesis-related genes, VEGF in particular, in the risk of prostate cancer and response to treatment are few and quite frequently in disagreement with each other. Potential reasons are as follows: (1) small cohort of patients, (2) criteria of disease stratification, (3) ethnic stratification, (4) retrospective design, (5) choice of polymorphism, and (6) lack of validation of techniques for genome analysis.

A study examined the association between 58 SNPs in nine angiogenesis-related candidate genes, namely epidermal growth factor (EGF), lymphotoxin-α (LT-α), hypoxia inducible factor-1α (HIF-1α), HIF-1α subunit inhibitor (HIF-1αN), metalloproteinase-2 (MMP2), MMP9, endothelial nitric oxide synthase (NOS3), inducible nitric oxide synthase (NOS2A), and VEGF, and the risk of overall and advanced prostate cancer in a large cohort of prostate cancer patients ($n=1,425$) and controls ($n=1,453$) [16]. No associations were found between either SNPs in VEGF, HIF-1α, or NOS3, nor SNPs in EGF, LT-α, HIF-1αN, MMP9, or NOS2A and prostate cancer [16]. In the MMP2 gene, three intronic SNPs, all in linkage disequilibrium, were apparently associated with overall and advanced prostate cancer [16]. However, two of these SNPs (rs17301608 and rs11639960) were examined, and their association was not confirmed when the results of this study were pooled with those from the prostate, lung, colorectal, and ovary cohort study; neither SNP was associated with prostate cancer [16].

The single-gene approach in association studies of polygenic diseases is likely to provide limited value in predicting risk. The combined analysis of genetic variants that interact in the same pathway may amplify the effects of individual polymorphisms and enhance the predictive power. To evaluate higher order gene–gene interaction, a study has examined the contribution of four gene polymorphisms of factors involved in angiogenesis (VEGF -1154G>A, VEGF 634G>C, MMP9 1562C>T, and TSP1 8831A>G) in combination to the risk of prostate cancer [17]. For the combined analysis of VEGF and MMP9 SNPs, it was found a significant gene–dosage effect for increasing numbers of potential high-risk genotypes. Compared to referent group (low-risk genotypes), individuals with one (OR = 2.79), two (OR = 4.57), and three high-risk genotypes (OR = 7.11) had increasingly elevated risks (OR, odd ratio) of prostate cancer [17]. Similarly, gene–gene interaction of VEGF and thrombospondin-1 (TSP1) polymorphisms increased the risk of prostate cancer in additive manner (OR = 6.00, $P = 0.03$), although the TSP1 polymorphism itself was not associated with the risk [17]. In addition, the analysis of the synergistic effect of these polymorphisms, in relation to prostate cancer prognosis according to histopathological grade and clinical stage at diagnosis, revealed potential higher order gene–gene interactions between VEGF and TSP1 polymorphisms in increasing the risk of developing an aggressive phenotype disease [17]. Patients carrying three high-risk genotypes showed a 20-fold increased risk of high-grade tumor (OR = 20.75). These results suggest that the interaction between polymorphic genes increase the risk of prostate cancer and its aggressiveness [17].

Another study evaluated the role of the functional VEGF polymorphisms as genetic markers for prostate cancer susceptibility and prognosis. The study included 101 patients with prostate cancer and 100 age-matched healthy men. The VEGF genotypes -1154G>A were identified by allele-specific polymerase chain reaction, and the genotypes -634G>C and 936C>T were identified by restriction fragment length polymorphism-polymerase chain reaction [18]. The study found a negative association between VEGF -1154G>A genotype and prostate cancer risk (OR = 0.27). Furthermore, the presence of the VEGF -1154A allele appeared to be associated with an increased risk of higher tumor grade (OR = 0.37) [18]. A significant increased risk of prostate cancer was associated with the VEGF -634 (GC + CC) combined genotype (OR = 1.95). The VEGF -634C allele was associated with the aggressive phenotype of prostate cancer as defined by the high histological grade (OR = 3.48). On the contrary, the VEGF -1154A/-634G haplotype was negatively associated with prostate cancer risk (OR = 0.48) and high tumor grade compared to low grade (OR = 0.37) [18]. Therefore, in this study, genetic variations in the VEGF may predict not only prostate cancer risk but also tumor aggressiveness [18] (Table 21.1).

A study investigated the potential association between DNA sequence variations in VEGF –460 gene region and occurrence of sporadic prostate cancer patients in the Turkish population. Two cohorts of 133 sporadic prostate cancer patients and 157 healthy controls were examined. Genotypes were determined by restriction fragment length polymorphism-polymerase chain reaction analysis. The distribution of genotype and allele frequencies of the polymorphism did not

Table 21.1 VEGF polymorphisms and prostate cancer

Polymorphisms	Risk (OR)		References
101 Patients vs. 74 controls			
-1154**G**[a]>A plus MMP9 1562C>**T**	1 Risk genotype	(2.79)	[17]
-634G>**C**	2 Risk genotypes	(4.57)	
	3 Risk genotypes	(7.11)	
Plus TSP1 8831A>**G**	3 Risk genotypes	(20.75)	
101 Patients vs. 100 controls			
-1154**G**>A	AA genotype	(0.27)	[18]
	-1154A/-634G	(0.37)	
-634G>**C**	GC + CC 1.95		
133 Patients vs. 157 controls			
-460C>T	No association		[19]
247 Patients vs. 263 controls			
-1154**G**>A	AA genotype	(0.45)	[20]
IL8 251A>**T**	TT genotype	(0.66)	
IL10 1082**A**>G	AA genotype	(1.78[b])	
64 Controls			
–2578C>A, –2498C>T, –1498C>T, –634G>C, –7C>T, 936C>T, 1612G>A	No association		[21]

[a]In boldface, high risk alleles

[b]Associated with PSA levels

show a statistically significant difference between patients and controls [19]. Furthermore, classification of patients by tumor-lymph nodes-metastasis stage, Gleason scores, and PSA levels did not demonstrate significant differences among the VEGF –460C>T genotypes. This negative study demonstrated that the VEGF –460C>T polymorphism in men is not associated with sporadic prostate cancer at least in the Turkish population [19].

Polymorphisms in the promoter regions of cytokine genes may influence prostate cancer development *via* regulation of the antitumor immune response and/or pathways of tumor angiogenesis. Prostate cancer patients (247) and 263 healthy controls were genotyped for interleukin (IL)-1β 511C>T, IL-8 251A>T, IL-10 1082A>G, tumor necrosis factor (TNF)-α 308A>G, and VEGF -1154A>G single nucleotide polymorphisms [20]. IL-8 TT and VEGF AA genotypes were decreased in patients compared with controls (23.9 versus 32.3%, OR=0.66 and 6.3 versus 12.9%, OR=0.45, respectively), whereas the IL-10 AA genotype was significantly increased in patients compared with controls (31.6 versus 20.6%, OR=1.78) [20]. Stratification according to prognostic indicators showed significant association between IL-8 genotype and log PSA level. Therefore, these results suggest that single nucleotide polymorphisms associated with differential production of IL-8, IL-10, and VEGF are risk factors for prostate cancer, possibly acting via their influence on angiogenesis [20].

A haplotype represents a linear arrangement of alleles at different SNPs on a single chromosome, or part of a chromosome. The pair of haplotypes is called a diplotype and the observed phenotype of a diplotype is called a genotype. A case–control study addressed the role of VEGF single nucleotide polymorphisms and haplotypes in prostate cancer by including 702 prostate cancer patients and 702 male age-matched healthy control subjects. Seven VEGF candidate polymorphisms (–2578C>A, –2498C>T, –1498C>T, –634G>C, –7C>T, 936C>T, and 1612GA) were determined and VEGF plasma levels and genotypes were analyzed in a group of 64 healthy men [21]. Haplotype analysis showed two separate blocks of high-linkage disequilibrium, formed by five polymorphisms upstream of the coding sequence (–2578C>A, –2498C>T, –1498C>T, –634G>C, and –7C>T) and two polymorphisms downstream of the coding sequence (936C>T and 1612G>A). None of the single polymorphisms or haplotypes was significantly associated with the presence of prostate cancer [21]. In a multivariate regression analysis including age, VEGF genotypes, and haplotypes as covariates and VEGF plasma level as dependent variable, none of the VEGF polymorphisms or haplotypes was a significant predictor of VEGF plasma levels [21]. The present data suggest that polymorphisms or haplotypes in the VEGF gene do not modify the risk of prostate cancer [21].

Genetic Variants of Endostatin Gene and Prostate Cancer

Endostatin is an important molecule and one of the most potent inhibitors of angiogenesis. Lower level or impaired function of endostatin is associated with a higher risk of developing malignant solid tumors and with a worse prognosis of the disease. The missense change D104N (aspartic acid [D] to asparagine [N]), which corresponds to amino acid position 1437 and nucleotide 4349G>A of the cDNA medium form of collagen XVIII, leads to the creation of a restriction site for MseI [22]. The association study between the coding single nucleotide polymorphism (D104N) in endostatin and prostate cancer revealed that heterozygous N104 individuals have a 2.5 times increased chance of developing prostate cancer as compared with homozygous D104 subjects (OR, 2.4). Modeling of the endostatin mutant showed that the N104 protein is stable [22]. These results together with the observation that residue 104 is evolutionary conserved suggest that: (a) the DNA segment containing this residue might include a novel interaction site to a yet unknown receptor and (b) the presence of N104 impairs the function of endostatin [22].

The same D104N polymorphism was analyzed in the tissues from 98 Caucasian prostate cancer patients. The frequencies of homozygous 4349G/G (104D/D) and heterozygous 4349G/A (104D/N) were 83.67% and 16.33%, respectively; no individuals were found to be homozygous for 4349A/A (104N/N) [23]. Analyses of genotype frequencies by Fisher's exact test showed that the genotype of D104N was not significantly related to tumor grade, PSA, and clinical stage [23]. There was no difference in relapse-free survival or overall survival between patients with 104D/N and those with 104D/D. The study concluded

Table 21.2 Endostatin, HIF, MMP1 and TNF polymorphisms and prostate cancer

Gene	Polymorphisms	Risk (OR)	References
Endostatin	*181 Patients vs. 198 controls*	DN heterozygous (2.4)	[22]
	4349G>**A** (D104**N**)		
	98 Patients	No association	[23]
	4349G>**A** (D104**N**)		
HIF	*1,072 Patients vs. 1271 controls*	No association	[25]
	P582S (C>T), A588T (G>A)		
MMP1	*55 Patients vs. 43 controls*	No association	[31]
	-1607insG (1G/2G)		
TNF	*2,321 Patients vs. 2560 controls*	No association	[32]
	rs1799964, rs1800630		
	rs1799724, rs1800629		
	rs361525, rs1800610		

In boldface, high risk alleles

that endostatin polymorphism was not associated with the aggressiveness of prostate cancer in Caucasian patients [23] (Table 21.2).

Genetic Variants of HIF Gene and Prostate Cancer

HIF-1α regulates cellular responses to hypoxia and is rapidly degraded under normoxia through von Hippel-Lindau (VHL) mediated ubiquitination. Although HIF-1α stabilization appears to be the molecular basis for VHL-associated cancers, stabilizing mutations in HIF-1α have not been reported. A study examined metastatic androgen-independent prostate cancers for mutations in the oxygen-dependent domain (ODD) of HIF-1α by PCR amplification and DNA sequencing [24]. A somatic proline to serine mutation in codon 582 (P582S) was identified in one sample. Transfection studies with a HIF-1α regulated reporter gene showed increased transcriptional activity that correlated with higher mutant HIF-1α protein expression [24]. It was found that increased expression of the P582S mutant induced by iron chelation, which blocks proline hydroxylation of wild-type HIF-1α, was markedly attenuated. The mutant also showed increased stability under normoxic versus hypoxic conditions. The P582S HIF-1α is a stable variant and HIF-1α mutation is a mechanism for enhancing HIF-1α activity in human cancer. Therefore, this variant may increase tumor susceptibility or cause more aggressive biological behavior [24].

A second study examined a cohort of prostate cancer patients ($n = 1,072$ incident cases) and 1,271 controls

for the prevalence of two nonsynonymous polymorphisms (P582S C>T and A588T G>A) in the coding region of HIF-1α gene, which have been associated with enhanced stability of the protein and androgen-independent prostate cancer. The study also investigated the levels of insulin-like growth factor binding protein (IGFBP)-3, which is more abundantly expressed in hypoxia-related inflammatory angiogenesis and recent in vivo data suggest that IGFBP-3 has direct IGF-independent inhibitory effects on angiogenesis [25]. Neither the P582S nor the A588T polymorphism was associated with the risk of overall or metastatic/fatal prostate cancer. However, the study found that among men with the homozygous CC wildtype (but not CT/TT) of the HIF-1α P582S, higher IGFBP-3 levels were associated with a 28% lower risk of overall prostate cancer and a 53% lower risk of metastatic and fatal prostate cancer [25]. The occurrence of A588T polymorphism in the population of patients enrolled in this study was too rare to assess interactions. Therefore, the two HIF-1α gene polymorphisms selected in this study were not directly associated with prostate cancer, although the authors suggested that the interaction between the P582S polymorphism and IGFBP-3 merits further evaluation in mechanistic studies [25].

Genetic Variants of PDGF and PDGFR Gene and Prostate Cancer

Although there are no studies published thus far on the role of genetic variants of PDGF and PDGFR-α/-β in the progression of prostate cancer, several direct evidences are in favor of its involvement. Therefore, variability in PDGF production or PDGFR expression may play an important role in prostate cancer biology.

In vitro, prostate carcinoma cell lines DU-145 and PC-3 express both PDGFR-α and PDGFR-β genes. Concomitantly, these cells synthesize and secrete PDGF-like proteins [26]. Both DU-145 and PC-3 cell lines appear to lack receptors for PDGF as indicated by their inability to mitogenically respond to PDGF and receptor binding of ^{125}I-labeled PDGF [26]. Production of PDGF-like proteins by human prostate carcinoma cells may play an important role in a paracrine mode in the organization of the extracellular matrix of the malignant tissue and stimulate the development of angiogenesis [26].

A study analyzed the combined VEGF (SU5416) and PDGF (SU6668) receptor tyrosine kinase inhibition with irradiation in human endothelial (HUVEC) and prostate cancer (PC3) cells in vitro and in vivo. Combined inhibition of VEGF and PDGF signaling resulted in enhanced apoptosis, reduced cell proliferation, and clonogenic survival as well as reduced endothelial cell migration and tube formation compared with single pathway inhibition. These effects were further enhanced by additional irradiation. Likewise, in PC3 tumors grown subcutaneously (s.c.) on BALB/c nu/nu mice, dual inhibition of VEGF and PDGF signaling significantly increased tumor growth delay than in each monotherapy. Radiation at approximately 20% of the dose necessary to induce local tumor control exerts similar tumor growth-inhibitory effects as the antiangiogenic drugs given at their maximum effective dose. Addition of radiotherapy to both mono- as well as dual-antiangiogenic treatments markedly increased tumor growth delay. With respect to tumor angiogenesis, radiation further decreased microvessel density (CD31 count) and tumor cell proliferation (Ki-67 index) in all drug-treated groups. Of note, the slowly growing PC3 tumor responded well to the antiangiogenic drug treatments. Interestingly, radiation induced up-regulation of all four isoforms of PDGF in endothelial cells resulting in a prosurvival effect of radiation. The addition of SU6668 attenuated this undesirable paracrine radiation effect, which may rationalize the combined application of radiation with PDGF signaling inhibition to increase antitumor effects in prostate cancer [27].

The factors regulating the bone tropism of disseminated prostate cancer cells are still vaguely defined.

Prostate cancer cells that metastasize to the skeleton respond to human bone marrow with a robust stimulation of the phosphatidylinositol 3-kinase/Akt pathway, whereas prostate cells that lack bone-metastatic potential respond negligibly [28]. The majority of this Akt activation is dependent on PDGFRα signaling. Low concentrations of PDGF-AA and PDGF-BB found in bone marrow aspirates do not account for the high levels of PDGFRα signaling. Additionally, neutralization of PDGF binding using PDGFRα-specific antibody failed to produce a significant inhibition of bone marrow-induced Akt activation [28]. However, the inhibitory effect of the antibody antagonized that of AG1296. The study concluded that PDGFRα is activated by multiple soluble factors contained within human bone marrow, in addition to its natural ligands, and this trans-activation is dependent on receptor localization to the plasma membrane. Therefore, PDGFRα expression may provide selected prostate phenotypes with a growth advantage within the bone microenvironment [28].

To further assess the role of PDGF and its receptors in cancer biology and aggressiveness, a study selected multidrug-resistant human PC-3MM2 prostate cancer cells (PC-3MM2-MDR cells) by culturing them in increasing concentrations of paclitaxel [29]. PC-3MM2-MDR cells were implanted orthotopically into one tibia of 80 nude mice. Two weeks later, the mice were randomly assigned to receive vehicle control, paclitaxel, imatinib (an inhibitor of PDGFR), or imatinib plus paclitaxel for 10 weeks. The results showed that PC-3MM2-MDR cells were resistant to paclitaxel and imatinib in vitro [29]. Treatment of implanted mice with imatinib plus paclitaxel led to statistically significant decreases in bone tumor incidence, median tumor weight, bone lysis, and the incidence of lymph node metastasis. Treatment with imatinib alone had similar effects, and imatinib treatment also inhibited phosphorylation of PDGFR on tumor cells and tumor-associated endothelial cells and increased the level of apoptosis of endothelial cells, but not tumor cells [29]. Treatment with imatinib alone or in combination with paclitaxel decreased mean vessel density, which was followed by apoptosis of tumor cells. These interesting results provide evidence that tumor-associated endothelial cells, rather than tumor cells themselves, appear to be the target for imatinib in prostate cancer bone metastasis [29].

Despite these promising preclinical data, the crucial issue is the selection of patients who may benefit from treatment with anti-PDGFR drugs. A study characterized the expression of PDGFR-β in a wide spectrum of prostate cancer samples to provide a rational basis to treatment strategy [30]. A survey of five published prostate expression array studies, including 100 clinically localized prostate cancers, did not identify tumors with increased PDGFR-β expression level. Protein expression of PDGFR-β, as determined by immunohistochemistry, revealed 5% of clinically localized prostate cancers and 16% of metastatic prostate cancer cases to show moderate or strong expression [30]. To develop a strategy to detect patients most likely to benefit from anti-PDGF treatment, cDNA expression array data from 10,000 transcripts for PDGFR-β expression were examined and tumors were stratified based on PDGFR-β expression level [30]. Performing a supervised analysis to identify potential comarkers of PDGFR-β in prostate cancer, a set of genes were identified whose expression was associated with PDGFR-β status including early growth response 1 (Egr1), an upstream effector of PDGF (4.2-fold upregulation), alpha-methylacyl-CoA racemase, as well as v-Maf and neuroblastoma suppressor of tumorigenicity (both with a 2.2-fold downregulation) [30]. This study suggests that only a small subset of prostate cancers is likely to benefit from treatment with tyrosine kinase inhibitors of PDGFR.

Genetic Variants of MMP and TNF Gene and Prostate Cancer

Metalloproteinase-1 (MMP1) promoter displays polymorphic variants (1G/2G); this variation is a single nucleotide polymorphism (SNP) located at −1607 bp, where an insertion of a guanine base (G) creates the sequence of 5′-GGAT-3′, the core binding site for members of the Ets family of transcription factors. A study on prostate carcinoma risk in the Turkish population analyzed a small cohort of 55 prostate cancer patients and 43 healthy controls and demonstrated that the frequency of 1G/2G genotypes in prostate cancer patients was similar to that of the controls [31]. Compared with the 1G/1G genotype, neither the 2G/2G nor a combination with the 1G/2G genotype significantly modified the risk of developing prostate cancer and metastasis. In addition, the frequencies of genotypes were not significantly different among patients

stratified by family history of prostate cancer [31]. Therefore, the 2G allele of the MMP1 promoter polymorphism does not apparently modify the risk of prostate cancer, at least in the Turkish population [31] although these data should be taken with caution owing to the small cohort of patients examined.

Inflammation has been hypothesized to increase prostate cancer risk. Tumor necrosis factor (TNF) is an important mediator of the inflammatory process, but the relationship between TNF variants and prostate cancer remains unclear. Therefore, a study investigated the associations between TNF single nucleotide polymorphisms (rs1799964, rs1800630, rs1799724, rs1800629, rs361525, rs1800610) and prostate cancer risk among 2,321 cases and 2,560 controls from two nested case-control studies within the Prostate, Lung, Colorectal, and Ovarian (PLCO) Cancer Screening Trial and the Cancer Prevention Study II Nutrition Cohort [32]. No TNF SNP was associated with prostate cancer risk in PLCO, while in the Nutrition Cohort, associations were significant for two highly correlated variants (rs1799724 and rs1800610) [32]. In pooled analyses, no single SNP was associated with prostate cancer risk. After adjustment for multiple testing, no SNP was associated with prostate cancer risk in either cohort individually or in the pooled analysis [32]. Haplotypes based on five TNF SNPs did not vary by case/control status in PLCO but showed marginal associations in the Nutrition Cohort. Therefore, despite some results are suggestive of a borderline role of haplotype, overall no firm association has been found between TNF variants and prostate cancer risk [32].

Conclusions

The development and progression of prostate cancer has biologically and genetically bases that remained a mystery. A man's risk of developing prostate cancer is influenced by both genetic and environmental factors. Single nucleotide polymorphisms in angiogenesis-dependent genes may affect to some extent the individual predisposition to developing cancer and may also affect disease progression. Polymorphisms in the angiogenic genes/factors may in part explain the variation in tumor angiogenesis observed among individuals. However, angiogenesis is a multifactorial process regulated by a plethora of factors and attempts to correlate prostate cancer risk and progression to specific angiogenic genotypes have been disappointing, although these studies have had the merit of having increased our knowledge on the biology of this complex disease. Well designed, large case–control studies are necessary to establish associations between polymorphisms and cancer, but as yet there are few such studies. Individual polymorphisms, even if proven to be functional, may only contribute to (and not solely determine) the heritable variation in protein levels and/or function. Many protein molecules acting along different carcinogenic pathways influence the development and spread of tumors, and hence the final outcome. It is therefore possible that specific combinations of polymorphisms within one or several genes will have a greater impact on the final phenotype than the individual polymorphisms.

At the present time, polymorphisms in the VEGF, MMP and PA system and TNF genes seem to be promising in the quest for markers influencing the severity and extent of tumor angiogenesis. In parallel with the search for functional polymorphisms in angiogenesis related genes, epidemiological studies to detect associations of gene polymorphisms with disease phenotypes are desired.

References

1. van Moorselaar RJ, Voest EE. Angiogenesis in prostate cancer: its role in disease progression and possible therapeutic approaches. Mol Cell Endocrinol 2002;197:239–50.
2. Longoria RL, Cox MC, Figg WD. Antiangiogenesis: a possible treatment option for prostate cancer? Clin Genitourin Cancer 2005;4:197–202.
3. Aragon-Ching JB, Dahut WL. The role of angiogenesis inhibitors in prostate cancer. Cancer J 2008;14:20–5.
4. Di Lorenzo G, Figg WD, Fossa SD, et al. Combination of bevacizumab and docetaxel in docetaxel-pretreated hormone-refractory prostate cancer: a phase 2 study. Eur Urol 2008;54:1089–94.
5. Figg WD, Dahut W, Duray P, et al. A randomized phase II trial of thalidomide, an angiogenesis inhibitor, in patients with androgen-independent prostate cancer. Clin Cancer Res 2001;7:1888–93.
6. Figg WD, Arlen P, Gulley J, et al. A randomized phase II trial of docetaxel (taxotere) plus thalidomide in androgen-independent prostate cancer. Semin Oncol 2001;28:62–6.
7. Dahut WL, Gulley JL, Arlen PM, et al. Randomized phase II trial of docetaxel plus thalidomide in androgen-independent prostate cancer. J Clin Oncol 2004;22:2532–9.
8. Aragon-Ching JB, Li H, Gardner ER, Figg WD. Thalidomide analogues as anticancer drugs. Recent Patents Anticancer Drug Discov 2007;2:167–74.
9. Shah SR, Tran TM. Lenalidomide in myelodysplastic syndrome and multiple myeloma. Drugs 2007;67:1869–81.
10. Wilhelm S, Carter C, Lynch M, et al. Discovery and development of sorafenib: a multikinase inhibitor for treating cancer. Nat Rev Drug Discov 2006;5:835–44.
11. Steinbild S, Mross K, Frost A, et al. A clinical phase II study with sorafenib in patients with progressive hormone-refractory prostate cancer: a study of the CESAR Central European Society for Anticancer Drug Research-EWIV. Br J Cancer 2007;97:1480–5.
12. Chi KN, Ellard SL, Hotte SJ, et al. A phase II study of sorafenib in patients with chemo-naive castration-resistant prostate cancer. Ann Oncol 2008;19:746–51.
13. Dahut WL, Scripture C, Posadas E, et al. A phase II clinical trial of sorafenib in androgen-independent prostate cancer. Clin Cancer Res 2008;14:209–14.
14. Ryan CJ, Stadler WM, Roth B, et al. Phase I dose escalation and pharmacokinetic study of AZD2171, an inhibitor of the vascular endothelial growth factor receptor tyrosine kinase, in patients with hormone refractory prostate cancer (HRPC). Invest New Drugs 2007;25:445–51.
15. Balasubramanian SP, Brown NJ, Reed MW. Role of genetic polymorphisms in tumour angiogenesis. Br J Cancer 2002;87:1057–65.
16. Jacobs EJ, Hsing AW, Bain EB, et al. Polymorphisms in angiogenesis-related genes and prostate cancer. Cancer Epidemiol Biomarkers Prev 2008;17:972–7.
17. Sfar S, Saad H, Mosbah F, Chouchane L. Combined effects of the angiogenic genes polymorphisms on prostate cancer susceptibility and aggressiveness. Mol Biol Rep 2009;36(1):37–45.
18. Sfar S, Hassen E, Saad H, Mosbah F, Chouchane L. Association of VEGF genetic polymorphisms with prostate carcinoma risk and clinical outcome. Cytokine 2006;35:21–8.
19. Onen IH, Konac E, Eroglu M, Guneri C, Biri H, Ekmekci A. No association between polymorphism in the vascular endothelial growth factor gene at position -460 and sporadic prostate cancer in the Turkish population. Mol Biol Rep 2008;35:17–22.
20. McCarron SL, Edwards S, Evans PR, et al. Influence of cytokine gene polymorphisms on the development of prostate cancer. Cancer Res 2002;62:3369–72.
21. Langsenlehner T, Langsenlehner U, Renner W, et al. Single nucleotide polymorphisms and haplotypes in the gene for vascular endothelial growth factor and risk of prostate cancer. Eur J Cancer 2008;44:1572–6.
22. Iughetti P, Suzuki O, Godoi PH, et al. A polymorphism in endostatin, an angiogenesis inhibitor, predisposes for the development of prostatic adenocarcinoma. Cancer Res 2001;61:7375–8.
23. Li HC, Cai QY, Shinohara ET, et al. Endostatin polymorphism 4349G/A(D104N) is not associated with aggressiveness of disease in prostate cancer. Dis Markers 2005;21:37–41.
24. Fu XS, Choi E, Bubley GJ, Balk SP. Identification of hypoxia-inducible factor-1alpha (HIF-1alpha) polymorphism as a mutation in prostate cancer that prevents normoxia-induced degradation. Prostate 2005;63:215–21.
25. Li H, Bubley GJ, Balk SP, et al. Hypoxia-inducible factor-1alpha (HIF-1alpha) gene polymorphisms, circulating

insulin-like growth factor binding protein (IGFBP)-3 levels and prostate cancer. Prostate 2007;67:1354–61.

26. Sitaras NM, Sariban E, Bravo M, Pantazis P, Antoniades HN. Constitutive production of platelet-derived growth factor-like proteins by human prostate carcinoma cell lines. Cancer Res 1988;48:1930–5.

27. Timke C, Zieher H, Roth A, et al. Combination of vascular endothelial growth factor receptor/platelet-derived growth factor receptor inhibition markedly improves radiation tumor therapy. Clin Cancer Res 2008;14:2210–9.

28. Dolloff NG, Russell MR, Loizos N, Fatatis A. Human bone marrow activates the Akt pathway in metastatic prostate cells through transactivation of the alpha-platelet-derived growth factor receptor. Cancer Res 2007;67:555–62.

29. Kim SJ, Uehara H, Yazici S, et al. Targeting platelet-derived growth factor receptor on endothelial cells of multidrug-resistant prostate cancer. J Natl Cancer Inst 2006;98: 783–93.

30. Hofer MD, Fecko A, Shen R, et al. Expression of the platelet-derived growth factor receptor in prostate cancer and treatment implications with tyrosine kinase inhibitors. Neoplasia 2004;6:503–12.

31. Albayrak S, Canguven O, Goktas C, Aydemir H, Koksal V. Role of MMP-1 1G/2G promoter gene polymorphism on the development of prostate cancer in the Turkish population. Urol Int 2007;79:312–5.

32. Danforth KN, Rodriguez C, Hayes RB, et al. TNF polymorphisms and prostate cancer risk. Prostate 2008;68:400–7.

Part IV
Bone Metastasis

Chapter 22
Pathophysiology of Prostate Cancer Bone Metastasis

Evan T. Keller and Christopher L. Hall

Abstract Prostate cancer (CaP) is the most frequently diagnosed cancer in men and the second leading cause of cancer death among men in the United States. The most common site of CaP metastasis is the bone with skeletal metastases identified in virtually all patients dying from CaP. Skeletal metastasis in CaP patients results in bone pain, impaired mobility, pathological fracture, spinal cord compression, and symptomatic hypercalcemia. The mechanisms through which CaP metastasizes to and interacts with bone are not well-defined. There are both osteolytic and osteoblastic components of CaP metastasis. A variety of factors including receptor activator of NFkB ligand (RANKL), interleukin-6 (IL-6), matrix metalloproteinases (MMPs), and parathyroid hormone-related protein (PTHrP) have been implicated in the osteolytic activity of CaP. In terms of osteoblastic metastasis, many proteins including bone morphogenetic proteins (BMPs), Wnts, and endothelin-1 (ET-1) have been implicated as CaP-produced osteoblastic factors. Once in the bone microenvironment, the CaP cells interact with the bone resulting in an overall balance that shifts the CaP from an osteolytic to an osteoblastic activity. Understanding the mechanisms through which CaP metastasizes and interacts with bone will hopefully lead to therapies for CaP bone metastasis.

Keywords Prostate cancer • Bone metastasis • RANKL • Bone morphogenetic protein

E.T. Keller (✉)
Department of Urology, University of Michigan,
Ann Arbor, MI, USA
e-mail: etkeller@umich.edu

Introduction

Prostate cancer (CaP) is the most frequently diagnosed cancer in men and the second leading cause of cancer death among men in the United States [1]. The most common site of CaP metastasis is the bone with skeletal metastases identified in virtually all patients dying from CaP [2]. Skeletal metastasis in CaP patients results in bone pain, impaired mobility, pathological fracture, spinal cord compression, and symptomatic hypercalcemia [3]. Significant advances in the diagnosis and management of primary CaP have been made that have improved cure rates; however, once disease becomes advanced, it remains incurable. In the case of metastatic disease, most therapies are palliative and include hormonal therapy, pharmacological management of bone pain, radiotherapy for pain and spinal cord compression. It is critical that a solid understanding of the pathophysiology of CaP skeletal metastatic process is developed to provide the basis for creating strategies to prevent or diminish their occurrence and associated complications.

Bone Biology

An understanding of the basic components and functions of bone is critical to provide a basis for understanding bone metastasis. The skeleton functions as a framework for the body, the main site for hematopoiesis, a reservoir for calcium, and a structure for muscle attachments. The skeleton is divided into the appendicular skeleton consisting of the limbs and the axial skeleton consisting of the skull, vertebral column, ribs, and sternum. The skeleton is a dynamic organ and is constantly

W.D. Figg et al. (eds.), *Drug Management of Prostate Cancer*,
DOI 10.1007/978-1-60327-829-4_22, © Springer Science+Business Media, LLC 2010

remodeling in response to stress placed on it [4]. A typical bone consists of both a cortical (also known as compact bone) component and a trabecular (also known as spongy or cancellous bone) component (Fig. 22.1). Cortical bone is made of concentric layers of bone that forms a hard outer shell and typically found in the shafts of appendicular bone. Trabecular bone consists of struts of bone found within the concentric bone shell and found in through the metaphyses and epiphyses of bones.

Bone is a very active substance that is composed of mineralized and nonmineralized components [5]. Collagen is the main protein constituent of the unmineralized extracellular matrix (also known as osteoid) and is considered to provide the framework for mineralization. Other proteins that contribute to the osteoid include osteopontin, bone sialoprotein (BSP), osteonectin, and alkaline phosphatase (BAP) [6, 7]. Bone mineral consists of primarily calcium and phosphate that forms an organized crystalline structure called hydroxyapatite. When bone is initially formed, the collagen fibers are laid down in a disorganized interwoven fashion forming what is termed as woven bone [8]. As bone matures, the collagen fibrils become lined up in a parallel fashion forming lamellar bone [9]. Woven bone is not as strong in terms of biomechanical properties as lamellar bone [10]. As bone becomes more mineralized, its strength increases up to a point, but

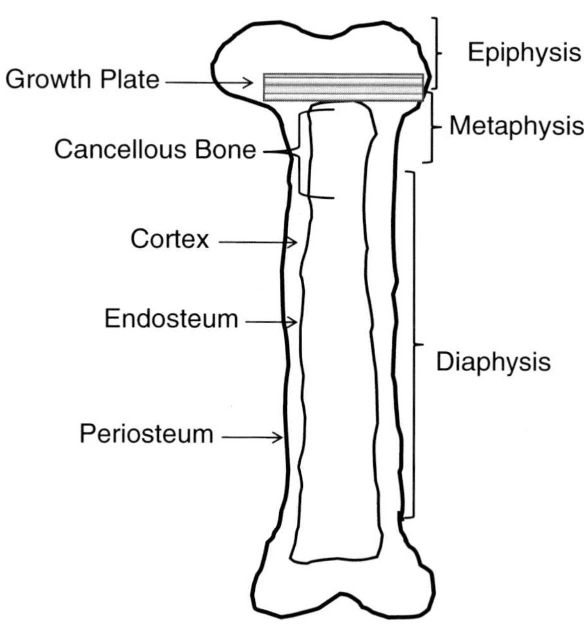

Fig. 22.1 Anatomy of bone. Longitudinal section of a long bone

further mineralization beyond an optimal level reduces bone elasticity leading to the inability of the bone to respond to certain stresses which then results in fragile bone that is predisposed to fracture [11].

The key cells that are involved in bone production and remodeling are the osteoblasts and osteoclasts. Osteoblasts are the cells that lay down collagen matrix and promote mineralization. Osteoblast production requires specific transcription factors. RUNX2 (also called Cbfa1 and OSF2), a member of the runt/Cbfa family of transcription factors, was first identified as the nuclear protein binding to an osteoblast-specific cis-acting element activating the expression of osteocalcin [12]. RUNX2 was shown to regulate the expression of all the major genes expressed by osteoblasts and be a key regulator of osteoblast differentiation in vivo [13].

As opposed to osteoblasts that produce mineralized matrix, osteoclasts are multinucleated cells responsible for bone resorption that dissolve the mineralized hydroxyapatite and degrade nonmineralized bone matrix [14]. They are derived from the colony-forming unit granulocyte-macrophage (CFU-GM) hematopoietic precursor cells. Several factors promote osteoclastogenesis including growth factors and cytokines. Both colony stimulating factor (CSF-1) and interleukins-1 and -6 (IL-1 and IL-6) expand the osteoclast precursor pool. TNF-alpha promotes conversion of the promonocyte to a committed osteoclast precursor [15].

Although several factors promote osteoclastogenesis, one factor that is required for production of mature osteoclasts is receptor activator of nuclear factor kappa B ligand (RANKL). A member of the tumor necrosis factor family, RANKL is initially expressed by bone marrow stromal cells, osteoblasts, and activated-T cells. RANKL is most commonly a membrane anchored molecule; however, a small fraction of RANKL is released through proteolytic cleavage from the cell surface as a soluble 245 amino acid homotrimeric molecule (sRANKL) [16]. Both soluble and membrane bound RANKL promote osteoclast formation and activation by binding to RANK on the osteoclast precursor membrane that has the characteristics of a monocyte [17]. RANKL binding to RANK induces NFkappaB and Fos activation [18].

In addition to RANKL and RANK, another key modulator of osteoclastogenesis is osteoprotegerin (OPG) (also known as osteoclastogenesis inhibitory factor-OCIF) [19, 20]. OPG serves as a decoy receptor that binds RANKL and thus blocks its ability to bind to

RANK and induce osteoclastogenesis. In contrast to RANKL and RANK, whose expression is mainly restricted at low levels to the skeletal and immune systems, OPG is expressed in a variety of tissues, such as liver, lung, heart, kidney, stomach, intestines, skin, and calvaria in mice and lung, heart, kidney, and placenta in humans. In bone, OPG is mainly produced by osteoblastic lineage cells, and its expression increases as the cells become more differentiated [21]. Several factors including, 1,25-dihydroxyvitamin D3, interleukin-1-β (IL-1-β), tumor necrosis factor-α (TNF-α), and bone morphogenetic protein 2 (BMP-2) induce OPG mRNA expression in human osteoblast cell lines [22]. Administration of recombinant OPG to normal rodents resulted in increased bone mass [19] and completely prevented ovariectomy-induced bone loss without apparent adverse skeletal and extraskeletal side effects [19]. It appears that the balance of the ratio of RANKL to OPG is very important in controlling the overall activity (i.e., lysis vs. no lysis) that will be observed.

When initiating bone resorption, osteoclasts become polarized, and three distinct membrane domains appear: a ruffled border, a sealing zone, and a functional secretory domain [14]. The actin cytoskeleton forms an attachment ring at the sealing zone that anchors the osteoclast to the bone matrix. The ruffled border appears inside the sealing zone and vesicle transport to the ruffled border delivers hydrochloric acid and proteases to an area between the ruffled border and the bone surface called the resorption lacuna [14]. In this extracellular compartment, crystalline hydroxyapatite is dissolved by acid, and a mixture of proteases degrades the organic matrix. The degradation products of collagen and other matrix components are endocytosed, transported through the cell, and exocytosed through a functional secretory domain [23].

Proteases that are important mediators of osteoclastic activity include cathepsin K and metalloproteinases. Cathepsin K can cleave bone proteins such as Type I collagen, osteopontin, and osteonectin [24]. Overexpression of cathepsin K in the mouse results in accelerated bone turnover [25], whereas knockout of cathepsin K results in retarded bone matrix degradation and osteopetrosis [26]. In addition to the proteases, acid is secreted from osteoclasts to resorb the mineralized matrix. Acid is believed to be secreted through vacuolar H(+)-ATPase-dependent pumps present on the osteoclasts ruffled membranes [27]. Several hormones regulate acid secretion, including parathyroid hormone, which increases acid secretion and calcitonin, which decreases acid secretion. Carbonic anhydrase II appears to be an important mediator of acid production because acetazolamide, a carbonic anhydrase inhibitor-based diuretic, can block bone resorption [28]. Another diuretic, indapamide, increased osteoblast proliferation and decreased bone resorption, at least in part, by decreasing osteoclast differentiation via a direct effect on hematopoietic precursors in vitro [29].

Bone Remodeling

Bone remodeling is the cyclical replacement of old bone by new bone. Remodeling serves to maintain bones' mechanical stability and allows it to perform its metabolic actions. In each cycle, a defined volume of bone is removed by osteoclastic resorption and subsequently replaced by osteoblastic formation at the same location. Remodeling is carried out by elongated structures known as basic multicellular units (BMU; sometimes called bone metabolic units) that travel through or across the surface of bone. In the human, each BMU lasts about 6 months, with continued sequential recruitment of new osteoclasts and osteoblasts [30]. The BMU is initiated by osteoclasts resorbing old bone followed by osteoblasts synthesizing new bone in the resorption lacunae (areas resorbed by osteoclasts).

Osteoblastic Bone Metastases

Many functions contribute to the ability of CaP cells to target to bone including homing and attachment to bone and invasion into bone. Once in the bone, CaP skeletal metastases are most often characterized as radiographically osteoblastic (i.e., increased bone density on the radiograph) as opposed to osteolytic. Other tumors, such as breast cancer, can form osteoblastic lesions; however, these occur less frequently [31]. In spite of the radiographic osteoblastic appearance, it is clear from histological evidence that CaP metastases form a heterogeneous mixture of osteolytic and osteoblastic lesions although osteoblastic lesions are predominate [32]. Recent evidence shows that osteoblastic metastases form on trabecular bone at sites of previous osteoclastic resorption, and that such resorption may be required for subsequent osteoblastic bone formation [33]. These findings suggest that CaP induces bone production through an overall increase in bone remodeling, which in the nonpathologic state is a balance between osteoclast resorption of bone, followed by osteoblast-mediated replacement of resorbed bone. In the case of CaP, it appears the induction of osteoblast-mediated mineralization outweighs the increase in osteoclast resorption resulting in an overall formation of osteoblastic lesions. The osteoblastic lesions result in overall weakening of the bone due to the production of woven bone and hypermineralization. Thus, the combination of underlying osteolysis and production of weak bone leads to a predisposition to fracture. The mechanisms through which CaP cells promote bone mineralization remain poorly understood.

CaP cells produce a variety of factors that have direct or indirect osteogenic properties (Table 22.1). Some of these factors, such as bone morphogenetic proteins (BMP) [34] and enodothlin-1 (ET-1) [35] may directly stimulate differentiation of osteoblast precursors to mature mineral-producing osteoblasts. Other factors such as parathyroid hormone-related protein (PTHrP) may work through inhibition of osteoblast apoptosis [36]. Additionally, there are proteins that may work indirectly to enhance bone production, such as the serine proteases, prostate specific antigen (PSA), and urinary plasminogen activator (uPA), which can activate latent forms of osteogenic proteins, such as transforming growth factor-β (TFG-β) [37]. Finally, some molecules, such as osteoprotegerin (OPG) [38] and ET-1 (in a dual role with its osteoblast-stimulating activity) [39] can enhance osteosclerosis through inhibiting osteoclastogenesis. In spite of this gamut of putative mediators of CaP-induced osteosclerosis, the authors

Table 22.1 Osteogenic factors produced by prostate cancer cells

Factor	References
Bone morphogenetic proteins (BMP)	[34, 96]
Endothelin-1 (ET-1)	[97-100]
Insulin-like growth factors (IGF)	[101, 102]
Interleukin-1 and -6	[103, 104]
Osteoprotegerin (OPG)	[38, 105]
Parathyroid hormone-related peptide (PTHrP)	[36, 106]
Transforming growth factor-β (TFG-β)	[107]
Urinary plasminogen activator (urokinase)	[108]
Vascular endothelial growth factor (VEGF)	[109]
Wnts	[110]

are unaware of in vivo studies that unequivocally demonstrate their role in this process. The large number of factors suggest that several of these osteogenic factors work in concert to produce maximal bone production.

Osteoclastic Bone Metastases

Osteolytic activity is a key component of CaP bone metastasis and is regulated by a critical factor, RANKL. Several lines of evidence support the role of RANKL in prostate cancer-mediated osteolysis. Although a bone metastatic prostate cancer cell line has been shown to express OPG [40], that same line overexpresses RANKL [41]. Additionally, in normal prostate, OPG protein was detected in luminal, epithelial, and stromal cells (5–65% and 15–70%, respectively), and RANKL immunoreactivity was observed in 15–50% of basal epithelial cells, 40–90% of luminal epithelial cells, and 70–100% of stromal cells [42]. OPG was not detected in eight of ten primary CaP specimens, but RANKL was heterogeneously expressed in 10 of 11 CaP specimens [42]. Importantly, the percentage of tumor cells expressing OPG and RANKL was significantly increased in all CaP bone metastases compared with nonosseous metastases or primary CaP. The presence of RANKL in CaP tissues has been shown to indicate poor prognosis [43, 44]. Serum OPG levels are elevated in patients with advanced prostate cancer compared to less advanced prostate cancer [45]. In one study, serum RANKL levels were not altered, although the RANKL–OPG was altered in these patients due to changes in OPG [46]. It is possible that RANKL is only expressed locally at the skeletal metastatic site and therefore not detectable in the serum. Regardless, taken together, these observations suggest that the RANKL–OPG axis may play an important role in prostate cancer bone metastases. Further support for this possibility was demonstrated by the observation that administration of OPG prevented establishment of mixed osteoblastic/osteolytic prostate cancer cells in the bones of SCID mice, although it had no effect on establishment of subcutaneous tumors in the same mice [41]. However, in another study, OPG administration did not prevent establishment of an osteoblastic prostate cancer tumor although it slowed the tumor growth [47]. OPG also diminished the progression of established osteoblastic prostate cancer in human bone implants in mice [48]. Taken together, these studies suggest that OPG can inhibit prostate tumor growth in bone.

Matrix metalloproteinases (MMPs), a family of enzymes whose primary function is to degrade the extracellular matrix, play a role in bone remodeling. This activity occurs in the absence of osteoclasts [49] suggesting that MMPs have a direct resorptive effect. Several have the ability to degrade the nonmineralized matrix of bone including MMP1, MMP9, and MMP13, which are collagenases. Other MMPs such as stromelysin (MMP3) activate MMP1. Through their proteolytic activity, MMPs contribute to metastatic invasion, including destruction of bone [50].

Prostate carcinomas and their cell lines express a large number of MMPs. Levels of MMP9 secretion in primary prostate cancer cultures increased with Gleason histological grade [51]. Active MMP9 species were detected in 15 cultures (31%) of primary prostate cancer tissues. The presence of the mineralized matrix has been shown to induce MMP9 expression from prostate carcinoma cells [52]. MMP12 has been shown to be upregulated in CaP, and knockdown of MMP12 inhibited the ability of a CaP cell line perform in vitro invasion [53].

The initial functional data that suggested CaP bone metastasis modulate bone remodeling through MMPs was provided by in vitro studies. Specifically, blocking MMP activity with 1,10-phenanthroline, a MMP inhibitor, diminished bone matrix degradation induced by PC-3 cells in vitro [54, 55]. Matrilysin (MMP7) has been shown to be upregulated in DU-145 prostate cancer cells and can enhance their invasive ability. Monoclonal antibody targeting the cytokine interleukin-6 (IL-6) has been shown to increase promatrilysin expression in DU-145 cultures [56]. This suggests that IL-6, which is increased in prostate cancer (reviewed in [57]), enhances prostate cancer invasion through production of MMP-7.

The importance of MMPs in bone metastasis has been further confirmed in vivo. An MMP inhibitor, batimistat, has been shown to inhibit development bone resorption in vitro and in vivo in murine models of breast [58] and CaP [59]. The mechanism through which CaP-produced MMPs induce bone resorption is not clear; however, it appears to involve induction of osteoclastogenesis as inhibition of MMPs reduced the number of osteoclasts associated with prostate tumor growth in human bone implants in mice [59].

Additionally, the bisphosphonate alendronate blocked MMP production from PC-3 cells [60]. This was associated with diminished establishment of bone metastasis in mice injected with PC-3 tumors [49].

PTHrP, a protein with limited homology to parathyroid hormone (PTH), was originally identified as a tumor-derived factor responsible for humoral hypercalcemia of malignancy (HHM). PTH and PTHrP bind to the same receptor (the PTH-1 receptor) and evoke the same biological activity due to similarities in their steric configurations at the region of 25–34 amino acids. Patients with solid tumors and hypercalcemia have increased serum PTHrP in 80% of the cases, emphasizing the impact of this peptide to increase bone resorption and renal tubular resorption of calcium [61]. Subsequent to its characterization in HHM, PTHrP was found to be produced by many normal tissues including, epithelium, lactating mammary gland, and cartilage where it has an autocrine, paracrine, or intracrine role [61].

PTHrP is an attractive candidate for influencing CaP growth. PTHrP is produced by normal prostate epithelial cells, from which CaP arises and PTHrP is found in the seminal fluid [62, 63]. PTHrP has been immunohistochemically identified in prostate carcinoma tissue in patients with clinically localized disease [64], is found in higher levels in prostate intraepithelial neoplasia than in normal prostate epithelium, is found in higher levels in prostate carcinoma than in benign prostatic hyperplasia [65, 66], and is found in human metastatic lesions in bone [67]. However, in some studies, expression of PTHrP receptor in prostate cancer appears to be more consistent than expression of PTHrP itself [68]. Overexpression of ras oncogene in immortalized prostate epithelial cells has been shown to promote PTHrP expression [69]. This may account for the increased expression of PTHrP as the cells progress to a malignant phenotype.

There is evidence that PTHrP can act as an autocrine growth factor for CaP cells in vitro [62] although it does not affect proliferation of normal prostate cells [70]. PTHrP production by primary prostatic tumors is associated with increased tumor size and rate of growth in an animal model [67] suggesting that PTHrP acts in an autocrine or intracrine mechanism to promote tumor growth. In contrast, in this same model and in an intracardiac injection model of CaP, PTHrP was not associated with an increase in metastatic potential [67, 71]. This suggests that PTHrP is important in the bone microenvironment where target cells with receptors are present (osteoblasts); it may play a critical role in the bone response to CaP. PTHrP expression has been localized to CaP tissues demonstrating it is present in the bone microenvironment [72]. Overexpression of PTHrP in CaP cells has been shown to induce osteolytic lesions in the bone of rats [73] although the level of expression may not directly correlate with the degree of osteolysis [71]. PTHrP also promotes monocytes activity at CaP sites, which can induce osteolytic activity [74]. All these data suggest that PTHrP has a critical role in the local bone microenvironment of metastatic prostate carcinoma; but what this precise role is has yet to be determined.

IL-6 belongs to the "interleukin-6 type cytokine" family that also includes leukemia inhibitory factor, interleukin-11, ciliary neurotrophic factor, cardiotrophin-1, and oncostatin M [75]. Many physiologic functions are attributed to IL-6 including promotion of antibody production from B lymphocytes, modulation of hepatic acute phase reactant synthesis, promotion of osteoclastic-mediated bone resorption, and induction of thrombopoiesis [76]. IL-6 mediates its activity through the IL-6 receptor complex, which is composed of two components; an 80 Kd transmembrane receptor (IL-6Rp80, IL-6R, α-subunit) that specifically binds IL-6, but has no signaling capability and a 130 Kd membrane glycoprotein (gp130) that mediates signal transduction following IL-6R binding [77]. In addition to the transmembrane IL-6R, a soluble form of IL-6R (sIL-6R) exists that is produced by either proteolytic cleavage of the 80 kDa subunit [78, 79] or differential splicing of mRNA [80]. Although the sIL-6R does not possess a transmembrane component, it can still bind to IL-6 and the ligand bound sIL-6R·IL-6 complex activates signal transduction and biological responses through membrane-bound gp130 [81].

Multiple studies have demonstrated that IL-6 is elevated in the sera of patients with metastatic prostate cancer [82-84]. Adler et al. [82] demonstrated that serum levels of IL-6 and transforming growth factor-β1 are elevated in patients with metastatic prostate cancer, and that these levels correlate with tumor burden as assessed by serum PSA or clinically evident metastases. In a similar fashion, Drachenberg et al. [85] reported elevated serum IL-6 levels in men with castrate-resistant prostate cancer compared to normal controls, benign prostatic hyperplasia, prostatitis, and

localized or recurrent disease. In an animal model, prostate tumor cells injected next to human bones implanted in the limb of mice demonstrated IL-6 expression [86]. In addition to IL-6, the IL-6R has been identified in human normal prostate and prostate carcinoma tissue [87, 88].

The secretion of IL-6 by prostate cancer cells in the bone microenvironment may impact bone remodeling (reviewed in [89]). IL-6 promotes osteoclastogenesis [90] most likely through increasing osteoclastogenic precursors. IL-6-mediated osteoclastogenesis is directly related to the level of gp130 present on the precursor cells [91]. It appears that IL-6-mediated osteoclastogenesis is independent of promoting RANKL expression [92]. However, IL-6 has been shown to potentiate PTHrP-induced osteoclastogenesis [93, 94]. Administration of anti-IL-6 antibody has been shown to diminish the growth of subcutaneously injected prostate cancer cells in nude mice, thus demonstrating the potential utility of this compound in clinical prostate cancer [95]. These results strongly suggest that IL-6 may serve as a therapeutic target for the osteolytic component of prostate cancer skeletal metastases.

Summary

Bone metastasis is a frequent and debilitating complication of men with CaP. The bone provides a unique environment that both fosters the development of metastases and responds to the CaP cells resulting in aberrant bone production that results in clinical symptoms. The interaction between the CaP cells and bone is complex (summarized in Fig. 22.2). The CaP cells induce bone resorption, which promotes CaP growth and changes them to an osteoblastic-inducing phenotype. A variety of factors participate in the induction of bone resorption. It appears that RANKL is a key factor induced by CaP cells, which results in osteoclastogenesis. Additionally, a large number of CaP-produced factors have been implicated as being osteoblastic. Most likely, several factors work in unison to produce the overall osteoblastic phenotype. It is hoped that as we learn more about the pathophysiology of bone metastasis, we will be able to develop therapies to target this process.

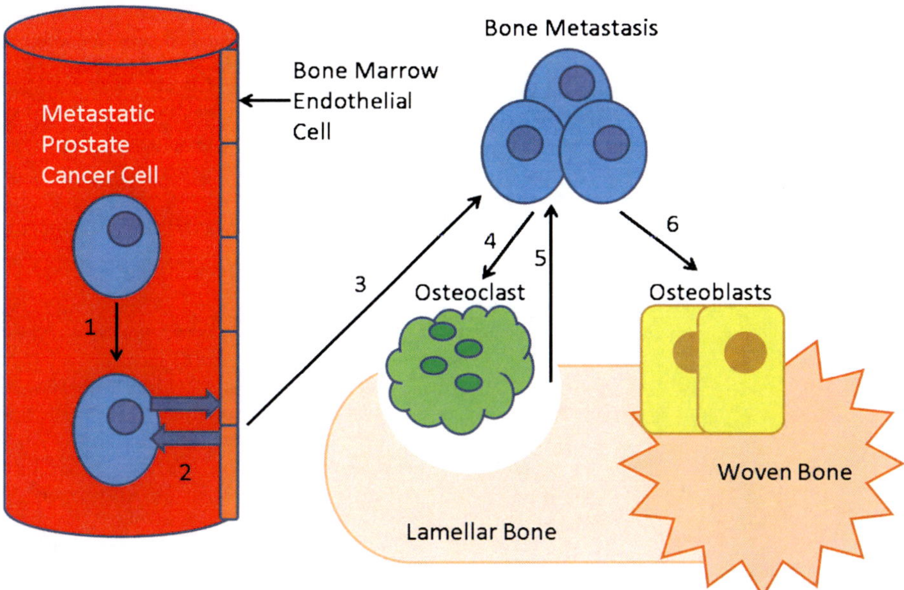

Fig. 22.2 Model of cross-talk between prostate carcinoma cells and the bone microenvironment. The bone produces chemotactic factors that attract prostate carcinoma cells to migrate (1) through the vascular system toward the skeleton. The bone marrow endothelial displays adhesion molecules that are complement those expressed by the prostate carcinoma cell, resulting in attachment of the cell (2). The prostate carcinoma cell extravasates and invades into the skeletal extracellular tissue (3), at which point it releases factors that stimulate osteoclastogenesis (4). The subsequent bone resorption is accompanied by release of growth factors that stimulate the prostate carcinoma proliferation (5). The progressing prostate carcinoma releases factors that promote osteoblast production and inhibit osteoblast apoptosis (6) resulting in production of woven bone and the characteristic osteosclerotic lesion. This process continues in a cyclical fashion with continued induction of osteoclastic activity, carcinoma cell proliferation, and bone production

References

1. Landis SH, Murray T, Bolden S, Wingo PA. Cancer statistics, 1999. CA Cancer J Clin 1999;49:8–31.
2. Shah RB, Mehra R, Chinnaiyan AM, et al. Androgen-independent prostate cancer is a heterogeneous group of diseases: lessons from a rapid autopsy program. Cancer Res 2004;64:9209–16.
3. Moul JW, Lipo DR. Prostate cancer in the late 1990s: hormone refractory disease options. Urol Nurs 1999;19: 125–31; quiz 32 3.
4. Augat P, Simon U, Liedert A, Claes L. Mechanics and mechano-biology of fracture healing in normal and osteoporotic bone. Osteoporos Int 2005;16(Suppl 2):S36–43.
5. Hasegawa K, Turner CH, Burr DB. Contribution of collagen and mineral to the elastic anisotropy of bone. Calcif Tissue Int 1994;55:381–6.
6. Pinero GJ, Farach-Carson MC, Devoll RE, Aubin JE, Brunn JC, Butler WT. Bone matrix proteins in osteogenesis and remodelling in the neonatal rat mandible as studied by immunolocalization of osteopontin, bone sialoprotein, alpha 2HS-glycoprotein and alkaline phosphatase. Arch Oral Biol 1995;40:145–55.
7. Romanowski R, Jundt G, Termine JD, von der Mark K, Schulz A. Immunoelectron microscopy of osteonectin and type I collagen in osteoblasts and bone matrix. Calcif Tissue Int 1990;46:353–60.
8. Oguma H, Murakami G, Takahashi-Iwanaga H, Aoki M, Ishii S. Early anchoring collagen fibers at the bone-tendon interface are conducted by woven bone formation: light microscope and scanning electron microscope observation using a canine model. J Orthop Res 2001;19:873–80.
9. Marotti G, Muglia MA, Palumbo C. Collagen texture and osteocyte distribution in lamellar bone. Ital J Anat Embryol 1995;100(Suppl 1):95–102.
10. Currey JD. The many adaptations of bone. J Biomech 2003;36:1487–95.
11. Currey JD. Tensile yield in compact bone is determined by strain, post-yield behaviour by mineral content. J Biomech 2004;37:549–56.
12. Schinke T, Karsenty G. Characterization of Osf1, an osteoblast-specific transcription factor binding to a critical cis-acting element in the mouse Osteocalcin promoters. J Biol Chem 1999;274:30182–9.
13. Ducy P. Cbfa1: a molecular switch in osteoblast biology. Dev Dyn 2000;219:461–71.
14. Vaananen HK, Zhao H, Mulari M, Halleen JM. The cell biology of osteoclast function. J Cell Sci 2000;113 (Pt 3):377–81.
15. Uy HL, Mundy GR, Boyce BF, et al. Tumor necrosis factor enhances parathyroid hormone-related protein- induced

hypercalcemia and bone resorption without inhibiting bone formation in vivo. Cancer Res 1997;57:3194–9.

16. Lum L, Wong BR, Josien R, et al. Evidence for a role of a tumor necrosis factor-alpha (TNF-alpha)- converting enzyme-like protease in shedding of TRANCE, a TNF family member involved in osteoclastogenesis and dendritic cell survival. J Biol Chem 1999;274:13613–8.

17. Shalhoub V, Elliott G, Chiu L, et al. Characterization of osteoclast precursors in human blood. Br J Haematol 2000;111:501–12.

18. Hofbauer LC, Heufelder AE. The role of osteoprotegerin and receptor activator of nuclear factor kappaB ligand in the pathogenesis and treatment of rheumatoid arthritis. Arthritis Rheum 2001;44:253–9.

19. Simonet WS, Lacey DL, Dunstan CR, et al. Osteoprotegerin: a novel secreted protein involved in the regulation of bone density. Cell 1997;89:309–19.

20. Tsuda E, Goto M, Mochizuki S, et al. Isolation of a novel cytokine from human fibroblasts that specifically inhibits osteoclastogenesis. Biochem Biophys Res Commun 1997;234:137–42.

21. Nagai M, Sato N. Reciprocal gene expression of osteoclastogenesis inhibitory factor and osteoclast differentiation factor regulates osteoclast formation. Biochem Biophys Res Commun 1999;257:719–23.

22. Hofbauer LC, Dunstan CR, Spelsberg TC, Riggs BL, Khosla S. Osteoprotegerin production by human osteoblast lineage cells is stimulated by vitamin D, bone morphogenetic protein-2, and cytokines. Biochem Biophys Res Commun 1998;250:776–81.

23. Roodman GD. Cell biology of the osteoclast. Exp Hematol 1999;27:1229–41.

24. Katunuma N. Mechanism and regulation of bone resorption by osteoclasts. Curr Top Cell Regul 1997;35:179–92.

25. Kiviranta R, Morko J, Uusitalo H, Aro HT, Vuorio E, Rantakokko J. Accelerated turnover of metaphyseal trabecular bone in mice overexpressing cathepsin K. J Bone Miner Res 2001;16:1444–52.

26. Gowen M, Lazner F, Dodds R, et al. Cathepsin K knockout mice develop osteopetrosis due to a deficit in matrix degradation but not demineralization. J Bone Miner Res 1999;14:1654–63.

27. Lee BS, Holliday LS, Ojikutu B, Krits I, Gluck SL. Osteoclasts express the B2 isoform of vacuolar H(+)-ATPase intracellularly and on their plasma membranes. Am J Physiol 1996;270:C382–8.

28. Lehenkari P, Hentunen TA, Laitala-Leinonen T, Tuukkanen J, Vaananen HK. Carbonic anhydrase II plays a major role in osteoclast differentiation and bone resorption by effecting the steady state intracellular pH and Ca^{2+}. Exp Cell Res 1998;242:128–37.

29. Lalande A, Roux S, Denne MA, et al. Indapamide, a thiazide-like diuretic, decreases bone resorption in vitro. J Bone Miner Res 2001;16:361–70.

30. Rodan GA. The development and function of the skeleton and bone metastases. Cancer 2003;97:726–32.

31. Munk PL, Poon PY, O'Connell JX, et al. Osteoblastic metastases from breast carcinoma with false-negative bone scan. Skeletal Radiol 1997;26:434–7.

32. Roudier M, Sherrard D, True L, et al. Heterogenous bone histomorphometric patterns in metastatic prostate cancer. J Bone Miner Res 2000;15S1:S567.

33. Carlin BI, Andriole GL. The natural history, skeletal complications, and management of bone metastases in patients with prostate carcinoma. Cancer 2000;88:2989–94.

34. Hullinger TG, Taichman RS, Linseman DA, Somerman MJ. Secretory products from PC-3 and MCF-7 tumor cell lines upregulate osteopontin in MC3T3-E1 cells. J Cell Biochem 2000;78:607–16.

35. Lalich M, McNeel DG, Wilding G, Liu G. Endothelin receptor antagonists in cancer therapy. Cancer Invest 2007;25:785–94.

36. Cornish J, Callon KE, Lin C, Xiao C, Moseley JM, Reid IR. Stimulation of osteoblast proliferation by C-terminal fragments of parathyroid hormone-related protein. J Bone Miner Res 1999;14:915–22.

37. Rabbani SA, Gladu J, Mazar AP, Henkin J, Goltzman D. Induction in human osteoblastic cells (SaOS2) of the early response genes fos, jun, and myc by the amino terminal fragment (ATF) of urokinase. J Cell Physiol 1997;172: 137–45.

38. Honore P, Luger NM, Sabino MA, et al. Osteoprotegerin blocks bone cancer-induced skeletal destruction, skeletal pain and pain-related neurochemical reorganization of the spinal cord. Nat Med 2000;6:521–8.

39. Chiao JW, Moonga BS, Yang YM, et al. Endothelin-1 from prostate cancer cells is enhanced by bone contact which blocks osteoclastic bone resorption. Br J Cancer 2000;83:360–5.

40. Lin DL, Tarnowski CP, Zhang J, et al. Bone metastatic LNCaP-derivative C4-2B prostate cancer cell line mineralizes in vitro. Prostate 2001;47:212–21.

41. Zhang J, Dai J, Qi Y, et al. Osteoprotegerin inhibits prostate cancer-induced osteoclastogenesis and prevents prostate tumor growth in the bone. J Clin Invest 2001;107:1235–44.

42. Brown JM, Corey E, Lee ZD, et al. Osteoprotegerin and rank ligand expression in prostate cancer. Urology 2001;57:611–6.

43. Perez-Martinez FC, Alonso V, Sarasa JL, et al. Receptor activator of nuclear factor-kappaB ligand (RANKL) as a novel prognostic marker in prostate carcinoma. Histol Histopathol 2008;23:709–15.

44. Chen G, Sircar K, Aprikian A, Potti A, Goltzman D, Rabbani SA. Expression of RANKL/RANK/OPG in primary and metastatic human prostate cancer as markers of disease stage and functional regulation. Cancer 2006;107:289–98.

45. Brown JM, Vessella RL, Kostenuik PJ, Dunstan CR, Lange PH, Corey E. Serum osteoprotegerin levels are increased in patients with advanced prostate cancer. Clin Cancer Res 2001;7:2977–83.

46. Jung K, Stephan C, Semjonow A, Lein M, Schnorr D, Loening SA. Serum osteoprotegerin and receptor activator of nuclear factor-kappa B ligand as indicators of disturbed osteoclastogenesis in patients with prostate cancer. J Urol 2003;170:2302–5.

47. Kiefer JA, Vessella RL, Quinn JE, et al. The effect of osteoprotegerin administration on the intra-tibial growth of the osteoblastic LuCaP 23.1 prostate cancer xenograft. Clin Exp Metastasis 2004;21:381–7.

48. Zhang J, Dai J, Yao Z, Lu Y, Dougall W, Keller ET. Soluble receptor activator of nuclear factor kappaB Fc diminishes prostate cancer progression in bone. Cancer Res 2003;63:7883–90.

49. Stearns ME, Wang M. Effects of alendronate and taxol on PC-3 ML cell bone metastases in SCID mice. Invasion Metastasis 1996;16:116–31.

50. John A, Tuszynski G. The role of matrix metalloproteinases in tumor angiogenesis and tumor metastasis. Pathol Oncol Res 2001;7:14–23.

51. Festuccia C, Bologna M, Vicentini C, et al. Increased matrix metalloproteinase-9 secretion in short-term tissue cultures of prostatic tumor cells. Int J Cancer 1996;69:386–93.

52. Festuccia C, Giunciuglio D, Guerra F, et al. Osteoblasts modulate secretion of urokinase-type plasminogen activator (uPA) and matrix metalloproteinase-9 (MMP-9) in human prostate cancer cells promoting migration and matrigel invasion. Oncol Res 1999;11:17–31.

53. Nabha SM, dos Santos EB, Yamamoto HA, et al. Bone marrow stromal cells enhance prostate cancer cell invasion through type I collagen in an MMP-12 dependent manner. Int J Cancer 2008;122:2482–90.

54. Duivenvoorden WC, Hirte HW, Singh G. Use of tetracycline as an inhibitor of matrix metalloproteinase activity secreted by human bone-metastasizing cancer cells. Invasion Metastasis 1997;17:312–22.

55. Sanchez-Sweatman OH, Orr FW, Singh G. Human metastatic prostate PC3 cell lines degrade bone using matrix metalloproteinases. Invasion Metastasis 1998;18:297–305.

56. Stratton MS, Sirvent H, Udayakumar TS, Nagle RB, Bowden GT. Expression of the matrix metalloproteinase promatrilysin in coculture of prostate carcinoma cell lines. Prostate 2001;48:206–9.

57. Smith PC, Hobish A, Lin D, Culig Z, Keller ET. Interleukin-6 and prostate cancer progression. Cytokine Growth Factor Rev 2001;12:33–40.

58. Lee J, Weber M, Mejia S, Bone E, Watson P, Orr W. A matrix metalloproteinase inhibitor, batimastat, retards the development of osteolytic bone metastases by MDA-MB-231 human breast cancer cells in Balb C nu/nu mice. Eur J Cancer 2001;37:106–13.

59. Nemeth JA, Yousif R, Herzog M, et al. Matrix metalloproteinase activity, bone matrix turnover, and tumor cell proliferation in prostate cancer bone metastasis. J Natl Cancer Inst 2002;94:17–25.

60. Stearns ME, Wang M. Alendronate blocks metalloproteinase secretion and bone collagen I release by PC-3 ML cells in SCID mice. Clin Exp Metastasis 1998;16:693–702.

61. Strewler GJ. The physiology of parathyroid hormone-related protein. N Engl J Med 2000;342:177–85.

62. Iwamura M, Abrahamsson PA, Foss KA, Wu G, Cockett AT, Deftos LJ. Parathyroid hormone-related protein: a potential autocrine growth regulator in human prostate cancer cell lines. Urology 1994;43:675–9.

63. Deftos LJ. Prostate carcinoma: production of bioactive factors. Cancer 2000;88:3002–8.

64. Iwamura M, di Sant'Agnese PA, Wu G, et al. Immunohistochemical localization of parathyroid hormone-related protein in human prostate cancer. Cancer Res 1993;53:1724–6.

65. Asadi F, Farraj M, Sharifi R, Malakouti S, Antar S, Kukreja S. Enhanced expression of parathyroid hormone-related protein in prostate cancer as compared with benign prostatic hyperplasia. Hum Pathol 1996;27:1319–23.

66. Iwamura M, Gershagen S, Lapets O, et al. Immunohistochemical localization of parathyroid hormone-related protein in prostatic intraepithelial neoplasia. Hum Pathol 1995;26:797–801.

67. Dougherty KM, Blomme EA, Koh AJ, et al. Parathyroid hormone-related protein as a growth regulator of prostate carcinoma. Cancer Res 1999;59:6015–22.

68. Iddon J, Bundred NJ, Hoyland J, et al. Expression of parathyroid hormone-related protein and its receptor in bone metastases from prostate cancer. J Pathol 2000;191:170–4.

69. Kremer R, Goltzman D, Amizuka N, Webber MM, Rhim JS. ras Activation of human prostate epithelial cells induces overexpression of parathyroid hormone-related peptide. Clin Cancer Res 1997;3:855–9.

70. Peehl DM, Edgar MG, Cramer SD, Deftos LJ. Parathyroid hormone-related protein is not an autocrine growth factor for normal prostatic epithelial cells. Prostate 1997;31:47–52.

71. Blomme EA, Dougherty KM, Pienta KJ, Capen CC, Rosol TJ, McCauley LK. Skeletal metastasis of prostate adenocarcinoma in rats: morphometric analysis and role of parathyroid hormone-related protein. Prostate 1999;39:187–97.

72. Perez-Martinez FC, Alonso V, Sarasa JL, et al. Immunohistochemical analysis of low-grade and high-grade prostate carcinoma: relative changes of parathyroid hormone-related protein and its parathyroid hormone 1 receptor, osteoprotegerin and receptor activator of nuclear factor-kB ligand. J Clin Pathol 2007;60:290–4.

73. Rabbani SA, Gladu J, Harakidas P, Jamison B, Goltzman D. Over-production of parathyroid hormone-related peptide results in increased osteolytic skeletal metastasis by prostate cancer cells in vivo. Int J Cancer 1999;80:257–64.

74. Lu Y, Xiao G, Galson DL, et al. PTHrP-induced MCP-1 production by human bone marrow endothelial cells and osteoblasts promotes osteoclast differentiation and prostate cancer cell proliferation and invasion in vitro. Int J Cancer 2007;121(4):724–33.

75. Sehgal P, Wang L, Rayanade R, Pan H, Margulies L. Interleukin-6 type cytokines. In: Mackiewicz A, Koji A, Sehgal P, eds. Annals of the New York Academy of Sciences. New York: New York Academy of Sciences; 1995:1–14.

76. Hirano T. The biology of interleukin-6. Chem Immunol 1992;51:153–80.

77. Taga T, Hibi M, Murakami M, et al. Interleukin-6 receptor and signals. In: Kishimoto T, ed. Interleukins: Molecular Biology and Immunology, Chem Immunol. Basel: Karger; 1992:181–204.

78. Mullberg J, Oberthur W, Lottspeich F, et al. The soluble human IL-6 receptor. Mutational characterization of the proteolytic cleavage site. J Immunol 1994;152:4958–68.

79. Rose-John S, Heinrich PC. Soluble receptors for cytokines and growth factors: generation and biological function. Biochem J 1994;300:281–90.

80. Lust JA, Donovan KA, Kline MP, Greipp PR, Kyle RA, Maihle NJ. Isolation of an mRNA encoding a soluble form of the human interleukin-6 receptor. Cytokine 1992;4:96–100.

81. Mackiewicz A, Schooltink H, Heinrich PC, Rose-John S. Complex of soluble human IL-6-receptor/IL-6 up-regulates expression of acute-phase proteins. J Immunol 1992;149: 2021–7.

82. Adler HL, McCurdy MA, Kattan MW, Timme TL, Scardino PT, Thompson TC. Elevated levels of circulating interleukin-6 and transforming growth factor-beta1 in patients with metastatic prostatic carcinoma. J Urol 1999;161:182–7.

83. Hoosien N, Abdul M, McCabe R, et al. Clinical significance of elevation in neuroendocrine factors and interleukin-6 in metastatic prostate cancer. Urol Oncol 1995;1:246–51.

84. Twillie DA, Eisenberger MA, Carducci MA, Hseih WS, Kim WY, Simons JW. Interleukin-6: a candidate mediator of human prostate cancer morbidity. Urology 1995;45:542–9.

85. Drachenberg DE, Elgamal AA, Rowbotham R, Peterson M, Murphy GP. Circulating levels of interleukin-6 in patients with hormone refractory prostate cancer. Prostate 1999;41:127–33.

86. Tsingotjidou AS, Zotalis G, Jackson KR, et al. Development of an animal model for prostate cancer cell metastasis to adult human bone. Anticancer Res 2001;21:971–8.

87. Siegsmund MJ, Yamazaki H, Pastan I. Interleukin 6 receptor mRNA in prostate carcinomas and benign prostate hyperplasia. J Urol 1994;151:1396–9.

88. Hobisch A, Rogatsch H, Hittmair A, et al. Immunohistochemical localization of interleukin-6 and its receptor in benign, premalignant and malignant prostate tissue. J Pathol 2000;191:239–44.

89. Ershler WB, Keller ET. Age-associated increased interleukin-6 gene expression, late-life diseases, and frailty [In Process Citation]. Annu Rev Med 2000;51:245–70.

90. Jilka RL, Passeri G, Girasole G, et al. Estrogen loss upregulates hematopoiesis in the mouse: a mediating role of IL-6. Exp Hematol 1995;23:500–6.

91. O'Brien CA, Lin SC, Bellido T, Manolagas SC. Expression levels of gp130 in bone marrow stromal cells determine the magnitude of osteoclastogenic signals generated by IL-6-type cytokines. J Cell Biochem 2000;79:532–41.

92. Hofbauer LC, Lacey DL, Dunstan CR, Spelsberg TC, Riggs BL, Khosla S. Interleukin-1beta and tumor necrosis factor-alpha, but not interleukin- 6, stimulate osteoprotegerin ligand gene expression in human osteoblastic cells. Bone 1999;25:255–9.

93. Greenfield EM, Shaw SM, Gornik SA, Banks MA. Adenyl cyclase and interleukin 6 are downstream effectors of parathyroid hormone resulting in stimulation of bone resorption. J Clin Invest 1995;96:1238–44.

94. de la Mata J, Uy HL, Guise TA, et al. Interleukin-6 enhances hypercalcemia and bone resorption mediated by parathyroid hormone-related protein in vivo. J Clin Invest 1995;95:2846–52.

95. Smith PC, Keller ET. Anti-interleukin-6 monoclonal antibody induces regression of human prostate cancer xenografts in nude mice. Prostate 2001;48:47–53.

96. Bentley H, Hamdy FC, Hart KA, et al. Expression of bone morphogenetic proteins in human prostatic adenocarcinoma and benign prostatic hyperplasia. Br J Cancer 1992;66:1159–63.

97. Nelson JB, Hedican SP, George DJ, et al. Identification of endothelin-1 in the pathophysiology of metastatic adenocarcinoma of the prostate. Nat Med 1995;1:944–9.

98. Nelson JB, Carducci MA. The role of endothelin-1 and endothelin receptor antagonists in prostate cancer. BJU Int 2000;85(Suppl 2):45–8.

99. LeRoy BE, Sellers RS, Rosol TJ. Canine prostate stimulates osteoblast function using the endothelin receptors. Prostate 2004;59:148–56.

100. Jimeno A, Carducci M. Atrasentan: targeting the endothelin axis in prostate cancer. Expert Opin Investig Drugs 2004;13:1631–40.

101. Pirtskhalaishvili G, Nelson JB. Endothelium-derived factors as paracrine mediators of prostate cancer progression. Prostate 2000;44:77–87.

102. Perkel VS, Mohan S, Baylink DJ, Linkhart TA. An inhibitory insulin-like growth factor binding protein (In-IGFBP) from human prostatic cell conditioned medium reveals N-terminal sequence identity with bone derived In-IGFBP. J Clin Endocrinol Metabol 1990;71: 533–5.

103. Taguchi Y, Yamamoto M, Yamate T, et al. Interleukin-6-type cytokines stimulate mesenchymal progenitor differentiation toward the osteoblastic lineage. Proc Assoc Am Physicians 1998;110:559–74.

104. Le Brun G, Aubin P, Soliman H, et al. Upregulation of endothelin 1 and its precursor by IL-1beta, TNF-alpha, and TGF-beta in the PC3 human prostate cancer cell line. Cytokine 1999;11:157–62.

105. Guise TA. Molecular mechanisms of osteolytic bone metastases. Cancer 2000;88:2892–8.

106. Karaplis AC, Vautour L. Parathyroid hormone-related peptide and the parathyroid hormone/parathyroid hormone-related peptide receptor in skeletal development. Curr Opin Nephrol Hypertens 1997;6:308–13.

107. Killian CS, Corral DA, Kawinski E, Constantine RI. Mitogenic response of osteoblast cells to prostate-specific antigen suggests an activation of latent TGF-beta and a proteolytic modulation of cell adhesion receptors. Biochem Biophys Res Commun 1993;192:940–7.

108. Goltzman D, Karaplis AC, Kremer R, Rabbani SA. Molecular basis of the spectrum of skeletal complications of neoplasia. Cancer 2000;88:2903–8.

109. Dai J, Kitagawa Y, Zhang J, et al. Vascular endothelial growth factor contributes to the prostate cancer-induced osteoblast differentiation mediated by bone morphogenetic protein. Cancer Res 2004;64:994–9.

110. Hall CL, Bafico A, Dai J, Aaronson SA, Keller ET. Prostate cancer cells promote osteoblastic bone metastases through Wnts. Cancer Res 2005;65:7554–60.

Chapter 23
Radiopharmaceuticals

Oliver Sartor and Damerla R. Venugopal

Abstract Bone-targeted radiopharmaceuticals have an established role as safe and effective agents for the treatment of men with bone-metastatic castration-resistant prostate cancer (CRPC). Three FDA approved radiopharmaceuticals are available for use by clinicians including [153]samarium-EDTMP, [89]strontium chloride, and [32]phosphorus. Data from placebo-controlled randomized trials support the palliative use of these compounds but no consensus currently exists regarding how these compounds should be sequenced with other agents known to be active in the CRPC patient. Multiple factors, including market forces, have limited current use. Newer bone-targeted isotopic therapies are currently under development and large phase III multinational placebo-controlled trials in bone-metastatic CRPC patients are currently being planned for [223]radium. Combinations of radiopharmaceuticals and chemotherapy have yielded promising survival results in small randomized studies, but confirmation of survival benefit in larger studies has yet to occur. Various combinations of radiopharmaceuticals and chemotherapy are currently under active investigation.

Keywords Radiopharmaceuticals • [153]Samarium-EDTMP • [89]Strontium chloride • [223]Radium • [32]Phosphorus • Palliation • Prostate cancer • Bone metastases • Bone-targeted therapy

O. Sartor (✉)
Departments of Medicine and Urology, Tulane Medical School, New Orleans, LA, USA
e-mail: osartor@tulane.edu

Introduction

Bone targeted therapy with radio-isotopes began nearly 60 years ago with the pioneering studies of Friedell and Storaasli [1] using [32]phosphorus (^{32}P) for patients with bone-metastatic breast cancer. Studies in patients with bone-metastatic prostate cancer using radioactive phosphates date to the late 1950s [2]. Today, metastatic bone lesions can be targeted using several distinct FDA-approved radiopharmaceuticals including [153]samarium lexidronam ([153]Sm ethylenediaminetetramethylenephosphonic acid or [153]Sm-EDTMP), [89]Strontium chloride (^{89}Sr), and [32]P. Each of these agents varies in their physical properties and mechanisms of bone-targeting, sharing in common only the relatively selective delivery of beta particles to bone metastatic lesions.

Bone metastases are the most significant clinical manifestation for the vast majority of metastatic castration-resistant prostate cancer (CRPC) patients. The American Cancer Society current estimates for prostate cancer mortality rates indicate that approximately 28,660 deaths will occur in 2008 [3]. The vast majority of these patients will have bone-metastases at the time of death. A variety of contemporary clinical trials systematically assessing both bone and soft tissue disease [4, 5] demonstrate that bone metastases are radiographically detected in the 84–92% of patients whereas measureable soft tissue disease (predominantly lymph node) is present in 39–44% of patients. Perhaps more importantly, in these large multi-institutional chemotherapy studies, over one third of these patients had bone pain that interfered with function at the beginning of therapy [5]. Thus from both radiographic and symptomatic perspective, bone metastases are highly prevalent and clinically significant in patients with metastatic CRPC.

W.D. Figg et al. (eds.), *Drug Management of Prostate Cancer*,
DOI 10.1007/978-1-60327-829-4_23, © Springer Science+Business Media, LLC 2010

It has long been appreciated that prostate cancer cells are osteotropic though the exact mechanism for this tropism is debated. This topic is the subject of considerable ongoing investigation [6]. One of the attractive features regarding bone-targeted therapies in metastatic prostate cancer is the fact that the ratio of bone to soft tissue metastases is remarkably high in comparison to other solid tumors. Thus, bone-targeted agents have the capacity to treat not only the most clinically relevant aspect of metastatic prostate cancer but frequently the only clear radiographic manifestation of the disease. Such is not the case for other common metastatic malignancies such as lung cancer, colon cancer, breast cancer, etc., which typically have bone metastases as only one feature of widespread metastatic disease.

Another relatively unique aspect of prostate bone metastases is that osteoblastic growth pattern strongly predominates. Though many types of cancers may have osteoblastic manifestations, prostate cancer is the most consistent in forming osteoblastic patterns. Given that current bone-targeted radiopharmaceuticals selectively target the stroma of osteoblastic rather than osteolytic lesions, this provides a particular rationale for their utilization in patients with bone-metastatic CRPC.

Clinical Manifestations of Bone Metastases

Clinical manifestations of bone metastases include both focal and systemic symptoms. Pain is the most common focal complaint but both pathologic fractures and cord compression are significant complications of bone metastases and these symptoms represent a source of significant morbidity in the CRPC patient. Pathologic fractures, cord compression, radiation to bone, surgery to bone, and/or a change in antineoplastic therapy secondary to bone pain have been termed as skeletal-related events (SREs). Though this particular grouping may be debatable in its utility, the Food and Drug Administration (FDA) has accepted SREs as a relevant endpoint in selected registrational clinical trials [7] and thus SREs are commonly evaluated in current clinical trials evaluating patients with bone metastatic disease.

It should be noted that evaluating various bone pains in older men with prostate cancer is not simplistic. Epidemiology studies indicate that there are over 60 million visits each year for back pain alone in the United States [8]. Various musculoskeletal pains (arthritis, muscular spasms, sciatica, etc.) are common in this setting, and new pains cannot readily be ascribed to cancer without careful questioning and radiologic investigation. In the absence of radiographic metastases, pain can typically be attributed to noncancerous causes. In the presence of radiographic evidence of metastatic cancer, pain may or may not be causally related. Data indicate that bone metastases can typically be detected by bone scan approximately 4 months before symptoms are present [9], thus the simple presence of bone metastases does not imply that pain is derived from imaged lesions.

The measurement of pain due to bone metastases is not distinct from that of other malignant-induced pain. A variety of pain scales have been utilized in clinical trials (the McGill-Melzack Questionnaire, Brief Pain Inventory (BPI), Visual Analog Scale (VAS), Pain Descriptor Scales, etc.) and though a thorough review of this topic is relevant, it is beyond the scope of this particular chapter. Suffice it to say that pain assessments should be patient reported, repetitive, and quantitative. Regardless, as particular clinical trials are reviewed herein, the particulars of how pain was measured in that trial will be discussed as an understanding of pain assessment is critical to interpretation. Too often ignored in this context is analgesic consumption. Trials measuring pain and pain relief also require careful and repetitive measurement of analgesic utilization.

Systemic complications related to bone metastatic spread include both hypercalcemia and anemia. Hypercalcemia, a common manifestation of certain osteolytic bone tropic diseases such as multiple myeloma, is uncommon in patients with prostate cancer presumably due to relatively osteoblastic nature of prostatic metastases. Anemia in the advanced prostate cancer patient is a topic of considerable complexity. Direct invasion of marrow, androgen deprivation therapy, disseminated intravascular coagulation (DIC), proinflammatory cytokines, and chemotherapy are implicated in the anemia of prostate cancer patients [10, 11]. Though etiologies are often multifactorial, the prognostic importance of anemia in advanced disease is well documented and confirmed in multivariate analyses [12, 13]. Patients with significant anemia have a significantly shorter life-expectancy than those with normal or near-normal hemoglobin. Asthenia, loss of stamina, loss of appetite, weight loss, and occasionally fever are not specific manifestations of bone-metastatic disease, but are not uncommon in patients with advanced prostate cancer.

Physical Properties and Mechanisms of Targeting of Bone-Targeted Radiopharmaceuticals

Radiopharmaceuticals have often been reviewed in overly simplistic terms. In actuality, the agents used to date vary widely in particle emissions, half-life, and energy (see Table 23.1). The three currently available isotopes in the United States are all beta (β) emitters but the energy, half-life, and typical bone penetration depth of these agents are quite distinct as shown in Table 23.1. ^{153}Sm-EDTMP has both the lowest average energy for the beta emission (0.22 MeV) and the shortest physical half life (1.9 days) of the currently available bone-targeted isotopes. ^{89}Sr has a much longer half life (50.5 days) and is associated with a higher energy beta emission (0.58 MeV). ^{32}P has the highest energy beta (and hence the greatest degree of bone penetration) with an average energy of 0.71 MeV and a 14 day half life. ^{223}Radium (^{223}Rd) is the first bone-targeted alpha-emitter to enter advanced clinical trials. It has a physical half-life of 11.4 days with a complex decay chain that includes radon, polonium, lead, bismuth, and thallium radioactive isotopes. Alpha particle emitters such as ^{223}Rd are less penetrant in tissue (range typically <100 μm) than β-emitters but considerably more cytotoxic to the tumor cells and supportive stromal cells due to their high linear energy transfer [14].

After their intravenous administration, the bone-targeted radionuclides are preferentially incorporated into the sites of bone metastases at rates 2–120 times greater than that present in normal bone [15, 16]. ^{32}P tracks and deposits in inorganic phosphate containing complexes in the hydroxyapatite crystal contained abundantly in the areas of remodeled diseased bone and has been a relatively forgotten isotope despite early studies of efficacy [2, 17]. ^{153}Sm chelated to EDTMP homes to sites of new bone formation where it binds to newly deposited osteoid, which is abundantly deposited in the osteoblastic lesions associated with metastatic

Table 23.1 Physical properties of radionuclides used for treatment of metastatic bone pain

Radionuclide	Half-life	Average/maximum MeV	Bone penetration (mm)
^{32}P	14.3 days	0.7/1.7(β)	2.7
^{89}Sr	50.5 days	0.58/1.46(β)	2.4
^{153}Sm	1.9 days	0.23/0.8(β,γ)	0.55
^{223}Rd[a]	11.4 days	6/9(α,γ)	0.0001

[a]Not currently FDA approved

bone disease [16]. Without the EDTMP and its phosphonic acid groups, ^{153}Sm will not concentrate in bone. ^{89}Sr and ^{223}Rd [15, 18] are calcium homologues and are deposited in regions of newly formed bone where there is active calcium deposition. Once embedded in the bone mineral matrix, radionuclides cause direct DNA damage to both tumor and other adjacent cells including the various aspects of tumor-associated stroma (fibroblasts, endothelial cells, etc.). Because stromal-tumor interactions have been linked to cancerous growth, the importance of stromal alteration should not be underestimated as changes in the tumor microenvironment may have important therapeutic implications (Table 23.1)

A variety of non-FDA approved isotopic preparation have been used in various clinical trials, however, the vast majority of these compounds are not being currently developed for therapeutic use and thus coverage in this review will be limited. These compounds include several preparations of rhenium (^{186}Re-1,1-hydroxyethylidene diphosphonate also known as ^{186}Re-HEDP or ^{186}Re-etidronate, ^{188}Re-HEDP), tin in the form of ^{117}Sn(4+)diethylenetriaminepentaacetic acid (^{117}Sn-DTPA), ^{85}strontium, and ^{166}holmium in the form of ^{166}Ho-Labeled 1,4,7,10-tetraazacyclododecane-1,4,7,10-tetramethylenephosphonate (^{166}Ho-DOTMP).

Current Guidelines

Current National Cancer Comprehensive (NCCN) guidelines recommend systemic radionuclide therapy for the palliation of bone pain on disease progression despite androgen deprivation therapies (V.1.2009) but neither the NCCN or other guidelines have been clear in terms of how these and other active agents might be sequenced in prostate patients with metastatic castrate-refractory disease. Both current guidelines and FDA labels limit the use of bone seeking radio-isotopes to monotherapies indicated explicitly for bone pain palliation, however, the field is evolving rapidly and multiple clinical trials [19–22] have attempted to use combined modality therapy to change utilization of these isotopes from the strictly palliative uses that are indicated in the clinic today.

Current Indications and Contraindications for Radionuclide Therapy

Current indications for bone seeking radionuclide therapy (Table 23.2) involves the clear demonstration of pain attributable to bone metastatic disease. The presence of positive imaging studies are key to making a firm diagnosis of metastatic bone pain, and all clinical trials published to date evaluating this class of agents have required confirmation of bone metastases by the presence of radiographic imaging. Isotopic bone scan findings are typically used as the imaging modality, with equivocal bone scan findings being resolved by additional standard imaging modalities. The osteoblastic lesions detected by bone scan provide confirmation that a radiopharmaceutical targetable lesion is present. Little experience with radiopharmaceuticals is available for patients with osteolytic lesions that are bone scan negative, such as the nonbisphosphonate treated typical multiple myeloma patients. Laboratory findings are rarely specific and are not typically used in bone pain diagnosis though an elevated bone alkaline phosphatase can provide a confirmatory finding. N-telopeptide and other markers of bone turnover have not been used clinically in this setting (Table 23.2).

Once the presence of painful bone metastases is ascertained, the patient is a potential candidate for bone-seeking radiopharmaceutical therapy. Whether this approach is optimal, however, depends on the availability and potential applicability of other therapeutic choices. For the prostate cancer patient who is hormone-therapy naïve, the first choice of therapy is standard androgen deprivation therapy. For patients with significant elements of symptomatic soft-tissue metastases, the limitation of bone-targeted therapies is readily apparent. For unifocal bone disease, external beam

Table 23.2 Current Indications and contraindications for bone-seeking radiopharmaceuticals in prostate cancer

Indications
- Osteoblastic lesions on bone scans
- Bone pain from multifocal disease
- Hormone refractory disease
- Bone pain poorly controlled with conventional analgesics or analgesic intolerance

Relative contraindications
- Present or impending pathological fracture or spinal cord compression
- A significant soft tissue component of pain
- Single site of bone metastases
- Pure osteolytic bone lesions

Absolute contraindications
- Negative bone scan
- Severe marrow failure
- Severe renal insufficiency

radiation provides a reasonable and highly effective alternative in the vast majority of patients [23, 24]. If cord compression, pathologic fracture, or a high risk of pathologic fracture is suspected, alternative therapies to radiopharmaceuticals should be sought. Taken together, individuals with castrate-refractory multifocal metastatic bone disease with a minimum of soft-tissue symptoms are typically ideal for radiopharmaceutical consideration. From a safety perspective, adequate hematological status and the excretion of the particular isotope should be considered prior to finalizing decisions. ^{153}Sm-EDTMP is excreted via the urine and ^{89}Sr is excreted via both the urine and stool. Consequently, consideration of creatinine clearance as well as hematological parameters is needed prior to the administration of radiopharmaceuticals.

Overview of Randomized and Repeat-Dosing Studies with ^{89}Strontium

The vast majority of the trials published with ^{89}Sr have been small, retrospective, nonrandomized, and/or reported only in abstract form. A recent review identified 38 observational studies using ^{89}Sr for the management of metastatic bone cancer. These observational trials will not be assessed and covered in this chapter given the inconclusive nature of these types of trials. In this synopsis, larger randomized trials and studies of repeated doses are emphasized.

In a comprehensive study performed by the European Organization for Research and Treatment of Cancer (EORTC), ^{89}Sr was compared to local field radiation therapy in patients with bone-metastatic symptomatic CRPC [25]. A total of 203 patients were randomized between a single dose of 150 MBq (~4 mCi) ^{89}Sr and external beam radiation. External beam treatment planning was left to the individual center. Some patients received single doses as low as 4 Gy, whereas other patients received as much as 43 Gy in multiple fractions. The median dose/schedule was 20 Gy spread over 5 fractions. Pain was assessed by a 5 point World Health Organization (WHO) scale evaluating pain in terms of the type and frequency of analgesia required (nonopiate or opiate, regular or nonregular). Subjective pain responses using the analgesia-requirement scale were recorded in approximately one third of each patient treatment group, however, no comprehensive pain management plan was implemented across the trial sites. Time to subjective progression was approximately 3 months in each arm. Duration of pain response in responding patients was approximately 4.5 months for each treatment. There were no statistically significant differences in either the time to subjective progression or duration of pain response in responding patients. PSA declines of $\geq 50\%$ were recorded in 13% of the isotope-treated patients and 10% of the external beam radiation-treated patients. Pain flare was reported in 18.4% of the isotope group as compared to 8.2% of the external beam group. The survival of ^{89}Sr treated patients was compromised as compared to those receiving local field radiotherapy alone (median of 7.2 versus 11.0 months). This survival impairment was statistically significant ($p=0.0457$). Toxicities were relatively mild, with grade 3 thrombocytopenia was recorded in only one patient. Though the decrement in survival has not been reported in other trials, this does represent one of the largest trials evaluating ^{89}Sr to date.

In the largest prospective randomized trial evaluating radiopharmaceuticals in symptomatic and bone metastatic CRPC, 284 men in the UK were randomized between single dose [89]Sr (200 MBq) and external beam radiation [26]. In this particular study, endpoints were clearly defined and included pain at the index site, appearance of new painful sites, a requirement for additional palliative external beam radiation, and survival. The external beam radiation was either focal or hemi-body. Interestingly, the intravenous radioisotope and the two forms of external beam radiation had no significant differences in pain relief at the index site (61–66% of patients experienced relief), however, in the ^{89}Sr arm, there were fewer new painful sites as compared to those patients who received the focal external beam radiation. In addition, fewer patients treated with the radioisotope (as compared to focal therapy) required subsequent radiation (2 patients vs. 12), indicating potential benefit of systemic treatment. Survival was quite short (~21 weeks) but equal in each treatment arm. Clinically significant toxicity was minor; however, both platelets and white blood cells fell by an average of 30–40% after ^{89}Sr administration.

In a double-blind placebo-controlled randomized trial in 126 patients performed in Canada combining adjuvant radiopharmaceutical therapy with external beam radiation to bone, patients with painful bone metastatic CRPC were randomized to single dose placebo or ^{89}Sr after local field radiotherapy was administered to the most significant site of pain [27]. In these studies, strontium was given as a single injection of 400 Mbq (10.8 mCi). This represents a dose that is 2.5 times higher than that of the FDA approved dose (4 mCi) in the United States. Endpoints included analgesic consumption, new sites of painful metastatic bone disease, survival, and a reduction of pain at the primary sites of metastatic bone pain. Using these parameters, there was a significant reduction in analgesic use at 3 months in patients assigned to [89]Sr. In the isotope-treated group, 17% of patients were able to discontinue analgesics as compared to only 2% in the control group. In addition, there were significantly fewer new sites of active pain at 3 months. A quality-of-life analysis demonstrated a statistically significant improvement in ^{89}Sr treated patients with regard to alleviating pain and improving physical activity. There were no differences between the treatment arms in either survival or pain reduction at the index site. Toxicity in the form of grade 4 thrombocytopenia was noted in 10.4% of patients treated with [89]Sr. Time to platelet recovery was not specified in this manuscript.

With regard to smaller randomized trials, Lewington et al. [28] compared ^{89}Sr to placebo in 32 patients with bone-metastatic CRPC. All patients had evidence of pain from the metastatic disease. The patients were evaluated after a single dose using a single time point (5 weeks after dosing). Of the 32 patients, only 26 were evaluable. The study concluded that ^{89}Sr led to an improvement in pain relief, however, the methodology of pain assessment and time points were limited and there was no quantitative assessment of analgesia requirements.

In another small randomized study involving 49 patients with metastatic CRPC, the [89]Sr (2 mCi) or placebo was administered at monthly intervals for three doses [29]. In this particular trial, no significant differences were noted in pain variation but analgesic consumption was not monitored. The authors concluded that bone pain relief did not occur at this dose/schedule of ^{89}Sr, however, the radiopharmaceutical group had a longer survival than did the placebo group. These survival results have not been replicated.

Studies on repeated doses of ^{89}Sr have been reported by Kasalicky and Krajska [30]. In this study, 36% of the patients had prostate cancer (lung, breast, and others were also included). A total of 76 patients had two or more doses (2–5 doses were administered). The mean interval between doses was not specified. Typical graded adverse event reporting (common toxicity criteria) was not done in this Czech Republic study but toxicity was limited. No patient had a platelet or leukocyte decrease of >50% from baseline on repeated dosing. Palliative responses were not assessed in a blinded fashion and no placebo controls were utilized. Mild improvement was noted in 41% of patients and substantial or complete improvement was noted in 47.5%.

Pons et al. [31] retreated 16 patients with a mean interval between the first and second doses of 7 months. Though not blinded, they reported that pain relief in the retreated patients was excellent as "good clinical response" was obtained in 63% of cases. Three patients received a third dose. Significant toxicity was not reported.

Overview of Randomized and Repeat-Dose Studies with [153]Samarium-EDTMP

Two prospective placebo-controlled randomized multi-institutional double-blind phase III trials have been performed testing the efficacy of 153Sm-EDTMP in comparison to placebo. No trials have compared this isotope to external beam radiation or another isotope. The first of these trials [32] was not completely prostate cancer focused, though 68% of the 118 patients enrolled had prostate cancer. The remaining enrolled patients had breast cancer (18%) or a variety of miscellaneous malignancies. All enrolled patients had painful bone scan-positive metastatic disease and were randomly assigned to 153Sm-EDTMP at one of two doses (0.5 or 1 mCi/kg) or a similar but nonradioactive compound (152Sm-EDTMP). Pain scores were assessed both by a daily patient recorded pain diary and a global physician assessment. The treatment was unblinded at the end of 4 weeks for any patient not responding to treatment and those patients receiving placebo and who continued to meet eligibility requirements were given the opportunity to crossover to a 1 mCi/kg dose of the radiopharmaceutical. This trial design had the advantage of allowing patients to crossover but as a consequence of removing all nonresponding patients 4 weeks posttreatment, statistically valid comparisons beyond the 4 week time period were not able to be made with regard to placebo. As measured by patient reported pain scores, the 1 mCi/kg dose had improved pain relative to the placebo group at weeks 1–4. Seventy-two percent of test group patients who received 1 mCi/kg had significantly reduced pain scores within 4 weeks after treatment. This response lasted for 16 weeks in 43% of the 1 mCi/kg dosed cohort. The decline in pain scores was also associated with a parallel analgesic consumption decrease. The 0.5 mCi/kg was less effective in pain palliation; in the FDA reviews, the 1 mCi/kg dose was approved for the palliation of pain due to bone metastases. Transient grade 3 platelet and leukocyte declines were observed in 3% and 14% of patients of the higher dose subgroup of radio-active isotope arm, typically recovering to baseline by about 8 weeks. Median platelet nadir was 45% of baseline, and median WBC decline was 51% of baseline.

Results of the second multi-institutional placebo-controlled randomized trial of 153 Sm were published by Sartor and colleagues [33]. This trial exclusively treated patients diagnosed with prostate cancer. A total of 152 bone-metastatic CRPC patients were randomized in a 2:1 ratio to 152samarium-EDTMP ($n = 51$) or a 1 mCi/kg dose of 153Sm-EDTMP ($n = 101$) and were followed up to 16 weeks. Again the crossover design of allowing nonresponders to be unblinded after 4 weeks was utilized, compromising statistical analysis beyond the 4 week time point. Response endpoints were subject's recording of pain intensity twice daily by patients using a VAS pain assessment as well as a

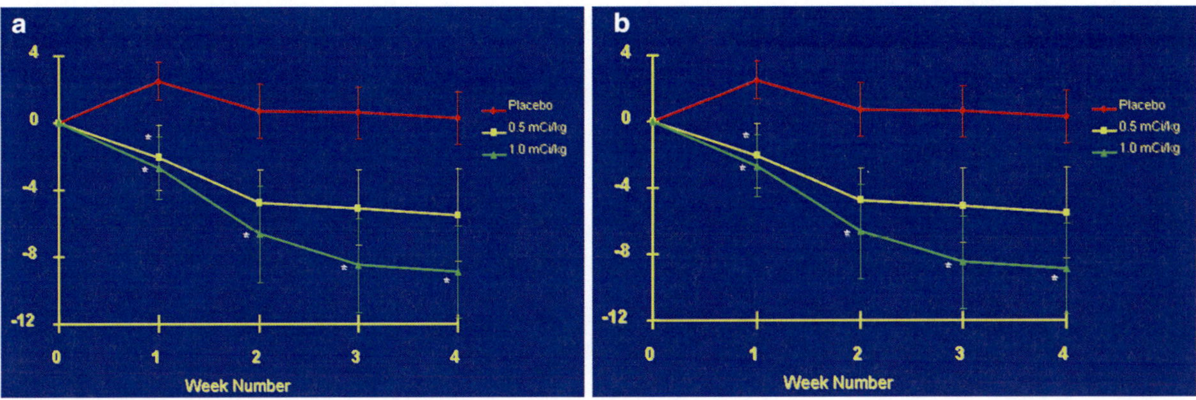

Fig. 23.1 Change from baseline in the VAS pain scores in the placebo-controlled randomized prostate cancer [153]Sm-EDTMP phase III trials published by Sartor et al. [33]. Reproduced with permission from Elsevier, copyright 2004

pain descriptor scale. Analgesic consumption was also tracked daily. Patients were contacted weekly and analgesic adjustments were made as needed, thus ongoing pain management was a part of the trial design. Significant reductions in pain scores were observed at weeks 3 and 4 (Fig. 23.1) in the radiopharmaceutical-treated group. The mean platelet and white blood count nadir was 127,000/μL and 3,800/μL, respectively. Decreases in white blood cell and platelet counts generally began within 1 or 2 weeks after dose administration, with the nadirs occurring by 3–5 weeks and recovery to normal levels by approximately week 8. No grade 4 white blood cell or platelet toxicity was noted. Grade 2, or less, toxicities were noted in 95% of the patients treated during the blinded phase of the trial.

Sartor and colleagues [34] also published results of concerning repetitive dosing in a cohort of 202 patients with 77% of the study group having been diagnosed metastatic prostate cancer. The aim was to assess the safety of repeat administration of 153Sm-EDTMP in patients who had been previously entered on randomized trials. Patients were not formally required to have repeat dosing but were potentially offered repeat dosing if they were deemed to have benefited from the original radiopharmaceutical dosing and continued to meet the trials eligibility criteria. Pain was assessed at baseline, and again at weeks 4 and 8, by a VAS score but the participants were not blinded nor treated with a placebo when receiving repeated doses, thus pain assessments were suboptimal. A total of 55 patients of the 202 were given repeated treatment with the 1 mCi/kg dosing schema. Grade 3 platelet declines occurred in 11%, 12%, and 17% of patients after the first, second, and

third doses, respectively. Grade 3 leukopenia occurred in less than 7% of the initial and repeat dose patients and was not associated with repeat dosing. In terms of efficacy, decreases in pain scores were documented in 70%, 63%, and 80% of patients at week 4 after the first, second, or third dose administration. After the second dose of the isotope, pain score reductions were statistically significant at week 4 and week 8. For patients who received three doses, pain score reduction were significant at week 4 but not week 8.

The safety and tolerability of repetitive doses of the bone seeking radiopharmaceutical 153Sm-EDTMP were investigated in men with hormone-naive prostate cancer metastatic to bone, and it concluded that the feasible dose and schedule for repeated doses of the isotope was 2 mCi/kg given every 16 weeks for three doses [35]. In this study, beginning shortly after androgen deprivation was initiated in patients with androgen-sensitive bone metastatic prostate cancer, 4 planned doses q 12 weeks were planned. The first cohort of six patients received 153Sm-EDTMP at 2 mCi/kg per dose; three patients completed all four doses and three received three doses, however, there were seven episodes of grade 3 neutropenia and one each of grade 3 and 4 thrombocytopenia. Of six patients in the second cohort (153samarium 2.5 mCi/kg per dose), only one received all four doses. Four events of grade 3 neutropenia and 2 events of grade 3 thrombocytopenia were reported. The 12-week dose schedule resulted in persistent low-grade thrombocytopenia and/or leukopenia, which prevented timely administration of the four planned doses. As a result, the dose of 153Sm-EDTMP was decreased to 2 mCi/kg for a total of three doses administered every 16 weeks. Five of six patients in this cohort received all three doses of 153 Sm. There were seven episodes of reversible grade 3 neutropenia. For all 18 patients on the study, there were no drug-related serious adverse events or grade 4 nonhematologic toxicities.

Additional studies of repeat dose 153Sm-EDTMP have also been administered in CRPC patients in combination with docetaxel chemotherapy by Morris et al. [19]. Interestingly, in this study, the 1 mCi/kg doses were administered q 6 weeks with less toxicity than expected. See the section below on combination therapies for a more extensive review of this trial.

^{223}Radium: An Isotope in Current Development

After preclinical studies in rats [18], the safety of ^{223}Rd was tested by Nilsson and colleagues [36] in a single dose, phase I clinical trial consisting of 25 patients with bone metastatic breast and prostate cancer. Toxicity and adverse were analyzed over an 8-week period. The increasing dosages for each group of five patients were 46, 93, 163, 213, and 250 kBq/kg. At 1, 4, and 8-week postadministration, 52%, 60%, and 56% of patients reported improvement of pain index scores using the pain scale derived from the European Organization for Research and Treatment of Cancer (EORTC) QLQ-C 30 Questionnaire. Toxicity was minimal at these doses though diarrhea was noted in 10/25 patients and a transient bone pain "flare" was noted in 9/25 patients. Transient myelosuppression in the patients was within acceptable ranges and surprisingly mild at these dosages (grade 3 neutropenia in 1/5 patients at the highest dose and 0/5 patients with grade 3 thrombocytopenia).

In addition, Nilsson and colleagues [37] recently published the results of their phase II randomized placebo-controlled multicenter trial investigating ^{223Rd} in symptomatic metastatic castrate-refractory prostate cancer patients. This trial, though relatively small, will be covered in detail as it is the first randomized trial for an alpha-particle emitter. All patients in both placebo ($n=30$) and ^{223}Rd arms ($n=33$) were bone-metastatic (as assessed by bone scan) and were castrate-refractory. All patients received palliative external beam radiation to the most painful site (not exceeding an area of

400 cm^2) followed by treatment with placebo or isotope. The test group received four doses of a 50 kBq/kg injection of ^{223}Rd every 4 weeks over a 12 week period. Bone markers and PSA were followed every 2 weeks until 4 weeks after the last injection, and then at 6, 9, and 12 months. SREs and bone-alkaline phosphatase (bALP) were co-primary end points. Secondary endpoints consisted of time to PSA progression, toxicity effects, and overall survival. A variety of bone metabolic markers were assessed. Pain was assessed by a Norwegian version of the BPI scale every 2 weeks. The bALP decreased in the test group by 65.6% and increased by 9.3% in the control group. Median time to first SRE was 14 weeks in the ^{223}Rd treated patients and 11 weeks in the placebo arm. Median change in PSA at 4 weeks post last injection (relative to baseline) was −24% in the radioisotope group and +45% in the placebo group. Median time to PSA progression was 26 weeks for the ^{223}Rd arm compared to 8 weeks in the placebo arm. Median overall survival was 65.3 weeks for the isotopic arm and 46.4 weeks for control arm ($p=0.066$, see Fig. 23.2). This prolongation of survival was provocative as the baseline characteristics appeared to be balanced.

Phase III trials of ^{223}Rd are now ongoing in Europe and will soon be expanded to Asia, South America, and Canada. The phase III trial ALSYMPCA (*AL*pharadin in *SYM*ptomatic *P*rostate *CA*ncer) study is targeted to bone-metastatic CRPC patients who are not candidates for chemotherapy. Approximately, 750 patients are expected to be enrolled in this pivotal trial which is powered for a primary endpoint of overall survival. Phase I/II trials looking at the efficacy of the combination of ^{223}Rd with radio-sensitizing chemotherapeutic agents are also in the planning stage.

Comparison Trials Using Various Radiopharmaceuticals

Baczyk et al. [38] have published the only direct comparison randomized trial between ^{89}Sr and ^{153}Sm. This trial was performed in Poland at a single institution and involved 100 patients, 60% with prostate cancer and 40 with breast cancer. Prior treatments were not specified (including hormonal therapies). ^{89}Sr was used at a dose of 150 MBqs, and ^{153}Sm-EDTMP was used at a dose of 37 MBq/kg. A 10 point VAS pain score was utilized in

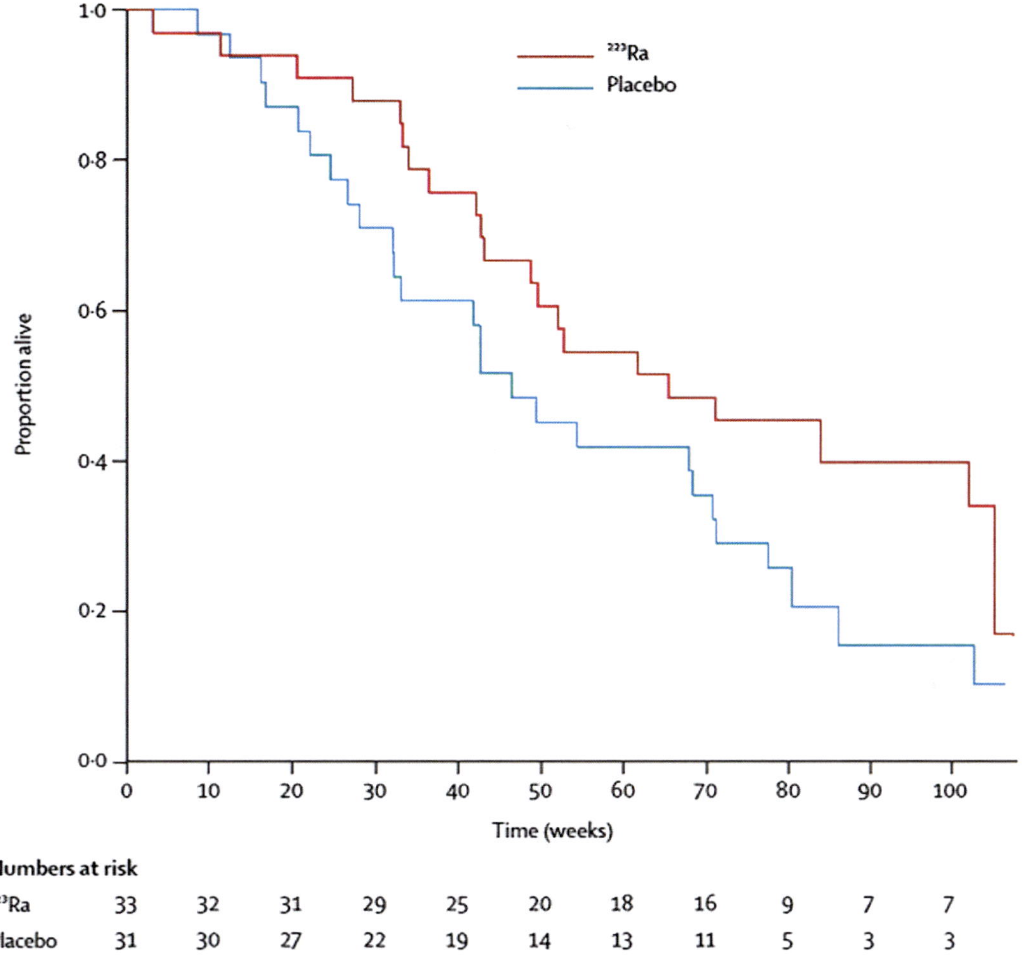

Numbers at risk										
²²³Ra	33	32	31	29	25	20	18	16	9	7	7
Placebo	31	30	27	22	19	14	13	11	5	3	3

Fig. 23.2 Overall survival for bone-metastatic CRPC patients in the randomized phase II trial comparing ²²³Rd and placebo [37]. Reproduced with permission from Elsevier, copyright 2007

combination with assessment of analgesic consumption. A median baseline VAS score was 7 (range 5–10). A "complete effect" was recorded if the VAS scores posttreatment were 0–1; partial effects were recorded if VAS scores of 2–4. Responses were measured at a single time point, 2 months after treatment. In the prostate cancer patients, no responses were recorded in 20% of patients in each arm whereas 33% of the ⁸⁹Sr and 40% of the ¹⁵³Sm-EDTMP patients had a complete response. The remaining patients had partial effects, thus the overall positive effect as measured by the VAS scores at 2 months postdosing was 80% in both arms. Analgesic consumption at 2 months postdosing was –45% and –55% in the samarium and strontium arms, respectively. Adverse events were not specifically recorded, however, five cases of "severe pancytopenia" were

encountered including three patients treated with ⁸⁹Sr and two patients treated with ¹⁵³Sm-EDTMP.

A single institutional trial comparing ⁸⁹Sr and ³²P was published from India [39]. Thirty-one patients with skeletal metastases were treated with ³²P (16 patients) or ⁸⁹Sr (15 patients). Oral ³²P was administered as a 12 mCi dose, and ⁸⁹Sr was as a 4 mCi (148 MBq) dose. Baseline pain scores of "5–10" were required pretherapy. Posttherapy, absence of pain was seen in 7/16 ³²P-treated patients and in 7/15 ⁸⁹Sr patients. A decline in pain scores of 50% or better were observed in 14/16 patients given ³²P and 14/15 patients administered ⁸⁹Sr. Mean duration of pain relief was ~10 weeks for both isotopes. There were no significant differences in terms of toxic effects, and no patients had significant neutropenia. Though this setting was relatively small, it did not demonstrate significant differences between the older and newer isotopes.

Liepe and Kotzerke [40] evaluated ^{188}Re-HEDP, ^{186}Re-HEDP, ^{153}Sm-EDTMP, and ^{89}Sr effects on pain in a single institution trial in Germany consisting of 79 patients (18 breast cancer and 61 CRPC patients). The study was nonrandomized, but VAS scores and analgesic use were obtained weekly. A total of 31 patients were treated with ^{188}Re-HEDP, 15 patients each with ^{186}Re-HEDP and ^{153}Sm-EDTMP, and 18 patients with ^{89}Sr. Analysis of responses were somewhat hampered by the lack of blinding, the lack of placebo, the lack of randomization, and the fact that breast and prostate cancer patients were not distinctly divided. Differences between the isotopes in terms of response rate or response duration were not apparent. Approximately 70% of patients in all groups had a pain response, and approximately 15% of the patients in each group were rendered pain free. Toxicities were restricted to hematological effects (though a pain flare was noted in 19% of patients). Only one patient had a grade 3 thrombocytopenia, and no patients had grade 3 neutropenia.

Combinations of Radiopharmaceuticals and Chemotherapy

^{89}Sr has been evaluated in several distinct CRPC trials in combination with chemotherapy. The largest and the most promising trial was a single institution randomized phase II study by Tu et al. [21] consisting of ^{89}Sr in combination with weekly doxorubicin. A total of 103 bone metastatic CRPC patients received induction KAVE chemotherapy, and 72 patients were subsequently randomized. The KAVE chemotherapy consisted of ketoconazole, adriamycin, vinblastine, and estramustine. Only those patients who were able to tolerate KAVE and those without progressive cancer were eligible for ^{89}Sr (4 mCi) or placebo in combination with doxorubicin for six doses (20 mg/m^2/week). In the subset of patients randomized to ^{89}Sr, a significantly prolonged median progression-free survival (13 vs. 7 months) and median overall survival (28 vs. 19 months) were observed. Grade 4 neutropenia was more common in the ^{89}Sr group, while the incidence of grade 4 thrombocytopenia was similar. Further multi-institutional randomized studies are underway using a similar design (MDA-3410/CTSU) to confirm these

important findings, but no results to date have been reported and the rate of accrual has been slower than expected.

Monotherapy with ^{89}Sr (150 MBq) was compared to a combination of ^{89}Sr and low dose cisplatin in 70 patients with CRPC patients reporting painful bone metastases [22]. The cisplatin was administered as three separate infusions (50 mg/m^2 total dose) over 11 days (before and after ^{89}Sr). In this single institution study, prespecified study endpoints were bone pain palliation at 2 months, new onset bone pain, radiographic progression of bone metastases, and survival. Bone pain improved at 2 months in 91% of those with combined modality therapy as compared to 63% in the monotherapy arm. The median survival without new painful sites was 4 months versus 2 months favoring combination therapy. Bone disease progression was observed in 27% of patients in arm the combined treatment arm as compared to 64% of patients in the ^{89}Sr alone arm. There were no statistically differences in survival. Neither thrombocytopenia nor neutropenia was problematic, no grade 3 toxicities in either realm were observed.

Morris et al. [19] recently presented initial findings of their phase I trial combining ^{153}Sm-EDTMP and docetaxel in metastatic CRPC. Cohorts of 3–6 patients were treated in a dose-escalating fashion. Prior treatment with taxanes was not an exclusion criteria. Cohorts are defined by dose escalations of docetaxel at 65, 70, 75, 75, and 75 mg/m^2 and ^{153}Sm-EDTMP was administered at 0.5, 0.5, 0.5, 0.75, and 1 mCi/kg. Each cycle was 6 weeks, except cohort 6, which explores a q 9 week cycle for the isotope. Docetaxel was given on day 1 and 22 and isotope on day −1 to 1 of each cycle. No dose limiting toxicity was reached though 6 of 28 patients came off study for prolonged thrombocytopenia. It was concluded that coadministration of docetaxel and ^{153}Sm-EDTMP was surprisingly well tolerated even with full doses of both drugs (1 mCi/kg of isotope and 75 mg/m^2 of docetaxel) with each drug administered in a repetitive fashion. Interestingly, some patients who were docetaxel resistant coming into the protocol were able to respond (by PSA criteria) to combination therapy, suggesting the possibility of synergy between these two agents. Additional studies, with randomization, will be necessary to understand the therapeutic potential of this combination.

In a distinct trial design reminiscent of the ^{89}Sr study by Tu et al. [21], patients with bone metastatic

CRPC achieving a response or stabilization after four cycles of docetaxel and estramustine were given "consolidation" docetaxel at a dose of 20 mg/m²/week for 6 weeks in combination with ^{153}Sm-EDTMP (1 mCi/kg). A total of 43 patients were included in this trial [20]. A PSA response was obtained in 77%, and the pain response rate was 69%. At least five of the six planned weekly injections of docetaxel were administered to 34 patients (81%). The consolidation docetaxel-^{153}Sm-EDTMP regimen was well tolerated with no febrile neutropenia, and only two episodes (5%) of rapidly reversible grade 3 thrombocytopenia occurred. The median survival was 29 months, the 1-year survival rate was 77%, and the 2-year survival rate was 56%. This survival exceeds expectations but confirmation in larger, multi-institutional randomized studies will be required for full credibility.

Current Utilization of Radiopharmaceuticals

Though the use of the radiopharmaceuticals are FDA approved and supported by prospective randomized placebo-controlled trials, their use has been more limited than expected based on these data. The reasons for limited use are multifactorial and in part involve a variety of market forces. Reimbursement of chemotherapeutic agents and radiopharmaceuticals are distinct, and some authors have made note that this could be a contributing factor impairing isotopic utilization [41]. Further, despite some evidence to the contrary [42], concerns that radiopharmaceuticals may interfere with subsequent chemotherapy dosing have been cited as a potentially limiting reason for using these agents.

References

1. Friedell HL, Storaasli JP. The use of radioactive phosphorus in the treatment of carcinoma of the breast with widespread metastases to bone. Am J Roentgenol Radium Ther 1950;64:559–75.
2. Kaplan E, Fels, IG, Kotlowski BR, et al. Therapy of carcinoma of the prostate metastatic to bone with P³² labeled condensed phosphate. J Nucl Med 1960;1:1–13.
3. Jemal A, Siegel R, Ward E, et al. Cancer statistics, 2008. CA Cancer J Clin 2008;58:71–96.
4. Tannock IF, de Wit R, Berry WR, et al. Docetaxel plus prednisone or mitoxantrone plus prednisone for advanced prostate cancer. N Engl J Med 2004;351:1502–12.
5. Petrylak DP, Tangen CM, Hussain MH, et al. Docetaxel and estramustine compared with mitoxantrone and prednisone for advanced refractory prostate cancer. N Engl J Med 2004;351:1513–20.
6. Loberg RD, Logothetis CJ, Keller ET, Pienta KJ. Pathogenesis and treatment of prostate cancer bone metastases: targeting the lethal phenotype. J Clin Oncol 2005;23:8232–41.
7. Saad F, Gleason DM, Murray R, et al. A randomized, placebo-controlled trial of zoledronic acid in patients with hormone-refractory metastatic prostate carcinoma. J Natl Cancer Inst 2002;94:1458–68.
8. Licciardone JC. The epidemiology and medical management of low back pain during ambulatory medical care visits in the United States. Osteopath Med Prim Care 2008;2:11.
9. Newling DW, Denis L, Vermeylen K. Orchiectomy versus goserelin and flutamide in the treatment of newly diagnosed metastatic prostate cancer. Analysis of the criteria of evaluation used in the European Organization for Research and Treatment of Cancer – Genitourinary Group Study 30853. Cancer 1993;72(12 Suppl):3793–8.
10. Strum SB, McDermed JE, Scholz MC, et al. Anaemia associated with androgen deprivation in patients with prostate cancer receiving combined hormone blockade. Br J Urol. 1997;79:933–41.
11. Spivak JL. The anaemia of cancer: death by a thousand cuts. Nat Rev Cancer 2005;5:543–55.
12. Halabi S, Small EJ, Kantoff PW, et al. Prognostic model for predicting survival in men with hormone-refractory metastatic prostate cancer. J Clin Oncol 2003;21:1232–7; erratum in: J Clin Oncol 2004;22:3434.
13. Beer TM, Tangen CM, Bland LB, et al. Prognostic value of anemia in newly diagnosed metastatic prostate cancer: a multivariate analysis of southwest oncology group study 8894. J Urol 2004;172:2213–7; erratum in: J Urol 2005;174:1156.
14. Ritter MA, Cleaver JE, Tobias CA. High-LET radiations induce a large proportion of non-rejoining DNA breaks. Nature 1977;266:653–5.
15. Ben-Josef E, Maughan RL, Vasan S, Porter AT. A direct measurement of strontium-89 activity in bone metastases. Nucl Med Commun 1995;16:452–6.
16. Goeckeler WF, Edwards B, Volkert WA, et al. Skeletal localization of samarium-153 chelates: potential therapeutic bone agents. J Nucl Med 1987;28:495–504.
17. Vinjamuri S, Ray S. Phosphorus-32: The forgotten radiopharmaceutical? Nucl Med Commun 2008;29:95–7.
18. Henriksen G, Breistøl K, Bruland ØS, et al. Significant anti-tumor effect from bone-seeking, alpha-particle-emitting (223)Ra demonstrated in an experimental skeletal metastases model. Cancer Res 2002;62:3120–5.
19. Morris MJ, Pandit-Taskar N, Carrasquillo J, et al. Phase I Study of Samarium-153 Lexidronam (153Sm-EDTMP) with Docetaxel in castration-resistant metastatic prostate cancer. J Clin Oncol 2009;27:2436–42.
20. Fizazi P, Beuzeboc J, Lumbroso, et al. A prospective Phase II trial of consolidation Docetaxel and Samarium-153 in patients with bone metastases from castration resistant prostate cancer. J Clin Oncol 2009;27:2429–35.

21. Tu SM, Millikan RE, Mengistu B, et al. Bone-targeted therapy for advanced androgen-independent carcinoma of the prostate: a randomized Phase II trial. Lancet 2001;357: 336–41; erratum in: Lancet 2001;357:1210.

22. Sciuto R, Festa A, Rea S, et al. Effects of low-dose cisplatin on 89Sr therapy for painful bone metastases from prostate cancer: a randomized clinical trial. J Nucl Med 2002;43:79–86.

23. Steenland E, Leer JW, van Houwelingen H, et al. The effect of a single fraction compared to multiple fractions on painful bone metastases: a global analysis of the Dutch Bone Metastasis Study. Radiother Oncol 1999;52:101–9; erratum in: Radiother Oncol 1999;53:167; Leer J [corrected to Leer JW]; van Mierlo T [corrected to van Mierlo I].

24. Wu JS, Monk G, Clark T, et al. Palliative radiotherapy improves pain and reduces functional interference in patients with painful bone metastases: a quality assurance study. Clin Oncol (R Coll Radiol) 2006;18:539–44.

25. Oosterhof GO, Roberts JT, de Reijke TM, et al. Strontium (89) chloride versus palliative local field radiotherapy in patients with hormonal escaped prostate cancer: a phase III study of the European Organisation of Research and Treatment of Cancer, Genitourinary Group. Eur Urol 2003;44:519–26.

26. Quilty PM, Kirk D, Bolger JJ, et al. A comparison of the palliative effects of strontium-89 and external beam radiotherapy in metastatic prostate cancer. Radiother Oncol 1994;31:33–40.

27. Porter AT, McEwan AJ, Powe JE, et al. Results of a randomized phase-III trial to evaluate the efficacy of strontium-89 adjuvant to local field external beam irradiation in the management of endocrine resistant metastatic prostate cancer. Int J Radiat Oncol Biol Phys 1993;25:805–13.

28. Lewington VJ, McEwan AJ, Ackery DM, et al. A prospective, randomised double-blind crossover study to examine the efficacy of strontium-89 in pain palliation in patients with advanced prostate cancer metastatic to bone. Eur J Cancer 1991;27:954–8.

29. Buchali K, Correns HJ, Schuerer M, et al. Results of a double blind study of 89-strontium therapy of skeletal metastases of prostatic carcinoma. Eur J Nucl Med 1988;14:349–51.

30. Kasalický J, Krajská V. The effect of repeated strontium-89 chloride therapy on bone pain palliation in patients with skeletal cancer metastases. Eur J Nucl Med 1998;25:1362–7.

31. Pons F, Herranz R, Garcia A, et al. Strontium-89 for palliation of pain from bone metastases in patients with prostate and breast cancer. Eur J Nucl Med 1997;24:1210–4.

32. Serafini AN, Houston SJ, Resche I, et al. Palliation of pain associated with metastatic bone cancer using samarium-153 lexidronam: a double-blind placebo-controlled clinical trial. J Clin Oncol 1998;16:1574–81.

33. Sartor O, Reid RH, Hoskin PJ, et al. Quadramet 424Sm10/11 Study Group. Samarium-153-Lexidronam complex for treatment of painful bone metastases in hormone-refractory prostate cancer. Urology 2004;63:940–5.

34. Sartor O, Reid RH, Bushnell DL, et al. Safety and efficacy of repeat administration of samarium Sm-153 lexidronam to patients with metastatic bone pain. Cancer 2007;109: 637–43.

35. Higano CS, Quick DP, Bushnell D, Sartor O. Safety analysis of repeated high doses of samarium-153 lexidronam in men with hormone-naive prostate cancer metastatic to bone. Clin Genitourin Cancer 2008;6:40–5.

36. Nilsson S, Larsen RH, Fossa SD, et al. First Clinical Experience with α emitting radium-223 in the treatment of skeletal metastases. Clin Cancer Res 2005;11:4451–59.

37. Nilsson S, Franzén L, Parker C, et al. Bone-targeted radium-223 in symptomatic, hormone-refractory prostate cancer: a randomised, multicentre, placebo-controlled phase II study. Lancet Oncol 2007;8:587–94.

38. Baczyk M, Czepczyński R, Milecki P, et al. 89Sr versus 153Sm-EDTMP: comparison of treatment efficacy of painful bone metastases in prostate and breast carcinoma. Nucl Med Commun 2007;28:245–50.

39. Nair N. Relative efficacy of 32P and 89Sr in palliation in skeletal metastases. J Nucl Med 1999;40:256–61.

40. Liepe K, Korzerke J. A comparative study of 188Re-HEDP, 186Re-HEDP, 153 Sm-EDTMP and 89Sr in the treatment of painful skeletal metastases. Nucl Med Commun 2007;28: 623–30.

41. Berenson A. Market Forces Cited in Lymphoma Drugs' Disuse. New York Times, July 14, 2007 (http://www.nytimes.com/2007/07/14/health/14lymphoma.html, referenced 1/5/09).

42. Tu SM, Kim J, Pagliaro LC, et al. Therapy tolerance in selected patients with androgen-independent prostate cancer following strontium-89 combined with chemotherapy. J Clin Oncol 2005;23:7904–10.

Chapter 24
Bisphosphonates for Prevention and Treatment of Bone Metastases

Philip J. Saylor and Matthew R. Smith

Abstract Most men with advanced prostate cancer develop bone metastases. The most common sites of bone metastases from prostate cancer are the spine, pelvis, and ribs. Though they typically have a sclerotic or osteoblastic appearance when imaged, these metastases feature excess activity by both osteoblasts and osteoclasts. Pathologic osteoclast activation is associated with skeletal complications, disease progression, and death. The clinical burden of bone metastases is high as they commonly present with pain but can also present with spinal cord compression, fractures, and myelophthisis.

Zoledronic acid is a potent intravenous bisphosphonate. In men with castration-resistant prostate cancer and bone metastases, zoledronic acid decreases the risk of disease-related skeletal complications. There is limited information about the optimal frequency and duration of therapy for men with castration-resistant disease and bone metastases. The role of zoledronic acid and other bisphosphonates in androgen-sensitive disease or for prevention of bone metastases is unknown. Further clinical trials are needed to establish its optimal frequency, dose, and duration of therapy.

Denosumab is a fully human monoclonal antibody against receptor activator of nuclear factor-kappa-B ligand (RANKL). Denosumab is currently under investigation in three major prostate cancer trials that are designed to evaluate its ability to prevent fractures, bone metastases, and disease-related skeletal events.

Keywords Prostate cancer • Bone metastases • Osteoclast • Bisphosphonate • Skeletal-related events • Denosumab • Odanacatib

P.J. Saylor (✉)
Department of Medicine, Division of Hematology/Oncology,
Massachusetts General Hospital Cancer Center, Boston, MA, USA
e-mail: psaylor@partners.org

Normal Bone Physiology

Healthy bone is maintained by a dynamic and ongoing process of remodeling throughout the skeleton. This process depends on a balance between bone resorption by osteoclasts and new bone formation by osteoblasts. Osteoclasts are tissue-specific macrophages that grow and differentiate from monocyte/macrophage progenitors. Osteoclasts resorb bone by binding to it and creating a sealed resorption vacuole into which they secrete protons and lytic enzymes. The two most active enzymes within this acidified compartment are tartrate-resistant acid phosphatase (TRAP) and cathepsin [1].

The receptor activator of nuclear factor-kappa-B (RANK) signaling pathway is central to regulation of both immature and mature osteoclasts, though at least 24 additional genes or loci have been shown to be involved in osteoclast regulation. The pathway consists of RANK ligand (RANKL) and its two receptors: RANK and osteoprotegerin. Osteoprotegerin competitively inhibits RANK activation by acting as a decoy receptor for RANKL. Activation of RANK by RANKL on the surface of osteoclast precursors leads to gene expression and cellular differentiation to mature multi-nucleated osteoclasts. Similar RANK activation on mature osteoclasts leads to longer survival and an increase in bone resorption.

Pathophysiology of Osteoblastic Bone Metastases

Bone biopsies in men with metastatic prostate cancer show evidence of a high turnover state with activation of both osteoclasts and osteoblasts in the areas involved

W.D. Figg et al. (eds.), *Drug Management of Prostate Cancer*,
DOI 10.1007/978-1-60327-829-4_24, © Springer Science+Business Media, LLC 2010

with tumor. As osteoclasts erode normal trabecular bone, osteoblasts replace it with sclerotic woven bone. Though woven bone characteristically appears dense or blastic when imaged, such blastic metastases considerably weaken the structural integrity of the bone and increase fracture risk [2].

Several urine and serum laboratory markers are elevated in the presence of bone metastases as a reflection of bone resorption and formation. Urinary N-telopeptide (NTx) is a marker of collagen breakdown by osteoclasts. Bone-specific alkaline phosphatase (BAP) is a marker of osteoblast function. Both NTx and BAP have been found to be significantly elevated in patients with bone metastases from prostate cancer [3]. Correlation between serum alkaline phosphatase (AP) and BAP is strong, making the more available AP a practical alternative to measuring the bone-specific isoform [4].

These lab tests can be used to estimate prognosis and monitor response to therapy. Binary (high vs. low) classification of resorption (NTx) and formation (BAP) markers in patients with solid tumors metastatic to bone has demonstrated that high initial levels correlate with adverse outcomes such as skeletal-related events, clinical bone disease progression, and death. Markers of resorption fall substantially in response to osteoclast inhibition or to RANKL inhibition [5]. Bone metabolism markers have been used to guide decisions about dose and schedule selection in early phase clinical trials but are not yet used to make treatment decisions in routine clinical practice.

Clinical Manifestations of Bone Metastases

Pain is easily the most frequent clinical manifestation of bone metastases, though they can also cause fractures or spinal cord compression. Androgen deprivation therapy (ADT), the mainstay of treatment for metastatic prostate cancer, accelerates bone turnover [6, 7], decreases bone mineral density (BMD) [6–11], and contributes to fracture risk [12–14]. Fracture is most common in the vertebral bodies but can also be observed in the pelvis, ribs, or long bones. Hypocalcemia due to calcium deposition in newly formed bone is common but is usually asymptomatic. Finally, androgen deprivation routinely causes a mild normocytic anemia [15].

Bisphosphonates

Bisphosphonates are chemically similar to inorganic pyrophosphate, a necessary component of normal bone [16]. A central carbon binds to the two phosphate groups and to the two organic side chains that identify each particular bisphosphonate. Their therapeutic benefits seem to stem from a combination of this affinity for bone and their effects on the osteoclasts themselves.

The negatively charged phosphate groups have strong affinity for cations such as calcium and therefore are easily incorporated into bone, though the strength of this affinity varies considerably from one bisphosphonate to the next. Bisphosphonates are chemically resistant to hydrolysis and exert potent inhibitory and even proapoptotic effects on the osteoclasts that encounter them at highest concentration and ingest them by endocytosis [17]. Nitrogen-containing bisphosphonates (alendronate, risedronate, ibandronate, zoledronic acid) inhibit farnesyl pyrophosphate synthase, a branch-point enzyme in the mevalonate pathway that is important to osteoclast function, though other cellular pathways are likely involved [18].

Potency of osteoclast inhibition can be estimated by farnesyl pyrophosphate synthase inhibition, a property that orders the available bisphosphonates as follows: etidronate = clodronate $<<<$ pamidronate $<$ alendronate $<$ ibandronate $<$ risedronate $<$ zoledronic acid [18]. Zoledronic acid is the most potent of the available bisphosphonates, at least 100 times more potent than clodronate or pamidronate in preclinical models.

Bisphosphonates in Metastatic Bone Disease

In 1995, pamidronate was approved by the Food and Drug Administration to prevent disease-related skeletal complications in patients with bone metastases from breast cancer and bone disease from multiple myeloma. In 2002, zoledronic acid was approved for the prevention of skeletal complications in patients with myeloma bone disease and bone metastases from solid tumors including breast, lung, and prostate cancer. This approval of zoledronic acid was based on the results of three large randomized controlled trials that included over 3,000 patients with a variety of malignancies [19–21]. In prostate cancer specifically, it was shown to reduce skeletal-related events (SREs) in the setting of castration-resistant metastatic disease [21]. Zoledronic acid is not approved for treatment of hormone-sensitive metastatic disease or for treatment of men without bone metastases.

Bisphosphonates in the Treatment of Castration-Resistant Prostate Cancer

In the USA, zoledronic acid is approved for the prevention of SREs in men with prostate cancer and bone metastases who have failed first line hormone therapy (castration-resistant metastatic disease). The Zometa 039 study established its efficacy in this setting where comparably designed trials with pamidronate and clodronate had failed to demonstrate benefit (Table 24.1).

Zometa 039 was a randomized, placebo controlled trial that enrolled 643 patients with castration-resistant prostate cancer and asymptomatic or minimally symptomatic bone metastases. Subjects were randomized to placebo or to one of two doses of zoledronic acid (4 or 8 mg every 3 weeks for 15 months). Primary therapy for the prostate cancer was as chosen by the treating physicians, and androgen deprivation was continued throughout. The primary efficacy endpoint was the proportion of patients who experienced at least one SRE during the study period. SREs included pathologic bone fractures, spinal cord compression, surgery or radiation to bone, and antineoplastic therapy to treat bone pain [21].

Though the trial began with two-dose cohorts for zoledronic acid, concern about renal toxicity led to two protocol modifications prior to completion. First, the infusion time was lengthened from 5 to 15 min. Second, the 8-mg group was dose reduced to 4 mg. Of the 643 patients enrolled, 14 experienced grade 3 serum increases in creatinine (7 in the 4-mg group, 5 in the 8/4-mg group, 2 in the placebo group); none required dialysis.

At the 15-month conclusion of the trial, patients treated with 4-mg zoledronic acid had fewer SREs (33.2%) than patients who received placebo (44.2%) ($P=0.02$). See Fig. 24.1 for a combined analysis of SRE prevention in this trial and another similar trial. Zoledronic acid treatment at 4 mg also lengthened median time to first SRE from 321 to 488 days ($P=0.009$) [22]. Though the study was not designed to assess differences in overall survival, there was a non-significant improvement in median survival from 464 to 546 days ($P=0.091$) in the 4-mg group compared with placebo. Follow-up at 24 months showed durable benefit as the risk of SREs was reduced by 36% compared with placebo ($P=0.002$) [22]. This trial led to the approval of zoledronic acid for the treatment of castration-resistant prostate cancer metastatic to bone.

Combined analysis was performed on two multicenter, randomized, placebo-controlled trials (Protocol 032 and INT 05) that evaluated pamidronate (90 mg given intravenously every 3 weeks for 27 weeks). Together, the trials enrolled 350 patients. Efficacy was assessed with self-reported pain score, analgesic use, and proportion of patients with a SRE. There were no statistically significant differences in these endpoints between the treatment and placebo groups. Urinary bone resorption markers did decline with treatment, though less so than has typically been observed with zoledronic acid treatment. For example, NTx levels fell approximately 50% from baseline with pamidronate treatment but fell by more than 70% on treatment in the Zometa 039 study. Lack of pamidronate efficacy in this study may be at least partially due to less potent osteoclast inhibition [23].

Table 24.1 Notable randomized controlled trials using bisphosphonates for metastatic prostate cancer

Study	n	Study population	Arms	Outcome
Zometa 039	643	Asymptomatic or minimally symptomatic, castration-resistant	Zoledronic acid vs. placebo, every 3 weeks	Significant decrease in skeletal-related events, trend toward improved survival
Study 032/INT	350	Symptomatic, castration-resistant	Pamidronate vs. placebo, every 3 weeks	No significant difference in pain, analgesic use, or skeletal-related events
NCIC Pr06	204	Symptomatic, castration-resistant	Mitoxantrone and prednisone ± clodronate, every 3 weeks IV	No significant difference in palliative response (pain scores or analgesic use)
MRC Pr05	311	Androgen-sensitive	Daily oral clodronate vs. placebo	Trend toward improved bone progression-free survival ($P=0.066$)

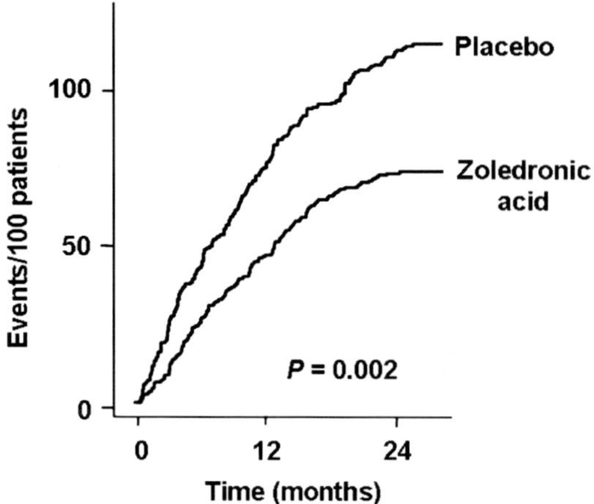

Fig. 24.1 Cumulative incidence of skeletal-related events [28] The survival-adjusted cumulative incidence of skeletal-related events was significantly reduced by 35.3% by treatment with 4-mg zoledronic acid compared with placebo in two large prospective randomized controlled trials [20, 21]

The National Cancer Institute of Canada Pr06 (NCIC Pr06) evaluated patients with castration-resistant prostate cancer and symptomatic bone metastases. They were randomized in this double-blind, controlled trial to mitoxantrone and prednisone with or without the addition of clodronate (1,500 mg intravenously every 3 weeks). Mitoxantrone was given 12 mg/m^2 intravenously every 3 weeks and prednisone was given 5 mg twice daily. The primary endpoint was palliative response, defined as either a two-point pain reduction by the present pain intensity index or a 50% decrease in analgesic use. The majority (77%) of the 209 patients had mild pain scores at baseline. There was no statistically significant difference in achievement of the primary endpoint between the study group (46%) and the control group (39%) (P=0.54). Secondary endpoints such as survival, quality of life, and progression-free survival (PFS) were also statistically unchanged between the groups [24].

Bisphosphonates in the Treatment of Androgen-Sensitive Prostate Cancer

The only completed trial to examine bisphosphonates in androgen-sensitive prostate cancer is the MRC PR05 trial that compared oral sodium clodronate (2,080 mg/day) to placebo for men with bone metastases. It was a double-blind, placebo-controlled trial and enrolled

311 patients for a maximum of 3 years of study-directed treatment. The primary endpoint was symptomatic bone PFS. Symptomatic bone PFS is a similar endpoint to SREs but requires that the event be clinically appreciated rather than simply an imaging finding. Overall survival was a secondary endpoint. After a median of 59 months, the treatment group showed nonsignificant improvements in overall survival (HR 0.80, 95% CI 0.62–1.03, P=0.082) and in symptomatic bone PFS (HR 0.79, 95% CI 0.61–1.02, P=0.066). Patients in the treatment group had a higher incidence of gastrointestinal adverse events (HR 1.71, 95% CI 1.21–2.41; P=0.002) [25]. Interestingly, subgroup analysis suggested that earlier start of this therapy improved efficacy.

CALGB/CTSU 90202 is a currently enrolling randomized, double-blind, placebo-controlled phase III trial comparing early to standard zoledronic acid for the prevention of SREs in men with androgen-sensitive prostate cancer metastatic to bone. All patients are started on zoledronic acid within 3 months of initiation of androgen deprivation. This will be an important trial as it is well designed and examines a high risk but previously understudied population (hormone sensitive) while making use of a more potent bisphosphonate than was used in the MRC PR05 trial. The goal accrual is 680 patients.

Bisphosphonates for the Prevention of Bone Metastases

Two randomized controlled trials have evaluated bisphosphonates for prevention of bone metastases in prostate cancer; neither showed significant benefit.

First, the Medical Research Council Pr04 trial enrolled 508 men with nonmetastatic prostate cancer and randomized them to daily oral clodronate (2,080 mg/daily) or to placebo for a maximum of 5 years. The patients were followed for a median of nearly 10 years. All men had locally advanced (T2–T4) prostate cancer and a negative bone scan at enrollment. The treatment group showed no sign of benefit. There was a nonsignificant increase in new bone metastases (80 events with clodronate, 68 events with placebo; HR=1.22; 95% CI 0.88–1.68) and no change in overall survival (130 deaths with clodronate and 127 deaths with placebo, HR=1.02, 95% CI=0.80–1.30). Clodronate was well tolerated with only mild increases in gastrointestinal problems and increased lactate dehydrogenase levels [26]. Though the trial was well designed and follow-up was excellent, it was likely hurt by the use of clodronate, a comparatively weak bisphosphonate.

Second, Zometa 704 was designed to evaluate the ability of zoledronic acid to delay the time to first bone metastasis in patients with castration-resistant prostate cancer. Progression during ADT prior to study enrollment was defined as three consecutive rises in PSA at least 2 weeks apart from one another, initial PSA rise within 10 months of study entry, or last PSA at least 150% of the nadir value. Subjects were randomized to either zoledronic acid (4 mg intravenously every 4 weeks) or to placebo. Unfortunately, the study was placed on hold in September 2002 due to low event rate after accruing 398 of the planned 991 patients. It was eventually terminated. The study and control groups had similar time to first metastases but the low event rate and the low accrual both conspired against thorough evaluation.

Though the Zometa 704 trial was ended early, analysis of the 201 patients in the placebo group did yield interesting information about the natural history of PSA-only recurrent prostate cancer. Median bone metastasis-free survival was 30 months, and at 2-year follow-up 33% of patients had developed a bone metastasis. The most powerful predictors of time to first metastasis and overall survival were baseline PSA (if >10 ng/mL, relative risk 3.18) and PSA velocity. Median time to first bone metastasis and overall survival had not been reached [27].

Though results of both trials were disappointing, they have strongly influenced the design of subsequent studies. The low event rate and long metastasis-free survival, even with castration-resistant prostate cancer, have led investigators to plan for higher enrollment and longer follow-up to achieve adequate statistical power. As an example, the three current denosumab trials (Table 24.2) are planned to accrue over 4,500 patients in all.

Bisphosphonates: Safety

Current clinical trial evidence supports the use of zoledronic acid (4 mg intravenously every 3–4 weeks) to reduce the risk of SREs in men with castration-resistant prostate cancer and bone metastases [28]. Androgen-sensitive disease is an area of ongoing investigation and is currently without clear evidence to support bisphosphonate treatment. Widespread and increasingly long courses of bisphosphonate treatment have led to a better understanding of their toxicities.

The two most common side effects of bisphosphonate therapy are an acute phase reaction and hypocalcemia. This acute phase reaction is generally a self-limited flu-like illness that starts within a day of the infusion and may include nausea/vomiting and fever [29]. Calcium and vitamin D supplementation are recommended during bisphosphonate treatment to prevent symptomatic hypocalcemia. The two most feared complications of bisphosphonate use are acute renal failure and osteonecrosis of the jaw (ONJ).

Renal toxicity has been observed to range in severity from a transient asymptomatic creatinine elevation to permanent dialysis dependence. In one early series, patients who developed renal failure during bisphosphonate treatment underwent kidney biopsies, which showed evidence of acute tubular necrosis with tubular cell degeneration, loss of brush border, and apoptosis [30]. In another series of 72 cases of FDA-reported adverse events with the 4 mg/15 min infusion combination, the effected patients began with a mean baseline creatinine of 1.7 mg/dL (range 0.6–5.2) and developed renal failure an average of 56 days after initiation of zoledronic acid use (range: 1–51 months) [31]. Among

Table 24.2 Current randomized controlled trials of denosumab for prostate cancer

Study/purpose	n	Study population	Arms	Endpoint(s)
Amgen protocol 138: fracture prevention	1,468	Current androgen deprivation therapy; no metastases	Denosumab vs. placebo	Incident vertebral fractures, bone mineral density
Amgen protocol 147: metastasis prevention	1,400	Castration-resistant, high risk but no bone metastases	Denosumab vs. placebo	Bone metastasis-free survival
Amgen protocol 103: prevention of skeletal complications	1,700	Castration-resistant, bone metastases	Denosumab vs. zoledronic acid	Skeletal-related events

patients who developed renal failure, about one-quarter experienced the deterioration of renal function after the first dose.

The zoledronic acid package insert specifies that single doses should not exceed 4 mg and that the infusion duration should be no less than 15 min. It also recommends that if the baseline creatinine was normal but increased 0.5 mg/dL or was abnormal and increased 1.0 mg/dL within 2 weeks of zoledronic acid dosing, the drug should be held until creatinine is within 10% of its initial value. The most recent update of the document includes recommended starting dose reductions for calculated creatinine clearances of less than 60 mL/min [32].

ONJ presents clinically in bisphosphonate-treated patients as nonhealing areas of exposed and necrotic bone in the maxillofacial region. Much descriptive literature has been published since the first recognized cases of ONJ in 2003 and 2004 [33, 34]. It is exceedingly rare with the use of oral bisphosphonates (e.g., 0.7/100,000 person/years of exposure for alendronate according to Merck [35]). Published retrospective studies of ONJ incidence with intravenous bisphosphonates show estimates ranging from 0.8 to 12% [36]. Another large retrospective analysis of patients treated with intravenous bisphosphonates showed that dose and duration of treatment were higher in patients with ONJ ($P<0.0001$). Finally, multivariate Cox proportional hazards regression analysis has showed dental extractions ($P<0.0001$) and treatment with zoledronic acid ($P=0.0004$) to be significant risk factors for ONJ [37].

The optimal duration of bisphosphonate therapy in patients with bone metastases from prostate cancer has not yet been defined. Relevant clinical trials have included up to 24 months of treatment. Practice guidelines for duration of therapy for prostate cancer do not yet exist.

The American Association of Oral and Maxillofacial Surgeons wrote a position paper about bisphosphonate-related ONJ [35]. It recommends oral examination and optimization prior to initiation of treatment (with extraction of nonrestorable teeth and 14–21 day wait until the extraction site has mucosalized), discontinuation of therapy for 3 months on either side of elective dental surgery, and avoidance of invasive procedures if possible. In patients with established ONJ, treatment depends on severity of the lesion. Early lesions seem to benefit from oral antimicrobial rinses such as chlorhexidine 0.12%. Intermediate disease is managed with the addition of systemic antibiotic therapy. Advanced disease usually causes pain and is managed with surgical debridement and antibiotic therapy. Others have suggested that resolution with antibiotic therapy alone is rare and that early conservative surgical therapies such as laser treatment may be more broadly indicated [38].

Future Directions in Bone-Targeted Therapy for Prostate Cancer

Though zoledronic acid is the only drug currently approved for the management of prostate cancer bone metastases, there are a variety of nonbisphosphonate bone-targeted drugs currently in development. The two that are in phase III study are the monoclonal antibody RANK-ligand inhibitor denosumab.

Denosumab: RANK-Ligand Inhibitor in Current Clinical Trials

The role of receptor activator of nuclear factor-kappa-B ligand (RANKL) in osteoclast differentiation, function, and survival makes it a rational target for drug development in osteoclast-mediated diseases. Denosumab is a fully human monoclonal antibody against RANKL and has shown promise in early clinical trials for both benign and malignant bone disease. It is administered subcutaneously and inhibits RANKL by binding avidly and specifically to it. Even a single dose has been shown to promptly decrease the bone turnover marker NTx in 84% of patients and for up to 6 months [5]. In an early trial of denosumab in myeloma and breast cancer patients, the highest two doses suppressed NTx levels within 1 day and sustained this suppression for 84 days. Mean denosumab half-lives were 33.3 and 46.3 days for those two highest doses [39].

Denosumab has preliminarily been shown to be effective in the treatment of postmenopausal bone loss and in the treatment of bone lesions caused by breast cancer or multiple myeloma. It is currently under development for three distinct indications in the management of prostate cancer: prevention of bone loss and fractures during ADT (discussed in the following section), prevention of bone metastases in castration-resistant prostate cancer, and prevention of SREs in castration-resistant prostate cancer with bone metastases. Over 4,500 patients are involved in these three clinical trials (see Table 24.2).

Amgen protocol 147 is enrolling men with prostate cancer and rising PSA despite ADT but without bone metastases. The study involves only subjects at high risk for the development of bone metastases based on PSA ≥ 8 ng/dL and/or PSA doubling time ≤ 10 months. Subjects are randomized to denosumab or placebo. The study is planned to accrue 1,400 patients. The primary study endpoint is bone metastasis-free survival.

Amgen protocol 103 is a study of men with prostate cancer metastatic to bone and disease progression despite ADT. Subjects are assigned to denosumab or zoledronic acid, the current standard therapy for prevention of skeletal complications in this setting. The primary endpoint is time to first SRE (pathological fracture, radiation to bone, surgery to bone, or spinal cord compression). The study is planned to accrue 1,700 patients and is designed to demonstrate that denosumab is not inferior to zoledronic acid.

Denosumab seems to hold much promise in the treatment of prostate cancer, though it requires further evaluation of both efficacy and toxicity. In contrast to zoledronic acid, denosumab has not been associated with renal toxicity or ONJ. Ongoing and future clinical trials will define the efficacy and safety of denosumab.

Prevention of Osteoporosis and Fractures During ADT

Fractures are a substantial burden to men worldwide [40]. For example, one-third of all hip fractures occur in men [41]. The most common causes of acquired osteoporosis in men are hypogonadism, chronic glucocorticoid therapy, and alcohol abuse [42]. The leading cause of hypogonadism in men is ADT for prostate cancer.

ADT is the mainstay of treatment for metastatic prostate cancer [43] and is accomplished by either bilateral orchiectomies or by administration of a GnRH agonist. GnRH agonist therapy is also often given to men concurrently with primary radiation for locally advanced disease and to men with recurrent nonmetastatic prostate cancer. BMD falls during ADT, a change

that correlates with rising fracture risk [44]. ADT increases the risk for fractures in men [12, 13].

Several bisphosphonates have been shown to increase BMD and decrease markers of bone metabolism in men receiving ADT for prostate cancer. Among these are pamidronate [45, 46], zoledronic acid [47, 48], and alendronate [49]. Several additional classes of drugs have been studied or are currently under study. Raloxifene and toremifene, both selective estrogen receptor modulators, have been shown to increase BMD and decrease markers of bone metabolism in men receiving ADT for prostate cancer [50, 51].

Until recently, however, there was limited data about the prevention of osteoporotic fractures in men receiving ADT for prostate cancer. Phase III trials to assess the impact of toremifene and denosumab on BMD and incident fractures have been completed. Final results are pending. Denosumab is being studied (Amgen protocol 138) in men with prostate cancer who are receiving current ADT and are at increased risk for fracture based on older age and/or low BMD. Subjects are randomized to denosumab or placebo. The study has accrued 1,468 patients. Study endpoints are incident fractures and change in BMD.

Toremifene, the selective estrogen receptor modulator, is being studied in a multicenter phase III fracture prevention study in which men 50 years or older are randomized to receive 80 mg daily oral toremifene or placebo. The trial has enrolled 1,392 men and is powered to examine fracture prevention. Planned interim analysis of the first 197 subjects showed that the treatment arm enjoyed significant increases in BMD at all examined skeletal sites [52].

Conclusion

Bone metastases are a common feature of advanced prostate cancer. They contribute significantly to the clinical burden of the disease as they frequently cause pain and can also cause fractures and spinal cord compression. Bisphosphonates were the first class of drugs to gain FDA approval for the management of bone metastases. Specifically, zoledronic acid is the standard-of-care for the prevention of SREs due to bone metastases in castration-resistant prostate cancer. The role of bisphosphonates in the management of nonmetastatic disease or androgen-sensitive metastatic disease is currently under study. Bisphosphonates are generally well tolerated but do cause risk for a variety of side effects both common (self-limited acute phase reaction) and rare-but-morbid (ONJ, acute renal failure). Two bone-targeted investigational agents are currently in phase III clinical trials. Denosumab, a human monoclonal antibody targeting RANKL, is under study in three distinct clinical trials for the prevention of bone loss and fractures during ADT, the prevention of bone metastases in castration-resistant prostate cancer, and the prevention of SREs in castration-resistant prostate cancer with bone metastases.

References

1. Boyle WJ, Simonet WS, Lacey DL. Osteoclast differentiation and activation. Nature 2003;423(6937):337–42.
2. Clarke NW, McClure J, George NJ. Osteoblast function and osteomalacia in metastatic prostate cancer. Eur Urol 1993;24(2):286–90.
3. Demers LM, Costa L, Lipton A. Biochemical markers and skeletal metastases. Cancer 2000;88(12 Suppl):2919–26.
4. Cook RJ, Coleman R, Brown J, et al. Markers of bone metabolism and survival in men with hormone-refractory metastatic prostate cancer. Clin Cancer Res 2006;12(11 Pt 1):3361–7.
5. Bekker PJ, Holloway DL, Rasmussen AS, et al. A single-dose placebo-controlled study of AMG 162, a fully human monoclonal antibody to RANKL, in postmenopausal women. J Bone Miner Res 2004;19(7):1059–66.
6. Maillefert JF, Sibilia J, Michel F, Saussine C, Javier RM, Tavernier C. Bone mineral density in men treated with synthetic gonadotropin-releasing hormone agonists for prostatic carcinoma. J Urol 1999;161(4):1219–22.
7. Smith MR, McGovern FJ, Zietman AL, et al. Pamidronate to prevent bone loss during androgen-deprivation therapy for prostate cancer. N Engl J Med 2001;345(13):948–55.
8. Berruti A, Dogliotti L, Terrone C, et al. Changes in bone mineral density, lean body mass and fat content as measured by dual energy X-ray asbsorptiometry in patients with prostate cancer without apparent bone metastases given androgen deprivation therapy. J Urol 2002;167(6):2361–7; discussion 7.
9. Daniell HW, Dunn SR, Ferguson DW, Lomas G, Niazi Z, Stratte PT. Progressive osteoporosis during androgen deprivation therapy for prostate cancer. J Urol 2000;163(1):181–6.
10. Diamond T, Campbell J, Bryant C, Lynch W. The effect of combined androgen blockade on bone turnover and bone mineral densities in men treated for prostate carcinoma: longitudinal evaluation and response to intermittent cyclic etidronate therapy. Cancer 1998;83(8):1561–6.
11. Smith MR, Eastham J, Gleason DM, Shasha D, Tchekmedyian S, Zinner N. Randomized controlled trial of zoledronic acid to prevent bone loss in men receiving androgen deprivation therapy for nonmetastatic prostate cancer. J Urol 2003;169(6):2008–12.
12. Shahinian VB, Kuo YF, Freeman JL, Goodwin JS. Risk of fracture after androgen deprivation for prostate cancer. N Engl J Med 2005;352(2):154–64.
13. Smith MR, Lee WC, Brandman J, Wang Q, Botteman M, Pashos CL. Gonadotropin-releasing hormone agonists and fracture risk: a claims-based cohort study of men with nonmetastatic prostate cancer. J Clin Oncol 2005;23(31):7897–903.
14. Smith MR, Boyce SP, Moyneur E, Duh MS, Raut MK, Brandman J. Risk of clinical fractures after gonadotropin-releasing hormone agonist therapy for prostate cancer. J Urol 2006;175(1):136–9; discussion 9.
15. Strum SB, McDermed JE, Scholz MC, Johnson H, Tisman G. Anaemia associated with androgen deprivation in patients with prostate cancer receiving combined hormone blockade. Br J Urol 1997;79(6):933–41.
16. Santini D, Vespasiani Gentilucci U, Vincenzi B, et al. The antineoplastic role of bisphosphonates: from basic research to clinical evidence. Ann Oncol 2003;14(10):1468–76.
17. Fisher JE, Rogers MJ, Halasy JM, et al. Alendronate mechanism of action: geranylgeraniol, an intermediate in the mevalonate pathway, prevents inhibition of osteoclast formation, bone resorption, and kinase activation in vitro. Proc Natl Acad Sci U S A 1999;96(1):133–8.
18. Russell RG, Xia Z, Dunford JE, et al. Bisphosphonates: an update on mechanisms of action and how these relate to clinical efficacy. Ann N Y Acad Sci 2007;1117:209–57.
19. Rosen LS, Gordon D, Kaminski M, et al. Zoledronic acid versus pamidronate in the treatment of skeletal metastases in patients with breast cancer or osteolytic lesions of multiple myeloma: a phase III, double-blind, comparative trial. Cancer J 2001;7(5):377–87.
20. Rosen LS, Gordon D, Tchekmedyian S, et al. Zoledronic acid versus placebo in the treatment of skeletal metastases in patients with lung cancer and other solid tumors: a phase III, double-blind, randomized trial–the Zoledronic Acid Lung Cancer and Other Solid Tumors Study Group. J Clin Oncol 2003;21(16):3150–7.
21. Saad F, Gleason DM, Murray R, et al. A randomized, placebo-controlled trial of zoledronic acid in patients with hormone-refractory metastatic prostate carcinoma. J Natl Cancer Inst 2002;94(19):1458–68.
22. Saad F, Gleason DM, Murray R, et al. Long-term efficacy of zoledronic acid for the prevention of skeletal complications in patients with metastatic hormone-refractory prostate cancer. J Natl Cancer Inst 2004;96(11):879–82.
23. Small EJ, Smith MR, Seaman JJ, Petrone S, Kowalski MO. Combined analysis of two multicenter, randomized, placebo-controlled studies of pamidronate disodium for the palliation of bone pain in men with metastatic prostate cancer. J Clin Oncol 2003;21(23):4277–84.
24. Ernst DS, Tannock IF, Winquist EW, et al. Randomized, double-blind, controlled trial of mitoxantrone/prednisone and clodronate versus mitoxantrone/prednisone and placebo in patients with hormone-refractory prostate cancer and pain. J Clin Oncol 2003;21(17):3335–42.
25. Dearnaley DP, Sydes MR, Mason MD, et al. A double-blind, placebo-controlled, randomized trial of oral sodium clodronate for metastatic prostate cancer (MRC PR05 Trial). J Natl Cancer Inst 2003;95(17):1300–11.
26. Mason MD, Sydes MR, Glaholm J, et al. Oral sodium clodronate for nonmetastatic prostate cancer--results of a

randomized double-blind placebo-controlled trial: Medical Research Council PR04 (ISRCTN61384873). J Natl Cancer Inst 2007;99(10):765–76.

27. Smith MR, Kabbinavar F, Saad F, et al. Natural history of rising serum prostate-specific antigen in men with castrate nonmetastatic prostate cancer. J Clin Oncol 2005;23(13):2918–25.

28. Major PP, Cook RJ, Chen BL, Zheng M. Survival-adjusted multiple-event analysis for the evaluation of treatment effects of zoledronic Acid in patients with bone metastases from solid tumors. Support Cancer Ther 2005;2(4):234–40.

29. Zojer N, Keck AV, Pecherstorfer M. Comparative tolerability of drug therapies for hypercalcaemia of malignancy. Drug Saf 1999;21(5):389–406.

30. Markowitz GS, Fine PL, Stack JI, et al. Toxic acute tubular necrosis following treatment with zoledronate (Zometa). Kidney Int 2003;64(1):281–9.

31. Chang JT, Green L, Beitz J. Renal failure with the use of zoledronic acid. N Engl J Med 2003;349(17):1676–9; discussion 9.

32. Zometa. Full prescribing information. Novartis Pharmaceuticals Corporation. Rev: October 2009.

33. Marx RE. Pamidronate (Aredia) and zoledronate (Zometa) induced avascular necrosis of the jaws: a growing epidemic. J Oral Maxillofac Surg 2003;61(9):1115–7.

34. Ruggiero SL, Mehrotra B, Rosenberg TJ, Engroff SL. Osteonecrosis of the jaws associated with the use of bisphosphonates: a review of 63 cases. J Oral Maxillofac Surg 2004;62(5):527–34.

35. Advisory Task Force on Bisphosphonate-Related Ostenonecrosis of the Jaws, American Association of Oral and Maxillofacial Surgeons. American Association of Oral and Maxillofacial Surgeons position paper on bisphosphonate-related osteonecrosis of the jaws. J Oral Maxillofac Surg 2007;65(3):369–76.

36. Wang EP, Kaban LB, Strewler GJ, Raje N, Troulis MJ. Incidence of osteonecrosis of the jaw in patients with multiple myeloma and breast or prostate cancer on intravenous bisphosphonate therapy. J Oral Maxillofac Surg 2007;65(7):1328–31.

37. Hoff AO, Toth BB, Altundag K, et al. Frequency and risk factors associated with osteonecrosis of the jaw in cancer patients treated with intravenous bisphosphonates. J Bone Miner Res 2008;23(6):826–36.

38. Vescovi P, Manfredi M, Merigo E, Meleti M. Early surgical approach preferable to medical therapy for bisphosphonate-related osteonecrosis of the jaws. J Oral Maxillofac Surg 2008;66(4):831–2.

39. Body JJ, Facon T, Coleman RE, et al. A study of the biological receptor activator of nuclear factor-kappaB ligand inhibitor, denosumab, in patients with multiple myeloma or bone metastases from breast cancer. Clin Cancer Res 2006;12(4):1221–8.

40. Ebeling PR. Clinical practice. Osteoporosis in men. N Engl J Med 2008;358(14):1474–82.

41. Seeman E. The structural basis of bone fragility in men. Bone 1999;25(1):143–7.

42. Bilezikian JP. Osteoporosis in men. J Clin Endocrinol Metab 1999;84(10):3431–4.

43. Sharifi N, Gulley JL, Dahut WL. Androgen deprivation therapy for prostate cancer. JAMA 2005;294(2):238–44.

44. Greenspan SL. Approach to the prostate cancer patient with bone disease. J Clin Endocrinol Metab 2008;93(1):2–7.

45. Smith MR, McGovern FJ, Zietman AL, et al. Pamidronate to prevent bone loss in men receiving gonadotropin releasing hormone agonist therapy for prostate cancer. N Engl J Med 2001;345(13):948–55.

46. Diamond TH, Winters J, Smith A, et al. The antiosteoporotic efficacy of intravenous pamidronate in men with prostate carcinoma receiving combined androgen blockade: a double blind, randomized, placebo-controlled crossover study. Cancer 2001;92(6):1444–50.

47. Smith MR, Eastham J, Gleason D, Shasha D, Tchekmedyian S, Zinner N. Randomized controlled trial of zoledronic acid to prevent bone loss in men undergoing androgen deprivation therapy for nonmetastatic prostate cancer. J Urol 2003;169(6):2008–12.

48. Michaelson MD, Kaufman DS, Lee H, et al. Randomized controlled trial of annual zoledronic acid to prevent gonadotropin-releasing hormone agonist-induced bone loss in men with prostate cancer. J Clin Oncol 2007;25(9):1038–42.

49. Greenspan SL, Nelson JB, Trump DL, Resnick NM. Effect of once-weekly oral alendronate on bone loss in men receiving androgen deprivation therapy for prostate cancer: a randomized trial. Ann Intern Med 2007;146(6):416–24.

50. Smith MR, Fallon MA, Lee H, Finkelstein JS. Raloxifene to prevent gonadotropin-releasing hormone agonist-induced bone loss in men with prostate cancer: a randomized controlled trial. J Clin Endocrinol Metab 2004;89(8): 3841–6.

51. Steiner MS, Patterson A, Israeli R, Barnette KG, Boger R, Price D. Toremifene citrate versus placebo for treatment of bone loss and other complications of androgen deprivation therapy in patients with prostate cancer. Proc ASCO (abstract 4597) 2004.

52. Smith MR, Malkowicz SB, Chu F, et al. Toremifene increases bone mineral density in men receiving androgen deprivation therapy for prostate cancer: interim analysis of a multicenter phase 3 clinical study. J Urol 2008;179(1):152–5.

Chapter 25
Endothelin Receptors as Therapeutic Targets in Castration-Resistant Prostate Cancer

Joel B. Nelson

Abstract New, effective therapies for castration-resistant prostate cancer are needed to treat this lethal form of the disease. Through an understanding of the biology of endothelin-1 and the endothelin receptors (the endothelin axis) in prostate cancer, this axis has emerged as a promising target for therapeutic intervention. Clinical trials of potent, selective, or specific endothelin receptor A subtype (ET_A) antagonists have demonstrated clinical activity, but such agents have not yet been approved for the treatment of prostate cancer. These generally well-tolerated, oral agents are ideal for chronic administration. This chapter will discuss the biology of the endothelin axis, several of the preclinical observations supporting the therapeutic rationale, and some of the available clinical trial data on this promising new approach.

Keywords Bone metastases • Clinical trials • Endothelin receptors • Endothelin-1 • Prostate cancer

The Endothelin Axis

As a PhD project, a graduate student named Masashi Yanagisawa published a seminal paper in the journal Nature about the isolation and characterization of a new, 21-residue peptide produced by porcine aortic endothelial cells, called endothelin [1]. Endothelin is the most potent vasoconstrictor identified, at least ten times more potent than angiotensin II, and 100 times more potent, on a molar basis, than norepinephrine.

Since its discovery in 1988, there have been over 21,000 publications listing endothelin as a key word in the scientific literature. This peptide, now referred to as endothelin 1 (ET-1) (Fig. 25.1), is part of a family of similar peptides including ET-2, ET-3, and the sarafotoxins (isolated from the venom of the Israeli Burrowing Asp, atractaspis engaddensis) [2]. The 21 amino acid, active form of ET-1 is derived from a 39-amino acid precursor peptide, "big ET-1," following proteolytic cleavage of the C-terminal portion of the molecule by an endothelin-converting enzyme [3].

There are two endothelin receptors: endothelin receptor A (ET_A) and endothelin receptor B (ET_B), which are the members of the seven-transmembrane-segment G-protein-coupled superfamily. ET_A has a higher affinity to ET-1 and ET-2, and less for ET-3. ET_B binds all three endothelin ligands identically and plays an important role in ligand clearance. This differential function of the ET_A and ET_B receptors may be important in the activity of endothelin receptor antagonists as therapeutic agents. Although selective antagonists for the ET_A receptor have been developed, many also bind to the ET_B receptor; ET_A-specific or "pure" antagonists, such as ZD4054, do not bind to the ET_B receptor. Collectively, the ET family ligands and the ET receptors are termed the "ET axis."

Originally isolated from endothelial cells, it is now recognized that ET-1 is produced by a large variety of cells from a wide range of species: ET-1 has been identified in plasma, cerebrospinal fluid, urine, breast milk, and amniotic fluid [4]. An immunoreactive form of ET-1 was found in very large quantity in human seminal fluid from both intact and vasectomized men, where the testicular contribution to the ejaculate has been eliminated, indicating a prostatic and/or seminal vesicle source [5]. Indeed, the concentrations of ET-1 in the ejaculate are amongst the highest reported in any body fluid.

J.B. Nelson (✉)
Department of Urology, University of Pittsburgh,
Pittsburgh, PA, USA
e-mail: nelsonjb@UPMC.EDU

W.D. Figg et al. (eds.), *Drug Management of Prostate Cancer*,
DOI 10.1007/978-1-60327-829-4_25, © Springer Science+Business Media, LLC 2010

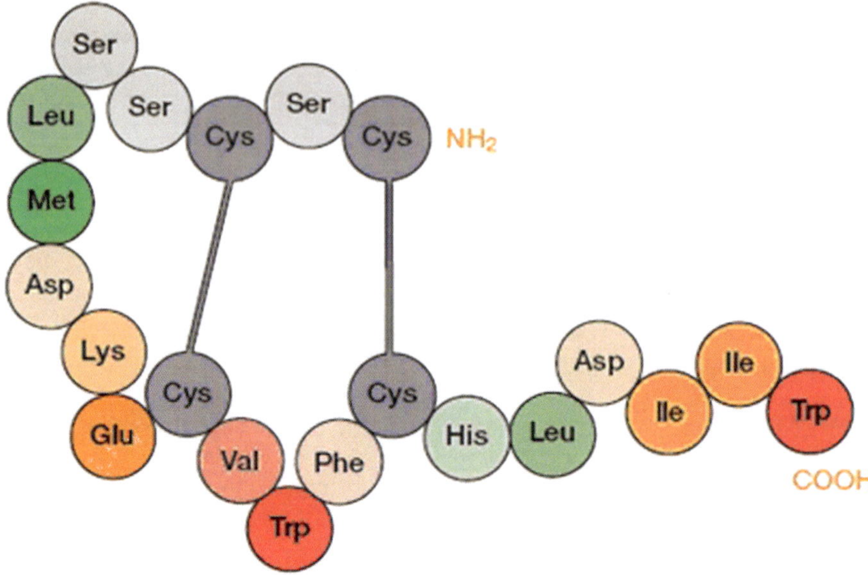

Fig. 25.1 Amino acid structure of endothelin-1 (ET-1). From Nelson [50]. With kind permission from Elsevier

Prostatic luminal epithelial cells produce ET-1, and it has been suggested that ET-1 may contribute to the contractility of the prostate stroma [6, 7]. ET-1 has a mitogenic effect on cultured smooth muscle cells from a human prostate [8]. The action of ET-1 on the prostate may be paracrine since both ET_A and ET_B receptors have been identified in the normal human prostate [6].

Endothelin-1 in Prostate Cancer

The difference in concentration of ET-1 in seminal fluid when compared with plasma is of a magnitude reminiscent of prostate-specific antigen (PSA), where concentrations in the semen are measured in the milligram range compared with nanogram quantities in circulation. Just as men with advanced prostate cancer have markedly elevated levels of PSA, was it possible that ET-1 levels would be increased in a similar fashion? To test this hypothesis, ET-1 plasma levels were measured in men with castration-resistant prostate cancer (CRPC) and compared with those from men with clinically localized disease and those without prostate cancer: as a group, men with CRPC had significantly higher ET-1 levels [9]. This increase in plasma ET-1 may only be the tip of the iceberg: local tissue concentrations of ET-1 are believed to be several fold higher than levels in circulation (where ET-1 half-life is 3.5 min), because of the homeostatic mechanisms controlling the concentrations of this most potent peptide [10]. The increase in ET-1 associated with CRPC may also reflect the loss of the expression and activity of the enzyme responsible for its cleavage, neutral endopeptidase 24.11 (NEP). In androgen-independent prostate cancer cell lines and prostate cancer samples from androgen ablated men, NEP is markedly reduced [11]. Every prostate cancer cell line studied expressed ET-1 mRNA and produced the protein [12]. In human tissue samples, ET-1 specific immunohistochemistry was observed in every primary prostate cancer and in primary and metastatic lesions obtained at autopsy from men dying from CRPC, and ET-1 expression was present almost without exception [13].

Secretion of ET-1 was also increased by cytokines and growth factors active in prostate stroma–epithelium interactions. Both ET-1 and its precursor big ET-1 were produced in greater quantities by the human PC3 and DU145 human prostate cancer cell lines in response to stimulation with interleukin-1α, interleukin-1β, tumor necrosis factor, transforming growth factor β-1, or epidermal growth factor [12, 14].

Endothelin Receptors in Prostate Cancer

In the normal prostate, both ET_A and ET_B receptors are expressed and are functional. Reflecting a tissue distribution seen in other organs – where ET_A receptors are concentrated in the stroma and ET_B receptors are concentrated on luminal cells – ET_A binding has been found predominant in the stromal component of the prostate, whereas ET_B binding is predominant in epithelial luminal cells [15]. However, unlike normal prostate epithelial cells, no ET_B binding could be detected in human prostate cancer cell lines [13]. This down regulation of ET_B receptor expression may reflect frequent somatic methylation of the ET_B receptor gene, *EDNRB*, observed in prostate cancer and, now, in a variety of malignancies. A CpG-rich sequence, referred to as a CpG island, is embedded in the 5′ regulatory region in *EDNRB*: somatic methylation of CpG islands in regulatory regions of genes has been associated with decreased transcriptional activity. In an initial study, this hypermethylation was found in 5/5 human prostate cancer cell lines, 15/21 primary prostate cancer tissues, and 8/14 prostate cancer metastases, or about 70% of the total number of samples examined [16]. In subsequent studies, *EDNRB* methylation was found to be associated with increased prostate cancer stage and grade [17]. *EDNRB* hypermethylation was not observed in normal tissues using southern-blot analysis but others have observed *EDNRB* methylation in benign prostatic hyperplasia (BPH) tissues using a more sensitive polymerase chain reaction approach, indicating the methylation status is not specific for prostate cancer and, therefore, would not be useful as a prostate cancer biomarker [16, 18]. *EDNRB* hypermethylation has also been observed in colon and bladder cancers, nasopharyngeal carcinoma, and lung cancer, suggesting ET_B silencing may have a more global role in carcinogenesis [19–21].

Increased ET_A expression has been associated with progression of prostate cancer. In the Dunning prostate cancer system, ET_A receptor binding was sevenfold higher in the metastatic MLL clone and threefold higher in the tumorigenic but nonmetastatic AT-1 clone, when compared with the nontumorigenic G clone [22]. ET_A expression by immunohistochemistry was studied in 51 human specimens: 71% were positive for ET_A expression, which increased to 100% in patients with bone metastasis. Gleason score 8–10 had particularly high rates of ET_A staining as did those cancer cells penetrating the prostatic capsule [23]. In a larger study examining 140 primary prostate cancers, high ET_A expression was observed in 72% of samples and this expression was significantly elevated with increased pathological stage and grade. Patients with PSA recurrence after prostatectomy had significantly greater ET_A expression in their primary tumors than

did patients who were disease-free at 5 years [24]. These findings suggest that the expression of the endothelin receptors may be useful prognosticators in prostate cancer and, importantly, guide selection of those who may benefit from receptor blockade.

Effects of Endothelin on Cancer Cells In Vitro

ET-1 is expressed by many epithelial carcinomas, and, in particular, those associated with a local desmoplastic stromal response (pancreatic, colon, breast, etc.) [25]. In addition, some cancer cells proliferated in a dose-dependent manner when stimulated by ET-1, most notably ovarian carcinoma, suggesting autocrine activity [26, 27]. Although ET-1 had a mitogenic effect in prostate cancer cell lines, the response was weak [9, 13]. The combination ET-1 and polypeptide growth factors, such as epidermal growth factor, greatly increased cellular proliferation compared with either factor alone [28]. This synergistic growth effect may be the result of transactivation of the peptide growth factor signaling pathway by ET-1 [29].

It has been postulated that defects in apoptosis are the central mechanism of CRPC progression. ET-1 inhibits apoptosis in a variety of benign and malignant cell lines, including prostate cancer. For example, treatment of the rat prostate cancer cell line MLL with paclitaxel easily induced apoptosis, but in the presence of ET-1, the amount of cell death is significantly reduced [22]. This anti-apoptosis effect of ET-1 is blocked by ET_A receptor antagonists, indicating that this is an ET_A receptor-mediated effect. In the human prostate cancer cell line PPC-1 transfected with an ET_A-over expression vector, ET-1 inhibited apoptosis in response to either paclitaxel or docetaxel, an effect blocked by an ET_A receptor antagonist [30]. In vivo, the combination of an ET_A receptor antagonist and docetaxel significantly inhibited tumor growth compared either with agent administered alone or with untreated controls. These findings have been supported by similar observations in other prostate cancer models using the combination of docetaxel and ET_A receptor antagonists, both in vitro and in vivo [31]. Likewise, ET_A receptor antagonists potentiate the cytotoxic effects of hypoxia-inducible factor inhibitor 2-methoxyestradiol in prostate cancer [32]. Collectively, these data strongly support the conduct of clinical trials examining the effects of combining ET_A receptor antagonists with certain cytotoxic chemotherapeutic agents.

What is the mechanism of ET-1-induced inhibition of apoptosis? ET-1 induces the expression of AKT, leading to the phosphorylation and inactivation of the proapoptotic protein, Bad [33]. ET-1 also reduced the expression of the proapoptotic proteins Bad, Bak, or Bax. On the contrary, reexpression of ET_B in prostate cancer induces apoptosis, increases expression of the same proapoptotic proteins, and increases sensitivity to paclitaxel.

Endothelin Axis and Bone Metastases

The classic response of bone to metastatic prostate cancer is mediated by osteoblasts. ET-1 is a potent stimulator of osteoblasts. Osteoblasts have high affinity ET_A receptors, at a density ($\sim 10^5$ per cell) greatly exceeding the density on prostate cancer cells [34]. The original hypothesis that ET-1 had a role in prostate cancer progression was largely based on its known effects on osteoblasts, as shown in a new-bone-forming model [9]. In an osteoblastic tumor model using the WISH cell line (a transformed human amnion cell line that induces a robust osteoblastic response), it was found that WISH produces large amounts of ET-1. Stable transfection of WISH with an ET-1 over expression cDNA construct generated clones producing 18-fold more bioactive ET-1. In this model, these ET-1-overexpressing clones produced significantly more new bone when implanted

in the lower leg of nu/nu mice [35]. These areas of new bone formation were significantly decreased in animals treated with a selective ET_A receptor antagonist. These findings have been supported by another in vivo model system, indicating the causal role of ET-1 in the pathogenesis of osteoblastic bone metastases in a breast carcinoma model [36]. Animals receiving an ET_A receptor antagonist had significantly less osteoblastic lesions than controls.

The possible role of ectopically secreted ET-1 from metastatic prostate cancer cells as an important factor in tumor growth in the bone microenvironment has led to a "vicious cycle" hypothesis of disease progression (Fig. 25.2). In this model, ET-1 stimulates the proliferation of osteoblasts, the deposition of new bone, and promotes the development of the osteoblastic lesion. In an attempt to maintain normal bone homeostasis, osteoclasts are activated to resorb bone. Since bone is a rich source of growth factors, this resorption releases these factors, making them accessible to prostate cancer cells and promoting their further growth. The use of ET_A receptor antagonists has been proposed as one mechanism to break this cycle.

ET Axis and Pain

The bite of the Israeli Burrowing Asp induces a dramatic local and systemic response, an effect mediated by the sarafotoxins within the venom. Since the sarafotoxins are members of the endothelin family, it is not

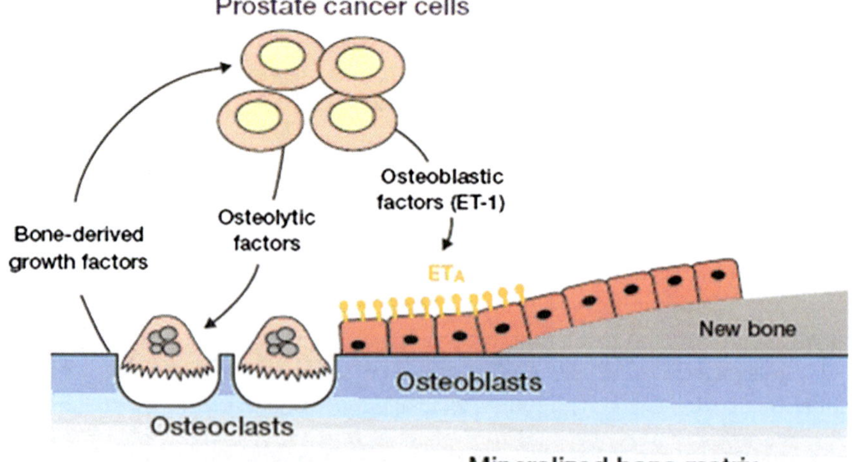

Fig. 25.2 Prostate cancer and bone interactions. This "vicious cycle" where ET-1 acting through the ET_A receptor stimulates osteoblasts, which, in turn, activate osteoclasts. The resorption of bone releases bone-derived growth factors, which stimulate prostate cancer proliferation. Strategic use of an ET_A receptor antagonist is one mechanism to block this cycle. From Nelson [50]. With kind permission from Elsevier

surprising that ET-1 induces hyperalgesia and pain in a variety of model systems, including a dramatic pain response in a man undergoing infusion of ET-1 into a brachial artery [37]. Men with advanced prostate cancer suffer considerably from tumor-induced pain, particularly in association with bone metastases: it is possible that some of the pain they experience is due to local ET-1 secretion by prostate cancer cells.

The mechanistic pattern of ET-1 induced pain appeared to be novel and unresponsive at usual doses to cyclooxygenase inhibitors such as indomethicin or ibuprofen, suggesting that agents specifically targeting ET-1 activity, such as ET_A antagonists, could be useful in alleviating pain [38]. As a mediator of pain, ET-1, acting through the ET_A receptor, had both direct effects on nerves and as a potentiator of other noxious stimuli [39]. In a new murine model of cancer pain, ET-1-producing tumors created within bone were significantly more painful than other, non-ET-1-producing tumors: local administration of an ET_A receptor antagonist significantly blocked this effect [40].

On the basis of the preclinical findings described earlier and the availability of potent and selective ET_A receptor antagonists, it was both reasonable and strategic to target ET-1 induced in men with prostate cancer [9].

Atrasentan (ABT-627)

Abbott Laboratories was one of the many pharmaceutical companies looking for new agents for cardiovascular disease, and developed ABT-627, which, at the time of disclosure, was the most potent and selective ET_A receptor antagonist described. ABT-627, or atrasentan, is a highly potent (Ki = 0.034 nM) and selective (1,800-fold) ET_A receptor antagonist, blocking the biological effects of ET-1 in a host of in vitro and in vivo model systems [41, 42]. Atrasentan was developed as an orally bioavailable agent with a half-life of 25 h, favoring once-per-day dosing. Single-dose pharmacokinetic studies with atrasentan in normal male volunteers demonstrated a terminal half-life range of 20–25 h with extensive tissue distribution. Consistent with its vasoactive nature, the most frequent adverse events were transient headache, rhinitis, and nausea. As seen throughout the subsequent trials in cancer, atrasentan did not induce hepatic or hematological toxicity [43].

Atrasentan: Phase I Trials

Two phase I clinical trials were performed to assess the safety and pharmacokinetics of atrasentan in men with CRPC and other patients with refractory adenocarcinomas [44, 45]. In both studies, patients were treated for 28 days with escalating oral atrasentan doses (2.5–95 mg) and were then eligible for an extension study. Similar to the phase I studies in normal males, the most common side effects were headache, rhinitis, and peripheral edema. In one trial, dose-limiting toxicity (headache) was seen at 75 mg [44]: in the other study, no maximum tolerated dose was found in the dose range studied (up to 95 mg) [45].

In men with CRPC, the PSA level was unchanged or dropped in 68% (15/22) during the 28-day exposure, with declines ranging from 5 to 95%. There was no obvious correlation between dose and PSA declines. In seven out of ten patients (70%) with narcotic-requiring pain, atrasentan reduced pain, as measured by the visual analog scale. These results, although not placebo-controlled and from short, open-label trials, were nevertheless compelling.

Atrasentan: Phase II Trials in Prostate Cancer

M96-500

On the basis of the preclinical findings implicating ET-1 in pain and the reduction in pain observed in some patients in the phase I clinical trials, a phase II trial was designed to study atrasentan in relieving prostate-cancer induced pain. In this double-blind, placebo-controlled study, 131 men with castration-resistant metastatic prostate cancer with disease-related pain requiring opioid analgesics were enrolled in three study groups: 43 were randomized to the placebo arm, 40 were randomized to the atrasentan 2.5 mg arm, and 48 were randomized to the atrasentan 10 mg arm. Eighty-one subjects (62%) discontinued study drug before the planned 84 days of treatment, reflecting high rates of disease progression. There was no statistically significant difference in response rates between placebo and atrasentan for the primary endpoint (pain relief at week 12). There was, however, a trend toward improvement in pain without increased analgesic consumption in atrasentan-treated patients: the average VAS pain score for subjects receiving atrasentan 10 mg decreased 8% from baseline, while the average VAS pain score for placebo subjects increased 8% from baseline. Statistically significant improvement was seen for the atrasentan 10 mg group vs. placebo ($p \leq 0.05$) at week 12 for two pain domains in the brief pain inventory (BPI): pain interference with relations with other people ($p = 0.031$), and worst pain in the last 24 h ($p = 0.030$).

M96-594

The efficacy of atrasentan in delaying disease progression was studied in a double-blind placebo-controlled Phase II trial in men with asymptomatic, hormone-refractory, metastatic prostate cancer [46]. In this international study, 288 men were randomized to receive daily oral doses of placebo, atrasentan 2.5 or 10 mg. The primary endpoint was time to disease progression, defined as new lesions, pain requiring opioids, disease-related symptoms requiring intervention. Secondary endpoints included time to PSA progression, changes in bone markers, and quality of life. Median time to disease progression was 183 days in the atrasentan 10 mg treated patients compared with 137 days for the placebo group ($p = 0.13$) in the intent-to-treat population. In the evaluable subset ($n = 244$), there was a significant ($p = 0.021$) delay in disease progression from 129 days (placebo) to 196 days (atrasentan 10 mg). There was a significant ($p = 0.002$) delay in PSA progression in the atrasentan 10 mg group: median time to PSA progression was more than twice (155 days) that of placebo (71 days). As observed in the previous trials, atrasentan was well tolerated, with headache, edema, and rhinitis being the most common side effects. Men reaching an endpoint were permitted to enter an open-label atrasentan study: this design with significant placebo crossover confounds any survival analysis. Markers of bone deposition (alkaline phosphatase, bone alkaline phosphatase) and bone resorption (N-telopeptides, C-telopeptides, and deoxypyridinoline) were also studied in this trial, based on the preclinical data implicating the ET axis in the osteoblastic response of bone to cancer [47]. At baseline, there were significant elevations in markers of both bone deposition and bone resorption, ranging from 1.4

to 2.7-fold above normal. Men on placebo had significant ($p < 0.001$) increases in both sets of markers, consistent with disease progression. In a dose-dependent fashion, men on atrasentan had a stabilization of these markers suggesting a disruption in the expected progression in bony sites. These finding were the first strong indication that atrasentan may be most active in men with bone-metastatic prostate cancer.

Atrasentan: Phase III Trials in Prostate Cancer

M00-211

A phase III trial of atrasentan was designed to essentially duplicate the time to disease progression phase II trial (M96-594), with a few notable differences. Given the increased response rate in the 10 mg atrasentan without an increase in side effects, the phase III trial had only placebo and 10 mg arms. The second difference was a mandated objective evaluation of disease progression to reduce, as much as possible, PSA bias. Therefore, unlike the phase II study, where radiographic imaging was performed for clinical indications only, in the phase 3 M00-211 study, bone scans and axial imaging were performed every 3 months. The primary endpoint (disease progression), secondary endpoints (PSA progression, markers of bone metabolism, quality of life), enrollment criteria (asymptomatic, metastatic CRPC) were otherwise the same.

In this multinational trial, a total of 809 men were enrolled (401 placebo, 408 atrasentan 10 mg) [48]. Atrasentan did not reduce the risk of disease progression relative to placebo (HR, 0.89; 95% confidence interval, 0.76–1.04; $p = 0.136$) (Fig. 25.3). The perprotocol analysis (329 placebo, 342 atrasentan 10 mg) was significantly in favor of atrasentan 10 mg (HR 1.26; 95% confidence intervals 1.06–1.50; $p = 0.007$). Secondary endpoints (PSA progression, bone marker progression, and certain quality of life tools) all significantly favored atrasentan 10 mg.

In a hypothesis-generating exercise, patients were stratified based on the characteristics of their metastatic disease at enrollment (bone only, bone and soft tissue, soft tissue only) to determine whether a particular disease presentation favored better response to atrasentan.

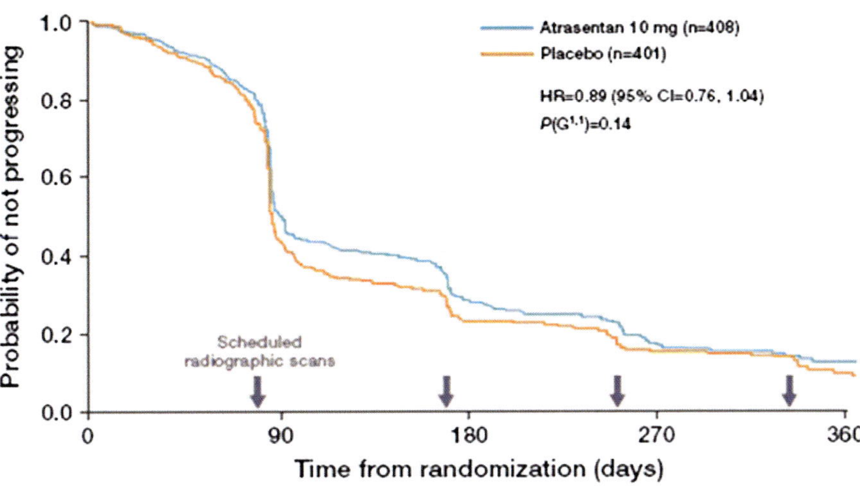

Fig. 25.3 Time to disease progression in a phase III study of atrasentan in men with metastatic castration-resistant prostate cancer (CRPC) (M00-211). Progression events cluster at the time of scheduled radiographic evaluations. Reproduced with permission from John Wiley & Sons, copyright 2008 [49]

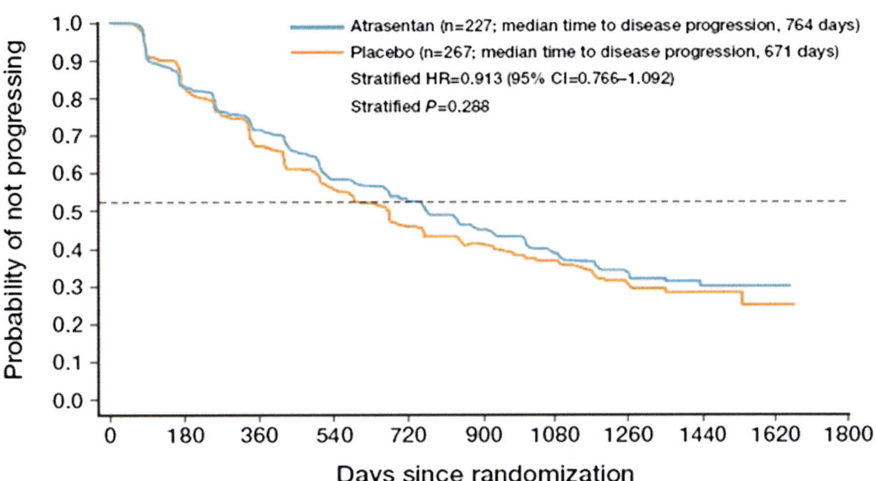

Fig. 25.4 Time to disease progression in a phase III study of atrasentan in men with nonmetastatic CRPC (M00-244). Median time to progression was 764 days with atrasentan and 671 days with placebo ($p = 0.288$). Reproduced with permission from John Wiley & Sons, copyright 2007 [48]

Consistent with the preclinical and earlier clinical trials, those men with bone metastases (with or without soft tissue metastases) enjoyed the most significant delays in disease progression compared with placebo-treated patients with the same characteristics. Since 85% of the men enrolled into this trial had bone metastases, this finding is pertinent to the large majority of CRPC patients, to the design of subsequent trials, and to the possible use of ET_A antagonists in this clinical setting.

M00-244

A double-blind, placebo-controlled trial (M00-244) was designed to determine whether atrasentan 10 mg can delay disease progression in men with rising PSA on hormonal therapy, but who do not yet have radiographic or clinical evidence of metastatic disease [49]. Of 941 men who met these criteria, 467 were randomized to receive atrasentan 10 mg and 474 to receive placebo. The primary endpoint was time to disease progression, defined as the onset of metastases. Secondary endpoints were time to PSA progression, change in bone alkaline phosphatase, PSA doubling time, and overall survival.

There was a 93-day delay in median time to disease progression with atrasentan compared with placebo (764 days vs. 671 days, respectively), but this difference was not significant (Fig. 25.4). There were large geographic differences in time to disease progression: in the United States, median time to disease progression was 590 days with atrasentan, compared with 847 days at non-United States sites (Canada, Europe, Africa).

A significantly higher percentage of atrasentan-treated patients discontinued prematurely compared with placebo (33.2 vs. 25.9%, respectively), an event significantly more common at United States sites (40.8%) than non-United States sites (21.9%). Atrasentan lengthened PSA doubling time and slowed the increase in bone alkaline phosphatase. Median survival was 1,477 days with atrasentan and 1,403 days with placebo: these data must be considered with caution, since 54% of placebo-treated patients subsequently enrolled in an open-label study and received atrasentan.

Ongoing Phase III Trial

The Southwestern Oncology Group (SWOG) has initiated a phase III study of docetaxel and atrasentan vs. docetaxel and placebo in men with CRPC. The primary endpoint of the trial is to compare overall survival and progression-free survival between the groups. The study is designed to enroll 930 men. It opened in August 2006 with an estimated primary completion date of June 2010. The trial is supported by the multiple preclinical observations about the synergistic effects of ET_A antagonists and cytotoxic chemotherapeutic agents.

Summary

The completed phase II and III trials of atrasentan in CRPC demonstrate a consistently modest effect favoring atrasentan. There have been repeated significant effects of atrasentan on attenuating markers of bone metabolism, supporting a mechanism of action targeting osseous prostate cancer metastases. Unfortunately, phase III trials were plagued by design (M00-211) and conduct (M00-244) flaws. Given the significant crossover of placebo-treated patients to receive atrasentan in open-label extension studies, an overall survival effect is not assessable. This final fact stands in stark contrast to the overall survival advantage recently observed in the phase II trial (Study 6) of the specific endothelin-A antagonist ZD4054, currently being developed by AstraZeneca, where crossover was not permitted [50].

Conclusions

The endothelin axis has emerged as a unique target for the treatment of castration-resistant prostate cancer, particularly for those with skeletal metastases. Preclinical studies of endothelin-1, the endothelin receptors ET_A and ET_B, indicate an important role in prostate cancer progression. Clinical trials of ET_A antagonists in CRPC support ongoing investigations of these agents. The consistency of findings in preclinical models and in phase I, phase II, and phase III clinical trials all support an ongoing investigation of agents designed to disrupt this axis. Although many questions remain unanswered, the ongoing phase III clinical trials will provide insights into the real benefits of this approach.

Acknowledgment Chapter reprinted from Nelson [51]. With kind permission from Elsevier.

References

1. Yanagisawa M, Kurihara H, Kimura S, et al. A novel potent vasoconstrictor peptide produced by vascular endothelial cells. Nature 1988;332:411–5.
2. Inoue A, Yanagisawa M, Kimura S, et al. The human endothelin family: three structurally and pharmacologically distinct isopeptides predicted by three separate genes. Proc Natl Acad Sci U S A 1989;86:2863–7.
3. Kimura S, Kasuya Y, Sawamura T, et al. Conversion of big endothelin-1 to 21-residue endothelin-1 is essential for expression of full vasoconstrictor activity: structure–activity relationships of big endothelin-1. J Cardiovasc Pharmacol 1989;13 Suppl 5:S5–7.
4. Battistini B, D'Orleans-Juste P, Sirois P. Biology of disease. Endothelins: circulating plasma levels and presence in other biologic fluids. Lab Invest 1993;68:600–28.
5. Casey ML, Byrd W, MacDonald PC. Massive amounts of immunoreactive endothelin in human seminal fluid. J Clin Endocrinol Metab 1992;74:223–5.
6. Prayer-Galetti T, Rossi GP, Belloni AS, et al. Gene expression and autoradiographic localization of endothelin-1 and its receptors A and B in the different zones of the normal human prostate. J Urol 1997;157:2334–9.
7. Lagenstroer P, Tang R, Shapiro E, Divish B, Opgenorth T, Lepor H. Endothelin-1 in the human prostate: tissue levels, source of production and isometric tension studies. J Urol 1993;150(2 Pt 1):495–9.
8. Saita Y, Yazawa H, Koizumi T, et al. Mitogenic activity of endothelin on human cultured prostatic smooth muscle cells. Eur J Pharmacol 1998;349:123–8.
9. Nelson JB, Hedican SP, George DJ, et al. Identification of endothelin-1 in the pathophysiology of metastatic adenocarcinoma of the prostate. Nat Med 1995;1:944–9.

10. Nelson JB, Opgenorth TJ, Fleisher LA, Frank SM. Perioperative plasma endothelin-1 and big endothelin-1 concentrations in elderly patients undergoing major surgical procedures. Anesth Analg 1999;88:898–903.

11. Papandreou CN, Usmani B, Geng Y, et al. Neutral endopeptidase 24.11 loss in metastatic human prostate cancer contributes to androgen-independent progression. Nat Med 1998;4:50–7.

12. Granchi S, Brocchi S, Bonaccorsi L, et al. Endothelin-1 production by prostate cancer cell lines is up-regulated by factors involved in cancer progression and down-regulated by androgens. Prostate 2001;49:267–77.

13. Nelson JB, Chan-Tack K, Hedican SP, et al. Endothelin-1 production and decreased endothelin B receptor expression in advanced prostate cancer. Cancer Res 1996;56:663–8.

14. Le Brun G, Aubin P, Soliman H, et al. Upregulation of endothelin 1 and its precursor by IL-1a, TNF-a, and TGF-B in the PC3 human prostate cancer cell line. Cytokine 1999;11:157–62.

15. Kobayashi S, Tang R, Wand B, et al. Localization of endothelin receptors in the human prostate. J Urol 1994;151:763–6.

16. Nelson JB, Lee W-H, Nguyen SH, et al. Methylation of the 5′ CpG island of the endothelin B receptor gene is common in human prostate cancer. Cancer Res 1997;57:35–7.

17. Yegnasubramanian S, Kowalski J, Gonzalgo ML, et al. Hypermethylation of CpG islands in primary and metastatic human prostate cancer. Cancer Res 2004;64:1975–86.

18. Jeronimo C, Henrique R, Campos PF, et al. Endothelin B receptor gene hypermethylation in prostate adenocarcinoma. J Clin Pathol 2003;56:52–5.

19. Pao MM, Tsutsumi M, Liang G, Uzvolgy E, Gonzales FA, Jones PA. The endothelin receptor B (EDNRB) promoter displays heterogeneous, site specific methylation patterns in normal and tumor cells. Hum Mol Genet 2001;10:903–10.

20. Lo K-W, Tsang Y-S, Kwong J, To K-F, Teo PML, Huang DP. Promoter hypermethylation of the EDNRB gene in nasopharyngeal carcinoma. Int J Cancer 2002;95:651–5.

21. Cohen AJ, Belinsky S, Franklin W, Beard S. Molecular and physiologic evidence for 5′ CpG island methylation of the endothelin B receptor gene in lung cancer. Chest 2002;121:27S–8.

22. Godara G, Cannon GW, Cannon GM, Bies RR, Nelson JB, Pflug B. Role of endothelin axis in progression to aggressive phenotype of prostate adenocarcinoma. Prostate 2005;65:27–34.

23. Gohji K, Kitazawa S, Tamada H, Katsuoka Y, Nakajima M. Expression of endothelin receptor A associated with prostate cancer progression. J Urol 2001;165:1033–6.

24. Godara G, Pecher S, Jukic DM, et al. Distinct patterns of endothelin axis expression in primary prostate cancer. Urology 2007;70:209–15.

25. Kusuhara M, Yamaguchi K, Nagasaki K, et al. Production of endothelin in human cancer cell lines. Cancer Res 1990;50:3257–61.

26. Schichiri M, Hirata Y, Nakajima T, et al. Endothelin-1 is an autocrine/paracrine growth factor for human cancer cell lines. J Clin Invest 1991;87:1867–71.

27. Nelson JB, Bagnato A, Battistini B, Nisen P. The endothelin axis: emerging role in cancer. Nat Rev Cancer 2003;3:110–6.

28. Brown KD, Littlewood CJ. Endothelin stimulates DNA synthesis in Swiss 3T3 cells. Synergy with polypeptide growth factors. Biochem J 1989;263:977–80.

29. Daub H, Weiss FU, Wallasch C, Ullrich A. Role of transactivation of the EGF receptor in signalling by G-protein-coupled receptors. Nature 1996;379:557–60.

30. Akhavan A, McHugh KH, Guruli G, et al. Endothelin receptor A blockade enhances taxane effects in prostate cancer. Neoplasia 2006;8:725–32.

31. Banerjee S, Hussain M, Wang Z, et al. In vitro and in vivo molecular evidence for better therapeutic efficacy of ABT-627 and taxotere combination in prostate cancer. Cancer Res 2007;67:3818–26.

32. Mabjeesh NJ, Shefler A, Amir S, Matzkin H. Potentiation of 2-methoxyestradiol-induced cytotoxicity by blocking endothelin A receptor in prostate cancer cells. Prostate 2008;68:679–89.

33. Nelson JB, Udan MS, Guruli G, Pflug BR. Endothelin-1 inhibits apoptosis in prostate cancer. Neoplasia 2005;7:631–7.

34. Takuwa Y, Ohue Y, Takuwa N, Yamashita K. Endothelin-1 activiates phospholipase C and mobilizes Ca^{++} from extra- and intracellular pools in osteoblastic cells. Am J Physiol 1989;257:E797–803.

35. Nelson JB, Nguyen SH, Wu-Wong JR, et al. New bone formation in an osteoblastic tumor model is increased by endothelin-1 overexpression and decreased by endothelin A receptor blockade. Urology 1999;53:1063–9.

36. Yin JJ, Mohammad KS, KaKonen SM, et al. A causal role of endothelin-1 in the pathogenesis of osteoblastic bone metastases. Proc Natl Acad Sci U S A 2003;100:10954–9.

37. Dahlof B, Gustafsson D, Hedner T, Jern S, Hansson L. Regional haemodynamic effects of endothelin-1 in rat and man: unexpected adverse reaction. J Hypertens 1990;8:811–7.

38. Raffa RB, Schupsky JJ, Lee DK, Jacoby HI. Characterization of endothelin-induced nociception in mice: evidence for a mechanistically distinct analgesic model. J Pharmacol Exp Ther 1996;278:1–7.

39. Davar G, Hans G, Fareed MU, Sinnott C, Strichartz G. Behavioral signs of acute pain produced by application of endothelin-1 to rat sciatic nerve. Neuroreport 1998;9:2279–83.

40. Peters CM, Lindsay TH, Pomonis JD, et al. Endothelin and the tumorigenic component of bone cancer pain. Neuroscience 2004;126:1043–52.

41. Opgenorth TJ, Adler AL, Calzadilla SV, et al. Pharmacological characterization of A-127722: an orally active and highly potent ETA-selective receptor antagonist. J Pharmacol Exp Ther 1996;276:473–81.

42. Verhaar MC, Grahn AY, van Weerdt AWM, et al. Pharmacokinetics and pharmacodynamic effects of ABT-627, an oral ETA selective endothelin antagonist, in humans. Br J Clin Pharmacol 2000;49:562–73.

43. Samara E, Dutta S, Cao G, Granneman GR, Dordal MS, Padley RJ. Single-dose pharmacokinetics of atrasentan, and endothelin-A receptor antagonist. J Clin Pharmacol 2001;41:397–403.

44. Carducci MA, Nelson JB, Bowling MK, et al. Atrasentan, an endothelin-receptor antagonist for refractory adenocarcinomas: safety and pharmacokinetics. J Clin Oncol 2002;20:2171–80.

45. Zonnenberg BA, Groenewegen G, Janus TJ, et al. Phase I dose-escalation study of the safety and pharmacokinetics of atrasentan: an endothelin receptor antagonist for refractory prostate cancer. Clin Cancer Res 2003;9:2965–72.

46. Carducci MA, Padley RJ, Breul J, et al. The effect of endothelin-A receptor blockade with atrasentan on tumor progression in men with hormone refractory prostate cancer: a randomized, placebo controlled trial. J Clin Oncol 2003;21:679–89.

47. Nelson JB, Nabulsi AA, Vogelzang NJ, et al. Suppression of prostate cancer induced bone remodeling by the endothelin receptor A antagonist atrasentan. J Urol 2003;169: 1143–9.

48. Carducci MA, Saad F, Abrahamsson P-A, et al. A phase 3 randomized controlled trial of the efficacy and safety of atrasentan in men with metastatic hormone-refractory prostate cancer. Cancer 2007;110:1959–66.

49. Nelson JB, Love W, Chin JL, et al. Phase 3, randomized controlled trial of atrasentan in patients with nonmetastatic hormone refractory prostate cancer. Cancer 2008;113(9): 2478–87.

50. James ND, Borre M, Zonnenberg B, et al. ZD4054, a potent, specific endothelin A receptor antagonist, improves overall survival in pain-free or mildly symptomatic patients with hormone-resistant prostate cancer (HRPC) and bone metastases. Eur J Cancer Suppl 2007;5:3. Abstract 3LB.

51. Nelson JB. Endothelin receptors as therapeutic targets in castration-resistant prostate cancer. Eur Urol Suppl 2009;8: 20–8.

Chapter 26
Calcitriol and Vitamin D Analogs

Ana R. Jensen, Russell Z. Szmulewitz, Tomasz M. Beer, and Edwin M. Posadas

Abstract Calcitriol (1,25-dihydroxycholecaliferol) is a synthetic analog of vitamin D that is physiologically active in absorption of calcium from the gastrointestinal tract. Recent clinical and laboratory developments have fueled enthusiasm for studying the role of vitamin D and its relationship to oncogenesis and malignant progression. There are epidemiological data pointing toward a link between vitamin D and prostate cancer as well as preclinical and clinical data linking antineoplastic activity of vitamin D receptor ligands with prostate cancer. As such, efforts have been geared toward the development of vitamin D receptor ligand-based therapy for early and advanced prostate cancer. In this chapter we will discuss the historic and current thoughts on the role that vitamin D may play in prostate cancer risk and treatment.

Keywords Vitamin D • Calcitriol • Vitamin D receptor

Epidemiology of Vitamin D and Prostate Cancer

Prostate Cancer Risk

A growing literature has identified vitamin D and calcium as risk factors for prostate cancer (CaP). Traditionally, a number of factors have been associated with increased risk of prostate cancer including advanced age, African genetic heritage, and residence in northern latitudes. These same factors have been associated with lower levels of vitamin D and have served as a rationale for the hypothesis that vitamin D played a critical role in the maintenance of the normal phenotype of prostate epithelial cells.

The evidence linking low vitamin D levels with prostate cancer has been mixed. The global pattern of greater risk in northern regions led investigators to suggest that reduced exposure to solar UV radiation and consequent reduction in endogenous vitamin D production may be associated with an increased risk of CaP [1]. A case-control study from the UK showed a reduced risk with greater UV exposure [2]. In a US study, there was only a weak link between average regional UV-B radiation and prostate cancer mortality [3]. Studies that examined 25-hydroxy vitamin D (25-OH vitamin D) levels in populations with a low prevalence of severe vitamin D deficiency did not reveal a relationship between vitamin D blood levels and prostate cancer risk [4–8]. Studies conducted in Nordic countries, where severe vitamin D deficiency is more common [9, 10], reported increased risk in men with the lowest vitamin D levels, although one of the studies [10] also suggested an increased risk at the highest levels. Two studies suggest that low 1,25-dihydroxy vitamin D (1,25-OH$_2$ vitamin D) levels were associated with an increased risk of aggressive prostate cancer [4, 5], but overall CaP risk was not associated with 1,25-OH$_2$ vitamin D in two recent, relatively small studies [6, 8]. To date, studies that examined dietary vitamin D intake have not revealed a protective effect from prostate cancer [11–15]. A meta-analysis of more than 26,000 patients in 45 studies published in 2008 did not show any strong protective effect associated with vitamin D consumption (RR = 1.16; 95% CI = 0.98–1.38) [16].

A number of studies have examined the role of dairy product consumption and prostate cancer risk that may be mediated through vitamin D. A 2004

E.M. Posadas (✉)
Section of Hematology/Oncology, Department of Medicine, University of Chicago, Chicago, IL 60637, USA
e-mail: eposadas@bsd.uchicago.edu

W.D. Figg et al. (eds.), *Drug Management of Prostate Cancer*,
DOI 10.1007/978-1-60327-829-4_26, © Springer Science+Business Media, LLC 2010

meta-analysis of 11 case control studies reported a combined odds ratio of 1.68 for high milk consumption and prostate cancer [17]. Giovanucci et al. have suggested that loss of 1-α hydroxylase activity in prostate cancer cells may explain these epidemiologic findings. Normal prostate epithelial cells or colon cancer cells [18, 19] express 1-α hydroxylase and can therefore convert 25-OH vitamin D to the active 1,25-OH_2 vitamin D. This activity can be lost when the cancer develops [20, 21]. The loss of this activity would be expected to render prostate cancer resistant to 25-OH vitamin D and dependent on circulating 1,25-OH_2 vitamin D for vitamin D receptor (VDR)-mediated activity. Circulating 1,25-OH_2 vitamin D levels are tightly controlled and largely unaffected by 25-OH vitamin D levels except for a severe deficiency state [22–25]. If this hypothesis proves correct, it would not be surprising that 25-OH vitamin D levels or behaviors that influence them (sunlight, vitamin D supplements) would have little effect on prostate cancer except in the extremes. At the same time, high milk and high calcium consumption are associated with a significant reduction in circulating 1,25-OH_2 vitamin D levels [26]. This reduction in circulating 1,25-OH_2 vitamin D levels could explain excess risk. Beer et al. showed that vitamin D receptors are universally expressed in human prostate cancer specimens and that preprostatectomy high-dose 1,25-OH_2 vitamin D treatment significantly reduces VDR expression in human prostate tumors [27]. This finding is consistent with the hypothesis advanced by Giovanucci.

VDR and binding protein (DBP) have also been implicated in the recognized racial disparities that exist in the population of men affected by CaP. In a case-control study of single nucleotide polymorphisms (SNPs) of VDR and DBP, African-American men who possessed at least one variant allele VDR-5132C had an increased risk of CaP (OR=1.83; 95% CI: 1.02, 3.31) [28]. The impact of VDR genetic variations is not limited to patients of African descent. Torkko et al. identified VDR mutations in concert with mutation in 5-α reductase that have been correlated with higher risk of CaP in Hispanic and non-Hispanic Caucasians [29]. These data and other studies of this nature point to the importance of vitamin D signaling in prostate cancer development, though much needs to be done to understand the final definitive pathways through which these risks are imparted.

Prostate Cancer Outcomes

Several investigators have recently reported that the season of diagnosis and treatment and vitamin D blood levels are important predictors of outcome in several cancer types including prostate cancer. Zhou et al. found that patients diagnosed and surgically treated for nonsmall cell lung cancer during the summer had a better relapse-free survival than patients diagnosed and treated in the winter. The greatest difference was seen when patients who had surgery in the summer and had a high intake of vitamin D were compared with patients operated on in the winter, who had low vitamin D intake (HR 0.33, 95% CI 0.15–0.74). A similar association for overall survival was also noted [30]. In a Norwegian study of 115,096 breast-, colon-, and prostate cancer patients, Robsahm et al. found that those diagnosed in the summer or fall had significantly lower case fatality rates than similar patients diagnosed in the winter and spring [31]. For CaP, the season of diagnosis was associated with a statistically significant 20–30% reduction in risk of death. Lagunova et al. performed a prostate cancer-specific analysis in the Norwegian population and showed a similar variation in relative risk favoring those patients diagnosed in the summer and fall over those diagnosed in the winter and spring [relative risk (RR) of death 0.8; 95% CI 0.75–0.85] [32]. The study controlled for UV exposure, rates of squamous cell carcinoma of the skin, and fish intake. Little variation was seen across age. The authors suggested that the effect may be related to variations in vitamin D intake and activity. There are no prospective studies of vitamin D supplementation or treatment with surgery or radiation for prostate cancer, but the emerging retrospective data are intriguing.

Mechanisms of Antineoplastic Activity in Preclinical Systems

Vitamin D Signaling

Vitamin D signaling involves both receptor-mediated genomic and nongenomic pathways. The VDR, the mediator of the classic genomic response, is a steroid hormone receptor and acts as a ligand-activated transcription factor [33]. It binds to the vitamin D response elements (VDRE) present in the regulatory region of many genes after forming a heterodimer with the retinoid-X receptor (RXR) and in some cases the retinoid A receptor (RAR) [34–36]. In the presence of coactivator complexes, the VDR heterodimer interacts with the RNA polymerase complex and initiates gene transcription. The number of genes that are recognized to have a functional VDRE is rapidly growing. Examples include a number of bone-associated genes such as osteocalcin [37], osteopontin [38], bone sialoprotein [39], receptor activator of NF-κB ligand (RANKL) [40], Runx2/Cbfa1 [41], tumor necrosis factor alpha [42], parathyroid hormone [43], parathyroid hormone-related protein [44], the insulin receptor [45], insulin-induced gene-2 [46], carbonic anhydrase II [47], human growth hormone [48], the calcium-binding proteins calbindin-D28k and D9k [49], fructose 1,6-bisphosphatase [50], the cell cycle regulators p21 [51], GADD45 [52], and IGFBP3 [53, 54], 25(OH)D3 24-hydroxylase [55], cytochrome P450 3A4 (CYP3A4) [56], organic anion transporter MRP3 [57], epidermal growth factor receptor (EGFR) [58], c-fos [59], phospholipase C [60], as well as a number of genes that regulate cell adhesion and differentiation such as fibronectin [61], β3 integrin [62], and involucrin [63]. Interestingly, several of these genes have been implicated in prostate cancer or prostate cancer metastases [64–66]. In addition to the classic genomic response, vitamin D also induces rapid nontranscriptional signals leading to increases in calcium and phosphate uptake in intestinal cells [67] and the opening of Ca^{2+}-dependent K^+- and voltage-gated calcium and chloride channels in kidney proximal tubules and skeletal muscle, respectively [68, 69]. Rapid vitamin D-induced nongenomic signals also include the regulation of protein kinase C [70–72], ras, and mitogen-activated protein kinase (MAPK) [70, 73–76], protein lipase A and prostaglandins [77, 78], cyclic AMP and protein kinase A [79, 80], phosphatidyl inositol 3-kinase/Akt [81, 82], and the ceramide pathway [83]. Ultimately these responses regulate cellular growth, differentiation, and apoptosis [73, 74, 84, 85]. They may also be mediated by the translocation of the VDR to the plasma membrane, cytosolic VDR, or by other unknown receptors [73, 86–91].

Spectrum of Activity

After Abe et al. reported that calcitriol induced terminal differentiation in myeloid leukemia cells [92], a number of investigators reported in vitro and/or in vivo activity in models of a broad range of human neoplasms including carcinoma of the bladder [93], breast [94], colon [95], endometrium [96], kidney [97, 98], lung [99], pancreas [100], prostate [101–107], sarcomas of the soft tissues [108], and bone [109, 110], neuroblastoma [111, 112], glioma [113], melanoma [114], squamous cell carcinoma [115, 116], and others. Vitamin D signaling is likely to be important throughout organ systems as VDR appears to be expressed in nearly all human tissues [117, 118].

Mechanisms of Antineoplastic Activity

Several mechanisms of activity have been demonstrated in preclinical systems, but given that vitamin D targets a broad range of genes, it is not surprising that the observed mechanisms vary under different experimental conditions and in different tumor models. It is likely that more than one of these mechanisms of activity is important in humans, and indeed different mechanisms may be important in different human diseases or at different stages of a human disease.

Differentiation and Inhibition of Proliferation

Inhibition of proliferation, which is associated with differentiation in some tumor models, has been extensively studied. In numerous cell lines, growth arrest in response to vitamin D occurs in the G1 phase of the cell cycle [51, 119–122]. In several tumor models, the G1 growth arrest has been linked to transcriptional activation of cyclin-dependent kinase (CDK) inhibitors p27[Kip1] and p21[Waf1] [51, 121]. These effects are not universally observed. For example, p21[Waf1] expression increases after 24 h and is reduced at 72 h in PC-3 prostate cancer cells, suggesting a biphasic, time-dependent response [123]. Induction of p27, which in contrast to p21 lacks a VDRE, appears to be mediated by NF-Y and SP1 [124, 125]. Thus, additional effects may take place at the level of protein stability [126, 127]. Dephosphorylation of the retinoblastoma protein in response to vitamin D has also been reported in both normal human keratinocytes [128] and several preclinical tumor models [115, 129–132]. Vitamin D has been shown to inhibit other mitogenic signals including the

ERK/MAPK pathway [73, 75], c-myc [133, 134], EGFR [135], and the insulin-like growth factor (IGF) system [136–138]. Vitamin D has also been shown to induce transforming growth factor-beta (TGFβ) [139, 140]. These effects vary across tumor models. While cell differentiation accompanies growth inhibition in some experimental systems, this association is not universal and differentiation can occur even in cells resistant to vitamin D-mediated growth arrest [141, 142]. Vitamin D inhibits fatty acid synthase (FAS) expression by stimulating the expression of long-chain fatty-acid-CoA ligase 3 (FACL3) in LNCaP cells. The upregulation of FACL3 and subsequent inhibition of FAS are involved in the antiproliferative effects of vitamin D [143]. Interestingly, the growth inhibitory effects of vitamin D on LNCaP cells are significantly attenuated by an inhibitor of FACL3 activity. Further, vitamin D is unable to regulate FACL3 expression in the absence of androgens, indicating that the upregulation of FACL3 expression by vitamin D is mediated through the androgen receptor (AR) signaling pathway [144]. Relevant to prostate cancer, androgen signaling may be important for vitamin D-mediated growth inhibition in human prostate cancer cells. In LNCaP cells and CWR22R cells, vitamin D induces AR expression. Vitamin D-mediated growth inhibition is reduced when AR signaling is blocked by antiandrogens, RNA interference, or targeted disruption of the AR [145].

Apoptosis

Vitamin D-induced apoptosis has been demonstrated in several prostate cancer models [146, 147]. Vitamin D has been reported to downregulate the antiapoptotic protein Bcl-2 in prostate cancer [146] and several other neoplastic cell types [75, 147–154]. In several cell lines, vitamin D-mediated apoptosis is independent of p53 status [150, 155, 156], although data about the role of p53 in this setting are not entirely consistent [149, 157]. In the CaP cell lines LNCaP and ALVA-31, as well as in the MCF-7 breast cancer cells, vitamin D stimulates cytochrome ***c release from mitochondria by a caspase-independent mechanism [146, 158]. Proapoptotic effects of vitamin D may also involve downregulation of the IGF receptor [159], upregulation of MEK kinase-1 [116], activation of the sphingomyelin-ceramide-ganglioside GD3 signaling pathway

[83], downregulation of Akt [160, 161], stimulation of TNF-α activity [162], induction of TGF-β signaling [163], and cytosolic calcium mobilization [164, 165]. Induction of ovarian cancer cell apoptosis by vitamin D is mediated through downregulation of telomerase [166]. Although proapoptotic activity has been demonstrated in multiple experimental systems, these effects are not universal and vitamin D-induced inhibition of apoptosis has also been described. For example, vitamin D inhibits ultraviolet B-induced apoptosis, Jun kinase activation, and interleukin-6 production in primary human keratinocytes [167].

Angiogenesis and Invasiveness

Several investigators have also reported antiangiogenic and anti-invasive effects of vitamin D in preclinical tumor models. Proliferation of tumor-derived endothelial cells [161] and sprouting and elongation of endothelial cells induced by vascular endothelial growth factor [168] are inhibited in in vitro models of angiogenesis. Antiangiogenic activity has been confirmed in mouse tumor models [168, 169]. Reduction of metastases with vitamin D therapy has been demonstrated in rodent models including those of prostate cancer [93, 101, 170], and reduced invasiveness has been shown in in vitro assays using prostate cancer [171–173], as well as a number of other tumor types [174, 175]. Serine proteinase and metalloproteinase inhibition [171, 173, 176], decreased α6 and β4 integrin expression [172], increased E-cadherin expression [177], and inhibition of tenascin-C [178] may explain the anti-invasive activity of vitamin D.

Preclinical Studies of Calcitriol and Vitamin D Analogs in Combination with Other Antineoplastic Agents

Steroids

The antineoplastic activity of vitamin D is enhanced by dexamethasone both in vitro and in vivo [159, 179]. In SCC cells, dexamethasone increases both VDR protein levels and ligand binding [179]. Dexamethasone increases both vitamin D-induced cell cycle arrest and apoptosis. Phospho-Erk1/2 and phospho-Akt levels and tumor-derived endothelial cell growth are suppressed more completely by the combination than by vitamin D alone [115, 160, 161, 179].

Cytotoxic Chemotherapy

Combinations of VDR ligands with several classes of chemotherapy drugs show additive or supra-additive activity in preclinical models. In prostate cancer models, enhanced activity of docetaxel [180], paclitaxel [123], platinum compounds [181], and mitoxantrone [182] has been reported. Animal model confirmation is available for paclitaxel and mitoxantrone [123, 182]. Similar results have been reported in several other tumor types [183–186]; however, the mechanisms of these interactions remain incompletely understood.

Retinoid Receptor Ligands

VDR forms heterodimers with RXR, thus synergistic growth inhibition by ligands for both receptors is expected [187, 188]. Synergistic induction of apoptosis [188] and inhibition of angiogenesis for vitamin D–retinoid combinations have also been reported [188]. Common effects on IGFBP-3 may explain synergistic growth inhibition for the combination of RAR and VDR ligands [189]. Recently, the combination of 9-cis retinoic acid with calcitriol has been shown to inhibit the human telomerase reverse transcriptase in prostate cancer cells. This effect is not seen when either agent is tested alone [190]. Common activation of target genes, such as p21 may also underlie interactions between retinoids and vitamin D.

Tamoxifen

VDR ligands significantly increase the inhibition of ***N-nitroso-N-methylurea (NMU)-induced mammary carcinogenesis by tamoxifen in Sprague–Dawley rats [191]. Both in vitro and in vivo data using MCF-7 cells demonstrate enhanced apoptosis with the combination

[192, 193]. Interestingly, recent results in MCF-7 cells suggest that sensitivity to vitamin D varies inversely with sensitivity to antiestrogens suggesting that sequential or concurrent use of these compounds would be of significant interest [194].

Nonsteroidal Anti-inflammatory Agents (NSAIDs)

Simultaneous treatment of LNCaP cells with VDR ligands along with ibuprofen resulted in additive suppression of growth in the absence of dihydrotestosterone (DHT) and synergistic growth inhibition in under DHT-stimulated conditions. Both decreased G1-S transition and enhanced apoptosis ***were reported [195]. cDNA analysis of LNCaP cells treated with calcitriol showed that the expression of prostaglandin synthesizing COX-2 gene is significantly decreased by calcitriol, while the prostaglandin inactivating 15-prostaglandindehydrogenase gene was upregulated [196]. The combination of calcitriol and nonsteroidal anti-inflammatory agents (NSAIDs) synergistically acted to inhibit LNCaP cell growth [197].

Radiation

p21 expression, known to be induced by vitamin D in a number of tumor models, has also been shown to sensitize cells to radiation therapy [198]. Potentiation of radiation-induced apoptosis with VDR ligands has been shown in several tumor models [199, 200] and in one analysis, increased ceramide generation may explain this interaction [201].

Clinical Trials of Calcitriol and Vitamin D Analogs

Calcitriol is clinically available and is indicated for patients who suffer from renal failure and therefore cannot adequately activate the storage form of vitamin D. The availability of this drug made it feasible for investigators to initiate studies in cancer. Because antineoplastic effects in vitro occur at significantly supraphysiologic concentrations (typically at or above 1 nM), dose escalation of calcitriol has been the goal of the phase I clinical programs.

Phase I Studies

The first clinical trials in prostate cancer were designed to build on standard replacement dosing of calcitriol. Using a daily administration schedule, Osborn et al. sought to dose escalate calcitriol in 11 patients with castration-resistant prostate cancer (CRPC). No prostate-specific antigen (PSA) responses were seen at doses that ranged from 0.5 to 1.5 µg daily. Further dose escalation was not pursued due to the risk of hypercalcemia [202]. Gross et al. took a similar approach to the study of seven patients with a rising PSA that had not been treated with castrate-sensitive patients. No PSA responses were seen; however, treatment appeared to favorably impact PSA kinetics (the PSA doubling time was reduced when compared with the same prior to treatment). Hypercalciuria was cited as the reason for avoiding doses above 2.5 µg/day [203].

Alternate Day Dosing

Subcutaneous administration every other day was the approach designed to test two hypotheses: that both the route and schedule of administration may reduce the calcemic toxicity of calcitriol. While hypercalcemia was the dose-limiting toxicity, this approach allowed significant escalation of the dose, with 10 µg daily being the highest dose tested [204]. Peak blood calcitriol concentrations of approximately 0.7 nM were observed at the 8-µg dose.

Weekly Dosing

In a dose-ranging study, weekly oral administration resulted in peak blood calcitriol concentrations of 3.7–6.0 nM without dose-limiting toxicity. Doses up to 2.8 µg/kg were examined; however, peak calcitriol concentrations (C_{max}) and the area under the

concentration curve (AUC) did not increase linearly at doses above 0.48 µg/kg [205]. This was the first study to report nonlinear pharmacokinetics with the commercially available formulation of calcitriol, a finding later confirmed by Muindi et al. [206]. This pharmacokinetic limitation, as well as the very large number of capsules required for treatment given the capsule sizes of 0.25 and 0.5 µg, later led to the development of a new high-dose formulation of calcitriol, DN-101. Administered as a single dose, DN-101 exhibits a dose-proportional increase in both C_{max} and AUC across a broad range of doses (15–165 µg). As a result, peak calcitriol concentrations achieved in this study were higher than in any previously reported study(14.9 nM at the 165-µg dose) [207]. In the preliminary report of the results with weekly dosing, grade 2 self-limited hypercalcemia was seen with repeat weekly dosing at 60 µg. Consequently, 45 µg weekly was recommended as the phase II weekly dose [208]. It is likely, however, that additional dose escalation on the weekly schedule would be feasible if either more conventional criteria for dose-limiting toxicity had been applied (grade 3 rather than grade 2 hypercalcemia) or if DN-101 were coadministered with an agent capable of reducing hypercalcemia.

Dosing 3 of Every 7 Days

Another approach to weekly dosing was administration of calcitriol for three consecutive days repeated every 7 days. In a phase I trial that combined calcitriol on this schedule with paclitaxel, daily doses up to 38 µg on three consecutive days every 7 days were administered without dose-limiting toxicity and produced a ***Cmax that ranged from 1.4 to 3.5 nM at the highest doses [207]. The same schedule of calcitriol was also evaluated in combination with zoledronate with dexamethasone added upon progression [209]. Daily calcitriol doses up to 30 µg for three consecutive days every 7 days were administered without dose-limiting toxicity and three patients had calcitriol dose reductions due to related laboratory abnormalities. There were no responses to calcitriol and zoledronate and one of seven patients responded when dexamethasone was added upon progression of the initial regimen.

Dosing Every 3 Weeks

If calcitriol is primarily used to modify tumor response to chemotherapy, even less frequent dosing may be useful, particularly when the chemotherapy regimen is dosed infrequently. Tiffany et al. tested 60 µg of calcitriol every 3 weeks 24 h before chemotherapy with docetaxel and estramustine [210]. The study used a dose de-escalation design and demonstrated that 60 µg can be safely administered on this schedule. Fifty-five percent of chemotherapy-naïve and 9% of patients previously treated with docetaxel-containing chemotherapy responded, but the study was not powered to show response.

The phase 1 efforts of a number of investigators clearly demonstrate that significant dose escalation of calcitriol with intermittent dosing is feasible. Indeed, most studies did not identify a maximum tolerated dose as dose escalation was limited by the number of capsules needed and by the nonlinear pharmacokinetics of the commercially available formulation of calcitriol. The DN-101 formulation overcomes both of these limitations and has been now studied the most extensively.

Phase II Studies

Single Agent Calcitriol

Weekly calcitriol has been tested as a single agent in castrate-sensitive prostate cancer and in combination with docetaxel in CRPC. In a nonrandomized study carried out in patients who had a biochemical progression after prostatectomy or radiation therapy, weekly calcitriol administered at a dose of 0.5 µg/kg was administered safely for a median of 10 months [211]. There were no confirmed PSA reductions in excess of 50%, but lesser PSA reductions as well as lengthening of the PSA doubling time when compared with pre-treatment conditions were observed.

Trump et al. performed another trial of calcitriol as a primary therapy for CRPC [212]. Calcitriol was administered orally on a weekly basis every Monday, Tuesday, and Wednesday (MTW) at a dosage of 8 µg for 4 weeks, 10 µg for the subsequent 4 weeks, and at 12 µg thereafter. Dexamethasone was administered orally each Sunday and MTW weekly at a dosage of 4 mg. Eight (19%) of 43 patients experienced a biochemical response (≥50%;

median decrease, 64%; range, 55–92%) persisting for ≥28 days. One patient experienced a decrease in PSA levels by 73%. However, persistent PSA decline was not assessed as the patient died 6 weeks after commencement of treatment due to a pulmonary embolism believed to be unrelated to treatment. Only four patients had a serum calcium level of >11.0 mg/dL. The biochemical response rate was similar to that of dexamethasone alone, but the regimen was well tolerated.

While these findings are suggestive of antitumor activity, a randomized trial would be needed to determine their clinical significance.

Combination with Docetaxel

These encouraging results led to the development of ASCENT (AIPC Study of Calcitriol Enhancing Taxotere), a placebo-controlled multi-institutional randomized study that randomized patients to weekly docetaxel (36 mg/m^2) with DN-101 45 µg or placebo [213, 214]. A total of 250 US and Canadian patients were entered. DN-101 was administered 24 h before docetaxel. This regimen was administered weekly for three consecutive weeks and repeated every 4 weeks. The primary end point of this study is a comparison of PSA response of >50% in the two arms. Within 6 months, PSA responses were seen in 58% in DN-101 patients and 49% in placebo patients ($P=0.16$). Overall, PSA response rates were 63% (DN-101) and 52% (placebo), $P=0.07$. Patients in the DN-101 group had a hazard ratio for death of 0.67 ($P=0.04$) in a multivariate analysis that included baseline hemoglobin and performance status. Beer et al. noted that median survival had not been reached in the DN-101 arm but estimated a median survival of 24.5 months compared with 16.4 months in the placebo arm. As the primary endpoint of this study was PSA response rate and not overall survival, a definitive phase III study (ASCENT-2) powered to evaluate survival was launched in 2006 and was closed to accrual in November 2007 with more than 900 of the intended 1,200 patients. Results from this trial are not yet publicly available. Because of advances in the field of chemotherapy for prostate cancer this study compared docetaxel administered weekly once with DN-101 to docetaxel administered every 3 weeks without DN-101. The trial was closed early by the DSMB due to an imbalance in the deaths.

An alternative calcitriol agent was reported in a phase II study by Attia et al. [215]. Patients with CRPC were randomized to receive docetaxel 35 mg/m² IV on days 1, 8, and 15 of a 28-day cycle either with or without doxercalciferol (1a-dihydroxyvitamin D2, Hectorol, Genzyme). This is an inactive prohormone that is hepatically metabolized and activated to 1α,25-dihydroxyvitamin D2 and 1α,24-dihydroxyvitamin D2 [216]. This agent has the advantage of less hypercalcemia as supported by early clinical studies [217]. Doxercalciferol was given at 10 µg orally, daily for 28 days. Seventy patients were randomized. PSA responses favored the doxercalciferol arm but did not meet statistical significance (46.7% vs. 39.5%, $P=0.560$). Median progression-free survival also did not differ significantly (6.17 months vs. 6.20 months, $P=0.764$).

Combinations with Carboplatin

A small phase II study also examined calcitriol 0.5 µg/kg in combination with carboplatin at an AUC dose of 7 (six in patients with prior radiation) dosed every 4 weeks [218]. The response rate was less than 10% and toxicity was unremarkable. It is not clear if this less encouraging result is related to the infrequent dosing schedule of calcitriol, to platinum resistance of prostate cancer, or due to chance given the small sample size ($n=17$).

A second phase II study was conducted with carboplatin, dexamethasone, and calcitriol by Flaig et al. [219]. In this study, men with CRPC were started on dexamethasone 1 mg daily. After 5 weeks, they were also given 0.5 µg of calcitriol provided their calcium remained <10.1 mg/dL. After 2 weeks of the additional calcitriol, carboplatin (AUC=2) administered weekly was begun. The regimen was not well tolerated by the initial group; thus, carboplatin dosing was changed to 4 weekly doses with 2 weeks of rest. Of the 34 patients treated, 13 showed PSA response. Of note, two patients died of cardiac complications and four experienced grade 3 neutropenia.

Combination with Mitoxantrone

Chan et al. have also tested the safety and efficacy of DN-101 with mitoxantrone [220]. DN-101 was given at a dose of 180 µg 24 h prior to mitoxantrone 12 mg/m² every 21 days with continuous oral prednisone for a maximum of 12 cycles. Five of 19 patients (26%; 95% confidence interval, CI, 9–51) achieved a ≥50% decline in PSA level. The median (95% CI) time to PSA progression was 16 (6–26) weeks. The overall median (95% CI) survival was 16 (6–26) months; 47 (21–73%) of patients achieved an analgesic response. Toxicity was similar to that expected with mitoxantrone and prednisone alone. The quality of life analysis suggested a decrease in physical functioning and increase in fatigue, insomnia, and diarrhea. The regimen is usable but will need to be evaluated further to determine if and when it should be employed in relationship to docetaxel-based chemotherapy.

Other Calcitriol Analogs

While much of the clinical testing of VDR ligands has been conducted with calcitriol, the naturally occurring ligand, another approach has been to develop calcitriol analogs designed to decouple antineoplastic activity from calcemic toxicity. The most common synthetic approach has been to modify the side chain of the calcitriol molecule and many such compounds have been chemically synthesized. Differences in protein binding, VDR affinity, and drug metabolism have all been cited as explanation for reduced calcemic activity [221–223]. Several of these compounds have entered clinical trials, some in prostate cancer. After phase I evaluation [224], Seocalcitol (EB1089) 10 µg daily was evaluated in phase II studies in pancreatic and hepatocellular carcinoma. No objective responses were seen in patients with pancreatic cancer [225], but two of 33 evaluable patients with unresectable hepatocellular carcinoma achieved complete remission that had endured beyond 29 months (last point of analysis) [226]. Three of the 14 patients with locally advanced or cutaneous metastatic adenocarcinoma of the breast responded to topical calcipotriol [227]. Two of 25 CRPC patients had objective partial responses in a phase I trial of 1-alphahydroxyvitamin D2 [228]. This study identified 12.5 µg as the phase II dose after encountering dose-limiting hypercalcemia and renal insufficiency. A follow-up phase II study examined this regimen in 26 patients with androgen-independent prostate cancer. As the investigators expected this analog to act primarily as a cytostatic agent, the trial's primary endpoint was progression-free survival.

Median time to progression was 12 weeks (mean 19 weeks) and one patient had stable disease for >2 years. The vitamin D3 analog ILX23-7553 has entered phase I clinical trials and was safe at doses up to 45 µg/m²/day for five consecutive days repeated every 14 days. The study was discontinued before dose-limiting toxicity was identified due to the number of capsules required. The authors suggest that further dose escalation should be pursued using a reformulated higher dose capsule [229].

Conclusions

There are intriguing epidemiological data and strong preclinical data that support targeting the VDR for cancer therapy in general and prostate cancer therapy, specifically. Most of the clinical trials conducted to date have examined supplementation with calcitriol, the naturally occurring ligand of the vitamin D receptor. Significant dose escalation of this compound is not feasible when it is dosed daily due to predictable hypercalcemia. Various intermittent dosing approaches have been developed and all demonstrate that intermittent dosing allows substantial escalation of the calcitriol dose and consequently of calcitriol exposure. An alternative approach is the development of calcitriol analogs that seek to uncouple antineoplastic activity from calcemic action. Several such analogs have entered clinical trials, but in prostate cancer have been less extensively studied than calcitriol. Single agent studies have largely focused on safety. Confirmed responses to single agent calcitriol or its analogs have been rarely reported. Stabilization of disease or apparent slowing of the rate of rise in serum PSA has been more often seen. While disease stabilization or PSA slowing are findings that are consistent with the hypothesis that VDR ligands are acting as cytostatic agents, the available studies are small and uncontrolled and are not sufficient to draw firm conclusions about the clinical meaning of these observations. Progress in single agent VDR ligand therapy will require a commitment to larger, randomized prospective clinical trials. A better understanding of the molecular determinants of response and resistance to calcitriol would also be helpful as it could allow for better selection of patients whose tumors are vulnerable to this class of agents. To date, phase I and II clinical data with calcitriol and other vitamin D analogs support its safety in concert with cytotoxic therapy. Impact on efficacy of therapy needs further testing at this time. Of these agents only DN-101 has reached phase III clinical testing. Despite the early closure of ASCENT-2, the final results may provide additional insight as to what role manipulation of vitamin D-oriented therapeutics may have in prostate cancer treatment.

References

1. Hanchette CL, Schwartz GG. Geographic patterns of prostate cancer mortality. Evidence for a protective effect of ultraviolet radiation. Cancer 1992;70(12):2861–9.
2. Luscombe CJ, et al. Prostate cancer risk: associations with ultraviolet radiation, tyrosinase and melanocortin-1 receptor genotypes. Br J Cancer 2001;85(10):1504–9.
3. Grant WB. An estimate of premature cancer mortality in the U.S. due to inadequate doses of solar ultraviolet-B radiation. Cancer 2002;94(6):1867–75.
4. Corder EH, et al. Vitamin D and prostate cancer: a prediagnostic study with stored sera. Cancer Epidemiol Biomarkers Prev 1993;2(5):467–72.
5. Gann PH, et al. Circulating vitamin D metabolites in relation to subsequent development of prostate cancer. Cancer Epidemiol Biomarkers Prev 1996;5(2):121–6.
6. Jacobs ET, et al. Plasma levels of 25-hydroxyvitamin D, 1,25-dihydroxyvitamin D and the risk of prostate cancer. J Steroid Biochem Mol Biol 2004;89–90(1–5):533–7.
7. Nomura AM, et al. Serum vitamin D metabolite levels and the subsequent development of prostate cancer (Hawaii, United States). Cancer Causes Control 1998;9(4):425–32.
8. Platz EA, et al. Plasma 1,25-dihydroxy- and 25-hydroxyvitamin D and subsequent risk of prostate cancer. Cancer Causes Control 2004;15(3):255–65.
9. Ahonen MH, et al. Prostate cancer risk and prediagnostic serum 25-hydroxyvitamin D levels (Finland). Cancer Causes Control 2000;11(9):847–52.
10. Tuohimaa P, et al. Both high and low levels of blood vitamin D are associated with a higher prostate cancer risk: a longitudinal, nested case-control study in the Nordic countries. Int J Cancer 2004;108(1):104–8.
11. Chan JM, et al. Dairy products, calcium, phosphorous, vitamin D, and risk of prostate cancer (Sweden). Cancer Causes Control 1998;9(6):559–66.
12. Chan JM, et al. Diet and prostate cancer risk in a cohort of smokers, with a specific focus on calcium and phosphorus (Finland). Cancer Causes Control 2000;11(9):859–67.
13. Giovannucci E, et al. Calcium and fructose intake in relation to risk of prostate cancer. Cancer Res 1998;58(3):442–7.
14. Kristal AR, et al. Associations of energy, fat, calcium, and vitamin D with prostate cancer risk. Cancer Epidemiol Biomarkers Prev 2002;11(8):719–25.
15. Park SY, et al. Calcium, vitamin D, and dairy product intake and prostate cancer risk: the Multiethnic Cohort Study. Am J Epidemiol 2007;166(11):1259–69.

16. Huncharek M, Muscat J, Kupelnick B. Dairy products, dietary calcium and vitamin D intake as risk factors for prostate cancer: a meta-analysis of 26,769 cases from 45 observational studies. Nutr Cancer 2008;60(4):421–41.

17. Qin LQ, et al. Milk consumption is a risk factor for prostate cancer: meta-analysis of case-control studies. Nutr Cancer 2004;48(1):22–7.

18. Cross HS, et al. 25-Hydroxyvitamin D(3)-1alpha-hydroxylase and vitamin D receptor gene expression in human colonic mucosa is elevated during early cancerogenesis. Steroids 2001;66(3–5):287–92.

19. Tangpricha V, et al. 25-Hydroxyvitamin D-1alpha-hydroxylase in normal and malignant colon tissue. Lancet 2001;357(9269):1673–4.

20. Chen TC, et al. Prostatic 25-hydroxyvitamin D-1alpha-hydroxylase and its implication in prostate cancer. J Cell Biochem 2003;88(2):315–22.

21. Hsu JY, et al. Reduced 1alpha-hydroxylase activity in human prostate cancer cells correlates with decreased susceptibility to 25-hydroxyvitamin D3-induced growth inhibition. Cancer Res 2001;61(7):2852–6.

22. Bouillon RA, et al. Vitamin D status in the elderly: seasonal substrate deficiency causes 1,25-dihydroxycholecalciferol deficiency. Am J Clin Nutr 1987;45(4):755–63.

23. Dandona P, et al. Low 1,25-dihydroxyvitamin D, secondary hyperparathyroidism, and normal osteocalcin in elderly subjects. J Clin Endocrinol Metab 1986;63(2):459–62.

24. Dubbelman R, et al. Age-dependent vitamin D status and vertebral condition of white women living in Curacao (The Netherlands Antilles) as compared with their counterparts in The Netherlands. Am J Clin Nutr 1993;58(1):106–9.

25. Lips P, et al. Vitamin D supplementation and fracture incidence in elderly persons. A randomized, placebo-controlled clinical trial. Ann Intern Med 1996;124(4):400–6.

26. Giovannucci E. Dietary influences of 1,25(OH)2 vitamin D in relation to prostate cancer: a hypothesis. Cancer Causes Control 1998;9(6):567–82.

27. Beer TM, et al. Randomized study of high-dose pulse calcitriol or placebo prior to radical prostatectomy. Cancer Epidemiol Biomarkers Prev 2004;13(12):2225–32.

28. Kidd LC, et al. Sequence variation within the 5′ regulatory regions of the vitamin D binding protein and receptor genes and prostate cancer risk. Prostate 2005;64(3):272–82.

29. Torkko KC, et al. VDR and SRD5A2 polymorphisms combine to increase risk for prostate cancer in both non-Hispanic White and Hispanic White men. Clin Cancer Res 2008;14(10):3223–9.

30. Zhou W, et al. Vitamin D is associated with improved survival in early-stage non-small cell lung cancer patients. Cancer Epidemiol Biomarkers Prev 2005;14(10):2303–9.

31. Robsahm TE, et al. Vitamin D3 from sunlight may improve the prognosis of breast-, colon- and prostate cancer (Norway). Cancer Causes Control 2004;15(2):149–58.

32. Lagunova Z, et al. Prostate cancer survival is dependent on season of diagnosis. Prostate 2007;67(12):1362–70.

33. Mangelsdorf DJ, et al. The nuclear receptor superfamily: the second decade. Cell 1995;83(6):835–9.

34. Carlberg C, Saurat JH. Vitamin D-retinoid association: molecular basis and clinical applications. J Investig Dermatol Symp Proc 1996;1(1):82–6.

35. Conde I, et al. Expression of vitamin D3 receptor and retinoid receptors in human breast cancer: identification of potential heterodimeric receptors. Int J Oncol 2004;25(4):1183–91.

36. Kliewer SA, et al. Retinoid X receptor interacts with nuclear receptors in retinoic acid, thyroid hormone and vitamin D3 signalling. Nature 1992;355(6359):446–9.

37. Nanes MS, et al. A single up-stream element confers responsiveness to 1,25-dihydroxyvitamin D3 and tumor necrosis factor-alpha in the rat osteocalcin gene. Endocrinology 1994;134(3):1113–20.

38. Koszewski NJ, Reinhardt TA, Horst RL. Vitamin D receptor interactions with the murine osteopontin response element. J Steroid Biochem Mol Biol 1996;59(5–6):377–88.

39. Kim RH, et al. Identification of a vitamin D3-response element that overlaps a unique inverted TATA box in the rat bone sialoprotein gene. Biochem J 1996;318(Pt 1):219–26.

40. Kitazawa R, Kitazawa S. Vitamin D(3) augments osteoclastogenesis via vitamin D-responsive element of mouse RANKL gene promoter. Biochem Biophys Res Commun 2002;290(2):650–5.

41. Drissi H, et al. 1,25-(OH)2-vitamin D3 suppresses the bone-related Runx2/Cbfa1 gene promoter. Exp Cell Res 2002;274(2):323–33.

42. Hakim I, Bar-Shavit Z. Modulation of TNF-alpha expression in bone marrow macrophages: involvement of vitamin D response element. J Cell Biochem 2003;88(5):986–98.

43. Hawa NS, O'Riordan JL, Farrow SM. Functional analysis of vitamin D response elements in the parathyroid hormone gene and a comparison with the osteocalcin gene. Biochem Biophys Res Commun 1996;228(2):352–7.

44. Falzon M. DNA sequences in the rat parathyroid hormone-related peptide gene responsible for 1,25-dihydroxyvitamin D3-mediated transcriptional repression. Mol Endocrinol 1996;10(6):672–81.

45. Maestro B, et al. Identification of a vitamin D response element in the human insulin receptor gene promoter. J Steroid Biochem Mol Biol 2003;84(2–3):223–30.

46. Lee S, et al. Identification of a functional vitamin D response element in the murine Insig-2 promoter and its potential role in the differentiation of 3T3-L1 preadipocytes. Mol Endocrinol 2005;19(2):399–408.

47. Quelo I, Machuca I, Jurdic P. Identification of a vitamin D response element in the proximal promoter of the chicken carbonic anhydrase II gene. J Biol Chem 1998;273(17):10638–46.

48. Seoane S, et al. Localization of a negative vitamin D response sequence in the human growth hormone gene. Biochem Biophys Res Commun 2002;292(1):250–5.

49. Gill RK, Christakos S. Identification of sequence elements in mouse calbindin-D28k gene that confer 1,25-dihydroxyvitamin D3- and butyrate-inducible responses. Proc Natl Acad Sci U S A 1993;90(7):2984–8.

50. Fujisawa K, et al. Identification of a response element for vitamin D3 and retinoic acid in the promoter region of the human fructose-1,6-bisphosphatase gene. J Biochem 2000;127(3):373–82.

51. Liu M, et al. Transcriptional activation of the Cdk inhibitor p21 by vitamin D3 leads to the induced differentiation of the myelomonocytic cell line U937. Genes Dev 1996;10(2):142–53.

52. Jiang F, et al. G2/M arrest by 1,25-dihydroxyvitamin D3 in ovarian cancer cells mediated through the induction of GADD45 via an exonic enhancer. J Biol Chem 2003; 278(48):48030–40.

53. Matilainen M, et al. Regulation of multiple insulin-like growth factor binding protein genes by 1alpha,25-dihydroxyvitamin D3. Nucleic Acids Res 2005;33(17): 5521–32.

54. Peng L, Malloy PJ, Feldman D. Identification of a functional vitamin D response element in the human insulin-like growth factor binding protein-3 promoter. Mol Endocrinol 2004; 18(5):1109–19.

55. Zierold C, Darwish HM, DeLuca HF. Identification of a vitamin D-response element in the rat calcidiol (25-hydroxyvitamin D3) 24-hydroxylase gene. Proc Natl Acad Sci U S A 1994;91(3):900–2.

56. Thompson PD, et al. Liganded VDR induces CYP3A4 in small intestinal and colon cancer cells via DR3 and ER6 vitamin D responsive elements. Biochem Biophys Res Commun 2002;299(5):730–8.

57. McCarthy TC, Li X, Sinal CJ. Vitamin D receptor-dependent regulation of colon multidrug resistance-associated protein 3 gene expression by bile acids. J Biol Chem 2005;280(24): 23232–42.

58. McGaffin KR, Chrysogelos SA. Identification and characterization of a response element in the EGFR promoter that mediates transcriptional repression by 1,25-dihydroxyvitamin D3 in breast cancer cells. J Mol Endocrinol 2005; 35(1):117–33.

59. Candeliere GA, et al. A composite element binding the vitamin D receptor, retinoid X receptor alpha, and a member of the CTF/NF-1 family of transcription factors mediates the vitamin D responsiveness of the c-fos promoter. Mol Cell Biol 1996;16(2):584–92.

60. Xie Z, Bikle DD. Differential regulation of vitamin D responsive elements in normal and transformed keratinocytes. J Invest Dermatol 1998;110(5):730–3.

61. Polly P, et al. Identification of a vitamin D3 response element in the fibronectin gene that is bound by a vitamin D3 receptor homodimer. J Cell Biochem 1996;60(3):322–33.

62. Cao X, et al. Cloning of the promoter for the avian integrin beta 3 subunit gene and its regulation by 1,25-dihydroxyvitamin D3. J Biol Chem 1993;268(36):27371–80.

63. Bikle DD, et al. The vitamin D response element of the involucrin gene mediates its regulation by 1,25-dihydroxyvitamin D3. J Invest Dermatol 2002;119(5):1109–13.

64. Deftos LJ, et al. Direct evidence that PTHrP expression promotes prostate cancer progression in bone. Biochem Biophys Res Commun 2005;327(2):468–72.

65. Lynch CC, et al. MMP-7 promotes prostate cancer-induced osteolysis via the solubilization of RANKL. Cancer Cell 2005;7(5):485–96.

66. Tenta R, et al. Bone microenvironment-related growth factors, zoledronic acid and dexamethasone differentially modulate PTHrP expression in PC-3 prostate cancer cells. Horm Metab Res 2005;37(10):593–601.

67. Nemere I, Yoshimoto Y, Norman AW. Calcium transport in perfused duodena from normal chicks: enhancement within fourteen minutes of exposure to 1,25-dihydroxyvitamin D3. Endocrinology 1984;115(4):1476–83.

68. De Boland AR, Boland RL. Non-genomic signal transduction pathway of vitamin D in muscle. Cell Signal 1994;6(7):717–24.

69. Edelman A, Garabedian M, Anagnostopoulos T. Mechanisms of 1,25(OH)2D3-induced rapid changes of membrane potential in proximal tubule: role of Ca2+-dependent K+ channels. J Membr Biol 1986;90(2):137–43.

70. Beno DW, et al. Protein kinase C and mitogen-activated protein kinase are required for 1,25-dihydroxyvitamin D3-stimulated Egr induction. J Biol Chem 1995;270(8): 3642–7.

71. de Boland AR, et al. Age-associated decrease in inositol 1,4,5-trisphosphate and diacylglycerol generation by 1,25(OH)2-vitamin D3 in rat intestine. Cell Signal 1996; 8(3):153–7.

72. de Boland AR, Morelli S, Boland R. 1,25(OH)2-vitamin D3 signal transduction in chick myoblasts involves phosphatidylcholine hydrolysis. J Biol Chem 1994;269(12):8675–9.

73. Capiati DA, et al. Inhibition of serum-stimulated mitogen activated protein kinase by 1alpha,25(OH)2-vitamin D3 in MCF-7 breast cancer cells. J Cell Biochem 2004;93(2): 384–97.

74. Gniadecki R. Activation of Raf-mitogen-activated protein kinase signaling pathway by 1,25-dihydroxyvitamin D3 in normal human keratinocytes. J Invest Dermatol 1996;106(6): 1212–7.

75. Park WH, et al. Induction of apoptosis by vitamin D3 analogue EB1089 in NCI-H929 myeloma cells via activation of caspase 3 and p38 MAP kinase. Br J Haematol 2000;109(3): 576–83.

76. Rossi AM, et al. MAPK inhibition by 1alpha,25(OH)2-vitamin D3 in breast cancer cells. Evidence on the participation of the VDR and Src. J Steroid Biochem Mol Biol 2004;89–90(1–5):287–90.

77. Bellido T, et al. Evidence for the participation of protein kinase C and 3′,5′-cyclic AMP-dependent protein kinase in the stimulation of muscle cell proliferation by 1,25-dihydroxy-vitamin D3. Mol Cell Endocrinol 1993;90(2):231–8.

78. Vazquez G, Boland R, de Boland AR. Modulation by 1,25(OH)2-vitamin D3 of the adenylyl cyclase/cyclic AMP pathway in rat and chick myoblasts. Biochim Biophys Acta 1995;1269(1):91–7.

79. Massheimer V, Boland R, de Boland AR. Rapid 1,25(OH)2-vitamin D3 stimulation of calcium uptake by rat intestinal cells involves a dihydropyridine-sensitive cAMP-dependent pathway. Cell Signal 1994;6(3):299–304.

80. Santillan GE, Boland RL. Studies suggesting the participation of protein kinase A in 1,25(OH)2-vitamin D3-dependent protein phosphorylation in cardiac muscle. J Mol Cell Cardiol 1998;30(2):225–33.

81. Hmama Z, et al. 1Alpha,25-dihydroxyvitamin D(3)-induced myeloid cell differentiation is regulated by a vitamin D receptor-phosphatidylinositol 3-kinase signaling complex. J Exp Med 1999;190(11):1583–94.

82. Lee JS, et al. Stable gene silencing in human monocytic cell lines using lentiviral-delivered small interference RNA. Silencing of the p110alpha isoform of phosphoinositide 3-kinase reveals differential regulation of adherence induced by 1alpha,25-dihydroxycholecalciferol and bacterial lipopolysaccharide. J Biol Chem 2004;279(10):9379–88.

83. Bektas M, Orfanos CE, Geilen CC, et al. Different vitamin D analogues induce sphingomyelin hydrolysis and apoptosis in the human keratinocyte cell line HaCaT. Cell Mol Biol (Noisy-le-grand) 2004;46(1):111–9.

84. Rebsamen MC, et al. 1Alpha,25-dihydroxyvitamin D3 induces vascular smooth muscle cell migration via activation of phosphatidylinositol 3-kinase. Circ Res 2002;91(1): 17–24.

85. Schwartz Z, et al. 1Alpha,25-dihydroxyvitamin D(3) and 24R, 25-dihydroxyvitamin D(3) modulate growth plate chondrocyte physiology via protein kinase C-dependent phosphorylation of extracellular signal-regulated kinase 1/2 mitogen-activated protein kinase. Endocrinology 2002;143(7):2775–86.

86. Erben RG, et al. Deletion of deoxyribonucleic acid binding domain of the vitamin D receptor abrogates genomic and nongenomic functions of vitamin D. Mol Endocrinol 2002;16(7):1524–37.

87. Huhtakangas JA, et al. The vitamin D receptor is present in caveolae-enriched plasma membranes and binds 1 alpha,25(OH)2-vitamin D3 in vivo and in vitro. Mol Endocrinol 2004;18(11):2660–71.

88. Mizwicki MT, et al. Evidence that annexin II is not a putative membrane receptor for 1alpha,25(OH)2-vitamin D3. J Cell Biochem 2004;91(4):852–63.

89. Norman AW, et al. Update on biological actions of 1alpha,25(OH)2-vitamin D3 (rapid effects) and 24R, 25(OH)2-vitamin D3. Mol Cell Endocrinol 2002;197(1–2): 1–13.

90. Norman AW, et al. Comparison of 6-s-cis- and 6-s-trans-locked analogs of 1alpha,25-dihydroxyvitamin D3 indicates that the 6-s-cis conformation is preferred for rapid nongenomic biological responses and that neither 6-s-cis-nor 6-s-trans-locked analogs are preferred for genomic biological responses. Mol Endocrinol 1997;11(10):1518–31.

91. Rohe B, et al. Identification and characterization of 1,25D3-membrane-associated rapid response, steroid (1,25D3-MARRS)-binding protein in rat IEC-6 cells. Steroids 2005;70(5–7):458–63.

92. Abe E, et al. Differentiation of mouse myeloid leukemia cells induced by 1 alpha,25-dihydroxyvitamin D3. Proc Natl Acad Sci U S A 1981;78(8):4990–4.

93. Konety BR, et al. Effects of vitamin D (calcitriol) on transitional cell carcinoma of the bladder in vitro and in vivo. J Urol 2001;165(1):253–8.

94. Colston KW, et al. Effects of synthetic vitamin D analogues on breast cancer cell proliferation in vivo and in vitro. Biochem Pharmacol 1992;44(4):693–702.

95. Cross HS, Huber C, Peterlik M. Antiproliferative effect of 1,25-dihydroxyvitamin D3 and its analogs on human colon adenocarcinoma cells (CaCo-2): influence of extracellular calcium. Biochem Biophys Res Commun 1991;179(1):57–62.

96. Yabushita H, et al. Vitamin D receptor in endometrial carcinoma and the differentiation-inducing effect of 1,25-dihydroxyvitamin D3 on endometrial carcinoma cell lines. J Obstet Gynaecol Res 1996;22(6):529–39.

97. Fujioka T, et al. Inhibition of tumor growth and angiogenesis by vitamin D3 agents in murine renal cell carcinoma. J Urol 1998;160(1):247–51.

98. Nagakura K, et al. Inhibitory effect of 1 alpha,25-dihydroxyvitamin D3 on the growth of the renal carcinoma cell line. Kidney Int 1986;29(4):834–40.

99. Higashimoto Y, et al. 1 Alpha,25-dihydroxyvitamin D3 and all-trans-retinoic acid inhibit the growth of a lung cancer cell line. Anticancer Res 1996;16(5A):2653–9.

100. Zugmaier G, et al. Growth-inhibitory effects of vitamin D analogues and retinoids on human pancreatic cancer cells. Br J Cancer 1996;73(11):1341–6.

101. Getzenberg RH, et al. Vitamin D inhibition of prostate adenocarcinoma growth and metastasis in the Dunning rat prostate model system. Urology 1997;50(6):999–1006.

102. Hedlund TE, Moffatt KA, Miller GJ. Vitamin D receptor expression is required for growth modulation by 1 alpha,25-dihydroxyvitamin D3 in the human prostatic carcinoma cell line ALVA-31. J Steroid Biochem Mol Biol 1996;58(3):277–88.

103. Peehl DM, et al. Antiproliferative effects of 1,25-dihydroxyvitamin D3 on primary cultures of human prostatic cells. Cancer Res 1994;54(3):805–10.

104. Schwartz GG, et al. Human prostate cancer cells: inhibition of proliferation by vitamin D analogs. Anticancer Res 1994;14(3A):1077–81.

105. Skowronski RJ, Peehl DM, Feldman D. Actions of vitamin D3, analogs on human prostate cancer cell lines: comparison with 1,25-dihydroxyvitamin D3. Endocrinology 1995;136(1):20–6.

106. Skowronski RJ, Peehl DM, Feldman D. Vitamin D and prostate cancer: 1,25 dihydroxyvitamin D3 receptors and actions in human prostate cancer cell lines. Endocrinology 1993;132(5):1952–60.

107. Zhuang SH, et al. Vitamin D receptor content and transcriptional activity do not fully predict antiproliferative effects of vitamin D in human prostate cancer cell lines. Mol Cell Endocrinol 1997;126(1):83–90.

108. Shabahang M, et al. The effect of 1,25-dihydroxyvitamin D3 on the growth of soft-tissue sarcoma cells as mediated by the vitamin D receptor. Ann Surg Oncol 1996;3(2):144–9.

109. Hara K, et al. Oral administration of 1 alpha hydroxyvitamin D3 inhibits tumor growth and metastasis of a murine osteosarcoma model. Anticancer Res 2001;21(1A):321–4.

110. Tokuumi Y. Correlation between the concentration of 1,25 alpha dihydroxyvitamin D3 receptors and growth inhibition, and differentiation of human osteosarcoma cells induced by vitamin D3. Nippon Seikeigeka Gakkai Zasshi 1995;69(4):181–90.

111. Celli A, Treves C, Stio M. Vitamin D receptor in SH-SY5Y human neuroblastoma cells and effect of 1,25-dihydroxyvitamin D3 on cellular proliferation. Neurochem Int 1999;34(2):117–24.

112. Veenstra TD, et al. Effects of 1,25-dihydroxyvitamin D3 on growth of mouse neuroblastoma cells. Brain Res Dev Brain Res 1997;99(1):53–60.

113. Naveilhan P, et al. Induction of glioma cell death by 1,25(OH)2 vitamin D3: towards an endocrine therapy of brain tumors? J Neurosci Res 1994;37(2):271–7.

114. Colston K, Colston MJ, Feldman D. 1,25-dihydroxyvitamin D3 and malignant melanoma: the presence of receptors and inhibition of cell growth in culture. Endocrinology 1981;108(3):1083–6.

115. Hershberger PA, et al. 1,25-Dihydroxycholecalciferol (1,25-D3) inhibits the growth of squamous cell carcinoma and down-modulates p21(Waf1/Cip1) in vitro and in vivo. Cancer Res 1999;59(11):2644–9.

116. McGuire TF, Trump DL, Johnson CS, et al. Vitamin D(3)-induced apoptosis of murine squamous cell carcinoma cells. Selective induction of caspase-dependent MEK cleavage and up-regulation of MEKK-1. J Biol Chem 2001;276(28):26365–73.

117. Berger U, et al. Immunocytochemical detection of 1,25-dihydroxyvitamin D receptors in normal human tissues. J Clin Endocrinol Metab 1988;67(3):607–13.

118. Holick MF. Vitamin D: a millennium perspective. J Cell Biochem 2003;88(2):296–307.

119. Campbell MJ, Koeffler HP. Toward therapeutic intervention of cancer by vitamin D compounds. J Natl Cancer Inst 1997;89(3):182–5.

120. Sheikh MS, Rochefort H, Garcia M. Overexpression of p21WAF1/CIP1 induces growth arrest, giant cell formation and apoptosis in human breast carcinoma cell lines. Oncogene 1995;11(9):1899–905.

121. Wang QM, Jones JB, Studzinski GP. Cyclin-dependent kinase inhibitor p27 as a mediator of the G1-S phase block induced by 1,25-dihydroxyvitamin D3 in HL60 cells. Cancer Res 1996;56(2):264–7.

122. Zhuang SH, Burnstein KL. Antiproliferative effect of 1alpha,25-dihydroxyvitamin D3 in human prostate cancer cell line LNCaP involves reduction of cyclin-dependent kinase 2 activity and persistent G1 accumulation. Endocrinology 1998;139(3):1197–207.

123. Hershberger PA, et al. Calcitriol (1,25-dihydroxycholecalciferol) enhances paclitaxel antitumor activity in vitro and in vivo and accelerates paclitaxel-induced apoptosis. Clin Cancer Res 2001;7(4):1043–51.

124. Huang YC, Chen JY, Hung WC. Vitamin D3 receptor/Sp1 complex is required for the induction of p27Kip1 expression by vitamin D3. Oncogene 2004;23(28):4856–61.

125. Inoue T, Kamiyama J, Sakai T. Sp1 and NF-Y synergistically mediate the effect of vitamin D(3) in the p27(Kip1) gene promoter that lacks vitamin D response elements. J Biol Chem 1999;274(45):32309–17.

126. Lin R, et al. Inhibition of F-Box protein p45(SKP2) expression and stabilization of cyclin-dependent kinase inhibitor p27(KIP1) in vitamin D analog-treated cancer cells. Endocrinology 2003;144(3):749–53.

127. Yang ES, Burnstein KL. Vitamin D inhibits G1 to S progression in LNCaP prostate cancer cells through p27Kip1 stabilization and Cdk2 mislocalization to the cytoplasm. J Biol Chem 2003;278(47):46862–8.

128. Kobayashi T, Hashimoto K, Yoshikawa K. Growth inhibition of human keratinocytes by 1,25-dihydroxyvitamin D3 is linked to dephosphorylation of retinoblastoma gene product. Biochem Biophys Res Commun 1993;196(1):487–93.

129. Fan FS, Yu WC. 1,25-Dihydroxyvitamin D3 suppresses cell growth, DNA synthesis, and phosphorylation of retinoblastoma protein in a breast cancer cell line. Cancer Invest 1995;13(3):280–6.

130. Hager G, et al. 1,25(OH)2 vitamin D3 induces elevated expression of the cell cycle-regulating genes P21 and P27 in squamous carcinoma cell lines of the head and neck. Acta Otolaryngol 2001;121(1):103–9.

131. Jensen SS, et al. Inhibitory effects of 1alpha,25-dihydroxyvitamin D(3) on the G(1)-S phase-controlling machinery. Mol Endocrinol 2001;15(8):1370–80.

132. Yen A, Varvayanis S. Late dephosphorylation of the RB protein in G2 during the process of induced cell differentiation. Exp Cell Res 1994;214(1):250–7.

133. Matsumoto K, et al. Growth-inhibitory effects of 1,25-dihydroxyvitamin D3 on normal human keratinocytes cultured in serum-free medium. Biochem Biophys Res Commun 1990;166(2):916–23.

134. Reitsma PH, et al. Regulation of myc gene expression in HL-60 leukaemia cells by a vitamin D metabolite. Nature 1983;306(5942):492–4.

135. Tong WM, et al. Growth regulation of human colon cancer cells by epidermal growth factor and 1,25-dihydroxyvitamin D3 is mediated by mutual modulation of receptor expression. Eur J Cancer 1998;34(13):2119–25.

136. Drivdahl RH, et al. IGF-binding proteins in human prostate tumor cells: expression and regulation by 1,25-dihydroxyvitamin D3. Prostate 1995;26(2):72–9.

137. Scharla SH, et al. 1,25-Dihydroxyvitamin D3 differentially regulates the production of insulin-like growth factor I (IGF-I) and IGF-binding protein-4 in mouse osteoblasts. Endocrinology 1991;129(6):3139–46.

138. Vink-van Wijngaarden T, et al. Inhibition of insulin- and insulin-like growth factor-I-stimulated growth of human breast cancer cells by 1,25-dihydroxyvitamin D3 and the vitamin D3 analogue EB1089. Eur J Cancer 1996;32A(5):842–8.

139. Haugen JD, et al. 1 Alpha,25-dihydroxyvitamin D3 inhibits normal human keratinocyte growth by increasing transforming growth factor beta 2 release. Biochem Biophys Res Commun 1996;229(2):618–23.

140. Wu Y, et al. 1 Alpha,25-Dihydroxyvitamin D3 increases transforming growth factor and transforming growth factor receptor type I and II synthesis in human bone cells. Biochem Biophys Res Commun 1997;239(3):734–9.

141. Elstner E, et al. 20-epi-vitamin D3 analogues: a novel class of potent inhibitors of proliferation and inducers of differentiation of human breast cancer cell lines. Cancer Res 1995;55(13):2822–30.

142. Studzinski GP, et al. Uncoupling of cell cycle arrest from the expression of monocytic differentiation markers in HL60 cell variants. Exp Cell Res 1997;232(2):376–87.

143. Qiao S, Tuohimaa P. Vitamin D3 inhibits fatty acid synthase expression by stimulating the expression of long-chain fatty-acid-CoA ligase 3 in prostate cancer cells. FEBS Lett 2004;577(3):451–4.

144. Qiao S, Tuohimaa P. The role of long-chain fatty-acid-CoA ligase 3 in vitamin D3 and androgen control of prostate cancer LNCaP cell growth. Biochem Biophys Res Commun 2004;319(2):358–68.

145. Bao BY, et al. Androgen signaling is required for the vitamin D-mediated growth inhibition in human prostate cancer cells. Oncogene 2004;23(19):3350–60.

146. Guzey M, Kitada S, Reed JC. Apoptosis induction by 1alpha,25-dihydroxyvitamin D3 in prostate cancer. Mol Cancer Ther 2002;1(9):667–77.

147. Modzelewski RA, Hershberger PA, Johnson CS, et al. Apoptotic effects of paclitaxel and calcitriol in rat dunning MLL and human PC-3 prostate tumors in vitro. Proc AACR 1999;40:580.

148. Elstner E, et al. Combination of a potent 20-epi-vitamin D3 analogue (KH 1060) with 9-cis-retinoic acid irreversibly inhibits clonal growth, decreases bcl-2 expression, and

induces apoptosis in HL-60 leukemic cells. Cancer Res 1996;56(15):3570–6.

149. James SY, Mackay AG, Colston KW. Effects of 1,25 dihydroxyvitamin D3 and its analogues on induction of apoptosis in breast cancer cells. J Steroid Biochem Mol Biol 1996;58(4):395–401.

150. Pepper C, et al. The vitamin D3 analog EB1089 induces apoptosis via a p53-independent mechanism involving p38 MAP kinase activation and suppression of ERK activity in B-cell chronic lymphocytic leukemia cells in vitro. Blood 2003;101(7):2454–60.

151. Sergeev INRW, Norman AW. 1,25-dihydroxyvitamin D3, intracellular Ca2+ and apoptosis in breast cancer cell lines. In: Norman AW, Bouillon R, Thomasset M, editors. Vitamin D chemistry, biology and clinical applications of the steroid hormone. Riverside, CA: University of California; 1997. p. 473–4.

152. Simboli-Campbell M, et al. 1,25-Dihydroxyvitamin D3 induces morphological and biochemical markers of apoptosis in MCF-7 breast cancer cells. J Steroid Biochem Mol Biol 1996;58(4):367–76.

153. Vandewalle B, Wattez N, Lefebvre J. Effects of vitamin D3 derivatives on growth, differentiation and apoptosis in tumoral colonic HT 29 cells: possible implication of intracellular calcium. Cancer Lett 1995;97(1):99–106.

154. Wagner N, et al. 1,25-Dihydroxyvitamin D3-induced apoptosis of retinoblastoma cells is associated with reciprocal changes of Bcl-2 and bax. Exp Eye Res 2003; 77(1):1–9.

155. Mathiasen IS, Lademann U, Jaattela M. Apoptosis induced by vitamin D compounds in breast cancer cells is inhibited by Bcl-2 but does not involve known caspases or p53. Cancer Res 1999;59(19):4848–56.

156. Polek TC, et al. p53 Is required for 1,25-dihydroxyvitamin D3-induced G0 arrest but is not required for G1 accumulation or apoptosis of LNCaP prostate cancer cells. Endocrinology 2003;144(1):50–60.

157. Galbiati F, et al. Molecular pathways involved in the antineoplastic effects of calcitriol on insulinoma cells. Endocrinology 2003;144(5):1832–41.

158. Narvaez CJ, Welsh J. Role of mitochondria and caspases in vitamin D-mediated apoptosis of MCF-7 breast cancer cells. J Biol Chem 2001;276(12):9101–7.

159. Xie SP, James SY, Colston KW. Vitamin D derivatives inhibit the mitogenic effects of IGF-I on MCF-7 human breast cancer cells. J Endocrinol 1997;154(3):495–504.

160. Bernardi RJ, et al. Combination of 1alpha,25-dihydroxyvitamin D(3) with dexamethasone enhances cell cycle arrest and apoptosis: role of nuclear receptor cross-talk and Erk/Akt signaling. Clin Cancer Res 2001;7(12):4164–73.

161. Bernardi RJ, et al. Antiproliferative effects of 1alpha,25-dihydroxyvitamin D(3) and vitamin D analogs on tumor-derived endothelial cells. Endocrinology 2002;143(7):2508–14.

162. Rocker D, et al. 1,25-Dihydroxyvitamin D3 potentiates the cytotoxic effect of TNF on human breast cancer cells. Mol Cell Endocrinol 1994;106(1–2):157–62.

163. Murthy S, Weigel NL. 1Alpha,25-dihydroxyvitamin D3 induced growth inhibition of PC-3 prostate cancer cells requires an active transforming growth factor beta signaling pathway. Prostate 2004;59(3):282–91.

164. Sergeev IN, Rhoten WB. Regulation of intracellular calcium in human breast cancer cells. Endocrine 1998;9(3):321–7.

165. Sergeev IN. Calcium as a mediator of 1,25-dihydroxyvitamin D3-induced apoptosis. J Steroid Biochem Mol Biol 2004;89–90(1–5):419–25.

166. Jiang F, et al. Induction of ovarian cancer cell apoptosis by 1,25-dihydroxyvitamin D3 through the down-regulation of telomerase. J Biol Chem 2004;279(51):53213–21.

167. De Haes P, et al. 1,25-Dihydroxyvitamin D3 inhibits ultraviolet B-induced apoptosis, Jun kinase activation, and interleukin-6 production in primary human keratinocytes. J Cell Biochem 2003;89(4):663–73.

168. Mantell DJ, et al. 1 Alpha,25-dihydroxyvitamin D(3) inhibits angiogenesis in vitro and in vivo. Circ Res 2000;87(3):214–20.

169. Majewski S, et al. Vitamin D3 is a potent inhibitor of tumor cell-induced angiogenesis. J Investig Dermatol Symp Proc 1996;1(1):97–101.

170. Yudoh K, Matsuno H, Kimura T. 1Alpha,25-dihydroxyvitamin D3 inhibits in vitro invasiveness through the extracellular matrix and in vivo pulmonary metastasis of B16 mouse melanoma. J Lab Clin Med 1999;133(2):120–8.

171. Schwartz GG, et al. 1 Alpha,25-dihydroxyvitamin D (calcitriol) inhibits the invasiveness of human prostate cancer cells. Cancer Epidemiol Biomarkers Prev 1997;6(9):727–32.

172. Sung V, Feldman D. 1,25-Dihydroxyvitamin D3 decreases human prostate cancer cell adhesion and migration. Mol Cell Endocrinol 2000;164(1–2):133–43.

173. Bao BY, Yeh SD, Lee YF. 1Alpha,25-dihydroxyvitamin D3 inhibits prostate cancer cell invasion via modulation of selective proteases. Carcinogenesis 2006;27(1):32–42.

174. Hansen CM, et al. 1 Alpha,25-dihydroxyvitamin D3 inhibits the invasive potential of human breast cancer cells in vitro. Clin Exp Metastasis 1994;12(3):195–202.

175. Young MR, et al. Treating tumor-bearing mice with vitamin D3 diminishes tumor-induced myelopoiesis and associated immunosuppression, and reduces tumor metastasis and recurrence. Cancer Immunol Immunother 1995;41(1):37–45.

176. Koli K, Keski-Oja J. 1Alpha,25-dihydroxyvitamin D3 and its analogues down-regulate cell invasion-associated proteases in cultured malignant cells. Cell Growth Differ 2000;11(4):221–9.

177. Campbell MJ, et al. Inhibition of proliferation of prostate cancer cells by a 19-nor-hexafluoride vitamin D3 analogue involves the induction of p21waf1, p27kip1 and E-cadherin. J Mol Endocrinol 1997;19(1):15–27.

178. Gonzalez-Sancho JM, Alvarez-Dolado M, Munoz A, et al. 1,25-Dihydroxyvitamin D3 inhibits tenascin-C expression in mammary epithelial cells. FEBS Lett 1998;426(2):225–8.

179. Yu WD, et al. Enhancement of 1,25-dihydroxyvitamin D3-mediated antitumor activity with dexamethasone. J Natl Cancer Inst 1998;90(2):134–41.

180. Beer TM, et al. Weekly high-dose calcitriol and docetaxel in advanced prostate cancer. Semin Oncol 2001;28(4 Suppl 15):49–55.

181. Moffatt KA, Johannes WU, Miller GJ. 1Alpha,25dihydroxyvitamin D3 and platinum drugs act synergistically to inhibit the growth of prostate cancer cell lines. Clin Cancer Res 1999;5(3):695–703.

182. Ahmed S, et al. Calcitriol (1,25-dihydroxycholecalciferol) potentiates activity of mitoxantrone/dexamethasone in an androgen independent prostate cancer model. J Urol 2002;168(2):756–61.

183. Light BW, et al. Potentiation of cisplatin antitumor activity using a vitamin D analogue in a murine squamous cell carcinoma model system. Cancer Res 1997;57(17):3759–64.

184. Wieder R, et al. 1,25-Dihydroxyvitamin D3 and all-trans retinoic acid promote apoptosis and sensitize breast cancer cells to the effects of chemotherapeutic agents. Proc Am Soc Clin Oncol 1998;17:107a.

185. Sundaram S, et al. The vitamin D3 analog EB 1089 enhances the antiproliferative and apoptotic effects of adriamycin in MCF-7 breast tumor cells. Breast Cancer Res Treat 2000;63(1):1–10.

186. Torres R, et al. Etoposide stimulates 1,25-dihydroxyvitamin D3 differentiation activity, hormone binding and hormone receptor expression in HL-60 human promyelocytic cells. Mol Cell Biochem 2000;208(1–2):157–62.

187. Koga M, Sutherland RL. Retinoic acid acts synergistically with 1,25-dihydroxyvitamin D3 or antioestrogen to inhibit T-47D human breast cancer cell proliferation. J Steroid Biochem Mol Biol 1991;39(4A):455–60.

188. Guzey M, Sattler C, DeLuca HF. Combinational effects of vitamin D3 and retinoic acid (all trans and 9 cis) on proliferation, differentiation, and programmed cell death in two small cell lung carcinoma cell lines. Biochem Biophys Res Commun 1998;249(3):735–44.

189. Peehl DM, Feldman D. Interaction of nuclear receptor ligands with the vitamin D signaling pathway in prostate cancer. J Steroid Biochem Mol Biol 2004;92(4):307–15.

190. Ikeda N, et al. Combination treatment with 1alpha,25-dihydroxyvitamin D3 and 9-cis-retinoic acid directly inhibits human telomerase reverse transcriptase transcription in prostate cancer cells. Mol Cancer Ther 2003; 2(8):739–46.

191. Anzano MA, et al. 1 Alpha,25-dihydroxy-16-ene-23-yne-26, 27-hexafluorocholecalciferol (Ro24-5531), a new deltanoid (vitamin D analogue) for prevention of breast cancer in the rat. Cancer Res 1994;54(7):1653–6.

192. Welsh J. Induction of apoptosis in breast cancer cells in response to vitamin D and antiestrogens. Biochem Cell Biol 1994;72(11–12):537–45.

193. Abe-Hashimoto J, et al. Antitumor effect of 22-oxa-calcitriol, a noncalcemic analogue of calcitriol, in athymic mice implanted with human breast carcinoma and its synergism with tamoxifen. Cancer Res 1993;53(11):2534–7.

194. Christensen GL, et al. Sequential versus combined treatment of human breast cancer cells with antiestrogens and the vitamin D analogue EB1089 and evaluation of predictive markers for vitamin D treatment. Breast Cancer Res Treat 2004;85(1):53–63.

195. Gavrilov V, Steiner M, Shany S. The combined treatment of 1,25-dihydroxyvitamin D3 and a non-steroid anti-inflammatory drug is highly effective in suppressing prostate cancer cell line (LNCaP) growth. Anticancer Res 2005;25(5):3425–9.

196. Moreno J, Krishnan AV, Feldman D. Molecular mechanisms mediating the anti-proliferative effects of vitamin D in prostate cancer. J Steroid Biochem Mol Biol 2005;97(1–2):31–6.

197. Moreno J, et al. Regulation of prostaglandin metabolism by calcitriol attenuates growth stimulation in prostate cancer cells. Cancer Res 2005;65(17):7917–25.

198. Hsiao M, et al. Functional expression of human p21(WAF1/CIP1) gene in rat glioma cells suppresses tumor growth in vivo and induces radiosensitivity. Biochem Biophys Res Commun 1997;233(2):329–35.

199. Dunlap N, et al. 1Alpha,25-dihydroxyvitamin D(3) (calcitriol) and its analogue, 19-nor-1alpha,25(OH)(2)D(2), potentiate the effects of ionising radiation on human prostate cancer cells. Br J Cancer 2003;89(4):746–53.

200. Polar MK, et al. Effect of the vitamin D3 analog ILX 23-7553 on apoptosis and sensitivity to fractionated radiation in breast tumor cells and normal human fibroblasts. Cancer Chemother Pharmacol 2003;51(5):415–21.

201. DeMasters GA, et al. Potentiation of cell killing by fractionated radiation and suppression of proliferative recovery in MCF-7 breast tumor cells by the vitamin D3 analog EB 1089. J Steroid Biochem Mol Biol 2004;92(5): 365–74.

202. Osborn JL, et al. Phase II trial of oral 1,25-dihydroxyvitamin D (calcitriol) in hormone refractory prostate cancer. Urol Oncol 1995;1(5):195–8.

203. Gross C, et al. Treatment of early recurrent prostate cancer with 1,25-dihydroxyvitamin D3 (calcitriol). J Urol 1998;159(6):2035–9. Discussion 2039–40.

204. Smith DC, et al. A phase I trial of calcitriol (1,25-dihydroxycholecalciferol) in patients with advanced malignancy. Clin Cancer Res 1999;5(6):1339–45.

205. Beer TM, Munar M, Henner WD. A phase I trial of pulse calcitriol in patients with refractory malignancies: pulse dosing permits substantial dose escalation. Cancer 2001;91(12):2431–9.

206. Muindi JR, et al. Pharmacokinetics of high-dose oral calcitriol: results from a phase 1 trial of calcitriol and paclitaxel. Clin Pharmacol Ther 2002;72(6):648–59.

207. Beer TM, et al. Pharmacokinetics and tolerability of a single dose of DN-101, a new formulation of calcitriol, in patients with cancer. Clin Cancer Res 2005;11(21):7794–9.

208. Beer TM, Javle MM, Henner WD and Trump DL. Pharmacokinetics (PK) and tolerability of DN-101, a new formulation of calcitriol, in patients with cancer. Proc Amer Assoc Cancer Res 2004;45:404.

209. Morris MJ, et al. High-dose calcitriol, zoledronate, and dexamethasone for the treatment of progressive prostate carcinoma. Cancer 2004;100(9):1868–75.

210. Tiffany NM, et al. High dose pulse calcitriol, docetaxel and estramustine for androgen independent prostate cancer: a phase I/II study. J Urol 2005;174(3):888–92.

211. Beer TM, et al. High-dose weekly oral calcitriol in patients with a rising PSA after prostatectomy or radiation for prostate carcinoma. Cancer 2003;97(5):1217–24.

212. Trump DL, et al. Phase II trial of high-dose, intermittent calcitriol (1,25 dihydroxyvitamin D3) and dexamethasone in androgen-independent prostate cancer. Cancer 2006;106(10):2136–42.

213. Beer TM, et al. Weekly high-dose calcitriol and docetaxel in metastatic androgen-independent prostate cancer. J Clin Oncol 2003;21(1):123–8.

214. Beer TM, et al. Double-blinded randomized study of high-dose calcitriol plus docetaxel compared with placebo plus

docetaxel in androgen-independent prostate cancer: a report from the ASCENT Investigators. J Clin Oncol 2007; 25(6):669–74.

215. Attia S, et al. Randomized, double-blinded phase II evaluation of docetaxel with or without doxercalciferol in patients with metastatic, androgen-independent prostate cancer. Clin Cancer Res 2008;14(8):2437–43.

216. Upton RA, et al. Pharmacokinetics of doxercalciferol, a new vitamin D analogue that lowers parathyroid hormone. Nephrol Dial Transplant 2003;18(4):750–8.

217. Sjoden G, et al. 1 Alpha-hydroxyvitamin D2 is less toxic than 1 alpha-hydroxyvitamin D3 in the rat. Proc Soc Exp Biol Med 1985;178(3):432–6.

218. Beer TM, Garzotto M, Katovic NM. High-dose calcitriol and carboplatin in metastatic androgen-independent prostate cancer. Am J Clin Oncol 2004;27(5): 535–41.

219. Flaig TW, et al. A phase II trial of dexamethasone, vitamin D, and carboplatin in patients with hormone-refractory prostate cancer. Cancer 2006;107(2):266–74.

220. Chan JS, et al. A phase II study of high-dose calcitriol combined with mitoxantrone and prednisone for androgen-independent prostate cancer. BJU Int 2008;102(11): 1601–6.

221. Kissmeyer AM, et al. Metabolism of the vitamin D analog EB 1089: identification of in vivo and in vitro liver metabolites and their biological activities. Biochem Pharmacol 1997;53(8):1087–97.

222. Bouillon R, et al. Non-hypercalcemic pharmacological aspects of vitamin D analogs. Biochem Pharmacol 1995;50(5):577–83.

223. Bouillon R, Okamura WH, Norman AW. Structure–function relationships in the vitamin D endocrine system. Endocr Rev 1995;16(2):200–57.

224. Gulliford T, et al. A phase I study of the vitamin D analogue EB 1089 in patients with advanced breast and colorectal cancer. Br J Cancer 1998;78(1):6–13.

225. Evans TR, et al. A phase II trial of the vitamin D analogue Seocalcitol (EB1089) in patients with inoperable pancreatic cancer. Br J Cancer 2002;86(5):680–5.

226. Dalhoff K, et al. A phase II study of the vitamin D analogue Seocalcitol in patients with inoperable hepatocellular carcinoma. Br J Cancer 2003;89(2):252–7.

227. Bower M, et al. Topical calcipotriol treatment in advanced breast cancer. Lancet 1991;337(8743):701–2.

228. Liu G, et al. Phase I trial of 1alpha-hydroxyvitamin d(2) in patients with hormone refractory prostate cancer. Clin Cancer Res 2002;8(9):2820–7.

229. Wieder R, et al. Pharmacokinetics and safety of ILX23-7553, a non-calcemic-vitamin D3 analogue, in a phase I study of patients with advanced malignancies. Invest New Drugs 2003;21(4):445–52.

Part V
Immunotherapy

Chapter 27

Cancer Immunology, Immunotherapeutics, and Vaccine Approaches

Ravi A. Madan, James L. Gulley, Jackie Celestin, Philip M. Arlen, and Jeffrey Schlom

Abstract Although most patients can be cured of their prostate cancer by initial definitive therapy, up to 40% of patients may have recurrent disease. For these patients, hormonal manipulations may provide initial benefit and chemotherapy has been demonstrated to extend survival when the disease is castration-resistant and metastatic. In spite of these therapeutic approaches, additional therapies are needed. Therapeutic cancer vaccines have been developed using several platforms to enhance immune targeting of prostate cancer cells and have shown promise in early clinical trials. There are several therapeutic cancer vaccine platforms for prostate cancer including vector-based, antigen-presenting cell pulsed and whole tumor-cell vaccines. Several phase II vaccine trials have demonstrated some degree of clinical benefit. Some of these trials, however, have underscored the need for new paradigms to be developed to evaluate the clinical benefit and utility of cancer vaccines. In addition, vaccines have demonstrated compatibility and synergy with standard therapies in both preclinical and clinical models. Several phase III trials with immunotherapies in prostate cancer are in late stages of planning or are ongoing. Future immunotherapy trials should focus on identifying appropriate patient populations most likely to benefit from vaccine therapy and appropriate trial endpoints.

Keywords Prostate cancer • Cancer vaccines • Immunotherapy

J.L. Gulley (✉)
Laboratory of Tumor Immunology and Biology, Medical Oncology Branch, National Cancer Institute, Bethesda, MD, USA
e-mail: gulleyj@mail.nih.gov

Rationale for Vaccines in the Treatment of Prostate Cancer

Although the US Food and Drug Administration's (FDA) approval of docetaxel for metastatic castration-resistant prostate cancer (CRPC) in 2004 was a significant advancement in the treatment of prostate cancer, additional therapies are still needed [1, 2]. When disease recurs after initial definitive therapy, sequential hormonal manipulations are often used prior to chemotherapy for metastatic CRPC [3]. Therapeutic cancer vaccines have been investigated in both castration-sensitive and castration-resistant disease to determine their role in this sequence of treatments or in combination with existing therapies.

In many ways, prostate cancer is an ideal candidate for treatments that stimulate the immune system to target cancer cells. In most instances, recurrent prostate cancer is detected by rising levels of serum prostate-specific antigen (PSA) when tumor volume is low and undetectable by imaging [3]. Prostate cancer often grows slowly, allowing time for the immune system to be stimulated and to mount an active immune response [4]. Several gene products are unique to prostate cancer cells, making them suitable targets for immunotherapy [5, 6]. Many patients with prostate cancer have low levels of cytolytic T cells capable of recognizing these tumor-associated antigens (TAAs), and this minimal response can be augmented with immune stimulation by therapeutic cancer vaccines [7]. Finally, because the prostate is a nonessential organ, targeting TAAs specific to prostatic tissue is unlikely to have a significant negative clinical impact.

W.D. Figg et al. (eds.), *Drug Management of Prostate Cancer*,
DOI 10.1007/978-1-60327-829-4_27, © Springer Science+Business Media, LLC 2010

Tumor-Associated Antigens As Targets of Immunotherapy

The ideal targets for cancer vaccines are TAAs that are unique to, or are overexpressed in, cancer cells relative to normal tissue. Prostate cancer cells express several such TAAs. PSA is a 34-kD protein uniquely expressed in prostate cancer cells and the nonessential epithelial cells within the prostate, making it the prime target for many prostate cancer vaccines [8, 9]. Prostate-specific membrane antigen (PSMA) is a 100-kD transmembrane glycoprotein that is principally expressed in both primary and metastatic prostate cancer cells [10]. An advantageous characteristic of PSMA is that androgen deprivation, which is fundamental to the treatment of prostate cancer, leads to increased PSMA expression [11]. Another TAA that has shown potential as a target of vaccines is prostatic acid phosphotase (PAP), a 102-kD glycoprotein overexpressed in prostate cancer cells that is believed to play a role in disease progression [12, 13].

Enhancing Antigen Presentation

Developing an effective prostate cancer vaccine presents several challenges. Although prostate cancer provides several TAAs as targets for vaccine therapy, they are commonly weakly immunogenic [7]. An effective vaccine strategy must overcome this obstacle (Table 27.1).

Cytokines have been found to effectively expand T-cell populations and to enhance the ability of antigen-presenting cells (APCs) to recognize TAAs. In an activated cellular immune response, APCs such as dendritic cells must be activated in order to process antigens, which are then presented to T cells in an immune context, leading to targeted cytolytic T cell-mediated destruction of tumor cells.

Granulocyte-macrophage colony-stimulating factor (GM-CSF) is commonly used as an adjuvant in immunotherapy. GM-CSF has been shown to increase immune response by stimulating the growth and maturation of APCs and helping them migrate to the vaccination site [14–16]. Some early trials tested GM-CSF as a single agent to see if it had clinical benefit as a nonspecific immune stimulant [17]. More recent studies have shown that injecting GM-CSF at the vaccination site enhances

Table 27.1 Modalities that synergize vaccine therapy

Method	Proposed mechanism
Cytokines	Traffic APCs to vaccination site; mature and activate APCs
Androgen-deprivation therapy	Traffic T cells to the prostate, enhance T-cell repertoire, and decrease immune tolerance of prostate cancer TAAs
Radiation	May upregulate MHC class I antigens, TAAs, and Fas ligand, all of which can enhance cytolytic T-cell activity
Chemotherapy	May enhance MHC class I and TAA expression. Chemotherapy-induced lysis of cells may expose an activated immune response to new TAAs for cytolytic T cells to target
Anti-CTLA-4 antibody	CTLA-4 is expressed on T cells as a way for the immune system to self-regulate immune responses. Blocking this molecule with an antibody can augment the effects of cytolytic T cell activity
Regulatory T-cell depletion	Regulatory T cells may suppress T-cell activation and proliferation in response to a vaccine. Using certain chemotherapy agents or monoclonal antibodies, it may be possible to selectively eliminate regulatory T cells and the barriers they pose to immune activation

APCs antigen-presenting cells; *ADT* androgen-deprivation therapy; *TAA* tumor-associated antigen; *MHC* major histocompatibility complex

targeted immune responses [18–20]. Other strategies use tumor cells transduced with the gene for GM-CSF to create GM-CSF-secreting whole tumor-cell vaccines [21].

Another mechanism to enhance APC activation of T cells is the use of costimulatory molecules. During the critical stage of antigen presentation, APCs present the antigen within its major histocompatibility complex (MHC) to the T cell via the T-cell receptor. The interaction of other accessory, or costimulatory, molecules is also necessary for T-cell activation, especially when the TAA is weakly immunogenic. The absence of costimulatory molecules with such weak antigens could lead to T-cell anergy and even apoptosis [22]. In poxviral-based cancer vaccines, transgenes for costimulatory molecules can be included with the TAA transgene within the vector. When such a poxviral-based vaccine infects APCs, it leads to expression of the TAA within the MHC for presentation to T cells. The vaccine's effects can be enhanced by including a transgene encoded for one or more costimulatory molecules, which are then expressed on the APC that is presenting the TAA [18, 19, 22].

Vaccines as Part of Combination Therapy for Prostate Cancer

Vaccine therapies are increasingly being investigated in combination with other therapies, potentially enhancing the treatment of both early- and late-stage prostate cancer. Some conventional therapies may actually enhance both the immune profile of tumors and cytolytic T-cell activity [23]. This can be particularly valuable in prostate cancer where, depending on the stage of disease, androgen-deprivation therapy (ADT), radiation, and chemotherapy all play a role.

Androgen-Deprivation Therapy

Patients with recurrent prostate cancer treated with hormonal manipulation alone often have asymptomatic disease. Here, the goal of therapy is to delay symptomatic disease that may require more aggressive therapies with greater toxicity [3]. Evidence suggests that ADT can enhance immune responses in these patients [24]. One study evaluated prostatic tissue before and after initiating ADT. T-cell infiltration of the prostate was seen within 1–3 weeks, and T cells isolated from the prostate exhibited a restricted receptor, indicating a local oligoclonal response [25]. In another study, the androgen receptor antagonist flutamide curtailed testosterone's potential for T-cell inhibition [26]. Other studies indicate that ADT decreases immune tolerance to prostate TAAs, promotes growth of the thymus (where T cells are produced), and enhances the T-cell repertoire [27–29]. All of these findings make combination therapy with ADT and vaccines an active and promising area of research.

Radiation Therapy

Local radiation of the prostate can be part of the initial definitive therapy of prostate cancer or part of a salvage regimen if the disease recurs after radical prostatectomy [30]. One potential drawback of radiation therapy is that some cells at the center of larger tumor masses may receive sublethal amounts of radiation, allowing them to survive initial definitive therapy.

Preclinical studies have demonstrated that low levels of radiation can upregulate certain membrane antigens, including MHC class I antigens, TAAs, and Fas ligand, which can enhance cytolytic T-cell activity potentially induced by a vaccine [31–33]. These effects of radiation on prostate cancer cells have led to studies of vaccines in the adjuvant setting, where patients with high-risk disease may benefit from enhanced immune surveillance [34].

Combination Chemotherapy

Chemotherapy is a noncurative treatment for most metastatic cancers, including prostate cancer, making its combination with vaccine potentially appealing if it can delay disease progression and increase overall survival. Certain chemotherapy agents have been shown to enhance expression of TAAs and MHC class I, both of which can make cancer cells more amenable to vaccine-induced cytolytic T-cell activity [35–38]. Additionally, an activated immune response triggered by a vaccine in the setting of chemotherapy-induced cell lysis may expose the immune system to a variety of antigens, leading to an immune response against TAAs not specifically targeted by the vaccine (antigen cascade) [34, 39]. Preclinical studies have further demonstrated other effects of chemotherapy that may increase the benefits of immune-mediated therapy. Doxorubicin has been shown to increase the number and activity of macrophages, while in vitro studies of docetaxel have demonstrated increases in proinflammatory cytokines [40–42]. Docetaxel has also been shown to enhance CD8 responses to vaccine, augmenting immune responses to TAAs specifically targeted by the vaccine in addition to other TAAs as part of an antigen cascade. Finally, docetaxel combined with vaccine has been shown to be more effective than either treatment alone in a murine tumor treatment model [39]. Other chemotherapeutic agents such as cyclophosphamide may enhance immune response and the benefits of vaccine by reducing the levels and inhibitory effects of regulatory T cells (Tregs) [43, 44].

The greatest potential drawback of combining chemotherapy with vaccine is that the cytotoxic effects of chemotherapy may kill the immune cells generated by the vaccine. However, recent clinical evidence indicates that some combinations of vaccine and chemotherapy may be compatible. A phase II trial combined docetaxel with a poxviral-based vaccine targeting PSA and compared the combination to the vaccine alone in patients with metastatic CRPC. After 3 months on study, the two groups showed equal immune responses to the vaccine, indicating that chemotherapy did not depress immune response to the vaccine [45].

Sequential Chemotherapy

There is mounting clinical evidence that vaccines may initiate a dynamic immune response to TAAs that could be augmented by subsequent chemotherapy. A phase I study treated 17 patients with a plasmid/microparticle-based vaccine targeting cytochrome P450B1, which is overexpressed in some tumors. The five patients who developed an immune response also had a longer than expected clinical response to salvage chemotherapy, some lasting up to 12 months [46]. In another study in nonsmall cell lung cancer, in which 29 patients were treated with an adenovirus-based vaccine targeting P53, a higher than expected proportion of patients (61.9%) had objective response to salvage chemotherapy initiated after vaccine treatments [47]. This phenomenon has also been seen in a prostate cancer trial. Of 34 patients with metastatic CRPC treated with the whole tumor-cell vaccine GVAX, 13 patients who went on to receive a taxane-based chemotherapy had a mean overall survival of 35.2 vs. 17.2 months for those who did not receive chemotherapy [48]. While these studies suggest a benefit for sequential vaccine followed by chemotherapy, further randomized studies designed to evaluate these treatments in these particular sequences are needed.

Anti-CTLA-4

For most weak antigens such as TAAs, a signal from the T-cell receptor is insufficient to optimally activate the T cell [49]. A second immune-enhancing signal mediated through CD28 on the T cell binding to B7 on the APC is required to activate the T cell specific for the target antigen. CTLA-4 is expressed on the surface of the T cell within 2–3 days following activation and also binds to B7. This high-affinity binding generates a negative signal, effectively halting an ongoing immune response. The key regulatory role of CTLA-4 is underscored in CTLA-4 knockout mice that cannot turn off immune responses and live only 2–3 weeks before succumbing to massive infiltration of organs by unchecked growth of autoreactive T cells [50]. Thus, antagonistic antibodies that prevent CTLA-4 signaling may enhance T-cell expansion.

Studies have shown the rejection of established tumors in murine models demonstrating the therapeutic potential of CTLA-4 blockade [51]. However, CTLA-4 blockade may also potentiate the growth of inhibitory Tregs. A recent study showed that anti-CTLA-4 monotherapy proportionally increased Tregs and effector T cells (Teffs) within the tumor, whereas CTLA-4 blockade with vaccine increased Teffs more than Tregs and, unlike CTLA-4 blockade alone, induced tumor rejection [52]. Furthermore, the quantity of tumor-specific Teffs may not be as important as the functional ability of those cells, for only high-avidity tumor-specific T cells can efficiently kill tumor cells [53]. Anti-CTLA-4 antibodies combined with vaccine not only increase the number of tumor-specific Teffs over vaccine alone, but, to a much greater magnitude, also increase the avidity of those T cells [54]. Several anti-CTLA-4 antibodies have been developed and preclinical models have demonstrated increased antitumor activity in the murine model, which can be enhanced by vaccines [54–56]. Several studies have evaluated anti-CTLA-4 antibodies in combination with a vaccine in the treatment of different malignancies, including prostate cancer [57–59].

Vaccine Approaches

Several different types of prostate cancer vaccine are currently in clinical development. Three vaccine types in particular represent different strategies that have been employed extensively in the clinical setting (Table 27.2).

Vector-Based Vaccines

The goal of targeted immune therapies is to focus the immune system on weakly immunogenic TAAs, such as PSA. Poxviral vaccines are able to deliver transgenes

Table 27.2 Three main vaccine approaches

Vaccine type	Mechanism of action
Vector-based	Poxviruses containing transgenes for TAAs and costimulatory molecules are injected subcutaneously. They infect APCs, leading to presentation of TAAs and costimulatory molecules in an immune context to T cells. These T cells are then activated and target TAAs on cancer cells
APC-pulsed	APCs are removed from a patient's circulation and exposed ex vivo to a specific TAA and cytokines for activation and maturation. These activated APCs are then re-infused into the blood stream where they activate T cells, leading to a targeted immune response. These treatments are patient-specific
Whole tumor-cell	Multiple allogeneic tumor cell lines are cultured ex vivo and then treated with lethal irradiation. The cells are then injected into subcutaneous sites where APCs process TAAs and activate T cells. Tumor cells may be transfected to express a cytokine such GM-CSF or other adjuvants may be used. This type of treatment is not patient-specific and does not define which TAA the T cells will target

APCs antigen-presenting cells; *TAA* tumor-associated antigen

for TAAs to APCs, where they are then processed and expressed on the APC surface within the MHC, leading to T-cell activation. Recombinant poxviral vectors are developed by first generating the recombinant plasmid containing the transgenes that will ultimately code for the selected proteins, in this case TAAs. The plasmid is then transfected into a permissive eukaryotic cell line, which is subsequently infected by wild-type poxviruses. As the poxviruses reproduce within the cell, a small proportion will contain the recombinant plasmid. Expression of certain markers included within the plasmid can help identify which poxviruses contain the recombinant plasmid. These particular poxviral vectors can then be isolated and amplified for use as a cancer vaccine [60].

There are many advantages to using a poxvirus as a delivery mechanism for cancer vaccines. Injecting the poxvirus into subcutaneous tissue results in an inflammatory response against foreign proteins. The ensuing chemotaxis sends APCs to the injection site. As a result, the recombinant protein product of the transgene contained within the poxvirus vector is significantly more immunogenic than the naked protein with an adjuvant [61, 62]. Several other factors make poxviruses ideal

delivery vehicles for vaccines. Poxviruses are extremely effective at infecting APCs, especially dendritic cells. When costimulatory molecules are also included within the poxvirus genome, the capability of cells to act as APCs is greatly enhanced [60, 63–65]. The large poxviral genome allows for the transfer of a large amount of DNA into host cells, which can include transgenes for costimulatory molecules in addition to multiple antigens [60, 66]. Vaccinia has been used safely in humans for over five decades, and all genes transported by the poxvirus are processed in the cell cytoplasm, eliminating the possibility of integration within or disruption of the host DNA. Furthermore, only poxviral enzymes are used in translation. Finally, poxviral vaccines are easily administered subcutaneously and require very little preparation.

A phase I study of a poxviral vaccine targeting PSA enrolled 42 patients with metastatic CRPC at five escalating doses. Patients were treated monthly for 3 months with recombinant vaccinia (rV)-PSA (containing the transgene for PSA). A cohort of patients also received GM-CSF at the vaccination site as part of an extension phase. The vaccine was well tolerated and reached no dose-limiting toxicity. The most common side effects were transient fever, fatigue, and injection-site reactions. In addition, three of five evaluable patients had increases in PSA-specific T cells, indicating that the vaccine had generated a targeted immune response [67].

A crucial factor in the effectiveness of poxviral vaccines is that different species of poxviruses allow for their sequential use for maximal immune response to transgene TAAs and clinical benefit. This feature was utilized to improve the poxviral vaccine targeting PSA [60]. Vaccinia is highly immunogenic and induces a robust immune response upon initial vaccination. Subsequent exposure to vaccinia, however, results in rapid neutralization by the host antibodies targeting viral coat proteins, which greatly reduces the ability of the vaccinia-based vaccine to infect APCs [67–69]. After priming with vaccinia, boosting with a second poxviral vector is required to sustain the immune response. Fowlpox-based vectors, which are also capable of infecting APCs, produce only early viral gene products, and not viral coat proteins. This characteristic prevents their replication in mammals and also prevents the host immune system from making significant quantities of neutralizing antibodies against fowlpox-based vaccines [70, 71]. This diversified prime and boost strategy was initially demonstrated in preclinical models and then in phase I human studies [71, 72]. A subsequent randomized trial targeting PSA showed that patients who received a vaccinia (rV-PSA) prime followed by fowlpox (rF-PSA) boosts had increased time to PSA progression compared with patients who received fowlpox alone or fowlpox before vaccinia [73, 74].

Several trials have employed a poxviral vaccine targeting PSA in combination with conventional therapies. Based on preclinical data suggesting that radiation may make tumor cells more susceptible to immune-mediated killing [31, 32], a study randomized 30 patients with localized prostate cancer 2:1 favoring vaccine plus radiation over radiation alone. Patients received an admixed priming vaccination [rV-PSA plus recombinant vaccinia containing the transgene for the costimulatory molecule B7.1 (rV-B7.1)]. Recombinant fowlpox (rF)-PSA was injected monthly as a booster, for a total of eight vaccines. All vaccines were given with low-dose IL-2 and GM-CSF as an immune adjuvant. Radiation therapy was given between months 4 and 6. Seventeen of 19 patients in the combination treatment arm completed all eight vaccinations and had a ≥3-fold increase in PSA-specific T cells after radiation, compared to no change in T cells in the radiation-only group ($p = 0.0005$) [34]. A follow-up study showed that metronomic doses of IL-2 produced similar levels of immune response to vaccine, with virtually none of the side effects associated with high-dose IL-2 [75]. A randomized phase II study is currently evaluating a next-generation poxviral vaccine containing three costimulatory molecules (see PSA-TRICOM below) in combination with Samarium-153 (Sm-153) vs. Sm-153 alone in patients with CRPC metastatic predominantly to bone. Sm-153, FDA-approved for palliation of pain in this setting, is composed of radioactive samarium and a tetraphosphate chelator that binds to metastatic lesions in bone. The goal of this study is to evaluate the benefits of low-level radiation to metastatic tumor sites provided by locally binding Sm-153 in the setting of an active immune response [76].

Another trial comparing hormonal therapy and a poxviral vaccine targeting PSA randomized 42 patients with nonmetastatic CRPC (stage D0.5) to initial treatment with nilutamide (an androgen receptor antagonist) or vaccine. Again, the vaccine regimen consisted of a prime with an admixture of rV-PSA and rV-B7.1 followed by monthly boosts of rF-PSA. Patients who had a rising PSA on either treatment, but no evidence of metastatic disease on imaging, could receive the other treatment in addition to their primary therapy. For patients randomized to the vaccine arm, median time to PSA progression was 9.9 months compared with 7.6 months for patients randomized to nilutamide. The results of this study suggested a benefit from combination therapy, especially when vaccine was started earlier. For the eight patients who were randomized to nilutamide and had vaccine added, median time to progression was 15.9 months after enrollment and 5.2 months after starting the combination. For the 12 patients who had vaccine first and nilutamide added, median time to progression was 25.9 months from enrollment and 13.9 months after starting the combination [77]. A subsequent survival analysis indicated a trend to improved overall survival in patients randomized to the vaccine arm compared with the nilutamide arm (median overall survival 5.1 vs. 3.4 years; $p = 0.13$). The survival benefit appeared to be greatest in patients with less aggressive disease (Gleason score ≤ 7; $p = 0.033$), lower PSA (<20 μg/mL; $p = 0.013$), and previous radiation therapy ($p = 0.018$). This survival trend associated with vaccine given earlier in treatment was also seen in patients who received both agents in combination. For patients who received vaccine first and had nilutamide added, the median overall survival was 6.2 vs. 3.7 years in patients randomized to nilutamide who had vaccine added ($p = 0.045$) [78]. A trial is currently accruing to confirm the benefits of androgen receptor antagonist (flutamide) in combination with a second-generation poxviral vaccine targeting PSA vs. androgen receptor antagonist alone in patients with nonmetastatic CRPC [79].

PSA-TRICOM

Further preclinical research with poxviral-based vaccines indicated that multiple costimulatory molecules could be delivered within a single vector. A construct containing a triad of costimulatory molecules called TRICOM includes transgenes for B7.1, intracellular adhesion molecule (ICAM)-1, and leukocyte function-associated antigen (LFA)-3. In vitro and in vivo studies have shown that TRICOM significantly enhances T-cell activation relative to just one or two costimulatory molecules [18, 19, 80]. A phase I study in patients with metastatic CRPC has shown that an rV-PSA-TRICOM prime followed by monthly boosts of rF-PSA-TRICOM was well tolerated. Furthermore, patients treated with PSA-TRICOM who were evaluable for immune response had an increase in PSA-specific T cells after treatment, and 9 of 15 patients had decreases in PSA velocity [81].

A pair of phase II studies has provided initial evidence for improved overall survival in patients treated with PSA-TRICOM. An industry-sponsored phase II trial employed PSA-TRICOM in 125 patients with metastatic CRPC and Gleason scores ≤7, randomized 2:1 in favor of vaccine vs. an empty fowlpox vector as control. Patients randomized to receive vaccine were given an rV-PSA-TRICOM prime with monthly boosts of rF-PSA-TRICOM, while control patients were given subcutaneous injections of fowlpox. The primary endpoint of the study was time to progression as measured by new or expanding lesions on bone scan and CT scan, respectively. The study failed to meet this primary endpoint, but median overall survival was 24.4 months in the vaccine arm compared with 16.3 months in the control arm, suggesting that although disease progression occurred at similar times in both groups, there appeared to be a long-term benefit for some patients treated with PSA-TRICOM [82].

In another phase II study of PSA-TRICOM at the National Cancer Institute (NCI), 32 patients with metastatic CRPC were treated with an rV-PSA-TRICOM prime and monthly boosts of rF-PSA-TRICOM. In that trial, 47% of patients had a decrease in PSA velocity, 38% had a PSA decline, 13 of 29 evaluable patients had a >2-fold increase in PSA-specific T cells, and five patients had a >6-fold increase in PSA-specific T cells which was associated with a trend to improved overall survival ($p=0.055$) [83]. The median overall survival of all patients enrolled was 26.6 months, which compares favorably to trials leading to approval for docetaxel in metastatic CRPC, where median survival was approximately 18 months [1, 2]. The overall survival of all patients was also compared with survival as predicted by the Halabi nomogram. The Halabi nomogram predicts survival based on seven baseline parameters (accounting for disease volume and aggressiveness) that were found to be significant based on an analysis of 1,101 patients with metastatic CRPC treated with chemotherapy or second-line hormonal therapy in Cancer and Leukemia Group B studies between 1991 and 2001 [84]. For patients with a predicted survival of <18 months, there was only a modest improvement after

treatment with PSA-TRICOM (14.6 vs. 12.3 months). When patients with better prognostic features (i.e., a predicted survival ≥18 months) were evaluated, there was a more pronounced improvement after treatment with PSA-TRICOM vs. that predicted with standard therapy, with a median overall survival not reached at 44.6 months vs. Halabi-predicted overall survival of 20.9 months. Although this was a small study, these results provide evidence that metastatic CRPC patients treated with a vaccine have an overall survival similar to the predicted survival of patients treated with chemotherapy or second-line hormone therapy. Furthermore, these data suggest that patients with more indolent disease may receive greater benefit from vaccine-mediated therapy than from chemotherapy or second-line hormone therapy. Follow-up studies are currently being designed to further test this hypothesis [83].

Antigen-Presenting Cell Vaccines: Sipuleucel-T

An alternative approach to vaccine therapy relies not on in vivo antigen stimulation, but on removing APCs, stimulating them with an antigen ex vivo, and then injecting the stimulated APCs back into the blood stream. The sipuleucel-T vaccine (Provenge®; Dendreon Corp., Seattle, WA) is developed from peripheral blood mononuclear cells exposed in vitro to a prostate cancer antigen in a process that takes under 48 h. Dendritic cells, T cells, B cells, and natural killer cells are selectively collected from patients by leukapheresis. These APCs are then processed and exposed ex vivo to PA2024, a recombinant fusion protein of human PAP and GM-CSF, which leads to APC activation and maturation. The excess antigen is then removed for the solution and the APCs are concentrated in 250 cc of Lactated Ringer's that can then be infused into the patient [85, 86].

A phase I study demonstrated the safety and efficacy of this approach in 12 evaluable patients with metastatic CRPC. Patients were given two infusions 1 month apart of autologous APCs exposed to PA2024 ex vivo, as described above. After the infusions, patients were given three escalating doses of subcutaneous PA2024 (0.3, 0.6, and 1.0 mg/injection) at 1-month intervals. The vaccine was well tolerated, with the main side effects being fevers, chills, fatigue, and injection-site reactions.

Three patients had PSA declines, and T-cell proliferation assays demonstrated up to a 10-fold increase from baseline in response to GM-CSF and PAP. The injections of PA2024, however, were not found to enhance cellular immune response [87].

A phase I/II study was also done in patients with nonmetastatic CRPC. Twelve patients were enrolled on the phase I-dose escalation portion (maximum doses 2×10^9 nucleated cells/m^2), and 19 patients were added in the phase II portion. Infusions were administered at weeks 0, 4, and 8 for all patients and at week 24 for patients who continued to have stable disease at that point. The infusions were well tolerated at all dose levels, with fever being the most frequent adverse event. Six patients had a >25% PSA decline, and three of these six had declines >50%. The median time to progression based on PSA was 12 weeks on phase I and 29 weeks on phase II, suggesting that patients did better with higher doses. An immune response to PAP was seen in 38% of patients, which also correlated with improved time to progression [88]. In another phase II trial in metastatic CRPC, 19 evaluable patients were given infusions of the sipuleucel-T vaccine on weeks 0 and 2 and injections of PA2024 (0.5 mg subcutaneously in each thigh) on weeks 4, 8, and 12. The treatment was well tolerated with only rare grade 3/4 infusion-associated toxicities (chills, fatigue, fever, malaise, emesis, dyspnea, and tachycardia). Three patients on this study had a >25% decrease in PSA, including one patient whose PSA dropped from 221 ng/mL to undetectable levels at 24 weeks. Median time to progression for all patients was 16.9 weeks. An immune analysis again showed increased responsiveness to PA2024 in vitro 4 weeks after initial treatment. The patient with the most significant drop in PSA had an increased immune response for 96 weeks after enrollment [89].

Two phase III placebo-controlled studies were done in patients with metastatic CRPC randomized 2:1 in favor of the sipuleucel-T vaccine, and results were encouraging but not definitive. In both studies, sipuleucel-T was administered on weeks 0, 2, and 4 and crossover was allowed for patients who progressed (defined as new lesions on imaging or increased pain) after 8 weeks. The primary endpoint of both studies was time to progression [90, 91]. The first trial to report results enrolled 82 patients on treatment and 45 patients on placebo (34 of whom would go on to receive sipuleucel-T as part of the crossover component). This trial failed to meet its primary endpoint, although time to progression favored the patients randomized to sipuleucel-T

(16.6 vs. 10 weeks; $p = 0.052$). Overall survival, however, showed a 4.5-month improvement in patients randomized to sipuleucel-T (25.9 vs. 21.4 months; $p = 0.01$). This overall survival benefit was even greater at 36 months, with estimated survival of 34% for the sipuleucel-T group vs. 11% for the placebo group ($p = 0.005$) [90]. When this phase III trial did not meet its primary endpoint of time to progression, but before survival benefit was seen, the second phase III trial was terminated early. When the 98 patients (65 treated with sipuleucel-T, 33 on placebo) in this second study were analyzed, no time to progression or survival benefit was seen [86, 91]. Given these varied results, the FDA has elected to await the results of an ongoing phase III trial that has already enrolled over 500 patients with metastatic CRPC. The endpoint of this study is overall survival, and it will be analyzed when 360 deaths have occurred. An interim analysis is expected in the fourth quarter of 2008 [92]. There is also an ongoing phase II study using this vaccine in the neoadjuvant setting, prior to radical prostatectomy in men with localized disease [93] (See Chapter 28: Sipuleucel-T for detailed information on this vaccine).

Whole Tumor-Cell Vaccines

GVAX

GVAX (Cell Genesys Inc., South San Francisco, CA) is an allogeneic cellular immunotherapy that is not patient-specific. GVAX consists of two prostate cancer cell lines (LNCaP and PC-3, derived from metastatic prostate cancer lesions) that have been transfected with a human gene that encodes GM-CSF. (This transfection was initially accomplished using a retroviral vector, but subsequent studies showed that an adenovirus vector results in increased secretion of GM-CSF.) After transfection, the cells are exposed to lethal levels of gamma radiation that denatures DNA and prevents cellular replication, while allowing GM-CSF secretion to continue. When injected into the patient, the cells cause a localized immune response, with the secreted GM-CSF as an adjuvant facilitating the attraction, maturation, and activation of APCs. These APCs then process TAAs and activate CD4$^+$ and CD8$^+$ T cells in local lymph nodes, leading to an antigen-specific T-cell response [21]. Since each patient's immune system processes whole tumor cells differently, the TAAs targeted may vary from patient to patient.

A phase I study first evaluated the concept of whole tumor-cell vaccines using autologous cells from 11 men who were found to have metastatic disease at radical prostatectomy. They were treated with autologous prostate cancer cells transfected to secrete GM-CSF and then irradiated. Eight of 11 patients had sufficient in vitro expansion of cultured cells to allow for treatment. The autologous cells were well tolerated, with injection-site reactions and flu-like symptoms the most common side effects. Although some patients showed evidence of B-cell and T-cell responses, the use of autologous cells proved to be too inefficient for further study [94].

Subsequent trials utilized the GM-CSF-secreting PC-3 and LNCaP cell lines. A phase I/II trial was done in patients with rising PSA after radical prostatectomy (castration-sensitive, nonmetastatic, or stage D0 prostate cancer). All 21 patients enrolled completed the course of 8 weekly intradermal injections (1.2×10^8 cells) of the whole tumor-cell vaccine (all doses contained equal parts of each cell line). Again, flu-like symptoms and injection-site reactions were the most common side effects. Clinically, one patient had a >50% PSA decline and 17 of 21 patients had decreases in PSA velocity 20 weeks after completing therapy ($p < 0.001$). From an immunologic standpoint, biopsies of the vaccination site showed that APCs had been recruited locally, while patients also had elevated levels of antibodies targeting five different antigens found on the allogeneic tumor cells. In addition, the best PSA response correlated with a high-titer antibody response to an LNCaP antigen [95].

Two dose-escalation studies of GVAX have been conducted. One study employed 5.0×10^8 cells as a priming dose and 1.0×10^8 as a booster every 2 weeks for up to 6 months. Twenty-one patients enrolled on study had nonmetastatic CRPC and 34 patients had asymptomatic metastatic CRPC. For patients with nonmetastatic CRPC, median time to PSA progression and progression of lesions on bone scan was 3.9 and 5.9 months, respectively. For patients with metastatic CRPC, time to PSA progression and progression of lesions on bone scan was 2.6 and 3.0 months, respectively. In the metastatic CRPC group, the last ten patients enrolled received 3.0×10^8 instead of 1×10^8 as a biweekly booster. The overall survival of the metastatic CRPC patients was 26.2 months; however, patients who received the high-dose booster lived 34.9 months compared with 24.0 months for patients who

received the lower dose, indicating that benefit may increase with higher doses of cells [48].

In a separate study of GVAX, 80 patients with metastatic CRPC were treated for 6 months at three different dose levels and schedules: low (1.0×10^8 or 2.0×10^8 monthly), medium (2.0×10^8 biweekly), or high (3.0×10^8 biweekly or 5.0×10^8 priming dose with 3.0×10^8 biweekly). A maximum tolerated dose was not reached and the previously seen side effects of flu-like symptoms, headache, and injection-site reactions were reported. One patient had a >50% decline in PSA lasting 3.9 months, and 15 patients had a stable PSA (<50% decline to <25% increase) for at least 90 days. No significant differences were seen in PSA responses among the different dose levels. Times to PSA progression were 2.8 months (low doses), 2.2 months (medium dose), and 2.5 months (high doses). Although 35% of all patients had stable disease, none had an objective response. Overall survival, however, was greater in the high-dose cohort: 35 vs. 23.1 months in patients treated with low doses and 20 months in those treated with the medium dose. Survival in the high-dose cohort also compared favorably to the Halabi predicted survival of 22.0 months [84, 96]. A study has also been done combining GVAX with the anti-CTLA-4 monoclonal antibody ipilimumab. Dosing of GVAX for this study was 5.0×10^8 as a prime, then 3.0×10^8 biweekly for 24 weeks, with escalating monthly doses of ipilimumab (0.3, 1, 3, or 5 mg/kg) for 24 weeks. In addition to injection-site reactions and flu-like symptoms, the combination was also associated with immune-mediated side effects, notably hypophysitis, in five of six patients at the higher dose levels. Immune breakthrough events correlated with clinical response as PSA declines > 50% were seen in these five patients, with durations of 6.7–23.1 months. Four patients also had stable bone scans for at least 3 months. Immunologic responses in the form of dendritic-cell and T-cell activation were also seen at the higher dose levels. Based on these preliminary findings, an expansion cohort of 16 patients will be enrolled to provide further safety and efficacy data [57, 58].

Two phase III trials with GVAX are currently underway. The endpoint for both studies is overall survival [97]. VITAL-1, a clinical trial that opened in 2004, is comparing GVAX to standard-of-care docetaxel and prednisone in patients with asymptomatic metastatic CRPC. VITAL-1 completed enrollment with about

600 patients. In 2005, VITAL-2 was opened for patients with metastatic CRPC who had disease-related pain. The 600 patients in this study were randomized to either GVAX and docetaxel or docetaxel and prednisone. A recent report indicated that this study has been stopped due to unforeseen toxicity in the vaccine plus chemotherapy arm; this is now being investigated.

ONY-P1

Another whole tumor-cell vaccine under clinical investigation is ONY-P1 (Onyvax Ltd., London, UK), which consists of three tumor cell lines (LNCaP, P4E6, and OnyCap-23) targeting prostate cancer TAAs. Initial studies showed that intraepidermal administration of this type of vaccine with a mycobacterial adjuvant is well tolerated and generates immune responses [98]. A later phase II study was done in 26 patients with CRPC without metastasis to the bone. The first two doses were administered biweekly with BCG as an adjuvant. Subsequently, the vaccine was given alone monthly for up to 12 months. Forty-two percent of patients had a statistically significant decline in PSA velocity, which correlated with an immune response [99]. A multi-center phase II placebo-controlled study with ONY-P1 has completed enrollment, and a second phase II study of ONY-P1 following limited ADT in castration-sensitive prostate cancer is ongoing at the NCI.

Future Directions

Regulatory T-Cell Depletion

Tregs help to regulate the body's immune response by maintaining a degree of self-tolerance and thereby decreasing autoimmunity [100–102]. Tregs, which make up 5–10% of circulating $CD4^+$ T cells, have the ability to suppress the activation and expansion of cytolytic T cells; thus, they can potentially limit the effectiveness of a vaccine designed to stimulate cytolytic T cells against TAAs [103, 104]. Furthermore, animal studies have shown that the number and activity of Tregs within tumors and peripheral blood increase with tumor burden [105, 106]. This has also been seen in human cancer patients, where higher levels of Tregs have also been correlated with poor outcome [107–110].

Experiments in preclinical models have demonstrated that selective removal of Tregs can enable a tumor-specific immune response [106, 111, 112]. Several methods of Treg depletion are under investigation [113]. Low doses of the chemotherapy agent cyclophosphamide have been shown to selectively decrease the number and function of Tregs while leaving cytolytic T cells unaffected [43, 114]. In addition, Tregs have been shown to express CD25, a high-affinity IL-2 receptor. In recent years, several antibodies have been developed to selectively target this marker, with the goal of neutralizing Tregs [109, 115–117]. As the understanding of the function of Tregs grows, new techniques may be developed to block their regulatory effects, thereby enhancing the effectiveness of vaccines in the treatment of cancer.

Evaluating Vaccines in the Clinical Setting

Objective evaluation of disease response in metastatic CRPC is difficult. About 60% of patients have metastasis only to bone, which is best visualized by whole-body scintigraphy. Unfortunately, complete responses with whole-body scintigraphy are rare, and there are no widely accepted criteria for partial responses. Moreover, increasing radionuclide uptake is associated with bone healing (possibly a therapeutic response), trauma, and progressive disease, further complicating interpretation. Only about 40% of patients have measurable soft tissue disease (mainly lymph node metastasis). Thus, standard evaluation paradigms may not be appropriate for vaccine-based treatment modalities. Standard chemotherapeutic agents are evaluated based on the response evaluation criteria in solid tumors (RECIST), where clinical benefit is evaluated strictly by tumor size [118, 119]. A review of the numerous trials of all three types of vaccines discussed here shows that clinical benefit as indicated by overall survival may be achieved in spite of early disease progression, which does not take into account a potentially burgeoning immune response [82, 90, 96] (Table 27.3).

One complicating factor in immunotherapy trials is that waxing/waning lymph nodes may represent vaccine-

Table 27.3 Vaccine trials showing improved survival in spite of lack of time to progression benefit

References	Vaccine	n	Patients	Results
[82]	PSA-TRICOM	125	mCRPC GS $\leq$ 7	Median OS was 24.4 mos for patients treated with vaccine compared to 16.3 mos for patients treated with an empty poxviral vector (randomized 2:1)
[90]	Sipuleucel-T	127	mCRPC	TTP favored vaccine (16.6 vs. 10 wks; $p=0.052$). Median OS favored vaccine 25.9 vs. 21.4 ($p=0.01$). At 36 mos, estimated OS was 34.1% for vaccine and 11% for placebo ($p=0.005$) (randomized 2:1)
[96]	GVAX	80	mCRPC	Study randomized patients to increasing dose levels and a dose effect was seen. OS favored high doses (35 mos) compared to medium (20 mos) and low doses (23.1 mos)

mCRPC metastatic castration-resistant prostate cancer; *GS* Gleason score; *OS* overall survival; *TTP* time to progression; *mos* months; *wks* weeks

driven therapeutic changes that can be misconstrued as progressive disease [120–122]. Furthermore, despite initial disease progression as measured by RECIST, subsequent therapies may exploit a smoldering immune response. Alternatively, ensuing therapies may enhance the immune response by eliminating Tregs or by exposing an active immune response to new TAAs through either chemotherapy-mediated cell lysis or treatment-induced tumor phenotypic alterations. To determine one potential clinical utility of vaccines, future clinical trials may need to randomize patients to vaccine followed by standard therapy compared with standard therapy alone to determine the benefits of sequential therapy [123], and employ survival as the primary endpoint.

Based on results of the clinical trials reviewed here, it appears that certain patients derive greater clinical benefit from prostate cancer vaccines than do other patients, a significant consideration in issues such as FDA approval and the design of future clinical trials. An instructive example is trastuzumab, an agent targeted against Her-2-positive breast cancer that likely would not have gained FDA approval had it been tested in patients with all types of breast cancer. Similarly, identifying the characteristic(s) of the subpopulation that will derive the greatest benefit from prostate cancer vaccines – whether that is disease burden, an aspect of the immune system, or a combination of both – must be the focus of future clinical trials. What seems clear is that the patient population classically represented in clinical trials – those previously treated with multiple therapies or who have a large disease burden – is not the appropriate population for clinically evaluating the effectiveness of a vaccine [124]. That is why prostate cancer, an often indolent disease

with a tumor marker (PSA) to detect low disease burden, may present a promising opportunity for defining the initial role of vaccines in cancer therapy.

References

1. Tannock IF, de Wit R, Berry WR, et al. Docetaxel plus prednisone or mitoxantrone plus prednisone for advanced prostate cancer. N Engl J Med 2004;351(15):1502–12.
2. Petrylak DP, Tangen CM, Hussain MH, et al. Docetaxel and estramustine compared with mitoxantrone and prednisone for advanced refractory prostate cancer. N Engl J Med 2004;351(15):1513–20.
3. Sharifi N, Gulley JL, Dahut WL. Androgen deprivation therapy for prostate cancer. JAMA 2005;294(2):238–44.
4. Coffey DS, Isaacs JT. Prostate tumor biology and cell kinetics – theory. Urology 1981;17 Suppl 3:40–53.
5. Rhodes DR, Barrette TR, Rubin MA, Ghosh D, Chinnaiyan AM. Meta-analysis of microarrays: interstudy validation of gene expression profiles reveals pathway dysregulation in prostate cancer. Cancer Res 2002;62(15):4427–33.
6. Fong L, Small EJ. Immunotherapy for prostate cancer. Semin Oncol 2003;30(5):649–58.
7. Chakraborty NG, Stevens RL, Mehrotra S, et al. Recognition of PSA-derived peptide antigens by T cells from prostate cancer patients without any prior stimulation. Cancer Immunol Immunother 2003;52(8):497–505.
8. Oesterling JE. Prostate specific antigen: a critical assessment of the most useful tumor marker for adenocarcinoma of the prostate. J Urol 1991;145(5):907–23.
9. Madan RA, Gulley JL, Arlen PM. PSA-based vaccines for the treatment of prostate cancer. Expert Rev Vaccines 2006;5(2):199–209.
10. Murphy GP, Elgamal AA, Su SL, Bostwick DG, Holmes EH. Current evaluation of the tissue localization and diagnostic utility of prostate specific membrane antigen. Cancer 1998;83(11):2259–69.

11. Wright Jr GL, Grob BM, Haley C, et al. Upregulation of prostate-specific membrane antigen after androgen-deprivation therapy. Urology 1996;48(2):326–34.

12. Veeramani S, Yuan TC, Chen SJ, et al. Cellular prostatic acid phosphatase: a protein tyrosine phosphatase involved in androgen-independent proliferation of prostate cancer. Endocr Relat Cancer 2005;12(4):805–22.

13. Vihko P, Virkkunen P, Henttu P, Roiko K, Solin T, Huhtala ML. Molecular cloning and sequence analysis of cDNA encoding human prostatic acid phosphatase. FEBS Lett 1988;236(2):275–81.

14. Disis ML, Bernhard H, Shiota FM, et al. Granulocyte-macrophage colony-stimulating factor: an effective adjuvant for protein and peptide-based vaccines. Blood 1996; 88(1):202–10.

15. Dranoff G, Jaffee E, Lazenby A, et al. Vaccination with irradiated tumor cells engineered to secrete murine granulocyte-macrophage colony-stimulating factor stimulates potent, specific, and long-lasting anti-tumor immunity. Proc Natl Acad Sci U S A 1993;90(8):3539–43.

16. Morrissey PJ, Bressler L, Park LS, Alpert A, Gillis S. Granulocyte-macrophage colony-stimulating factor augments the primary antibody response by enhancing the function of antigen-presenting cells. J Immunol 1987; 139(4):1113–9.

17. Small EJ, Reese DM, Um B, Whisenant S, Dixon SC, Figg WD. Therapy of advanced prostate cancer with granulocyte macrophage colony-stimulating factor. Clin Cancer Res 1999;5(7):1738–44.

18. Aarts WM, Schlom J, Hodge JW. Vector-based vaccine/cytokine combination therapy to enhance induction of immune responses to a self-antigen and antitumor activity. Cancer Res 2002;62(20):5770–7.

19. Grosenbach DW, Barrientos JC, Schlom J, Hodge JW. Synergy of vaccine strategies to amplify antigen-specific immune responses and antitumor effects. Cancer Res 2001;61(11):4497–505.

20. Kass E, Panicali DL, Mazzara G, Schlom J, Greiner JW. Granulocyte/macrophage-colony stimulating factor produced by recombinant avian poxviruses enriches the regional lymph nodes with antigen-presenting cells and acts as an immunoadjuvant. Cancer Res 2001;61(1): 206–14.

21. Ward JE, McNeel DG. GVAX: an allogeneic, whole-cell, GM-CSF-secreting cellular immunotherapy for the treatment of prostate cancer. Expert Opin Biol Ther 2007; 7(12):1893–902.

22. Wingren AG, Parra E, Varga M, et al. T cell activation pathways: B7, LFA-3, and ICAM-1 shape unique T cell profiles. Crit Rev Immunol 1995;15(3–4):235–53.

23. Gulley JL, Madan RA, Arlen PM. Enhancing efficacy of therapeutic vaccinations by combination with other modalities. Vaccine 2007;25 Suppl 2:B89–96.

24. Aragon-Ching JB, Williams KM, Gulley JL. Impact of androgen-deprivation therapy on the immune system: implications for combination therapy of prostate cancer. Front Biosci 2007;12:4957–71.

25. Mercader M, Bodner BK, Moser MT, et al. T cell infiltration of the prostate induced by androgen withdrawal in patients with prostate cancer. Proc Natl Acad Sci U S A 2001;98(25):14565–70.

26. Matejuk A, Hopke C, Vandenbark AA, Hurn PD, Offner H. Middle-age male mice have increased severity of experimental autoimmune encephalomyelitis and are unresponsive to testosterone therapy. J Immunol 2005;174(4): 2387–95.

27. Goldberg GL, Sutherland JS, Hammet MV, et al. Sex steroid ablation enhances lymphoid recovery following autologous hematopoietic stem cell transplantation. Transplantation 2005;80(11):1604–13.

28. Drake CG, Doody AD, Mihalyo MA, et al. Androgen ablation mitigates tolerance to a prostate/prostate cancer-restricted antigen. Cancer Cell 2005;7(3):239–49.

29. Sutherland JS, Goldberg GL, Hammett MV, et al. Activation of thymic regeneration in mice and humans following androgen blockade. J Immunol 2005;175(4):2741–53.

30. Lin AM, Small EJ. Prostate cancer update: 2007. Curr Opin Oncol 2008;20(3):294–9.

31. Chakraborty M, Abrams SI, Camphausen K, et al. Irradiation of tumor cells up-regulates Fas and enhances CTL lytic activity and CTL adoptive immunotherapy. J Immunol 2003;170(12):6338–47.

32. Garnett CT, Palena C, Chakraborty M, Tsang KY, Schlom J, Hodge JW. Sublethal irradiation of human tumor cells modulates phenotype resulting in enhanced killing by cytotoxic T lymphocytes. Cancer Res 2004;64(21):7985–94.

33. Friedman EJ. Immune modulation by ionizing radiation and its implications for cancer immunotherapy. Curr Pharm Des 2002;8(19):1765–80.

34. Gulley JL, Arlen PM, Bastian A, et al. Combining a recombinant cancer vaccine with standard definitive radiotherapy in patients with localized prostate cancer. Clin Cancer Res 2005;11(9):3353–62.

35. AbdAlla EE, Blair GE, Jones RA, Sue-Ling HM, Johnston D. Mechanism of synergy of levamisole and fluorouracil: induction of human leukocyte antigen class I in a colorectal cancer cell line. J Natl Cancer Inst 1995;87(7):489–96.

36. Fisk B, Ioannides CG. Increased sensitivity of adriamycin-selected tumor lines to CTL-mediated lysis results in enhanced drug sensitivity. Cancer Res 1998;58(21): 4790–3.

37. Aquino A, Prete SP, Greiner JW, et al. Effect of the combined treatment with 5-fluorouracil, gamma-interferon or folinic acid on carcinoembryonic antigen expression in colon cancer cells. Clin Cancer Res 1998;4(10):2473–81.

38. Matsuzaki I, Suzuki H, Kitamura M, Minamiya Y, Kawai H, Ogawa J. Cisplatin induces fas expression in esophageal cancer cell lines and enhanced cytotoxicity in combination with LAK cells. Oncology 2000;59(4):336–43.

39. Garnett CT, Schlom J, Hodge JW. Combination of docetaxel and recombinant vaccine enhances T-cell responses and antitumor activity: effects of docetaxel on immune enhancement. Clin Cancer Res 2008;14(11):3536–44.

40. Orsini F, Pavelic Z, Mihich E. Increased primary cell-mediated immunity in culture subsequent to adriamycin or daunorubicin treatment of spleen donor mice. Cancer Res 1977;37(6):1719–26.

41. Maccubbin DL, Wing KR, Mace KF, Ho RL, Ehrke MJ, Mihich E. Adriamycin-induced modulation of host defenses in tumor-bearing mice. Cancer Res 1992;52(13):3572–6.

42. Chan OT, Yang LX. The immunological effects of taxanes. Cancer Immunol Immunother 2000;49(4–5):181–5.

43. Lutsiak ME, Semnani RT, De Pascalis R, Kashmiri SV, Schlom J, Sabzevari H. Inhibition of CD4(+)25+ T regulatory cell function implicated in enhanced immune response by low-dose cyclophosphamide. Blood 2005;105(7):2862–8.

44. Ercolini AM, Ladle BH, Manning EA, et al. Recruitment of latent pools of high-avidity CD8(+) T cells to the antitumor immune response. J Exp Med 2005;201(10):1591–602.

45. Arlen PM, Gulley JL, Parker C, et al. A randomized phase II study of concurrent docetaxel plus vaccine versus vaccine alone in metastatic androgen-independent prostate cancer. Clin Cancer Res 2006;12(4):1260–9.

46. Gribben JG, Ryan DP, Boyajian R, et al. Unexpected association between induction of immunity to the universal tumor antigen CYP1B1 and response to next therapy. Clin Cancer Res 2005;11(12):4430–6.

47. Antonia SJ, Mirza N, Fricke I, et al. Combination of p53 cancer vaccine with chemotherapy in patients with extensive stage small cell lung cancer. Clin Cancer Res 2006;12(3 Pt 1):878–87.

48. Small EJ, Sacks N, Nemunaitis J, et al. Granulocyte macrophage colony-stimulating factor – secreting allogeneic cellular immunotherapy for hormone-refractory prostate cancer. Clin Cancer Res 2007;13(13):3883–91.

49. Mueller DL, Jenkins MK, Schwartz RH. Clonal expansion versus functional clonal inactivation: a costimulatory signalling pathway determines the outcome of T cell antigen receptor occupancy. Annu Rev Immunol 1989;7:445–80.

50. Waterhouse P, Penninger JM, Timms E, et al. Lymphoproliferative disorders with early lethality in mice deficient in CTLA-4. Science 1995;270(5238):985–8.

51. Leach DR, Krummel MF, Allison JP. Enhancement of antitumor immunity by CTLA-4 blockade. Science 1996;271(5256):1734–6.

52. Quezada SA, Peggs KS, Curran MA, Allison JP. CTLA4 blockade and GM-CSF combination immunotherapy alters the intratumor balance of effector and regulatory T cells. J Clin Invest 2006;116(7):1935–45.

53. Zeh III HJ, Perry-Lalley D, Dudley ME, Rosenberg SA, Yang JC. High avidity CTLs for two self-antigens demonstrate superior in vitro and in vivo antitumor efficacy. J Immunol 1999;162(2):989–94.

54. Hodge JW, Chakraborty M, Kudo-Saito C, Garnett CT, Schlom J. Multiple costimulatory modalities enhance CTL avidity. J Immunol 2005;174(10):5994–6004.

55. Egen JG, Kuhns MS, Allison JP. CTLA-4: new insights into its biological function and use in tumor immunotherapy. Nat Immunol 2002;3(7):611–8.

56. Allison JP, Chambers C, Hurwitz A, et al. A role for CTLA-4-mediated inhibitory signals in peripheral T cell tolerance? Novartis Found Symp 1998;215:92–8. Discussion 8–102, 86–90.

57. Gerritsen W, Van Den Eertwegh A, De Gruijl T, et al. A dose-escalation trial of GM-CSF-gene transduced allogeneic prostate cancer cellular immunotherapy in combination with fully human anti-CTL4 antibody (MDX-010, ipilimumab) in patients with metastatic hormone-refractory prostate cancer (mHRPC) [abstract]. ASCO Prostate Cancer Symposium 2007:262.

58. Gerritsen W, Van Den Eertwegh A, De Gruijl T. Expanded phase I combination trial of GVAX immunotherapy for prostate cancer and ipilimumab in patients with metastatic hormone-refractory prostate cancer (mHPRC) [abstract]. J Clin Oncol 2008;26(Suppl):5146.

59. Gulley J, Arlen P, Madan R, et al. Phase I trial of a PSA based vaccine and ipilimumab in patients (pts) with metastatic castrate resistant prostate cancer (CRPC) [abstract]. AACR-NCI-EORTC International Conference: Molecular Targets and Cancer Therapeutics Meeting Abstracts. October 2007:A142.

60. Essajee S, Kaufman HL. Poxvirus vaccines for cancer and HIV therapy. Expert Opin Biol Ther 2004;4(4):575–88.

61. Kass E, Schlom J, Thompson J, Guadagni F, Graziano P, Greiner JW. Induction of protective host immunity to carcinoembryonic antigen (CEA), a self-antigen in CEA transgenic mice, by immunizing with a recombinant vaccinia-CEA virus. Cancer Res 1999;59(3):676–83.

62. Kantor J, Abrams S, Irvine K, Snoy P, Kaufman H, Schlom J. Specific immunotherapy using a recombinant vaccinia virus expressing human carcinoembryonic antigen. Ann N Y Acad Sci 1993;690:370–3.

63. Hodge JW, Grosenbach DW, Rad AN, Giuliano M, Sabzevari H, Schlom J. Enhancing the potency of peptide-pulsed antigen presenting cells by vector-driven hyperexpression of a triad of costimulatory molecules. Vaccine 2001;19(25–26):3552–67.

64. Zhu M, Terasawa H, Gulley J, et al. Enhanced activation of human T cells via avipox vector-mediated hyperexpression of a triad of costimulatory molecules in human dendritic cells. Cancer Res 2001;61(9):3725–34.

65. Palena C, Zhu M, Schlom J, Tsang KY. Human B cells that hyperexpress a triad of costimulatory molecules via avipox-vector infection: an alternative source of efficient antigen-presenting cells. Blood 2004;104(1):192–9.

66. Moss B. Genetically engineered poxviruses for recombinant gene expression, vaccination, and safety. Proc Natl Acad Sci U S A 1996;93(21):11341–8.

67. Gulley J, Chen AP, Dahut W, et al. Phase I study of a vaccine using recombinant vaccinia virus expressing PSA (rV-PSA) in patients with metastatic androgen-independent prostate cancer. Prostate 2002;53(2):109–17.

68. Etlinger HM, Altenburger W. Overcoming inhibition of antibody responses to a malaria recombinant vaccinia virus caused by prior exposure to wild type virus. Vaccine 1991;9(7):470–2.

69. Kundig TM, Kalberer CP, Hengartner H, Zinkernagel RM. Vaccination with two different vaccinia recombinant viruses: long-term inhibition of secondary vaccination. Vaccine 1993;11(11):1154–8.

70. Konishi E, Pincus S, Paoletti E, Shope RE, Wason PW. Avipox virus-vectored Japanese encephalitis virus vaccines: use as vaccine candidates in combination with purified subunit immunogens. Vaccine 1994;12(7):633–8.

71. Hodge JW, McLaughlin JP, Kantor JA, Schlom J. Diversified prime and boost protocols using recombinant vaccinia virus and recombinant non-replicating avian pox virus to enhance T-cell immunity and antitumor responses. Vaccine 1997;15(6–7):759–68.

72. Marshall JL, Hoyer RJ, Toomey MA, et al. Phase I study in advanced cancer patients of a diversified prime-and-boost vaccination protocol using recombinant vaccinia virus and recombinant nonreplicating avipox virus to elicit anti-carcinoembryonic antigen immune responses. J Clin Oncol 2000;18(23):3964–73.

73. Kaufman HL, Wang W, Manola J, et al. Phase II randomized study of vaccine treatment of advanced prostate cancer (E7897): a trial of the Eastern Cooperative Oncology Group. J Clin Oncol 2004;22(11):2122–32.

74. Kaufman H, Wang W, Manola J, DiPaola R. Phase II prime/boost vaccination using poxviruses expressing PSA in hormone-dependent prostate cancer: follow-up clinical results from ECOG 7897 [abstract]. J Clin Oncol 2005;23(16S): 4501.

75. Lechleider RJ, Arlen PM, Tsang KY, et al. Safety and immunologic response of a viral vaccine to prostate-specific antigen in combination with radiation therapy when metronomic-dose interleukin-2 is used as an adjuvant. Clin Cancer Res 2008;14(16):5284–91.

76. Clinical Trials (PDQ). Samarium Sm 153 lexidronam pentasodium with or without vaccine therapy and GM-CSF in treating patients with prostate cancer and bone metastases. Available from:http://www.cancer.gov/search/ViewClinical Trials.aspx?cdrid=535561&version=patient&protocolsear chid=4937826. Accessed Jul 2008.

77. Arlen PM, Gulley JL, Todd N, et al. Antiandrogen, vaccine and combination therapy in patients with nonmetastatic hormone refractory prostate cancer. J Urol 2005;174(2):539–46.

78. Madan RA, Gulley JL, Schlom J, et al. Analysis of overall survival in patients with nonmetastatic castration-resistant prostate cancer treated with vaccine, nilutamide, and combination therapy. Clin Cancer Res 2008;14(14):4526–31.

79. Clinical Trials (PDQ). Flutamide with or without vaccine therapy in treating patients with nonmetastatic prostate cancer. Available from:http://www.cancer.gov/search/ ViewClinicalTrials.aspx?cdrid=535593&version=patient& protocolsearchid=4937826. Accessed Jul 2008.

80. Hodge JW, Sabzevari H, Yafal AG, Gritz L, Lorenz MG, Schlom J. A triad of costimulatory molecules synergize to amplify T-cell activation. Cancer Res 1999;59(22):5800–7.

81. Arlen PM, Skarupa L, Pazdur M, et al. Clinical safety of a viral vector based prostate cancer vaccine strategy. J Urol 2007;178(4 Pt 1):1515–20.

82. Kantoff P, Glode L, Tannenbaum S, Bilhartz D. Randomized, double-blind, vector-controlled study of targeted immunotherapy in patients with hormone-refractory prostate cancer [abstract]. J Clin Oncol 2005;24(18S):1501.

83. Madan R, Gulley J, Dahut W, et al. Overall survival (OS) analysis of a phase II study using a pox viral-based vaccine, PSA-TRICOM, in the treatment of metastatic, castrate-resistant prostate cancer (mCRPC): implications for clinical trial design [abstract]. J Clin Oncol 2008;16(20S):3005.

84. Halabi S, Small EJ, Kantoff PW, et al. Prognostic model for predicting survival in men with hormone-refractory metastatic prostate cancer. J Clin Oncol 2003;21(7):1232–7.

85. Rini BI. Technology evaluation: APC-8015, Dendreon. Curr Opin Mol Ther 2002;4(1):76–9.

86. Patel PH, Kockler DR. Sipuleucel-T: a vaccine for metastatic, asymptomatic, androgen-independent prostate cancer. Ann Pharmacother 2008;42(1):91–8.

87. Burch PA, Breen JK, Buckner JC, et al. Priming tissue-specific cellular immunity in a phase I trial of autologous dendritic cells for prostate cancer. Clin Cancer Res 2000;6(6):2175–82.

88. Small EJ, Fratesi P, Reese DM, et al. Immunotherapy of hormone-refractory prostate cancer with antigen-loaded dendritic cells. J Clin Oncol 2000;18(23):3894–903.

89. Burch PA, Croghan GA, Gastineau DA, et al. Immunotherapy (APC8015, Provenge) targeting prostatic acid phosphatase can induce durable remission of metastatic androgen-independent prostate cancer: a phase 2 trial. Prostate 2004; 60(3):197–204.

90. Small EJ, Schellhammer PF, Higano CS, et al. Placebo-controlled phase III trial of immunologic therapy with sipuleucel-T (APC8015) in patients with metastatic, asymptomatic hormone refractory prostate cancer. J Clin Oncol 2006;24(19):3089–94.

91. US Food and Drug Administration, Cellular, Tissue and Gene Therapies Advisory Committee. Sipuleucel-T briefing document. Dendreon Corporation. Available from:http:// www.fda.gov/ohrms/dockets/ac/07/briefing/2007- 4291B1_01.pdf. Accessed Jul 2008.

92. Dendreon expects interim data analysis for phase 3 PROVENGE IMPACT Trial in October. Available from:http://www.investor.dendreon.com/newsroom/ releasedetail.cfm?ReleaseID=323910&header=News. Accessed Aug 2008.

93. Clinical Trials (PDQ). Sipuleucel-T as neoadjuvant treatment in prostate cancer. Available from:http://www.cancer. gov/search/ViewClinicalTrials.aspx?cdrid=601177&versi on=HealthProfessional&protocolsearchid=5006778. Accessed Aug 2008.

94. Simons JW, Mikhak B, Chang JF, et al. Induction of immunity to prostate cancer antigens: results of a clinical trial of vaccination with irradiated autologous prostate tumor cells engineered to secrete granulocyte-macrophage colony-stimulating factor using ex vivo gene transfer. Cancer Res 1999;59(20):5160–8.

95. Simons JW, Carducci MA, Mikhak B, et al. Phase I/II trial of an allogeneic cellular immunotherapy in hormone-naive prostate cancer. Clin Cancer Res 2006;12(11 Pt 1): 3394–401.

96. Higano CS, Corman JM, Smith DC, et al. Phase 1/2 dose-escalation study of a GM-CSF-secreting, allogeneic, cellular immunotherapy for metastatic hormone-refractory prostate cancer. Cancer 2008;113:975–84.

97. Cell Genesys, Inc. GVAX immunotherapy for prostate cancer. Available from:http://www.cellgenesys.com/clinical-prostate-cancer.shtml. Accessed Aug 2008.

98. Eaton JD, Perry MJ, Nicholson S, et al. Allogeneic whole-cell vaccine: a phase I/II study in men with hormone-refractory prostate cancer. BJU Int 2002;89(1):19–26.

99. Michael A, Ball G, Quatan N, et al. Delayed disease progression after allogeneic cell vaccination in hormone-resistant prostate cancer and correlation with immunologic variables. Clin Cancer Res 2005;11(12):4469–78.

100. Sakaguchi S, Sakaguchi N, Asano M, Itoh M, Toda M. Immunologic self-tolerance maintained by activated T cells expressing IL-2 receptor alpha-chains (CD25). Breakdown of a single mechanism of self-tolerance causes various autoimmune diseases. J Immunol 1995;155(3):1151–64.

101. Morse MA, Clay TM, Mosca P, Lyerly HK. Immunoregulatory T cells in cancer immunotherapy. Expert Opin Biol Ther 2002;2(8):827–34.

102. Sakaguchi S. Regulatory T cells: key controllers of immunologic self-tolerance. Cell 2000;101(5):455–8.

103. Piccirillo CA, Shevach EM. Cutting edge: control of CD8+ T cell activation by CD4+CD25+ immunoregulatory cells. J Immunol 2001;167(3):1137–40.

104. Woo EY, Yeh H, Chu CS, et al. Cutting edge: regulatory T cells from lung cancer patients directly inhibit autologous T cell proliferation. J Immunol 2002;168(9):4272–6.

105. Fu T, Shen Y, Fujimoto S. Tumor-specific CD4(+) suppressor T-cell clone capable of inhibiting rejection of syngeneic sarcoma in A/J mice. Int J Cancer 2000;87(5):680–7.

106. Ghiringhelli F, Larmonier N, Schmitt E, et al. CD4+CD25+ regulatory T cells suppress tumor immunity but are sensitive to cyclophosphamide which allows immunotherapy of established tumors to be curative. Eur J Immunol 2004; 34(2):336–44.

107. Curiel TJ, Coukos G, Zou L, et al. Specific recruitment of regulatory T cells in ovarian carcinoma fosters immune privilege and predicts reduced survival. Nat Med 2004; 10(9):942–9.

108. Sato E, Olson SH, Ahn J, et al. Intraepithelial CD8+ tumor-infiltrating lymphocytes and a high CD8+/regulatory T cell ratio are associated with favorable prognosis in ovarian cancer. Proc Natl Acad Sci U S A 2005;102(51):18538–43.

109. Kawaida H, Kono K, Takahashi A, et al. Distribution of CD4+CD25 high regulatory T cells in tumor-draining lymph nodes in patients with gastric cancer. J Surg Res 2005;124(1):151–7.

110. Woo EY, Chu CS, Goletz TJ, et al. Regulatory CD4(+) CD25(+) T cells in tumors from patients with early-stage non-small cell lung cancer and late-stage ovarian cancer. Cancer Res 2001;61(12):4766–72.

111. Tanaka H, Tanaka J, Kjaergaard J, Shu S. Depletion of CD4+ CD25+ regulatory cells augments the generation of specific immune T cells in tumor-draining lymph nodes. J Immunother 2002;25(3):207–17.

112. Jones E, Dahm-Vicker M, Simon AK, et al. Depletion of CD25+ regulatory cells results in suppression of melanoma growth and induction of autoreactivity in mice. Cancer Immun 2002;2:1.

113. Schabowsky RH, Madireddi S, Sharma R, Yolcu ES, Shirwan H. Targeting CD4+CD25+FoxP3+ regulatory T cells for the augmentation of cancer immunotherapy. Curr Opin Investig Drugs 2007;8(12):1002–8.

114. Motoyoshi Y, Kaminoda K, Saitoh O, et al. Different mechanisms for anti-tumor effects of low- and high-dose cyclophosphamide. Oncol Rep 2006;16(1):141–6.

115. Strassburg A, Pfister ED, Arning A, Nashan B, Ehrich JH, Melter M. Basiliximab reduces acute liver allograft rejection in pediatric patients. Transplant Proc 2002;34(6): 2374–5.

116. Furtado GC, de Lafaille Curotto MA, Kutchukhidze N, Lafaille JJ. Interleukin 2 signaling is required for CD4(+) regulatory T cell function. J Exp Med 2002;196(6): 851–7.

117. Neuhaus P, Clavien PA, Kittur D, et al. Improved treatment response with basiliximab immunoprophylaxis after liver transplantation: results from a double-blind randomized placebo-controlled trial. Liver Transpl 2002;8(2): 132–42.

118. Therasse P, Arbuck SG, Eisenhauer EA, et al. New guidelines to evaluate the response to treatment in solid tumors. European Organization for Research and Treatment of Cancer, National Cancer Institute of the United States, National Cancer Institute of Canada. J Natl Cancer Inst 2000;92(3):205–16.

119. Therasse P, Eisenhauer EA, Verweij J. RECIST revisited: a review of validation studies on tumour assessment. Eur J Cancer 2006;42(8):1031–9.

120. Gulley JL, Arlen PM, Tsang KY, et al. Pilot study of vaccination with recombinant CEA-MUC-1-TRICOM poxviral-based vaccines in patients with metastatic carcinoma. Clin Cancer Res 2008;14(10):3060–9.

121. Jones RL, Cunningham D, Cook G, Ell PJ. Tumour vaccine associated lymphadenopathy and false positive positron emission tomography scan changes. Br J Radiol 2004;77(913):74–5.

122. Loveland BE, Zhao A, White S, et al. Mannan-MUC1-pulsed dendritic cell immunotherapy: a phase I trial in patients with adenocarcinoma. Clin Cancer Res 2006;12(3 Pt 1):869–77.

123. Schlom J, Arlen PM, Gulley JL. Cancer vaccines: moving beyond current paradigms. Clin Cancer Res 2007;13(13): 3776–82.

124. von Mehren M, Arlen P, Gulley J, et al. The influence of granulocyte macrophage colony-stimulating factor and prior chemotherapy on the immunological response to a vaccine (ALVAC-CEA B7.1) in patients with metastatic carcinoma. Clin Cancer Res 2001;7(5):1181–91.

Chapter 28
Sipuleucel-T: Autologous Cellular Immunotherapy for Metastatic Castration-Resistant Prostate Cancer

Celestia S. Higano

Abstract Few treatment options are currently available for patients with asymptomatic or minimally symptomatic metastatic castration-resistant prostate cancer (CRPC). Second line hormonal approaches are effective for a median of 3 months' time but have never been shown to prolong survival. Until recently, docetaxel was the only FDA-approved therapy for mCRPC that has been shown to extend survival. Sipuleucel-T is an autologous cellular immunotherapy treatment. In an initial Phase 3 study, a significant effect on the primary endpoint of time to disease progression was not demonstrated, but a 4.5-month improvement in median survival compared to control was observed. A subsequent phase III study of sipuleucel-T in 512 men with asymptomatic or minimally symptomatic CRPC, resulted in a 4.1-month improvement in median survival compared to control. The most common adverse events observed in sipuleucel-T treated patients in randomized trials have been chills, fatigue, fever, back pain, nausea, joint ache, and headache. The survival benefit, adverse event profile, and short course of treatment (4 weeks) associated with sipuleucel-T therapy make it an appealing treatment option for asymptomatic metastatic castrate resistant prostate cancer patients.

Keywords Autologous cellular immunotherapy • Castration-resistant • APC8015 • Hormone refractory • Immunotherapy • Prostate cancer • Provenge • Sipuleucel-T

C.S. Higano (✉)
University of Washington, Seattle Cancer Care Alliance,
Seattle, WA, USA
e-mail: thigano@u.washington.edu

Introduction

In 2009, prostate cancer is expected to claim the lives of 27,360 men in the USA, a statistic that is essentially unchanged from 1989 despite continued refinements in detection and treatment of this disease [1]. Each year brings the diagnosis of more than 192,000 new cases of prostate cancer, the second most common cause of cancer death in males [1]. As depicted in Fig. 28.1, first-line treatment for localized disease may consist of radical prostatectomy and/or radiation therapy [2]. If disease recurs, typically manifested by a rising prostate-specific antigen (PSA) without evidence of metastases on imaging studies, androgen deprivation may be initiated, either by orchiectomy or hormonal therapy with luteinizing hormone-releasing hormone agonists. Given sufficient time, most patients with hormone sensitive non-metastatic disease will progress to castration-resistant metastatic disease despite androgen deprivation.

Docetaxel (Taxotere®, Sanofi-Aventis, NY) is the first Food and Drug Administration (FDA)-approved agent to demonstrate a significant survival advantage in metastatic CRPC [3]. In the TAX327 study by Tannock and colleagues that formed the basis for approval [4], treatment with docetaxel and prednisone in a mixed population of symptomatic and asymptomatic patients resulted in a median survival benefit of 2.4 months when compared to mitoxantrone and prednisone. Serious adverse events were observed in 26% of patients. A supporting phase III trial of docetaxel and estramustine (Emcyt®, Pfizer, Inc, New York, NY) also demonstrated a median survival increase of 1.9 months compared to mitoxantrone and prednisone. Grade 3–5 toxicities were observed in 56% of patients [5].

Due to the toxicities of chemotherapy, many men with metastatic CRPC who do not have significant symptoms choose to delay or forgo chemotherapy despite the demonstration of survival benefit [7], particularly given that

W.D. Figg et al. (eds.), *Drug Management of Prostate Cancer*,
DOI 10.1007/978-1-60327-829-4_28, © Springer Science+Business Media, LLC 2010

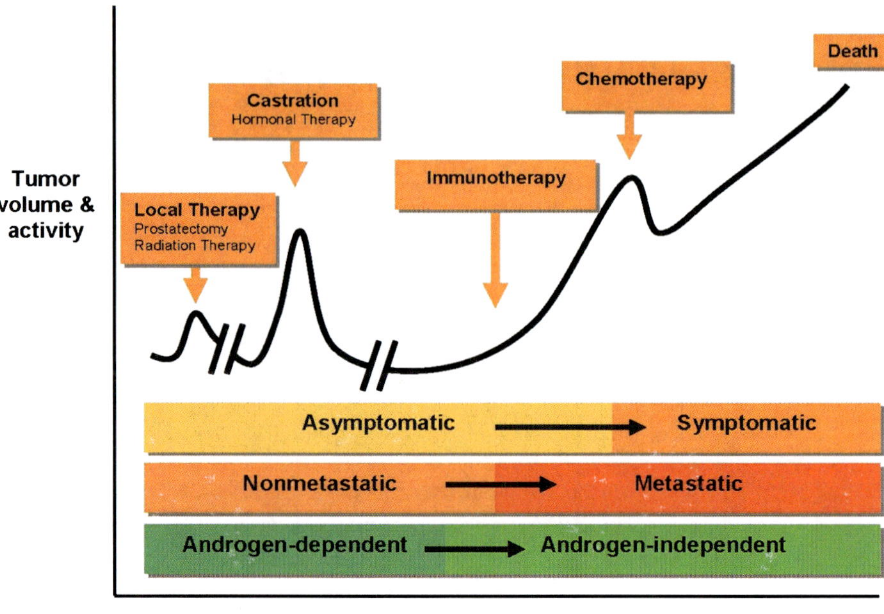

Fig. 28.1 Natural history of prostate cancer and common treatment options with proposed use of immunotherapy

there is no evidence that delaying administration of doc-etaxel is detrimental [6]. Men who have no or minimal symptoms due to metastatic CRCP make good subjects for the study of new agents with minimal toxicity. With respect to immunological approaches, this population is appropriate since it may take weeks to months for an immune response to be mounted.

Several immunologic approaches to prostate cancer are being studied [8]. Recently, Sipuleucel-T (Provenge®, APC8015; Dendreon Corporation, Seattle, WA, USA) an autologous cellular immunotherapy designed to treat prostate cancer, was approved by the FDA in April 2010 based on the results of a phase III trial in men with metastatic CRPC who had no or minimal symptoms [9]. Other active immunotherapy approaches for the treatment of prostate cancer include Prostvac VF (Bavarian Nordic, Kvistgaard, Denmark), a live attenuated virus encoding PSA and co-stimulatory molecules, and GVAX (BioSante Pharmaceuticals, Lincolnshire, IL), prostate cancer cell lines transfected with granulocyte macrophage-colony stimulating factor (GM-CSF) (see Chapter 29 on GVAX). This chapter will address the most recent clinical data on sipuleucel-T.

Sipuleucel-T Cellular Immunotherapy

Sipuleucel-T is an FDA approved autologous cellular immunotherapy product for the treatment of prostate cancer. Sipuleucel-T is an active immunotherapy which is dependent upon the effective presentation of a suitable target antigen to the immune system by antigen-presenting cells (APC). The sipuleucel-T product consists of autologous APCs loaded with a recombinant prostate antigen protein, PA2024, designed to stimulate a patient's own immunity to prostate cancer. PA2024 is a fusion protein composed of prostatic acid phosphatase (PAP) linked to GM-CSF. PAP is a prostate antigen that is expressed in more than 95% of prostate adenocarcinomas [10, 11] and has been shown to be an effective target antigen in experimental animal models [12, 13].

Preparation of sipuleucel-T involves harvesting peripheral blood mononuclear cells and loading them ex vivo with the PA2024 antigen (Fig. 28.2). The peripheral blood mononuclear cells include a large number of autologous APCs, in the range of 10^8–10^9 cells [14]. The ex vivo manufacturing process removes the APCs from the potentially immunosuppressive environment found in patients with advanced cancer and directly exposes them to PAP antigen, theoretically allowing for a more robust immune activation [15, 16]. Although the precise mechanism of action of sipuleucel-T is unknown, the activated autologous APCs that are infused back into the patient are thought to stimulate the immune system to attack and kill tumor cells.

Each lot of sipuleucel-T is prepared from the patient's own peripheral blood mononuclear cells obtained via a standard 1.5–2.0 blood volume leukapheresis

Fig. 28.2 Production of sipuleucel-T and its proposed mechanism of action for its effect on prostate cancer cells. A full course of therapy consists of a total of three leukapheresis procedures and product infusions, one each at weeks 0, 2, and 4

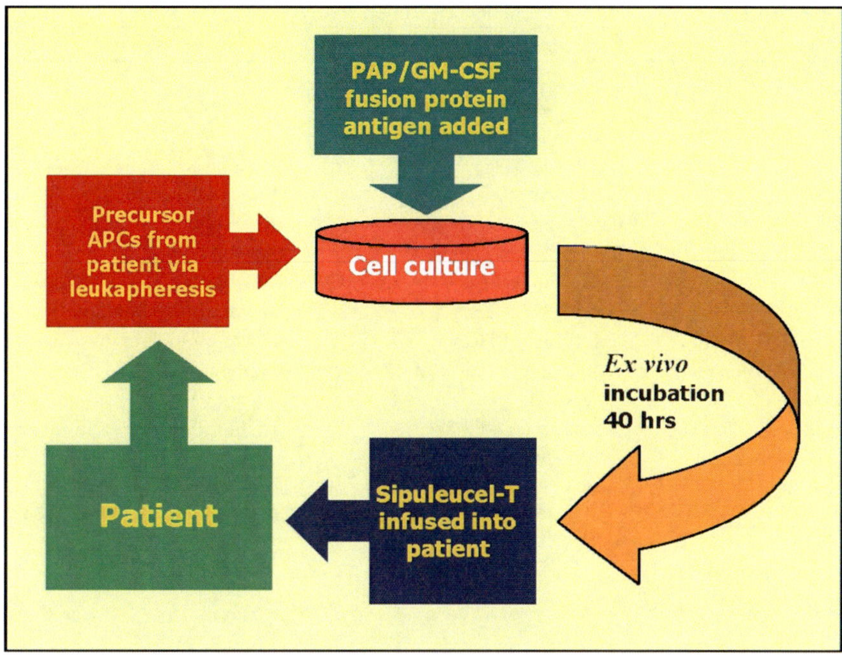

procedure as illustrated in Fig. 28.2. Autologous APCs are cultured ex vivo with PA2024 for approximately 40 h. Cells are washed, and the final cellular product is suspended in lactated ringer's solution and delivered for infusion approximately 3 days after completion of the leukapheresis. Sipuleucel-T is produced and administered intravenously at approximately weeks 0, 2, and 4.

Clinical Efficacy of Sipuleucel-T

Phase I/II Studies

Eight phase I/II studies (Table 28.1) have been conducted in 223 prostate cancer patients to evaluate safety and to explore dosing regimens for sipuleucel-T [14, 17–22]. Most were monotherapy treatments in CRPC, with the exception of the study by Beinart et al. [20] which evaluated sipulecuel-T in men with a rising PSA following definitive local therapy, and the study by Rini et al. [21] that evaluated sipuleucel-T in combination with bevacizumab in 22 androgen-sensitive prostate cancer patients with nonmetastatic, recurrent disease manifested by a rising PSA following definitive local therapy.

The ability of sipuleucel-T to stimulate an immune response was measured in several studies by T-cell proliferation and/or interferon-gamma enzyme-linked immunospot (ELISPOT) assay. In each of these studies, T-cell stimulation by the immunizing antigen was observed in 90–100% of patients treated with sipuleucel-T [14, 17, 21].

Completed Phase III Clinical Studies in CRPC

Completed phase III clinical studies of sipuleucel-T in metastatic CRPC involved treatment of a total of 737 patients in three trials (Table 28.1). D9901 and D9902A were identically designed, prospective, multicenter, randomized, double-blind, controlled studies in men with asymptomatic metastatic CRPC. The primary endpoint for these studies was time to disease progression (TTP), and a prespecified analysis of overall survival was to be performed after 36 months of follow-up. D9902B was a prospective, randomized, double blind, multi-center, controlled trial in men with symptomatic or minimally symptomatic metastatic CRPC. The primary efficacy endpoint for D9902B was overall survival.

D9901 Study

The D9901 (NCT00005947) study used a 2:1 enrollment scheme with 82 patients randomized to control consisting

Table 28.1 Clinical studies with sipuleucel-T in prostate cancer

Study	Phase	Description	N	Patient population	References
Studies with sipuleucel-T in castration-resistant prostate cancer					
D9610	I/II	Dose escalation, safety	31	Metastatic and nonmetastatic	Small et al. [14]
D9702	I/II	Dose escalation, safety	34	Metastatic	Burch et al. [18, 19]
D9801	I	Dose–response	15	Metastatic and nonmetastatic	Data on file[a]
D9906	I	Dose–response	18	Metastatic and nonmetastatic	Takaue et al.[17]
D9903	II	Cryopreserved product	56[b]	Asymptomatic metastatic	Data on file[a]
PB01	II	Cryopreserved product	28[c]	Asymptomatic metastatic	Data on file[a]
D9901	III	Safety and efficacy	127	Asymptomatic metastatic	Small et al. [9]
D9902A	III	Safety and efficacy	98	Asymptomatic metastatic	Higano et al. [22]
D9902B[c]	III	Safety and efficacy	512	Asymptomatic/minimally symptomatic	Kantoff et al. [23]
Studies with sipuleucel-T in nonmetastatic castration-sensitive prostate cancer					
D9905	II	Safety	19	Rising PSA after definitive local therapy	Beinart et al. [20]
P-16	II	Sipuleucel-T + bevacizumab	22	Rising PSA after definitive local therapy	Rini et al. [21]
P-11	III	Safety and efficacy	176	Rising PSA after radical prostatectomy and 3 months of hormonal therapy	Beer et al. [24]

[a]Dendreon Corporation, Seattle, WA

[b]Also enrolled in D9902A

[c]Also enrolled in D9902B

of mononuclear cells cultured without antigen; all 127 patients were included in the intent-to-treat (ITT) population. The primary endpoint was TTP on the basis of bone scan, computed tomography, or clinical events associated with progression. There was a 31% reduction in the risk of disease progression ($p=0.052$; log-rank; hazard ratio (HR) 0.69). The median TTP was 11.7 and 10.0 weeks in the treated and control groups, respectively [9]. In a 3-year ITT analysis, patients randomized to sipuleucel-T demonstrated a 41% decrease in the risk of death ($p=0.010$, log-rank; HR 0.58). The median overall survival was 25.9 months in the sipuleucel-T arm compared to 21.4 months for patients in the control arm (Fig. 28.3), a 4.5-month improvement. In addition, 34% of patients receiving sipuleucel-T were alive at 36 months compared to 11% of patients receiving control ($p=0.005$) (see Fig. 28.3). Finally, the treatment effect remained after adjustment for baseline prognostic factors (lactate dehydrogenase, PSA, number of bone metastases, body weight, and localization of disease.

Approximately 60% of these patients were subsequently treated with chemotherapy and similar numbers of each group (37% in the sipuleucel-T group and 49% in the control group) were treated specifically with docetaxel [9]. In addition, there was no evidence of a difference in the time to initiation of chemotherapy between the treatment arms, and the sipuleucel-T treatment effect persisted following adjustment for docetaxel use. Thus, the survival benefit observed in this study was not likely attributable to docetaxel or other subsequent chemotherapy.

A subset of patients in the D9901 study was assessed for immunological response to PA2024. Patients treated with sipuleucel-T treatment had an eightfold increase in T-cell stimulation to the immunizing antigen ($p<0.001$, Wilcoxon rank sum) compared to their baseline values [9].

D9902A Study

The D9902 study was identical in original design to the D9901 study. Based on the initial disease progression results from D9901, and prior to the availability of the overall survival results from D9901, enrollment in D9902 was halted at 98 patients (65 treated with sipuleucel-T and 33 treated with control). The study was renamed D9902A. There was no difference in TTP between the treatment arms. There was a 21% reduction in the risk of death for sipuleucel-T-treated patients relative to control, which was not statistically significant ($p=0.331$, log-rank; HR 0.79). The median survival was 19.0 months in the sipuleucel-T arm compared to 15.7 months in the control arm. The treatment effect remained after adjustment for baseline prognostic factors using an exploratory Cox multiple regression model developed on the D9901 data [22]. At 36 months post randomization,

Fig. 28.3 Overall Kaplan–Meier survival benefit from treatment with sipuleucel-T in the D9901 study. From Small et al. [9]. Reprinted with permission. ©2008 American Society of Clinical Oncology. All rights reserved

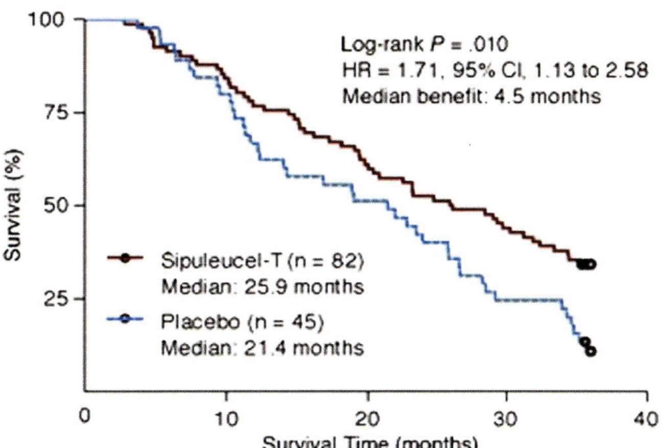

32% of the sipuleucel-T patients in D9902A were alive compared to 21% of the control-treated patients.

An exploratory integrated analysis of the data from D9901 and D9902A was performed based on the identical trial designs, eligibility criteria, and consistent treatment effects observed in the two studies. In this analysis, the reduction in the risk of death and survival benefit were maintained [22].

D9902B Study

The D9902B (NCT00065442) study used a 2:1 enrollment scheme, with 341 patients randomized to sipuleucel-T and 171 patients randomized to control; all 512 patients were included in the ITT population. The primary efficacy endpoint in D9902B was overall survival and the secondary efficacy endpoint was TTP by independent assessment of serial imaging studies. There was a 22.5% reduction in the risk of death (o=0.032; HR 0.775;) and a 4.1 month improvement in median survival (25.8 months for sipuleucel-T vs. 21.7 months for control) [23]. The median time to objective disease progression was 14.6 weeks (3.7 months) in the sipuleucel-T group and 14.4 weeks (3.6 months in the control (p=0.628; HR 0.951). In addition, 31.7% of patients receiving sipuleucel-T were alive at 36 months compared to 23.0% of patients for control. The treatment effect consistently favored the sipuleucel-T group in patient subgroups based on 20 baseline characteristics of the patients. The treatment effect was observed after adjustment for the presence or absence of docetaxel after sipuleucel-T (p=0.03; HR 0.78). Therapy with

sipuleucel-T was also associated with a positive overall survival effect in an analysis that included 18 additional deaths observed between the data-cutoff and study-completion dates, with a median of 36.5 months of follow-up (p=0.02; HR 0.76). Adverse events reported more frequently in the patients who received sipuleucel-T included chills, fever, and headache [23].

Developmental History of Sipuleucel-T in Metastatic CRPC

The original intent of the phase III studies, D9901 and D9902, was to evaluate the ability of sipuleucel-T to delay disease progression (TTP), the primary endpoint, in patients with asymptomatic metastatic CRPC. Additionally, there was a prespecified plan to analyze survival after all patients were followed for 36 months postrandomization. In 2002, when the primary analysis for study D9901 was performed, the disease progression endpoint was not met. Based on this result, D9902 enrollment was stopped early. The study remained blinded and was renamed D9902A. All subjects in both studies D9901 and D9902A continued to be followed for survival. From the knowledge gained in the analysis of D9901, a new phase III study was designed, D9902B, under a Special Protocol Assessment with the FDA. Following the availability of the overall survival results from D9901 and D9902A, a Biologics License Application was filed in 2006. In May 2007, the FDA requested additional clinical data from the D9902B trial prior to licensure of sipuleucel-T. In November 2009, Dendreon filed a supplement to the Biologics License

Application and received approval for licensure of sipuleucel-T by the FDA in April 2010 for the treatment of asymptomatic or minimally symptomatic metastatic CRPC.

Ongoing Randomized Study

One additional randomized study, P-11 is currently ongoing (Table 28.1). P-11 is a study of hormone-sensitive patients with nonmetastatic prostate cancer who experienced PSA elevation following radical prostatectomy [24]. P-11 has reached the enrollment goal and is closed to accrual, however, subjects continue to be followed for safety and the secondary endpoints of distant failure and survival. Endpoints in this trial include time to biochemical failure, PSA doubling time, safety, time to distant failure, and overall survival.

Safety and Tolerability

In phase I/II studies of sipuleucel-T, the maximum tolerated dose was not reached. The most common adverse events, reported in patients in the sipuleucel-T group at a rate $\geq 15\%$, were chills, fatigue, fever, back pain, nausea, joint ache, and headache [23]. In 67.4% of patients in the sipuleucel-T group, these adverse events were mild or moderate in severity. Severe (Grade 3) and life-threatening (Grade 4) adverse events were reported in 23.6% and 4.0% of patients in the sipuleucel-T group compared with 25.1% and 3.3% of patients in the control group. Fatal (Grade 5) adverse events were reported in 3.3% of patients in the sipuleucel-T group compared with 3.6% of patients in the control group. The most common ($\geq 2\%$) Grade 3–5 adverse events reported in the sipuleucel-T group were back pain and chills. Cerebrovascular events occurred in 3.5% of patients in the sipuleucel-T group compared to 2.6% of patients in the control group.

Discussion

The approach to the patient with metastatic CRPC with no or minimal symptoms remains individualized. Although docetaxel confers a modest survival benefit,

it can be associated with significant toxicities. Physicians and patients are often reluctant to proceed with chemotherapy despite the known survival benefit and therefore second-line hormonal manipulations are often used in this setting. Although PSA and some objective responses to second-line hormonal therapy have been reported, there is no evidence that survival is improved.

With FDA approval of sipuleucel-T approval, patients with no or minimal symptoms now have a therapeutic option that can prolong survival, is of short duration and low toxicity. Because the PSA does not usually decline nor do the imaging studies improve following treatment with sipulecuel-T, it may be difficult to determine whether an individual patient is benefiting from treatment with sipuleucel-T. With the development of improved biologic markers, it may become possible to better define those who are most likely to benefit from sipuleucel-T. At the present time, physicians should proceed with subsequent therapy appropriate for the patient's clinical condition, following treatment with sipuleucel-T. Currently available data suggests that administration of sipulecuel-T does not preclude subsequent chemotherapy [22, 23]. As sipuleucel-T is prescribed outside the clinical trial setting, there will be new lessons to be learned from the administration of immunotherapy in this population of prostate cancer patients. At one time, there was little enthusiasm for immunotherapy of solid tumors, and even less belief that such approaches would be beneficial in patients with metastatic disease. However, the results from the clinical trials of sipuleucel-T and other immunotherapeutic agents may change this paradigm. Results of the P-11 phase III trial of ADT induction followed by sipuleucel-T vs. control in men with hormone-sensitive biochemical relapse after prostatectomy will inform future studies in patients with low volume disease or those earlier in the natural history of the disease. In addition, sipuleucel-T may be of use in combination or in sequence with other active agents, as suggested by the pilot study combining sipuleucel-T with bevacizumab [21].

References

1. Jemal A, Siegel R, Ward E, et al. Cancer statistics. CA Cancer J Clin 2009;59:225–49.
2. Cookson MS, Aus G, Burnett AL, et al. Variation in the definition of biochemical recurrence in patients treated for localized

prostate cancer: the American Urological Association Prostate Guidelines for Localized Prostate Cancer Update Panel report and recommendations for a standard in the reporting of surgical outcomes. J Urol 2007;177:540–5.

3. Dagher R, Li N, Abraham S, Rahman A, Sridhara R, Pazdur R. Approval summary: Docetaxel in combination with prednisone for the treatment of androgen-independent hormone-refractory prostate cancer. Clin Cancer Res 2004;10:8147–51.

4. Tannock IF, de Wit R, Berry WR, et al. Docetaxel plus prednisone or mitoxantrone plus prednisone for advanced prostate cancer. N Engl J Med 2004;351:1502–12.

5. Petrylak DP, Tangen CM, Hussain MH, et al. Docetaxel and estramustine compared with mitoxantrone and prednisone for advanced refractory prostate cancer. N Engl J Med 2004;351:1513–20.

6. Berthold DR, Pond G, DeWit R, Eisenberger M, Tannock IF. Docetaxel plus prednisone or mitoxantrone plus prednisone for advanced prostate cancer: Updated survival of the TAX 327 study. ASCO Meeting Abstr 2007;25:50058.

7. Kirk TN, Moyad MA. National survey of advanced prostate cancer patients reveals disparity between perceptions and reality of treatment. J Clin Oncol (Meeting Abstracts) 2006;24:8590.

8. Drake, CG. Prostate cancer as a model for tumour immunotherapy. Nature Rev Immunol 2010;10:580–93.

9. Small EJ, Schellhammer PF, Higano CS, et al. Placebo-controlled phase III trial of immunologic therapy with sipuleucel-T (APC8015) in patients with metastatic, asymptomatic hormone refractory prostate cancer. J Clin Oncol 2006;24:3089–94.

10. Haines AM, Larkin SE, Richardson AP, Stirling RW, Heyderman E. A novel hybridoma antibody (PASE/4LJ) to human prostatic acid phosphatase suitable for immunohistochemistry. Br J Cancer 1989;60:887–92.

11. Goldstein NS. Immunophenotypic characterization of 225 prostate adenocarcinomas with intermediate or high Gleason scores. Am J Clin Pathol 2002;117:471–7.

12. Valone FH, Small E, MacKenzie M, et al. Dendritic cell-based treatment of cancer: closing in on a cellular therapy. Cancer J 2001;7 Suppl 2:S53–61.

13. Laus R, Yang D, Ruegg C. Dendritic cell immunotherapy of prostate cancer: preclinical models and early clinical experience. Cancer Res Ther Control 2001;11:1–10.

14. Small EJ, Fratesi P, Reese DM, et al. Immunotherapy of hormone-refractory prostate cancer with antigen-loaded dendritic cells. J Clin Oncol 2000;18:3894–903.

15. Rosenberg SA. Shedding light on immunotherapy for cancer. N Engl J Med 2004;350:1461–3.

16. Zou W. Immunosuppressive networks in the tumour environment and their therapeutic relevance. Nat Rev Cancer 2005;5:263–74.

17. Takaue Y, Tanosaki R, Tobisu K, Kakizoe T, Mizunuma Y, Yanagida M, Kawai H. Antigen-pulsed dendritic cell therapy for the treatment of hormone-refractory prostate cancer: a phase I trial of APC8015. Proc ASCO 2002;21:1881.

18. Burch PA, Breen JK, Buckner JC, et al. Priming tissue-specific cellular immunity in a phase I trial of autologous dendritic cells for prostate cancer. Clin Cancer Res 2000;6:2175–82.

19. Burch PA, Croghan GA, Gastineau DA, et al. Immunotherapy (APC8015, Provenge) targeting prostatic acid phosphatase can induce durable remission of metastatic androgen-independent prostate cancer: a Phase 2 trial. Prostate 2004;60:197–204.

20. Beinart G, Rini BI, Weinberg V, Small EJ. Antigen-presenting cells 8015 (Provenge) in patients with androgen-dependent, biochemically relapsed prostate cancer. Clin Prostate Cancer 2005;4:55–60.

21. Rini BI, Weinberg V, Fong L, Conry S, Hershberg RM, Small EJ. Combination immunotherapy with prostatic acid phosphatase pulsed antigen-presenting cells (provenge) plus bevacizumab in patients with serologic progression of prostate cancer after definitive local therapy. Cancer 2006;107:67–74.

22. Higano CS, Schellhammer PF, Small EJ, et al. Integrated data from 2 randomized, double-blind, placebo-controlled, phase 3 trials of active cellular immunotherapy with sipuleucel-T in advanced prostate cancer. Cancer 2009;115:3670–9.

23. Kantoff PW, Higano CS, Shore ND, et al. Sipuleucel-T Immunotherapy for Castration-Resistant Prostate Cancer. N Engl J Med 2010;363:411–422.

24. Beer TM, Bernstein GT, Corman JM, et al. Randomized trial of active cellular immunotherapy with sipuleucel-T in androgen dependent prostate cancer (ADPC). J Clin Oncol (Meeting Abstracts) 2007;25:5059.

Chapter 29
GM-CSF Gene-Transduced Prostate Cancer Vaccines: GVAX

Lalit R. Patel and Jonathan W. Simons

Abstract Prostate cancer offers both compelling and challenging problems for research and development of active specific immunotherapy using cancer vaccines. Vaccine strategies designed to break tolerance and generate a sustained, potent, antineoplastic immune response against prostate cancer represent a therapeutic strategy, which has emerged as a significant research enterprise over the past 15 years. Several approaches to prostate cancer immunotherapy have been investigated in the past decade, including defined peptide vaccines, dendritic cell-based vaccines, whole-tumor cell autologous and allogeneic vaccines, carbohydrate vaccines, and poxvirus vaccines. It is estimated that over 1,200 prostate cancer patients have been treated with investigational vaccines in Phase I, II, or III trials. This chapter will focus on a narrow segment of vaccine research: strategies employing GM-CSF gene-transduced whole prostate cancer cell vaccines (GVAX). Attention will be given to the preclinical rationale, clinical development, emerging body of knowledge on resistance mechanisms, clinical development challenges, and future directions for GVAX in particular. The extensive data with GVAX now in humans with advanced prostate cancer is likely to be instructive in the future research and development of antineoplastic immunotherapy for prostate cancer.

Keywords Prostate cancer • Vaccine • GVAX • GM-CSF • Immunotherapy

J.W. Simons (✉)
Prostate Cancer Foundation, Santa Monica, CA, USA
e-mail: jsimons@pcf.org

Introduction

All generalizations are false, including this one
  Mark Twain

Prostate cancer (CaP) is the most common noncutaneous neoplasm, and the second most common cause of cancer deaths in US men. New prostate cancer cases now account for a full third of all male cancer diagnoses and 10% of all deaths [1]. Fortunately, the death rate from prostate cancer has decreased over the last decade. Nevertheless, more than 28,000 US men are estimated to have died of advanced CaP in 2008 [2]. Prostate-specific antigen (PSA) screening is in part responsible for reducing the death rate and the increased diagnosis of localized disease. Unfortunately, even with digital rectal examination and PSA screening, up to 30–40% of patients have disease that recurs and metastasizes after local therapy. Progress in robotics in radical prostatectomy, IMRT (intensity-modulated radiation therapy) in radiation therapy, and in identifying patients who will benefit from watchful waiting [3–5] have all been important clinical advances. Yet new approaches to metastatic disease beyond the reach of local intervention are urgently needed.

Prostate cancer offers both compelling and challenging problems for research and development of active specific immunotherapy using cancer vaccines. Despite 40 years of testing, cytotoxic drugs have not conferred survival advantages in prostate cancer as they have in treatment of testicular cancer, lymphomas, breast cancer, and colon cancer. A theoretical advantage of CaP for immunotherapy is the relatively slower tumor cell growth in most cases and longer clinical course in which to study patients and their

W.D. Figg et al. (eds.), *Drug Management of Prostate Cancer*,
DOI 10.1007/978-1-60327-829-4_29, © Springer Science+Business Media, LLC 2010

immunity to their cancers. In concept, there is "time" to induce systemic immunity to prostate cancer in patients who have excellent performance status. A study of nearly 2,000 patients with good to moderate risk of disease and a biochemical recurrence of PSA following radical prostatectomy showed development of metastatic disease within 8 years [6]. Few situations in medical oncology offer so many patients such a significant interval for investigational therapeutics, if they are relatively well tolerated in the outpatient setting. For an effective immunotherapy, this period of time would be ideal for adjuvant immunotherapy – if an effective immunotherapy existed.

The standard of care for patients with recurrent prostate cancer is androgen deprivation therapy (ADT). The vast majority of ADT patients eventually become castration resistant. The median survival time of patients with castration-resistant prostate cancer (CRPC) may be improved from an average of about 12 months to about 17–18 months by the addition of antineoplastic chemotherapy with taxanes, and systemic ADT earlier in the disease course [7, 8]. Beyond "frontline" docetaxel-based chemotherapy for hormonal therapy refractory disease, the standard of care is treatment with investigational agents in clinical trials whenever clinically appropriate.

Vaccine strategies designed to break tolerance and generate a sustained, potent, antineoplastic immune response against prostate cancer represent a therapeutic strategy, which has emerged as a significant research enterprise over the past 15 years. A PubMed search shows 775 research reports on prostate cancer vaccines; to put the world-wide scope of the vaccine immunotherapy research activity into context, a literature search of "prostate cancer and p53 gene" generates 800 citations vs. 775 for prostate cancer vaccines.

Several approaches to prostate cancer immunotherapy have been investigated in the past decade, including defined peptide vaccines, dendritic cell-based vaccines, whole-tumor cell autologous and allogeneic vaccines, carbohydrate vaccines, and poxvirus vaccines. It is estimated that over 1,200 prostate cancer patients have been treated with investigational vaccines in Phase I, II, or III trials. This chapter will focus on a narrow segment of vaccine research: strategies employing GM-CSF gene-transduced whole prostate cancer cell vaccines (GVAX). Attention will be given to the preclinical rationale, clinical development, emerging body of knowledge on resistance mechanisms,

clinical development challenges, and future directions for GVAX in particular. As Churchill once observed, some generalizations for the future of treatment research in prostate cancer – made from the basic and clinical research experience using GVAX – are likely to be only partly true. Nevertheless, the extensive data with GVAX now in humans with advanced prostate cancer is likely to be instructive in the future research and development of antineoplastic immunotherapy for prostate cancer.

Preclinical Rationale for GM-CSF Genetically Transduced Vaccines

Tolerance is another word for indifference
 W. Somerset Maugham

Operationally, every CaP patient who succumbs to metastatic prostate cancer is the victim of genetically altered prostate cells, which have either escaped host immunity or induced immunologic tolerance or perhaps more precisely, "indifference." Immunologic "indifference" to metastatic prostate cancer is the threshold across which all forms of immunotherapy research must cross in the clinic. Research breaking immunologic "indifference" to prostate cancer cell-associated tumor antigens spurred the clinical development of GVAX.

Historically, vaccines are perhaps most familiar in the context of infectious disease, where their history is expansive. Although documentary evidence suggests the use of sheep pox inoculations as early as the sixteenth century among African nomadic herders, vaccination appears to have originated further east in China or India where variolation with powdered scabs may have been practiced as early as 1000 AD [9]. Vaccination against infectious disease typically involves the administration of attenuated whole pathogens or pathogen-derived immunogens with the intent to induce an immune response. The popular press, interest in prostate cancer vaccines, which has been disproportionate to objective clinical benefit, has been largely based on 100 years of vaccination for life-threatening illnesses.

Research on cancer vaccines is more recent. In 1957 Prehn and Main reported in the JNCI on an investigation with experimental whole cell tumor vaccines in mice to generate antitumor immune responses [10]. To the emerging field of cancer vaccines, the report was a seminal contribution. Prehn and Main demonstrated for the first time that the immunogenicity of whole cell tumor vaccines could be increased dramatically by prior gamma irradiation. Three decades prior to a molecular and cellular understanding of T-cell, B-cell, and innate immune responses to tumor-associated antigens, Prehn and Main demonstrated that autologous tumor cells could be used as immunogens. In 1975, Johns Hopkins researchers, Brannen and Coffey demonstrated that even in more advanced stages of disease, human prostate cancer cells possessed tumor-associated antigens that could be recognized within prostate cancer patients themselves [11]. A very small case series was reported from Hopkins using autologous prostate cancer cell plasma membranes in DTH (delayed-type hypersensitivity).

Autologous cancer cell vaccine development was explored intermittently throughout the twentieth century. Different bacterial adjuvants were used in some cases. Clinical responses to whole cell tumor vaccines were rare and often short lived as a generalization outside of melanoma. Prior to the cloning of cytokine genes and the use of recombinant cytokines with tumor vaccines, it was not possible to draw even beginning inferences on the mechanism of inducing antineoplastic immune responses. Viral "oncolysates" of tumor vaccines and combinations with BCG and C. parvum and other adjuvants were used as "activators" in what we now know as attempts to generate antigen presentation at vaccine sites.

Although cancer cells offer potentially unique tumor-associated antigens that may induce tumoricidal immunity, evasion of autologous host immune response is a common and perhaps central hallmark of cancer. Prostate cancer cells are, specifically, very poorly immunogenic and are poor at antigen presentation. Autoantibodies are not seen in prostate cancer patients. In addition, defects in the major histocompatibility (MHC) class I expression occur in 85% of primary tumors and 100% of metastases [12]. Along with others, we have defined antigen presentation defects in Class I MHC surface presentation [13]. Successful immunotherapy strategies against prostate cancer have to overcome the poor immunogenicity of this disease.

One method to optimize tumor antigen presentation is to employ cytokines involved in antigen recognition and response to drive prostate tumor-associated antigens to be presented better. Significant research screening cytokines head-to-head for their ability to increase the immunogenicity of poorly immunogenic tumors

was necessary to determine which cytokines to employ. Dranoff conducted the first systematic comparison of individual cytokines expressed by gene transfer in a melanoma tumor vaccine model. Compared to interleukin-2, interleukin-4, and other immunomodulatory molecules, granulocyte-macrophage colony-stimulating factor (GM-CSF) was the most potent cytokine signal tested for activation of antigen processing and presentation by dendritic cells (DCs) [14]. This work on the mechanism of action of GM-CSF gene-transduced tumor vaccines also implicated DCs as a critical component for induction of immunity to poorly immunogenic tumors. Paracrine GM-CSF secreted by GM-CSF gene-transduced tumors promotes migration of DCs to vaccination sites, activates the cellular machinery of antigen phagocytosis, and enhances antigen peptide presentation. DCs are the most potent antigen-presenting cells (APCs) in the immune system. GM-CSF, however, also has growth and maturational effects on multilineage progenitor cells, and activates other mature immune cells involved in antigen processing and presentation, such as macrophages and neutrophils [15]. APCs activated by GM-CSF enhance the immunogenicity of cancer vaccines by presenting cancer-associated antigens processed by the APCs to both CD4 (helper) and CD8 (cytolytic) T-cells in the draining lymph node of the vaccination sites [16]. The cytolytic T-cells generated by the active specific immunization with tumor-associated antigens then mount a systemic tumoricidal immune response, leave the draining lymph node of the vaccination site, and respond to metastatic cells elsewhere.

In the early 1990s, Dranoff et al. first characterized the promise of this approach using a murine model of melanoma [14]. The transduced vaccine conferred 100% protection, with vaccinated mice surviving both immediate (7 days after vaccination) and late (several months after vaccination) challenges. Mice vaccinated with the GM-CSF transduced vaccine were also able to reject preestablished tumors and to develop potent CD4+ and CD8+ T-cell-dependent systemic immunity against otherwise poorly immunogenic tumors. Irradiation of the gene-transduced vaccine was required to attenuate malignancy. Unirradiated GM-CSF gene-transduced murine tumor vaccines grew in the animal; however, irradiated GM-CSF gene-transduced poorly immunogenic tumor vaccines conferred the greatest antitumor immunity. Of note, lethal irradiation of vaccine also improved the immunogenicity of the vaccine. Extensive studies of

GM-CSF gene-transduced tumor vaccines induced similar immunologic memory, protective immunity, and curative effects in the Dunning models of prostate cancer [17–19]. In one study, animals injected with GM-CSF transduced cells performed significantly better than animals administered soluble GM-CSF in combination with cancer cell vaccine. These observations suggest that paracrine secretion of the GM-CSF at vaccination sites was a superior way to recruit DCs and other APCs in comparison to bolus systemic administration of GM-CSF.

Clinical Development of GM-CSF Genetically Transduced Vaccines

It ain't what you don't know that gets you into trouble. It's what you know for sure that just ain't so
    Mark Twain

The concept that *ex vivo* GM-CSF gene transduction of tumor cells could constitute antitumor immunotherapy was first explored in a Phase I trial in renal cell cancer. Renal cell carcinoma (RCC) was selected for the relative ease of generating an autologous tumor immunotherapy product, and the vaccine was engineered by transduction of patients' primary tumor cells (harvested at surgery) with GM-CSF [20]. The replication-defective retroviral vector MFG containing the human GM-CSF cDNA was used. This trial showed the approach to be safe, but only short-lived immunologic responses and one clinical response were noted in 18 patients. Compared to untransduced irradiated RCC vaccine injection sites, GM-CSF gene-transduced vaccines generated distinctive APCs at the vaccine sites identical to preclinical murine models of efficacy, and patients mounted significant delayed-type hypersensitivity (DTH) reactions to untransduced irradiated autologous tumor cells after vaccination. However, the proof-of-concept trial was clear that patients' autologous tumor cells were, in general, extremely variable in terms of viability of vaccine cell for irradiation, and transduction efficiency. Setting a fixed dose of vaccine cells and fixed secretion of GM-CSF for autologous vaccines for Phase II trials was deemed very difficult for multicenter clinical trials.

The immunogenicity of whole-tumor vaccines from prostate cancer was an open question and had never been tested. Autologous, irradiated GM-CSF gene-transduced vaccines for prostate cancer were initially investigated by Simons et al. [21]. This was also the first human gene therapy trial for prostate cancer. Surgically harvested prostate tumor cells from anatomic radical prostatectomies were placed in primary culture, irradiated, and engineered to secrete GM-CSF via the MFG replication-defective retrovirus.

In this initial Phase I human gene therapy trial, eight immunocompetent prostate cancer patients were treated with autologous, GM-CSF-secreting, irradiated tumor vaccines prepared from *ex vivo* retroviral transduction of surgically harvested cells. Expansion of primary cultures of autologous vaccine cells successfully met trial specifications in 8 of 11 cases (73%). The yields of the primary cell cultures limited the number of vaccination courses. Side effects were pruritis, erythema, and swelling at vaccination sites. Vaccine site biopsies demonstrated infiltrates of cells consistent with DCs and macrophages among prostate tumor vaccine cells after 3 days of vaccination. Vaccination activated new T-cell and B-cell immune responses against PCA antigens. T-cell responses, evaluated by assessing DTH reactions against untransduced autologous tumor cells, were evident in two of eight patients before vaccination and in seven of eight patients after treatment. Reactive DTH site biopsies manifested infiltrates of effector cells consisting of CD45RO+ T-cells, and degranulating eosinophils consistent with activation of both Th1 and Th2 T-cell responses. A distinctive eosinophilic vasculitis was evident near autologous tumor cells at vaccine sites, and at DTH sites. B-cell responses were also induced. Sera from three of eight vaccinated men contained new antibodies recognizing polypeptides of 26, 31, and 150 kDa in protein extracts from prostate cells. The 150-kDa polypeptide was expressed by LNCaP and PC-3 CaP cells, as well as by normal prostate epithelial cells, but not by prostate stromal cells. No antibodies against PSA were detected. These data suggest that both T-cell and B-cell immune responses to human CaP can be generated by treatment with irradiated, GM-CSF gene-transduced CaP vaccines. The numerous technical difficulties involved in the preparation and expansion of primary autologous prostate tumor cells, however, represent a significant limitation for clinical development of this approach. In this study, a sufficient volume of cells could not be harvested in three of 11 patients attempted. In addition, the individualized preparation of the vaccine was labor intensive and not robust enough for larger Phase II trials. Successful expansion of autologous prostate vaccine cells did not appear to be correlated with Gleason grade or obvious clinical factors. Furthermore, variability in the autologous cells precluded the development of vaccines with reproducible and robust immunogenicity between patients.

An approach to overcome the difficulties involved in engineering an autologous tumor vaccine emerged out of the observation that the immune system is not directly primed by antigen on tumor cells. Rather, these cells are phagocytosed and antigen is presented on professional antigen-presenting-cells from the host, i.e., DCs and macrophages. In other words, an irradiated GM-CSF gene-transduced tumor cell that expressed tumor-associated antigens shared by the metastatic cells in the patient could offer the "platform" for antigen loading without requiring the use of the patient's primary tumor as the antigen source. This concept led to the hypothesis that a cell-based immunotherapy product could be created by using allogeneic prostate cancer cell lines transduced to produce the appropriate stimulatory cytokine, i.e., GM-CSF. The use of allogeneic cells lines has been applied to a number of tumor types including pancreatic cancer, breast cancer and lung cancer as well as prostate cancer [22–25]. Furthermore, allogeneic vaccines can be developed from readily available established prostate cancer cell lines permitting vaccine manufacture on a large scale. An additional advantage of the allogeneic approach is that the tumor-associated antigens are processed within the autologous APCs to the autologous T-cells and B-cells via "cross priming." Patients therefore do not need to be HLA matched a priori for these GM-CSF gene-transduced, irradiated tumor vaccines in order to participate in larger Phase II or Phase III trials. Furthermore, with the ability to expand enormous quantities of *ex vivo* gene-transduced allogeneic tumor vaccines (which are stable in culture – unlike primary cultures of autologous cells), makes it possible to escalate the dose and repeated durations of vaccinations. In autologous GM-CSF gene-transduced tumor vaccine trials repeated "booster" vaccination was not possible in most patients because the supply of primary cultures of vaccine cells ran out.

An academic "proof of concept" Phase I/II trial for allogeneic GVAX for prostate cancer was conducted in the NCI S.P.O.R.E. in Prostate Cancer at Johns Hopkins [26]. The purpose of the single institution trial was to characterize the adverse effects, immunologic effects,

and clinical activity of immunotherapy with irradiated, allogeneic, prostate cancer cells expressing GM-CSF. Patients who were "hormone therapy naïve" who had recurrent CaP by biochemical relapse of PSA were selected. The Phase I/II trial was conducted in selected patients in the absence of radiologic metastases who were immunologically competent to mount DTH skin reactions to common microbial recall antigens. Patients were enrolled who had not received primary radiotherapy. Treatments were administered weekly via intradermal injections of $1.2 \times 10(8)$ GM-CSF gene-transduced, irradiated cancer cells ($6 \times 10(7)$ LNCaP cells and $6 \times 10(7)$ PC-3 cells) for 8 weeks. Both the cell lines were transduced with the MFG-GM-CSF vector. Patients were not given booster vaccinations. Twenty-one immunocompetent patients were treated. Toxicities included local injection-site reactions, pruritus, and flu-like symptoms. All who experienced toxicity were managed as outpatients. One patient had a partial PSA response of a 7-month duration. The same patient had elevated levels of CEA at the start of vaccination and CEA levels declined to normal intercurrent with the PSA response. This patient, along with all the vaccinated patients in the trial, did not mount anti-PSA antibodies or serologic signs of autoimmune disease. All patients were treated as outpatients only. At 20 weeks post-first treatment, 16 of 21 (76%) patients showed a statistically significant decrease in PSA velocity (slope) compared with prevaccination levels ($P < 0.001$). Injection-site biopsies showed intradermal infiltrates consisting of CD1a+ DCs and CD68+ macrophages, closely analogous to both previous clinical trials using autologous GM-CSF-transduced cancer cells and preclinical models. Posttreatment, patients developed new oligoclonal antibodies reactive against at least five identified antigens expressed by LNCaP or PC-3 cells. A high-titer antibody response (>1:250) against a 250-kDa antigen expressed on normal prostate epithelial cells was induced in a patient with partial PSA remission. Titers of this antibody decreased when treatment ended, and subsequent PSA relapse occurred. The nonpatient-specific prostate cancer immunotherapy had a favorable safety profile and is immunologically active. These findings warranted further evaluation of dose, schedule and assessment of efficacy.

Cell Genesys, South San Francisco, CA expanded from the academic proof of concept translational clinical development into a full-fledged clinical development program for GM-CSF gene-transduced irradiated whole prostate cancer cell vaccines. Vector improvements ensued, and an AAV based vector replaced the use of a replication-defective retroviral vector MFG [21, 27]. Furthermore, transfected allogeneic vaccine cells were expanded in large bioprocessor vats so patients could be vaccinated with single production "lots" under Good Manufacturing Practice. The company's IND-based GVAX vaccine was a combination of the two human prostate cancer cell lines PC-3 and LNCaP. These two cell lines were chosen in order to provide a potentially complementary source of potential tumor-associated antigens that might be expressed at metastatic sites. LnCaP as a cell line was derived from disease metastasis to a lymph node, and expresses a number of prostate epithelial antigens including PSMA and PSA. PC-3 is an androgen-refractory cell line derived from a bone metastasis and expresses several cancer-associated proteases [28]. Both cell lines were similarly transduced with an AAV-human GM-CSF cDNA vector and expressed high levels of paracrine, bioactive, human GM-CSF.

Expansion of Clinical Trials of GVAX from Academic Investigation

Phase II: G-9803 and G-0010

Two Phase II trials were conducted in CRPC patients with radiologically confirmed metastatic disease (metastatic CRPC) [26]. The first study (G-9803) administered GVAX in the outpatient setting, enrolling 34 patients who were selected for their excellent performance status and who had CRPC but were asymptomatic with their metastases. Multiple vaccinations were found to be very tolerable for outpatient treatment with no induction of autoimmune disease observed. Vaccine-site pruritis and erythema were the major consistent toxicity. The median survival for the GVAX-treated patients was 26.2 months, suggesting an improvement with vaccination in light of the 18-month median survival for patients with CRPC-receiving docetaxel. Comparing favorably at the time with palliative chemotherapy, this clinical result of median survival improvement exceeded expectations based on the natural history of the disease in this patient population, and stimulated interest in larger studies evaluating efficacy and increased vaccine dose. There was not, however, a high frequency of PSA responses

in the Phase II trial, even in patients whose survival appeared to be prolonged with time.

The Phase II study G-0010 in asymptomatic metastatic HRPC was subsequently initiated as a follow-up to the G-9803 study. The AAV-GM-CSF gene-transduced LnCAP and PC-3 combined allogeneic vaccine product was used at higher doses in this Phase II trial. The objective of the trial was to assess for an optimal dose for a Phase III efficacy evaluation trial. G-0010 enrolled 80 US patients who either received low-dose (200 million cells monthly), medium-dose (200 million cells biweekly), or high-dose (500 million cells as priming dose followed by 300 million cells biweekly) vaccine. Vaccine-specific antibodies were evaluated by Western blot analysis of vaccine lysates against the patient's sera collected before and after vaccination. Osteoclastic bone degradation in CRPC metastases was simultaneously assayed using the marker type 1 carboxy terminal telopeptide. Bone scans were obtained every 3 months. PSA was assayed at each treatment visit.

Of 19 patients, 6 (32%) in the high-dose GVAX group had PSA declines after repeated vaccinations. However, PSA continued to rise for the first 2 months before decreasing, even in apparent responders to vaccination. This "delayed" induction of apparent antineoplastic immune response pattern was consistent with the hypothesized kinetics of an immunotherapeutic effect that takes weeks to develop and requires multiple rounds of vaccination. In other words, multiple, repetitive vaccinations were required to present sufficient tumor-associated antigens to activate a T-cell and B-cell response – even in immunocompetent patients. Presumably, the low immunogenicity of human prostate cancer, even in the setting of paracrine expression of GM-CSF to activate DC antigen presentation, takes multiple doses. Unlike the immediate cytotoxic effects of chemotherapy, GVAX immunotherapy responses appeared later in the course of treatment. Consistent with this idea, patients showed biochemical evidence by PSA of tumor progression prior to arrest of progression, stabilization of PSA levels, and an objective response. Bone metastatic activity was assayed in this trial as a hypothesis of using type 1 carboxy terminal telopeptide as an intermediate endpoint of response. In 34 of 55 (62%) patients with osseous metastases stable or decreasing type 1 carboxy terminal telopeptide levels were observed, suggesting osteoclast inhibition in bone metastases. Patients were not allowed to use bisphosphonates or undergo hormone therapy changes while participating in this study, precluding changes in type 1 carboxy terminal telopeptide from being attributable to such treatment. Bone scans stabilized in 31 of 72 (43%) and apparently normalized in two cases.

The proportion of patients mounting *de novo* IgG antibody response to at least one prostate cell line increased with vaccine dose. In the highest vaccine-dose group, 87% of patients had an immune response compared with 72 and 40% in the medium and low-dose groups, respectively ($P=0.001$, Kendall tau-b). To the best of our knowledge, this was the first data in humans showing a dose–response relationship with activating B-cell responses to prostate cancer-associated antigens in a vaccine. Data from the 80 patients enrolled suggest that the vaccine was well tolerated, was immunogenic in a dose-dependent fashion, and had clinical activity. These observations complemented the median survival of 26.2 months observed in the earlier G-9803 study.

Safety Profile

In the Phase II trials described above, injection-site reaction was the most common adverse event, and was experienced by 100% of patients treated with intradermal injections of the GVAX® for prostate cancer [26]. Pruritus and erythema for 3–5 days were common low-grade adverse events postvaccination. Other side effects were consistent with an immunotherapy approach, and including fatigue, and flu-like symptoms that resolved with no active management after vaccination. No dose-limiting toxicity was observed. There was also no clinical or laboratory evidence of autoimmune disease in vaccinated patients despite prolonged vaccinations with irradiated allogeneic cells. Taken together, these two, small, highly selected Phase II trials suggested that larger efficacy evaluations for outpatient therapy were warranted, and provided the rationale for their design and implementation in future ongoing studies.

Phase III: Vital-1 and Vital-2

Subsequently, two Phase III trials were conducted that involved community practices as well as some academic centers. These two trials were entitled VITAL-1 and VITAL-2 and were a part of the sponsoring company's

Food and Drug Administration (FDA) registration strategy for GVAX. Patients in the VITAL-1 trial were enrolled in randomized open-label studies comparing vaccine to the standard-of-care chemotherapy regimen of docetaxel and prednisone. The primary objective of this study was to compare the duration of survival between the two treatment arms. The secondary objectives were the comparison between treatment arms of: (1) the proportion of patients who had a bone-related event including spinal cord compression, surgery to bone, local radiation therapy to bone, or skeletal fracture; (2) the proportion of patients who had a progression of bone metastases; and (3) time to onset of bone pain. The secondary objectives were intended to explore the impact of treatment on the significant morbidities that occur in advanced CRPC (i.e., complications of metastatic bony disease, and pain).

Data from both VITAL-1 and VITAL-2 were presented at the Genitourninary American Society of Clinical Oncology meeting in late February 2009, and are summarized below. Presented in abstract form, the data have not been peer-reviewed and published at the time this chapter was written. VITAL-1 was a Phase III clinical trial designed to compare GVAX immunotherapy (CG1940/CG8711) as a monotherapy for CaP against docetaxel chemotherapy plus prednisone in 600 patients with advanced castration-resistant metastatic disease. Enrollment began in 2004 and included only chemotherapy-naïve men without cancer-related pain requiring opioid analgesics were eligible.

In 2007, the VITAL-1 trial completed enrollment with 626 patients at 131 sites in North America and the European Union. A priming dose of GVAX was administered in the GVAX arm followed by routine "maintenance" vaccine treatments. The priming dose was a 500 million cells vaccination followed by 300 million cell booster GVAX doses every 2 weeks for 13 doses. Docetaxel (75 mg/m² q 3 weeks×9 cycles) plus prednisone (10 mg daily) was given in the control arm (D+P). The primary endpoint was superiority in overall survival in the GVAX arm. Of note, a positive trial for a survival advantage for GVAX compared with docetaxel would have been submitted to the FDA for approval. In January 2008, the independent data monitoring committee (IDMC) had completed a preplanned interim efficacy analysis for VITAL-1 and recommended that the study continue, providing no further information to the sponsoring company other than the recommendation to continue the trial. On 27 Aug 2008, the Company announced that it had requested the IDMC to conduct a previously unplanned futility analysis of VITAL-1. VITAL-1 was terminated in October 2008 based on the results of that analysis, which indicated that the trial had less than a 30% chance of meeting its predefined primary endpoint.

All 626 patients completed the initial 6-month treatment period. At the time of study termination the median follow-up was 66 weeks. Analysis of patient data from the trial revealed no imbalance in patient baseline characteristics. The Halabi predicted survival (HPS) was 16 months for the GVAX arm and the D+P arm suggesting a balance in both arms for adverse prognostic factors for CRPC. More than 45% of patients enrolled had aggressive disease at diagnosis with a primary biopsy of Gleason grade >8 pattern. The median number of GVAX treatment doses was 8 (range 1–51) for GVAX and 9 (1–16) for D+P. The frequency of Grade 3 or higher related adverse events was 8.8% for the GVAX arm vs. 43% for the D+P arm. The median survival was 20.7 months for patients on GVAX and 21.7 months on D+P, hazard ratio 1.03, 95% CI (0.83, 1.28), $P=0.78$, stratified log-rank test. The Kaplan–Meier (KM) curve showed GVAX crossing above the D+P survival curve at approximately 22 months in a small subset. In the subset of men with HPS >18 months ($n=264$), median survival was prolonged on GVAX (29.7 months) compared to D+P (27.1 months), HR 0.90 (0.61–1.33), $P=0.60$.

What was learned from this first multinational multicenter Phase III trial of GVAX? First, GVAX as a monotherapy does not appear to confer an antineoplastic immune response that can improve overall survival compared to standard-of-care palliative chemotherapy in most patients. At the dose and schedule chosen, single-agent GVAX treatment did not demonstrate a convincing and statistically superior overall survival compared to D+P. The observed, albeit not statistically significant, survival increase in a subset of patients with a HPS ≥18 months in VITAL-1 also suggests that this subset of patients may have a more favorable response to GVAX immunotherapy. What characteristics about patients in this subset predispose them to this response remains unknown as the trial was terminated. Treatment with GVAX, however, was generally very well tolerated in all patients treated in VITAL-1, and it had a side-effect profile favorable in comparison to that of standard-of-care palliative chemotherapy. This was particularly true for toxicities

of grade 3 and higher, which GVAX caused in appreciably less frequency (8.8% vs 43%).

Interestingly, a crossover exists in the final KM survival curves for the two treatment arms of VITAL-1, with the curve for GVAX patients crossing above the chemotherapy curve at approximately the same time median survival was reached in both treatment arms (~21 months). This has led some to hypothesize that a late favorable effect of GVAX may transpire that prolongs survival compared to chemotherapy in some patients. This finding, however, was not a primary endpoint of the trial as designed. Long-term follow-up is needed to interrogate the existence, nature, and duration of this putative "longer surviving tail" in the GVAX treatment arm of this study. Motivated in part by the unexpected KM crossover, Cell Genesys announced that it has recently taken steps to facilitate further studies of GVAX by academic investigators and the NCI.

VITAL-2 was a Phase III trial designed to compare GVAX immunotherapy in combination with docetaxel (G+D) to docetaxel plus prednisone (D+P) in CRPC patients with metastatic disease who were *symptomatic* with respect to cancer-related pain. The primary endpoint of the trial was also improvement in survival. VITAL-2 was initiated in June 2005 and had enrolled 408 patients at 115 clinical trial sites located in North America and the European Union prior to study termination. VITAL-2 trial was prematurely terminated on 27 Aug 2008 following the recommendation of the trial's IDMC, which observed in a routine safety review meeting an imbalance in deaths between the two treatment arms of the VITAL-2 study with more deaths occurring in the GVAX arm.

In contrast to the outpatient safety profile of VITAL-1, the VITAL-2 trial did raise a concern about safety in men with symptomatic pain from metastatic CaP. However, an updated analysis of adverse events showed no significant toxicities in the GVAX+Docetaxel arm that could explain the increased number of deaths in this arm. Eighty-five percent of deaths were reported as due to prostate cancer in both arms, but, at this writing, no trend has been found in this trial for the causes of death in the remaining 15% of mortalities. These observations are consistent with highly significant flaws in the study design of VITAL-2. The decision to omit concomitant prednisone in the G+D treatment arm was made to avoid the possible immunosuppressive effects of prednisone. This decision may have contributed to VITAL-2's unfavorable outcome, particularly when docetaxel is given with prednisone in the "control arm" of the trial. Considering how well GVAX was tolerated in VITAL-1 and in the Phase II setting, vaccination of patients with advanced symptomatic stage IV prostate cancer as opposed to men with less and asymptomatic tumor burdens may have been a factor. However, further analysis of VITAL-2 data have indicated that the imbalance in deaths between the two treatment arms decreased from 20 deaths at that the time of the IDMC's initial analysis (August 2008) to 9 deaths at the time of final analysis (December 2008).

Perhaps further academic investigations of GVAX, facilitated by Cell Genesys's recently announced efforts, will shed some light on this unresolved question of the effects of GVAX used in combination with docetaxel in men with advanced, metastatic CRPC. It is fair to say that both VITAL-1 and VITAL-2 clinical trials treated patients with disease burdens far greater than the patient populations vaccinated in the earlier clinical trials, and it is fair to say also that, as a monotherapy, allogeneic prostate GVAX does not confer a significant objective remission rate or survival advantage in CRPC.

Tumor Tolerance and Cancer Vaccine Resistance: New Frontiers

The new frontier for immunotherapy and vaccines for prostate cancer is the need to overcome a number of resistance pathways that have been identified since the entrance of GVAX into early clinical testing in 1995. While GM-CSF gene-transduced tumor cell vaccines enhance tumor antigen presentation, other forms of immune tolerance may not be overcome by even potent gene-transduced vaccines alone. Specifically, regulatory T-cells (T-regs) confer immune tolerance by suppressing the activity of their cytotoxic counterparts. While such tolerance from T-regs is required to protect healthy tissues from autoimmunity, an analysis of peripheral blood in 46 patients with epithelial malignancies showed an increase of T-reg-like CD4(+) CD25(+) cells when compared to samples from 34 healthy controls [29]. The same study also found that T-reg-like cells isolated from cancer patients inhibit natural-killer cell-mediated cytotoxicity. These observations suggest prostate cancers may avert tumoricidal immunity by exploiting T-reg-mediated immune tolerance. The specific T-reg mechanisms exploited by cancer must

accordingly be subverted before the full therapeutic effect of tumoricidal GM-CSF gene-transduced vaccinations can be realized in the clinic.

In addition to T-regs, the anticytotoxic T lymphocyte antigen CTLA-4 protein is perhaps the best-studied immune tumor evasion mechanism exploited by cancer. A regulator of T-cell proliferation and differentiation, CTLA-4 is expressed on the surface of T-regs and facilitates immune tumor evasion by tolerizing activated cytotoxic T-cells, suppressing their expansion, and altering differentiation [30]. These effects are partly induced by changes in glucose metabolism and PI3K/Akt signaling downstream of CTLA-4 ligation [31]. Preclinical evaluation of anti-CTLA-4 antibodies by Allison et al. show enhanced antitumor responses in several animal tumor models [32–34]. Synergy between immune modulation by CTLA-4 inhibition and immune priming with GVAX may translate into increased tumor vaccine efficacy in humans. A Phase I/II trial investigating this possibility using the CTLA-4 antibody MDX-010 in combination with GVAX is currently underway with over 20 CRPC patients at the Free University Cancer Center in Amsterdam. These data on the combination of CTLA-4 antibody and GVAX, however, have only been presented in abstract form at the time of this writing.

A similar strategy under evaluation is to combine GVAX with targeted inhibitors against programmed death 1 (PD1), a negative immune-modulating receptor ligated by B7-family members. Like CTLA-4, PD1 is a membrane protein expressed on T-cells following activation by an APC [35]. Ligation of PD1 by its ligand PD-L1 reduces the cytokine secretions and proliferation of T-cells [36], and induces their apoptosis [37]. PD1 ligation may also inhibit cytotoxic T-cell activity through changes in PI3K/Akt signaling and glucose metabolism, but appears to function through mechanisms distinct from those used by CTLA-4 in achieving the same effects [31]. The results of anti-PD-L1 antibody use in preclinical tumor models of multiple cancer types suggest successful, albeit transient, suppression of tumor tolerance [36, 38, 39]. Although it is aberrantly expressed, PD-1 expression correlates with disease progression, and associates with diminished survival in kidney and bladder cancer [40]. PD-L1 is poorly expressed in clinically localized prostate cancer [41]. To the best of our knowledge prostate cancer expression of PD-L1 has yet to be assessed in metastastatic sites. DCs responsible for presenting tumor antigens from engulfed cancer cells do express PD-L1 [42], suggesting the target may be very relevant to abrogating tumor antigen tolerance in prostate cancer patients treated with cellular cancer vaccines like GVAX.

In addition to CTLA-4 and PD-1, other members of the B7-family may provide a promising series of immune-modulating targets to inhibit in combination with vaccines that load APCs with prostate tumor-associated antigens. B7-H3 is of particular interest as it is over expressed in prostate cancer and correlates with tumor aggressiveness in localized prostate cancer [41]. While the precise function of B7-H3 and its mechanism of action are not fully characterized, it appears to enhance T-cell proliferation and promote immune response against allografts [43]. These observations suggest prostate cancer could be uniquely susceptible to tumoricidal immunity. However, the abundant expression of B7-H3 in lymphoid and nonlymphoid tissues also suggests a role in self-tolerance. In a study of DCs derived from C57BL/6 mice genetically transduced to produce a soluble mouse-B7-H3 human-IgG1-Fc fusion, transduced cells had no effect on cell cycling of T-cells, inhibited T-cell IL-2 and IFN-γ production, and significantly inhibited allogeneic immunogenicity in comparison to controls [44]. The conflicting results may be due to differences in methods and models. More importantly, T-cell tolerance is mediated by a combination of signals [45]. Thus the apparent bi-functionality of B7-H3 may be due to its interactions with a multitude of other B7-family immune modulators. Efforts to break tumor tolerance in prostate cancer patients will accordingly benefit from further study of the B7-family and the development of drugs targeting their cooperative immunosuppressive signaling.

Emerging evidence suggests that lymphocyte activation gene-3 (Lag-3) is another diversely active immune-modulating cell-surface molecule that is not of the B7-family, but may inhibit antineoplastic immunity in prostate cancer. A CD4 homolog selectively expressed on T-regs, Lag-3 binds the MHC class II receptor and appears to suppress effector T-cells [46]. Anterior chamber-associated immune deviation (ACAID) is an induced ocular pathology model of immune privilege. T-regs in ACAID mice were found to express Lag-3 in greater frequency and to have a greater ability to suppress effector T-cells in comparison to T-regs from non-ACAID controls [47]. It also appears that tissue-derived adenosine-mediated peripheral immune tolerance may

be caused in part by an increase in LAG-3(+) T-regs promoted by adenosine receptor ligation [48]. These observations suggest LAG-3 is an excellent candidate for making malignancies immune-privileged microenvironments. Elevated expression of LAG-3 observed on T-cells in antigen-expressing organs and tumors (including prostate cancer) further suggests a role in promoting tumor tolerance [49]. Antibodies targeting Lag-3 administered in combination with a recombinant vaccinia viral cancer vaccine in the TRAMP model of transgenic prostate cancer increased the number, restored cytotoxic activity, and caused prostatic accumulation of effector T-cells. More importantly, vaccinated mice when given the antibody displayed approximately 45% target-specific lysis on average as compared to vaccinated mice not given the antibody, which failed to mount a significant antitumor response [49]. While this finding is promising, it remains to be seen whether inhibition of Lag-3 will be as successful in the clinic or in combination with GVAX, anti-PD-1 or anti-CTLA-4 strategies.

Immune evasion to vaccination with GVAX may not solely be conferred by T-cell and APC-signaling molecules. Indoleamine 2,3 dioxygenase (INDO) is an inducible enzyme catalyzing the initial and rate-limiting step in the catabolism of tryptophan, causing it to passively immunize against microbes dependent upon external sources of this essential amino acid [50]. It also appears to function as a major immune modulator in tumor immunology. INDO is expressed by the human placenta [51] and when inhibited by 1-methyl-tryptophan (1MT) in fetal allograft murine models of pregnancy results in rejection and abortion of conceptuses [52], suggesting a natural role for the enzyme in fetal–maternal immune tolerance. The effect is achieved by inhibiting proliferation of T-cells, which develop G1-phase cell-cycle arrest in response to tryptophan shortage [53]. An expression analysis in human cancer cell lines and a broad panel of human tumor specimens including prostatic, colorectal, pancreatic, cervical, non-small-cell lung, ovarian, and head and neck carcinoma revealed constitutive expression of INDO in solid tumors of various stages. The same investigators who evaluated human cancers evaluated immunized mice bearing P815 tumors and found INDO expression by tumors conferred resistance to immune rejection [54]. INDO inhibition with 1MT, which entered Phase I clinical trials in 2007, slowed the growth of syngeneic mouse lung carcinoma [55] and retarded the growth of spontaneously arising mammary tumors in the MMTV-neu/HER2 transgenic mouse model of breast cancer [56]. In both models, antitumor efficacy of 1MT monotherapy was limited but enhanced by combination with cytotoxics. More interestingly, 1MT enhanced the antitumor efficacy of a DC/Lewis lung carcinoma (LLC) fusion vaccine applied to a murine LLC model [57]. These findings suggest a promise for combinations of INDO-targeting small molecules and GVAX in proof of concept clinical trials.

In addition to combining immunoregulatory therapies with vaccines, it may also be critical to investigate the therapeutic potential of targeting multiple effector T-cell suppressors to break tumor tolerance. Little is known about the synergy and overlap between immune modulators. The independent mechanisms used by PD1 and CTLA-4 to alter PI3K/Akt-signaling and glucose metabolism in activated T-cells suggests the possibility of synergy when therapeutically targeting both. Similarly, cotargeting CD4-family suppressor molecules and B7-family immune modulators may produce responses not achieved by monotherapy. Such cotargeting has yet to be evaluated in the preclinical and clinical setting. In the event a therapeutic window can be defined without the induction of autoimmunity, such combinations may be critical to breaking tumor tolerance barriers to successful cancer vaccine therapy.

Lastly, the late induction of apparent antineoplastic immune response patterns in Phase II trials of GVAX was itself hypothesis generating. This observation was consistent with the hypothesized kinetics of an immunotherapeutic effect that takes weeks to develop in most prostate cancer patients. A previously cited possibility is that multiple rounds of GVAX vaccination are required to present sufficient tumor-associated antigen to overcome a threshold for systemic antineoplastic response. Another possibility is antigen spreading might occur at the sites of metastasis after successful immunization transpires. Specifically, the cytotoxic response primed by GVAX vaccination may release tumor-associated antigens from lysed cancer cells at metastases. This additional priming at metastatic sites would provide APCs new combinations of tumor-specific epitopes, priming a sustained and more potent antineoplastic immune response. These hypothesized effects would also be manifested as a later induction of systemic antitumor responses in a clinical trial. Although highly speculative, the hypothesis of a delay in induction of immune responses in patients with advanced disease argues for combining vaccines and inhibitors of immune evasion with other cytotoxic therapies. Thus, the antitumor activity of vaccines may also be improved if given in combination with immune-modulating doses of chemotherapy or radiation therapy if given in the correct schedule. Consistent with this idea, data in several preclinical models have shown synergistic cytotoxic effects from immunotherapy with GM-CSF-secreting tumor cells in combination with chemotherapy [21, 58, 59]. Similarly, it was recently shown in the TRAMP model of prostate cancer that combining radiation therapy with a recombinant vaccinia viral anti-tumor vaccine provoked a tumoricidal immune response when either therapy alone did not [60]. Investigations probing the role of antigen spreading and the potential to enhance the immunogenicity of tumor vaccines by combination therapy with chemotherapy and radiation are warranted with vaccines like GVAX.

Conclusions, Observations, and Future Directions

Get your facts right first, then you can distort them as you please

Mark Twain

A number of important conclusions can be drawn from the experience with GVAX immunotherapy. First GM-CSF tumor vaccines do appear to break immunologic tolerance in men with advanced prostate cancer by both DTH assays and induction of new IgGs. Second, induction of immune responses to prostate cancer is insufficient to confer a large survival advantage in men with CRPC when GVAX is used as monotherapy at the one dose and schedule chosen for the VITAL-1 trial. It is unclear if subset analysis of the surviving "tail" in VITAL-1 will yield additional information on the unique characteristics of these patients in terms of their immune response. Certainly, the field would benefit from knowing what molecular factors underlie the immune response or resistance to treatment. Assessment of the role and expression of inhibitory factors including but not limited to CTLA-4, PD1, B7-H3, LAG3, and INDO which play a role in defining which patients received a survival advantage from GVAX would be of great interest. An important conclusion from the VITAL-2 trial in GVAX is that patients with far advanced prostate cancer and symptomatic bone pain from osseous metastasis are unlikely to be excellent candidates for efficacy evaluations of immunotherapy – until real efficacy has been demonstrated in other and earlier stages of the disease are confirmed. Whether or not the omission of prednisone in the GVAX arm of VITAL-2 contributed to the observed imbalance in deaths in VITAL-2 is also not known. The overall determination of whether GVAX is safe or unsafe in this very advanced population is simply clouded by the withdrawal of prednisone in these patients in the GVAX arm of the trial compared to the arm of patients that received continuous prednisone.

Translational science has demonstrated that GVAX is proof of concept for DC loading. Characterization of tumor-associated antigens observed after vaccination with GVAX is ongoing. Some of these antibodies may be part of the patients' allogeneic immune response. However, some of the IgGs may actually provide evidence that antineoplastic immune responses to antitumor antigens are adequately induced in patients, but insufficient to confer a prolonged survival advantage by themselves. Examples of GVAX-induced IgGs include antibodies directed against Filamin B and NY-ESO1 antigens.

It has also become abundantly clear that cotargeting combinations that permit better effector cell activation after vaccine-based immunotherapy is an important direction for the entire field. Anti-CTLA-4 antibody in combination with GVAX vaccination is being investigated in a Phase I/II trial at the VUMC. What could be contemplated – based on the data reviewed above – is that an ideal cotargeting strategy for immunotherapy of CRPC would be tested in patients with the earliest signs of PSA relapse, a lower tumor burden, and excellent performance status to permit long observation after treatment. This ideal strategy would consist of testing cohorts of patients to assess the correct combination of anti-CTLA-4, anti-LAG3, indo-1 inhibitor, and anti-PD-1 agents and would characterize toxicities with these potent combinations. Autoimmune toxicities are a great potential concern in these patients, and very careful clinical assessments of autoimmune events need to be conducted in these patients. However, short of well-designed Phase II trials testing these questions, it is unlikely that murine models are going to be as informative as translational clinical research trials in *Homo sapiens* with advanced prostate cancer.

The murine models that created the molecular immunology of prostate cancer have their limitations including the patient observation of GVAX-associated IgGs that are generated in patients with immune responses were not predicted, nor are the tumor-associated antigens found after GVAX were found in any of the preclinical models of prostate cancer. There is no substitute for *Homo sapiens* with prostate cancer as subjects of intelligently designed careful immunotherapy clinical trials.

Lastly, the experience of VITAL-2 and VITAL-1 suggest that more Phase II trials with molecular surrogates may be required to better define the right patient subsets for clinical benefit – before a large Phase III program is begun.

Over 800 prostate cancer patients have been vaccinated with GM-CSF gene-transduced prostate cancer vaccine cells. Unfortunately molecular data outside of academic centers does not exist for the great majority of patients now treated. It appears incumbent on investigators in academic centers, biotechnology, in government, and the pharmaceutical industry to work together to capture more molecular data in clinical development, including Phase III registration, in order to better elicit an understanding of treatment benefit when and if it is observed. That effort would further extend our understanding of the complexities of creating a sustained antineoplastic immune response that confers a survival advantage for patients.

Acknowledgment The authors acknowledge Rebecca Levine, of PCF, for her editorial and bibliographic assistance in the preparation of the manuscript.

References

1. Jemal A, Murray T, Ward E, et al. Cancer statistics. CA Cancer J Clin 2005;55(1):10–30.
2. SEER Cancer Statistics Review. National Cancer Institute. Bethesda, MD; 1975–2005.http://www.seer.cancer.gov/csr/1975_2005/. Accessed 13 Feb 2009.
3. Paulson DF, Moul JW, Walther PJ. Radical prostatectomy for clinical stage T1-2N0M0 prostatic adenocarcinoma: long-term results. J Urol 1990;144(5):1180–4.
4. Stamey TA, Yemoto CM, McNeal JE, Sigal BM, Johnstone IM. Prostate cancer is highly predictable: a prognostic equation based on all morphological variables in radical prostatectomy specimens. J Urol 2000;163(4):1155–60.
5. Dillioglugil O, Leibman BD, Kattan MW, Seale-Hawkins C, Wheeler TM, Scardino PT. Hazard rates for progression after radical prostatectomy for clinically localized prostate cancer. Urology 1997;50(1):93–9.

6. Pound CR, Partin AW, Eisenberger MA, Chan DW, Pearson JD, Walsh PC. Natural history of progression after PSA elevation following radical prostatectomy. JAMA 1999;281(17):1591–7.

7. Tannock IF, de Wit R, Berry WR, et al. Docetaxel plus prednisone or mitoxantrone plus prednisone for advanced prostate cancer. N Engl J Med 2004;351(15):1502–12.

8. Petrylak DP, Tangen CM, Hussain MH, et al. Docetaxel and estramustine compared with mitoxantrone and prednisone for advanced refractory prostate cancer. N Engl J Med 2004;351(15):1513–20.

9. Lombard M, Pastoret PP, Moulin AM. A brief history of vaccines and vaccination. Rev Sci Tech 2007;26(1):29–48.

10. Prehn RT, Main JM. Immunity to methylcholanthrene-induced sarcomas. J Natl Cancer Inst 1957;18(6):769–78.

11. Brannen GE, Gomolka DM, Coffey DS. Specificity of cell membrane antigens in prostatic cancer. Cancer Chemother Rep 1975;59(1):127–38.

12. Blades RA, Keating PJ, McWilliam LJ, George NJ, Stern PL. Loss of HLA class I expression in prostate cancer: implications for immunotherapy. Urology 1995;46(5):681–6. Discussion 686–7.

13. Sanda MG, Restifo NP, Walsh JC, et al. Molecular characterization of defective antigen processing in human prostate cancer. J Natl Cancer Inst 1995;87(4):280–5.

14. Dranoff G, Jaffee E, Lazenby A, et al. Vaccination with irradiated tumor cells engineered to secrete murine granulocyte-macrophage colony-stimulating factor stimulates potent, specific, and long-lasting anti-tumor immunity. Proc Natl Acad Sci U S A 1993;90(8):3539–43.

15. Warren TL, Weiner GJ. Uses of granulocyte-macrophage colony-stimulating factor in vaccine development. Curr Opin Hematol 2000;7(3):168–73.

16. Banchereau J, Steinman RM. Dendritic cells and the control of immunity. Nature 1998;392(6673):245–52.

17. Vieweg J, Rosenthal FM, Bannerji R, et al. Immunotherapy of prostate cancer in the Dunning rat model: use of cytokine gene modified tumor vaccines. Cancer Res 1994;54:1760–5.

18. Sanda MG, Ayyagari SR, Jaffee EM, et al. Demonstration of a rational strategy for human prostate cancer gene therapy. J Urol 1994;151(3):622–8.

19. Moody DB, Robinson JC, Ewing CM, Lazenby AJ, Isaacs WB. Interleukin-2 transfected prostate cancer cells generate a local antitumor effect in vivo. Prostate 1994;24(5):244–51.

20. Simons JW, Jaffee EM, Weber CE, et al. Bioactivity of autologous irradiated renal cell carcinoma vaccines generated by ex vivo granulocyte-macrophage colony-stimulating factor gene transfer. Cancer Res 1997;57(8):1537–46.

21. Simons JW, Mikhak B, Chang JF, et al. Induction of immunity to prostate cancer antigens: results of a clinical trial of vaccination with irradiated autologous prostate tumor cells engineered to secrete granulocyte-macrophage colony-stimulating factor using ex vivo gene transfer. Cancer Res 1999;59(20):5160–8.

22. Emens LA, Reilly RT, Jaffee EM. Breast cancer vaccines: maximizing cancer treatment by tapping into host immunity. Endocr Relat Cancer 2005;12(1):1–17.

23. Simons JW, Sacks N. Granulocyte-macrophage colony-stimulating factor-transduced allogeneic cancer cellular immunotherapy: the GVAX vaccine for prostate cancer. Urol Oncol 2006;24(5):419–24.

24. Laheru D, Jaffee EM. Immunotherapy for pancreatic cancer – science driving clinical progress. Nat Rev 2005;5(6):459–67.

25. Nemunaitis J, Sterman D, Jablons D, et al. Granulocyte-macrophage colony-stimulating factor gene-modified autologous tumor vaccines in non-small-cell lung cancer. J Natl Cancer Inst 2004;96(4):326–31.

26. Simons JW, Carducci MA, Mikhak B, et al. Phase I/II trial of an allogeneic cellular immunotherapy in hormone-naive prostate cancer. Clin Cancer Res 2006;12(11 Pt 1):3394–401.

27. Simons JW, Nelson WG, Nemunaitis J, et al. Phase II trials of a GM-CSF gene-transduced prostate cancer cell line vaccine (GVAX) in hormone refractory prostate cancer. Proc Am Soc Clin Oncol 2002;21:729.

28. Groh V, Li YQ, Cioca D, et al. Efficient cross-priming of tumor antigen-specific T cells by dendritic cells sensitized with diverse anti-MICA opsonized tumor cells. Proc Natl Acad Sci U S A 2005;102(18):6461–6.

29. Wolf AM, Wolf D, Steurer M, Gastl G, Gunsilius E, Grubeck-Loebenstein B. Increase of regulatory T cells in the peripheral blood of cancer patients. Clin Cancer Res 2003;9(2):606–12.

30. Walunas TL, Bluestone JA. CTLA-4 regulates tolerance induction and T cell differentiation in vivo. J Immunol 1998;160(8):3855–60.

31. Parry RV, Chemnitz JM, Frauwirth KA, et al. CTLA-4 and PD-1 receptors inhibit T-cell activation by distinct mechanisms. Mol Cell Biol 2005;25(21):9543–53.

32. Hurwitz AA, Foster BA, Kwon ED, et al. Combination immunotherapy of primary prostate cancer in a transgenic mouse model using CTLA-4 blockade. Cancer Res 2000;60(9):2444–8.

33. Kwon ED, Foster BA, Hurwitz AA, et al. Elimination of residual metastatic prostate cancer after surgery and adjunctive cytotoxic T lymphocyte-associated antigen 4 (CTLA-4) blockade immunotherapy. Proc Natl Acad Sci U S A 1999;96(26):15074–9.

34. Kwon ED, Hurwitz AA, Foster BA, et al. Manipulation of T cell costimulatory and inhibitory signals for immunotherapy of prostate cancer. Proc Natl Acad Sci U S A 1997;94(15):8099–103.

35. Freeman GJ, Long AJ, Iwai Y, et al. Engagement of the PD-1 immunoinhibitory receptor by a novel B7 family member leads to negative regulation of lymphocyte activation. J Exp Med 2000;192(7):1027–34.

36. Iwai Y, Ishida M, Tanaka Y, Okazaki T, Honjo T, Minato N. Involvement of PD-L1 on tumor cells in the escape from host immune system and tumor immunotherapy by PD-L1 blockade. Proc Natl Acad Sci U S A 2002;99(19):12293–7.

37. Dong H, Strome SE, Salomao DR, et al. Tumor-associated B7-H1 promotes T-cell apoptosis: a potential mechanism of immune evasion. Nat Med 2002;8(8):793–800.

38. Sun J, Xu K, Wu C, et al. PD-L1 expression analysis in gastric carcinoma tissue and blocking of tumor-associated PD-L1 signaling by two functional monoclonal antibodies. Tissue Antigens 2007;69(1):19–27.

39. Blank C, Brown I, Peterson AC, et al. PD-L1/B7H-1 inhibits the effector phase of tumor rejection by T cell receptor

(TCR) transgenic CD8+ T cells. Cancer Res 2004; 64(3):1140–5.

40. Inman BA, Sebo TJ, Frigola X, et al. PD-L1 (B7-H1) expression by urothelial carcinoma of the bladder and BCG-induced granulomata: associations with localized stage progression. Cancer 2007;109(8):1499–505.

41. Roth TJ, Sheinin Y, Lohse CM, et al. B7-H3 ligand expression by prostate cancer: a novel marker of prognosis and potential target for therapy. Cancer Res 2007;67(16):7893–900.

42. Martin-Orozco N, Wang YH, Yagita H, Dong C. Cutting edge: programmed death (PD) ligand-1/PD-1 interaction is required for CD8+ T cell tolerance to tissue antigens. J Immunol 2006;177(12):8291–5.

43. Wang L, Fraser CC, Kikly K, et al. B7-H3 promotes acute and chronic allograft rejection. Eur J Immunol 2005;35(2):428–38.

44. Xu J, Huang B, Xiong P, et al. Soluble mouse B7-H3 down-regulates dendritic cell stimulatory capacity to allogenic T cell proliferation and production of IL-2 and IFN-gamma. Cell Mol Immunol 2006;3(3):235–40.

45. Nurieva R, Thomas S, Nguyen T, et al. T-cell tolerance or function is determined by combinatorial costimulatory signals. EMBO J 2006;25(11):2623–33.

46. Huang CT, Workman CJ, Flies D, et al. Role of LAG-3 in regulatory T cells. Immunity 2004;21(4):503–13.

47. Zhu X, Yang P, Zhou H, et al. CD4+ CD25+ Tregs express an increased LAG-3 and CTLA-4 in anterior chamber-associated immune deviation. Graefe's Arch Clin Exp Ophthalmol 2007;245(10):1549–57.

48. Zarek PE, Huang CT, Lutz ER, et al. A2A receptor signaling promotes peripheral tolerance by inducing T-cell anergy and the generation of adaptive regulatory T cells. Blood 2008;111(1):251–9.

49. Grosso JF, Kelleher CC, Harris TJ, et al. LAG-3 regulates CD8+ T cell accumulation and effector function in murine self- and tumor-tolerance systems. J Clin Invest 2007;117(11):3383–92.

50. Munn DH, Zhou M, Attwood JT, et al. Prevention of allogeneic fetal rejection by tryptophan catabolism. Science 1998;281(5380):1191–3.

51. Kudo Y, Boyd CA, Spyropoulou I, et al. Indoleamine 2,3-dioxygenase: distribution and function in the developing human placenta. J Reprod Immunol 2004;61(2): 87–98.

52. Mellor AL, Sivakumar J, Chandler P, et al. Prevention of T cell-driven complement activation and inflammation by tryptophan catabolism during pregnancy. Nat Immunol 2001;2(1):64–8.

53. Munn DH, Shafizadeh E, Attwood JT, Bondarev I, Pashine A, Mellor AL. Inhibition of T cell proliferation by macrophage tryptophan catabolism. J Exp Med 1999;189(9): 1363–72.

54. Uyttenhove C, Pilotte L, Theate I, et al. Evidence for a tumoral immune resistance mechanism based on tryptophan degradation by indoleamine 2,3-dioxygenase. Nat Med 2003;9(10):1269–74.

55. Friberg M, Jennings R, Alsarraj M, et al. Indoleamine 2,3-dioxygenase contributes to tumor cell evasion of T cell-mediated rejection. Int J Cancer 2002;101(2): 151–5.

56. Muller AJ, DuHadaway JB, Donover PS, Sutanto-Ward E, Prendergast GC. Inhibition of indoleamine 2,3-dioxygenase, an immunoregulatory target of the cancer suppression gene Bin1, potentiates cancer chemotherapy. Nat Med 2005;11(3):312–9.

57. Ou X, Cai S, Liu P, et al. Enhancement of dendritic cell-tumor fusion vaccine potency by indoleamine-pyrrole 2,3-dioxygenase inhibitor, 1-MT. J Cancer Res Clin Oncol 2008;134(5):525–33.

58. Nigam A, Yacavone RF, Zahurak ML, et al. Immunomodulatory properties of antineoplastic drugs administered in conjunction with GM-CSF-secreting cancer cell vaccines. Int J Oncol 1998;12(1):161–70.

59. Emens LA, Jaffee EM. Leveraging the activity of tumor vaccines with cytotoxic chemotherapy. Cancer Res 2005;65(18):8059–64.

60. Harris TJ, Hipkiss EL, Borzillary S, et al. Radiotherapy augments the immune response to prostate cancer in a time-dependent manner. Prostate 2008;68(12): 1319–29.

Chapter 30
CTLA-4 Blockade for Prostate Cancer Treatment

Andrea L. Harzstark and Lawrence Fong

Abstract The immune system has demonstrated the ability to participate in cancer surveillance, but its role in promoting anticancer activity has only begun to be harnessed. Advances over the last 10 years have made the possibility of immunotherapy for the treatment of cancer a more realistic possibility. Prostate cancer is an ideal target for immunotherapy given its relatively slow growth rate and the time required to generate immune responses. This chapter will discuss an antibody to cytotoxic T lymphocyte antigen-4 (CTLA-4), which can dampen the restraints on T-cell activity to incite a T cell response to tumor, resulting in immune-mediated tumor regression, and the experience with this mechanism in treating advanced prostate cancer.

Keywords CTLA-4 • Ipilimumab • CTLA-4 blockade • Immunotherapy

Introduction

Successful immunotherapy requires the generation of an antigen-specific T cell response. The major components of this response are antigen-presenting cells (APCs), such as dendritic cells, monocytes and macrophages, and T lymphocytes. APCs digest tumor antigens and present them on major histocompatibility complex (MHC) molecules. They are then presented to T lymphocytes, where two independent signals are required for activation [1–3]. The first arises from the interaction between the MHC-bound antigen on the surface of the APC and the corresponding antigen-specific T-cell receptor. The second, or costimulatory signal, results from the interaction between B7.1 (CD80) and B7.2 (CD86), which are molecules present on the surface of APCs, with the T cell receptor CD28. This signal facilitates T-cell activation, promotes T-cell proliferation, and induces T-cell differentiation to the effector phenotype.

There is, however, an important mechanism that is thought to provide balance to this system by preventing too robust an immune response with possible resulting autoimmunity. After CD28 on the T-cell binds to the B7 ligands on the APC, resulting in T-cell activation, CTLA-4 (CD152) relocates to the surface of the T-cell (Fig. 30.1). CTLA-4 is a homolog of CD28 but binds to B7 with 50–200 times the affinity of CD28 [4]. Instead of providing a costimulatory signal, it provides an inhibitory signal to T cells. This serves to abrogate T-cell activation. Evidence of the clinical role of CTLA-4 in preventing too an robust immune response is provided by transgenic mice lacking the CTLA-4 receptor [5, 6]. These mice experience severe lymphoproliferative disorders, which result in multiorgan polyclonal lymphocytic infiltrates and death within 1 month. Further evidence is provided by the fact that mice that lack not only the CTLA-4 receptor but also the CD28 T-cell receptor do not experience the lymphoproliferative disorder [7]. This suggests that, without the costimulatory signal from CD28, there is no need for the inhibitory signal that CTLA-4 binding to B7 provides.

Preclinical

The above observations were taken into preclinical models for confirmation and exploration of clinical utility. It was observed that blockade of the CTLA-4

A.L. Harzstark (✉)
Department of Medicine, Division of Hematology/Oncology,
University of California San Francisco, San Francisco,
CA, USA
e-mail: andrea.harzstark@ucsf.edu

W.D. Figg et al. (eds.), *Drug Management of Prostate Cancer*,
DOI 10.1007/978-1-60327-829-4_30, © Springer Science+Business Media, LLC 2010

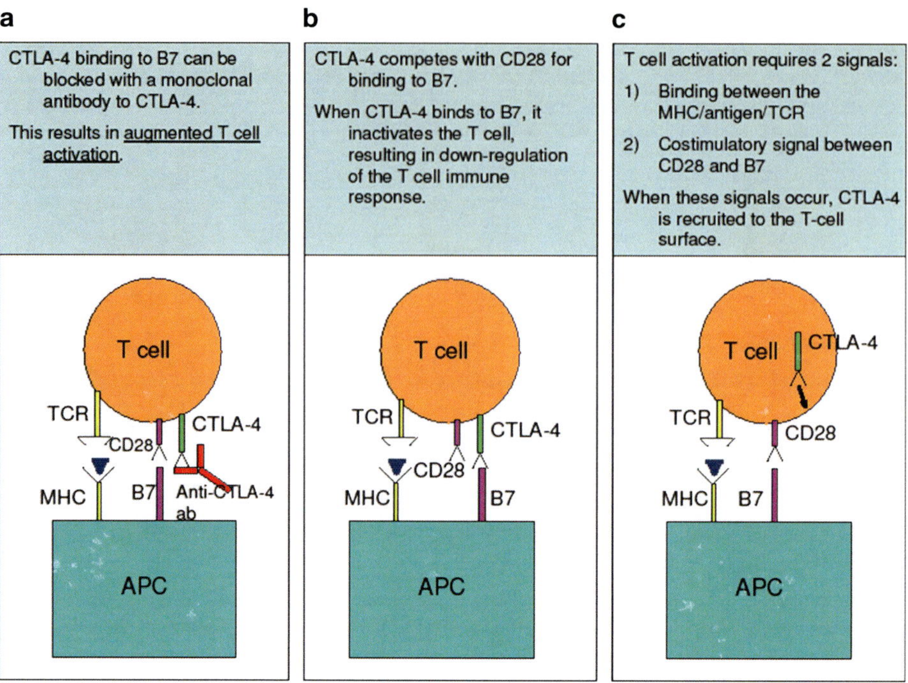

Fig. 30.1 Mechanism of T cell activation. (**a**) T cell activation requires two signals: (1) binding between the MHC/antigen/TCR; (2) costimulatory signal between CD28 and B7. When these signals occur, CTLA-4 is recruited to the T-cell surface. (**b**) CTLA-4 competes with CD28 for binding to B7. When CTLA-4 binds to B7, it inactivates the T cell, resulting in down-regulation of the T cell immune response. (**c**) CTLA-4 binding to B7 can be blocked with a monoclonal antibody to CTLA-4. This results in augmented T cell activation

receptor with an antibody promoted the regression of solid tumors in mice [8]. C57BL/6 mice were injected subcutaneously with tumor cells from TRAMP (transgenic adenocarcinoma of mouse prostate), followed by administration of an anti-CTLA-4 antibody in a proportion of mice. Nearly all of the mice administered anti-CTLA-4 antibody experienced partial or complete regression of subcutaneous TRAMP tumors. In addition, when mice with TRAMP tumors underwent surgical tumor removal, those administered anti-CTLA-4 antibody had metastatic outgrowth that was decreased by approximately 50% [9]. In these preclinical models, the only evidence of autoimmunity was the development of prostatitis and vitiligo.

Clinical

Given the success with CTLA-4 blockade in preclinical models, a fully humanized antibody was developed with the goal of using it in human anticancer therapy without generating antibodies to the therapy. The antibody ipilimumab (Bristol-Myers Squibb, New Jersey) targets the CTLA-4 receptor and has undergone extensive evaluation in melanoma and prostate cancer. For the purpose of this chapter, the discussion will focus on its evaluation in prostate cancer.

The first human study was done in 14 patients with metastatic castration-resistant prostate cancer (CRPC) [10]. Patients had a median age of 70, and a median prostate specific antigen (PSA) of 84.6 ng/mL; all 14 patients had evidence of bone metastases and, an additional four patients had soft tissue metastases, as well. In this study, patients received a single dose of 3 mg/kg of ipilimumab. It was well tolerated with a half-life of 12.5 ± 5.3 days. Two patients experienced PSA declines of at least 50%, lasting 60 and 135 days. These two patients underwent retreatment with a second dose of ipilimumab at the time of PSA progression but neither responded again. An additional eight out of 14 treated patients had a decline in PSA of <50%. Toxicity was reasonable with one patient experiencing a grade three rash/pruritis, which responded to systemic corticosteroids. This suggested that a single dose of ipilimumab was well tolerated and associated with some antitumor activity.

Combination Therapy

Repetitive doses have also been administered, both as monotherapy and in combination with other agents. Multiple studies have evaluated whether vaccination with tumor cells modified to express granulocyte-macrophage colony-stimulating factor (GM-CSF) can improve the effectiveness of CTLA-4 blockade. Treatment of TRAMP mice with a vaccine consisting of irradiated tumor cells modified to secrete GM-CSF resulted in a reduction in tumor incidence 2 months after treatment [11]. Treated mice were also found to have lower grade tumors with accumulation of inflammatory cells in interductal spaces.

GM-CSF is a growth factor for APCs and is able to induce PSA declines in patients with CRPC. Results from a phase I trial of GM-CSF in combination with escalating doses of ipilimumab have been reported [12]. GM-CSF was administered 250 μg/m^2/day SQ on days 1–14 of a 28-day cycle. Ipilimumab was administered as doses ranging from 0.5 to 10 mg/kg every 4 weeks, originally 4 times and eventually 6 times per patient. In the highest dose level reported to date (3 mg/kg), 50% of patients experienced PSA declines of at least 50%, and one patient experienced a partial radiographic response in liver metastases. Three of the 24 patients treated had grade three immune-related toxicities: grade three rash in one patient at a dosage of 1.5 mg/kg, grade three rash and panhypopituitarism in one patient at 3 mg/kg, and grade three colitis in one patient treated at 3 mg/kg. There was evidence of a dose–response relationship between anti-CTLA-4 antibody dosage and antigen-specific CD8+ T cells after treatment. In addition, an expansion of circulating CD4+ FoxP3+ regulatory T cells, which are thought to be immunosuppressive, was also seen with treatment. Once the maximum tolerated dose has been determined, a phase II expansion cohort and a randomized phase II study of ipilimumab monotherapy or in combination with GM-CSF is planned.

Ipilimumab has also been combined with the prostate cancer vaccine GVAX [13]. GVAX is a prostate cancer cell line modified to secrete GM-CSF and irradiated. A phase I/II study of GVAX in combination with ipilimumab is underway and has been reported. During the dose escalation portion of the study, 12 patients were treated with biweekly intradermal injections of GVAX and every 4 week doses of ipilimumab at a dosage of either 0.3 or 1 or 3 or 5 mg/kg. Median follow-up for these 12 patients is 21.2 months, and five of six patients treated at 3 or 5 mg/kg experienced grade two or three immune-related toxicities, including one patient with grade two or three hypophysitis and one patient with grade three alveolitis. Late onset PSA responses were seen in five patients, with durations of 6.7, 8.6, 9.5, 13.8 (ongoing), and 23.1 months. Four patients had stable disease by bone scan for at least 12 months. The expansion cohort consisted of 16 patients treated at a dosage of 3 mg/kg ipilimumab. Six patients have completed treatment; three have experienced immune-related toxicities, including one with grade one diarrhea, one with grade three adrenal insufficiency, and one with grade three hepatitis, which resolved with steroids. The median follow-up in the six patients who have completed treatment is 6.5 months; one patient has had a PSA decline of at least 50%, and three additional patients have had a stable PSA (including one patient with pain relief). Tumor-reactive antibodies induced by treatment have been identified using serologic analysis and include antibodies to filamin B, PSMA, and NY-ESO-1. Biopsies of injection sites have revealed evidence of T-cell infiltration. These results suggest that the use of CTLA-4 blockade in combination with other immunostimulatory therapies is promising and well tolerated. In addition, they provide proof of principle that an antigen-specific immune response can be generated.

However, the question arises as to whether there is a more effective way to improve antigen presentation to augment the immunostimulatory effects of CTLA-4 blockade. The cytotoxic effects of radiotherapy could potentially serve as a means of antigen priming, improving antigen presentation [14]. Radiation has long been known to have the ability to reduce tumor growth outside the field of radiation, which is known as the abscopal effect [15]. The biology of this is poorly understood, but it is thought to generate both tumor-specific antigen from dying cells and maturation stimuli necessary for the activation of tumor-specific T cells by dendritic cells [16, 17].

This theory was demonstrated in a study of mice with a syngeneic mammary carcinoma in both flanks who received radiation with or without a dendritic cell growth factor, Flt3-Ligand (Flt3-L) [17]. One tumor was irradiated and the effect on the other tumor was recorded. In mice who received radiation alone, the growth of the nonirradiated tumor was not impaired, while in mice who received Flt3-L, in addition to radiation, growth of the nonirradiated tumor was impaired. Growth of the nonirradiated tumor was not impaired in mice who received Flt3-L without radiation, suggesting radiation has the potential for additional benefit when combined with other agents. The dose of radiation (either two or six Gray) did not affect the results in this study. The effects were also noted to be tumor-specific; treatment with Flt-3 and radiation did not affect a second tumor of a different type. Demaria et al. have also shown that the combination of external beam radiation therapy (EBRT) and CTLA-4 blockade can be synergistic for inducing tumor responses in a murine model of an implantable breast cancer tumor line [17].

Based on the above results, a clinical trial for pre- and postchemotherapy patients with metastatic CRPC was launched, in which patients were treated with escalating doses of ipilimumab every 3 weeks for four doses at levels of 3, 5, and 10 mg/kg [18]. After the 10 mg/kg cohort was completed, a single fraction of radiation to up to three bony sites of disease was given within 24–48 h prior to initiating the first dose of ipilimumab. The primary endpoint was safety. Results for the first 26 patients have been reported to date, including eight, six, and six patients treated at the 3, 5, and 10 mg/kg dose levels, respectively, and six patients treated in the first radiation cohort. Nine patients experienced grade three or four immune-related toxicities, including diarrhea/colitis in six, hepatitis in two, and rash in one. Toxicities were responsive to immunosuppression. One patient died of opportunistic infections after 3 months of immunosuppression for colitis. Six patients (23%) experienced a PSA decline of at least 50% with a median duration of 140 days and a range from 49 to over 269 days. The median time for onset of response was 84 days with a range from 41 to 147, underscoring the need to allow for prolonged period until response is observed in studies of this agent. One of seven patients with measurable disease had a partial response in nodal metastases and the prostate and achieved an undetectable PSA after treatment with 10 mg/kg. All patients who experienced responses also experienced immune-related toxicities. Phase III evaluation of ipilimumab in combination with radiation is underway.

from exuberant activity of the immune system causing self-directed immune activity. In melanoma, these events have been demonstrated to correlate with tumor regression [19]. Attia et al. evaluated 56 patients with metastatic melanoma, 29 of whom were treated with ipilimumab 3 mg/kg every 3 weeks and 27 of whom were treated with ipilimumab 3 mg/kg initially followed by 2 mg/kg every 3 weeks. All the patients also received vaccination with two modified HLA-A*0201-restricted peptides from the gp100 melanoma-associated antigen, gp100:209–217(210 M) and gp100:280–288(288 V). Two patients had complete responses, which were ongoing at the time of report at 30 and 31 months and five patients had partial responses, lasting four, six, and ongoing at 25, 26, and 34 months. The overall objective response rate for the cohort was 13%. Fourteen patients experienced grade three or four IRAEs. Five (36%) out of the 14 patients who experienced these toxicities had a clinical response, compared to only two (5%) responses in the 42 patients without autoimmune toxicity ($P = 0.008$). This correlation demonstrates a relationship between IRAEs and activity in melanoma. A similar relationship in prostate cancer has not been definitively demonstrated but is hypothesized to exist, as well.

The mechanism for these toxicities has been demonstrated to be immune in nature with colonoscopies performed on patients with enterocolitis demonstrating increases in intraepithelial lymphocytes, increases in CD3 and CD8 T-cell markers, as well as increases in CD3+ CD4+ lymphocytes and eosinophils [19]. Similarly, biopsy of areas involved by dermatitis revealed papillary dermal edema, at times with pervascular lymphocytic infiltrates, which was CD3+ CD8+ and CD3+ CD4+. Liver biopsy revealed acute hepatitis with a predominantly lymphocytic infiltrate in a lobular pattern of inflammation and predominantly CD4+ cells in the periportal regions and CD8+ cells in the hepatic lobules. Most of the noncancer-bearing organs targeted by T cells for the toxicities observed (colon, duodenum, liver, eye, and pituitary) do not express the gp100 antigen, suggesting that the autoimmunity was not a result of the peptide vaccination, but rather the result of broken self-tolerance induced by CTLA-4 blockade.

Toxicity (and Response)

Immune-related toxicities have been termed immune-related adverse events (IRAEs) and are thought to result

Future Directions

Recently, immunogenic prostate tumor antigens identified by CTLA-4 blockade have been reported. Using the

TRAMP model, CTLA-4 in vivo blockade was administered in combination with a GM-CSF expressing TRAMP-C2 cell vaccine to generate an anti-TRAMP tumor response in nontransgenic, syngeneic C57BL/6 mice [20]. Tumor-specific T cells were isolated, and the first T-cell-defined TRAMP tumor antigen was expression cloned. It has been named *Spas-1* (stimulator of prostatic adenocarcinoma-specific T cells-1), and its expression is found to be increased in advanced primary TRAMP tumors. Immunization with dendritic cells pulsed with a peptide containing its immunodominant epitope SNC9-Ha resulted in protection against TRAMP-C2 tumor challenge, suggesting that this is a potentially attractive target antigen for the development of antigen-targeted immunotherapies, likely in combination with CTLA-4 directed therapy. SPAS-1 has a human ortholog known as SH3GLB2, which is known to be immunogenic in humans in vitro. The future for CTLA-4 blockade is likely to be in combination with other agents, such as vaccination with a SH3GLB2 containing peptide, with the hope of generating a more specific response.

In addition, CTLA-4 blockade will likely be combined with therapies that attempt to uncouple antitumor activity from toxicity. CD4+ regulatory T cells (Tregs) are a naturally occurring subpopulation of T cells with immunosuppressive function. Tregs prevent autoimmunity but can also inhibit rejection of transplants, regulate the immune response to infectious diseases, and suppress antitumor responses. Although present in mice and humans, at approximately 3–10% of all CD4+ T cells, Tregs have been shown to accumulate in blood and tumor sites in murine cancer models and cancer patients. The presence of Tregs within tumors has been shown to be inversely correlated with survival in ovarian cancer patients [21]. Treg depletion can induce tumor rejection in some murine tumor models [22]. The addition of Treg depletion to treatment with CTLA4 blockade can enhance antitumor immunity in mouse models [23]. Treatment with anti-CTLA4 antibody has been demonstrated to expand Tregs in vivo in prostate cancer patients. Depletion of Tregs may therefore enhance the antitumor immune responses induced with CTLA4 blockade in cancer patients.

Naturally occurring Tregs constitutively express CD25, a component of the high-affinity IL2 receptor, on their cell surface. Denileukin diftitox (Ontak, Ligand Pharmaceuticals) is an IL2-fusion toxin that is FDA-approved for use in treatment of cutaneous T-cell Lymphoma (CTCL), an IL2 receptor-expressing malignancy. Denileukin diftitox has been shown to reduce Tregs in tissue culture and in vivo in renal cell and ovarian cancer patients [24, 25]. Similarly, metronomic chemotherapy, specifically, oral cyclophosphamide, has demonstrated the ability to deplete Tregs in advanced cancer patients [26]. A better understanding of the role of Tregs and the utilization of methods to deplete them may make use of CTLA-4 blockade, a more realistic clinical possibility.

There have been recent strides in understanding the role of Tregs with the demonstration that anti-CTLA-4 antibody does not deplete human regulatory T cells in vivo; instead, it may mediate its effects through the activation of effector T cells [27]. Tregs constitutively express higher levels of CTLA-4 that translocate to the cell surface than effector T cells, and therefore, they may be more strongly regulated by the inhibitor effects of CTLA-4 than effector T cells. Lower antibody doses may actually result in the expansion of regulatory T cells, with expansion of effector T cells only at a higher threshold antibody dosage. This may make it possible to modulate the immune response to CTLA-4 blockade in the future using antibody dosage.

Conclusions

Much remains to be learned about the role of the immune system in cancer treatment and what stage of disease is the best place for application for these agents. In addition, the clinical trials community is learning how to design trials around immunologic agents, which may require additional time to demonstrate responses. Advances are being made in many of these issues, and if the toxicity of CTLA-4 blockade can be managed without compromising efficacy, the potential of CTLA-4 blockade for anticancer therapy is likely to be harnessed for clinical benefit.

References

1. Frauwirth KA, Thompson, CB. Activation and inhibition of lymphocytes by costimulation. J Clin Invest 2002;109(3): 295–9.
2. Chambers C, Kuhns MS, Egen JG, Allison JP. CTLA-4-mediated inhibition in regulation of T cell responses: mechanisms and manipulation in tumor immunotherapy. Annu Rev Immunol 2001;19:565–94.
3. Chen L. Co-inhibitory molecules of the B7-CD28 family in the control of T-cell immunity. Nat Rev Immunol 2004;4(5):336–47.

4. Thompson RH, Allison JP, Kwon ED. Anti-cytotoxic T lymphocyte antigen-4 (CTLA-4) immunotherapy for the treatment of prostate cancer. Urol Oncol 2006;24(5):442–7.

5. Waterhouse P, Penninger JM, Timms E, Wakeham A. Lymphoproliferative disorders with early lethality in mice deficient in Ctla-4. Science 1995;270(5238):985–8.

6. Tivol EA, Borriello F, Schweitzer AN, Lynch WP, Bluestone JA, Sharpe AH. Loss of CTLA-4 leads to massive lymphoproliferation and fatal multiorgan tissue destruction, revealing a critical negative regulatory role of CTLA-4. Immunity 1995;3(5):541–7.

7. Mandelbrot DA, McAdam AJ, Sharpe AH. B7-1 or B7-2 is required to produce the lymphoproliferative phenotype in mice lacking cytotoxic T lymphocyte-associated antigen 4 (CTLA-4). J Exp Med 1999;189(2):435–40.

8. Kwon ED, Hurwitz AA, Foster BA, et al. Manipulation of T cell costimulatory and inhibitory signals for immunotherapy of prostate cancer. Proc Natl Acad Sci U S A 1997;94(15):8099–103.

9. Kwon ED, Foster BA, Hurwitz AA, et al. Elimination of residual metastatic prostate cancer after surgery and adjunctive cytotoxic T lymphocyte-associated antigen 4 (CTLA-4) blockade immunotherapy. Proc Natl Acad Sci U S A 1999;96(26):15074–9.

10. Small EJ, Tchekmedyian NS, Rini B, et al. A pilot trial of CTLA-4 blockade with human anti-CTLA-4 in patients with hormone-refractory prostate cancer. Clin Cancer Res 2007;13(6):1810–5.

11. Hurwitz AA, Kwon ED, Truong T, Choi EM, Greenberg NM, Burg MB, Allison JP. Combination immunotherapy of primary prostate cancer in a transgenic mouse model using CTLA-4 blockade. Cancer Res 2000;60(9):2444–8.

12. Fong L, et al. Combination immunotherapy with GM-CSF and CTLA-4 blockade for hormone refractory prostate cancer: balancing the expansion of activated effector and regulatory T cells. J Clin Oncol 2007 ASCO Annual Meeting Proceedings 2007;25(18S):3001.

13. Gerritsen W, van den Eertwegh AJ, T. de Gruijl T, et al. Expanded phase I combination trial of GVAX immunotherapy for prostate cancer and ipilimumab in patients with metastatic hormone-refractory prostate cancer (mHRPC). Proc Am Soc Clin Oncol 2008:Abstr 5146.

14. Friedman EJ. Immune modulation by ionizing radiation and its implications for cancer immunotherapy. Curr Pharm Des 2002;8(19):1765–80.

15. Mole RH. Whole body irradiation; radiobiology or medicine? Br J Radiol 1953;26(305):234–41.

16. Demaria S, Ng B, Devitt ML, et al. Ionizing radiation inhibition of distant untreated tumors (abscopal effect) is immune mediated. Int J Radiat Oncol Biol Phys 2004;58(3):862–70.

17. Demaria S, Yang AM, Devitt ML, Babb JS, Allison JP, Formenti SC. Immune-mediated inhibition of metastases after treatment with local radiation and CTLA-4 blockade in a mouse model of breast cancer. Clin Cancer Res 2005;11(2 Pt 1):728–34.

18. Beer TM, Slovin SF, Higano CS, et al. Phase I trial of ipilimumab (IPI) alone and in combination with radiotherapy (XRT) in patients with metastatic castration resistant prostate cancer (mCRPC). Proc Am Soc Clin Oncol 2008:Abstr 5004.

19. Attia P, Phan GQ, Maker AV, et al. Autoimmunity correlates with tumor regression in patients with metastatic melanoma treated with anti-cytotoxic T-lymphocyte antigen-4. J Clin Oncol 2005;23(25):6043–53.

20. Fasso M, Waitz R, Hou Y, et al. SPAS-1 (stimulator of prostatic adenocarcinoma-specific T cells)/SH3GLB2: a prostate tumor antigen identified by CTLA-4 blockade. Proc Natl Acad Sci U S A 2008;105(9):3509–14.

21. Kryczek I, Wei S, Zhu G, et al. Relationship between B7-H4, regulatory T cells, and patient outcome in human ovarian carcinoma. Cancer Res 2007;67(18):8900–5.

22. Imai H, Saio M, Nonaka K, et al. Depletion of CD4+ CD25+ regulatory T cells enhances interleukin-2-induced antitumor immunity in a mouse model of colon adenocarcinoma. Cancer Sci 2007;98(3):416–23.

23. Tuve S, Chen B-M, Liu Y, et al. Combination of tumor site-located CTL-associated antigen-4 blockade and systemic regulatory T-cell depletion induces tumor-destructive immune responses. Cancer Res 2007;67(12):5929–39.

24. Morse MA, Hobeika AC, Osada T, et al. Depletion of human regulatory T cells specifically enhances antigen-specific immune responses to cancer vaccines. Blood 2008;112(3):610–8.

25. Dannull J, Su Z, Rizzieri D, et al. Enhancement of vaccine-mediated antitumor immunity in cancer patients after depletion of regulatory T cells. J Clin Invest 2005;115(12):3623–33.

26. Ghiringhelli F, Menard C, PE Puig PE, et al. Metronomic cyclophosphamide regimen selectively depletes CD4+ CD25+ regulatory T cells and restores T and NK effector functions in end stage cancer patients. Cancer Immunol Immunother 2007;56(5):641–8.

27. Kavanagh B, O'Brien S, Lee D, et al. CTLA4 blockade expands FoxP3+ regulatory and activated effector CD4+ T cells in a dose-dependent fashion. Blood 2008;112(4):1175–83.

Part VI
Prevention

Chapter 31
Prostate Cancer Chemoprevention Strategies

Howard L. Parnes, Margaret G. House, and Joseph A. Tangrea

Abstract Carcinogenesis is the multistep process by which normal cells undergo malignant transformation. The clinical expression of cancer may be prevented or delayed either by risk factor modification, such as quitting smoking, or by the administration of drugs to prevent or delay the clinical expression of the malignant phenotype. This chapter focuses on the latter approach, often referred to as "chemoprevention." Specifically, it addresses the two key issues distinguishing cancer prevention from cancer treatment agent development: selection of study endpoints and patient cohorts. In addition, a comprehensive update is provided of recently completed and ongoing phase 1, 2, and 3 prostate cancer prevention clinical trials conducted under the auspices of the Division of Cancer Prevention, NCI.

Keywords Chemoprevention • Agent development • Study endpoints • Patient cohorts • PCPT • SELECT • REDUCE

Abbreviations

8-OH-dG	8-Hydroxydeoxyguanosine is a marker of oxidative DNA damage
AR	Androgen receptor
Bax	A proapoptotic gene
Bcl-2	An anti-apoptotic proto-oncogene
Caspase-3	Caspases are critical effectors of apoptosis
cd31	Membrane protein cell–cell interactions, adhesion
CDC6	Cell division cycle 6 protein
CgA	Chromogranin A may be useful in establishing a prostate cancer diagnosis, determining prognosis, and predicting response to treatment
COX	Cyclooxygenase
DFMO	α-Difluoromethylornithine
DHCR24	Also known as seladin-1 is an anti-apoptotic protein
DHT	Dihydrotestosterone
DIM	3,3′-Di-indolylmethane
DNA	Deoxyribonucleic acid
E	Estradiol
ELISA	Enzyme-linked immunosorbent assay
HGPIN	High-grade prostatic intraepithelial neoplasia
IGF	Insulin-like growth factor
IGFBP3	Insulin-like growth factor binding protein 3
IHC	Immunohistochemistry
Ki-67	A marker of cellular proliferation
KLK2	Kallikrein-related peptidase 2 serum levels of human kallikrein increase with progression from benign prostate epithelium to primary cancer and metastatic disease
M30	A marker of apoptosis
MIB-1	A monoclonal antibody that detects the Ki-67 antigen
MMP	Matrix metalloproteinase
mRNA	Messenger ribonucleic acid
NF-κB	Nuclear factor-kappa B
ODD	Oxidative DNA damage
p21	A cyclin-dependent kinase cell cycle control
p27	A cyclin-dependent kinase inhibitor cell cycle control
P53	A tumor suppressor gene
Par-4	Protease activated receptor 4
PCNA	Proliferating cell nuclear antigen
PG	Prostaglandin

H.L. Parnes (✉)
Prostate and Urologic Cancer Research Group, NCI-Division of Cancer Prevention, Center for Cancer Research, National Cancer Institute, Bethesda, MD, USA
e-mail: parnesh@mail.nih.gov

W.D. Figg et al. (eds.), *Drug Management of Prostate Cancer*,
DOI 10.1007/978-1-60327-829-4_31, © Springer Science+Business Media, LLC 2010

PIN	Prostatic intraepithelial neoplasia
PPE	Polyphenon E
PSA	Prostate-specific antigen
PSAV	Prostate-specific antigen velocity
PTEN	A tumor suppressor gene
qRT-PCR	Reverse transcriptase-polymerase chain reaction
Se	Selenium
Se-met	Selenomethionine
SHBG	Sex hormone binding globulin
T	Testosterone
TGF-β	Transforming growth factor-beta 2
TUNEL	Terminal deoxynucleotidyl transferase (TdT)-mediated dUTP nick-end labeling
VEGF	Vascular endothelial growth factor

Introduction

Carcinogenesis

Carcinogenesis is the multistep process by which normal cells undergo malignant transformation. It is characterized by genetic and epigenetic alterations that disrupt the regulatory pathways controlling cell growth, apoptosis, and differentiation [1–3]. The observation that premalignant, noninvasive lesions often precede invasive carcinoma by decades suggests the possibility of intervening before the malignant phenotype is established [4, 5]. This may be achieved by modifying behaviors, for example, smoking cessation, or through "chemoprevention," the administration of natural or synthetic agents to reverse, inhibit, slow, or prevent the development of cancer [6].

Chemoprevention

Despite the advances in the treatment and the widespread adoption of PSA screening, prostate cancer remains the second leading cause of cancer death in the US males. Although screening clearly improves prostate cancer *survival*, which is subject to substantial lead-time and length bias, its impact on prostate cancer *mortality* is not known. This critical issue is the subject of two randomized, controlled clinical trials, and the results of which are eagerly anticipated. Even if shown to reduce prostate cancer mortality, population screening for prostate cancer will be associated with treatment-related morbidity as well as substantial financial costs. Given the inherent risks of screening, the nonmodifiable nature of the major prostate cancer risk factors (age, race, and family history), the difficulty of determining which cancers require treatment and the long natural history of this disease, prevention may be the best strategy to reduce the burden of prostate cancer.

Prostate Cancer Prevention Clinical Trials

Chemoprevention Agent Development

As the target population for cancer prevention drug therapy does not have overt disease and would likely require an extended period of treatment, chemoprevention agents must meet a very high standard with regard to toxicity, convenience, and cost. It is, therefore, not surprising that the majority of agents currently being studied for this purpose are bioactive dietary didid components. Examples include soy, lycopene, vitamins D and E, green tea catechins, and 3,3'-diindolyomethane (DIM). Supporting evidence for these and other agents has come from epidemiological observations, clinical trials, and experimental animal models [7].

Trial Endpoints

Chemoprevention agent development poses a number of challenges not faced in cancer treatment drug development. The major issues in this regard are the identification of study cohorts and the selection of endpoints. Given the long natural history of prostate cancer, one must rely upon intermediate endpoints, for example, biomarkers of response, to obtain preliminary evidence of efficacy [8]. The major categories of biomarkers include histopathologic markers (e.g., high-grade prostatic intraepithelial neoplasia or HGPIN), tissue-based markers of proliferation and apoptosis (Ki-67 and TUNEL assays, respectively), and serum markers (e.g., PSA) [9]. The reliance on intermediate endpoints requires that studies be well controlled, preferably placebo-controlled, as comparisons of intermediate endpoints before and after an uncontrolled intervention can be difficult to interpret.

Study Cohorts

Although appropriate cohorts for cancer treatment trials are readily defined, identifying cohorts for prostate cancer prevention studies poses a challenge. Even though the obvious answer would seem to be individuals who are at high risk of developing prostate cancer, the fact remains that all men are at substantial risk of this disease.

Given the importance of tissue-based intermediate endpoint biomarkers in the evaluation of putative cancer prevention agents, the ideal candidate for a prostate cancer chemoprevention trial is a man in whom prostate tissue will be obtained during the course of standard management. Examples include men with (1) HGPIN, (2) a positive family history, (3) an elevated PSA with a negative biopsy, (4) prostate cancer being followed with "watchful waiting" (more properly referred to as "active surveillance"), and (5) men with prostate cancer scheduled for surgery, i.e., preprostatectomy cohort. The NCI is currently supporting prostate cancer chemoprevention studies in each of these cohorts (Table 31.1).

Table 31.1 Completed phase II chemoprevention trials: selected results NCI-sponsored prostate cancer prevention trials

Study design	Cohort	Agent	Endpoints	Sample size	Status
Phase II, placebo control	Preprostatectomy	Lycopene (30 or 60 mg) 6 weeks	Tissue, serum lycopene levels DHT, T, PSA Ki-67, TUNEL	8/75	Ongoing [15]
Phase II, placebo control	Watchful waiting	Lycopene (30 mg) vs. Omega-3 fatty acids (1 g) 3 months	Gene expression IGF-1, COX-2 Clinical progression	85/180	Ongoing [16]
Phase II, placebo control	Watchful waiting	Isoflavones (80 mg) 3 months	Isoflavone levels, PSA T, E, SHBG	53/148	Study completed: No effect on PSA, T, E, or SHBG [17]
Phase II, placebo control	High-risk, postradical prostatectomy	Soy protein 20 g (24 mg genistein and 40 mg total isoflavones) 24 months	Two year PSA failure rate Time to PSA failure	161/284	Ongoing [18]
Phase II, placebo control	Preprostatectomy	Genistein (150, 300, 600 mg) 2–6 weeks	Oxidative stress (ODD) Plasma, tissue levels	34/80	Study completed: Preliminary results – no change in oxidative stress biomarkers; paradoxical increase in IGF-1 in 600 mg group; increase in plasma and tissue genistein levels in treated patients [19]
Phase II, placebo control	Preprostatectomy	Genistein (2 mg/kg/day) 1–2 months	Morphology (adhesion) Gene expression PSA, T, PCNA, apoptotic index	37/80	Accrual completed: Preliminary results – altered expression of motility genes [20]
Phase III, placebo control	Elevated PSA/ negative biopsy	Se-yeast (200, 400 µg) Up to 57 months	Prostate cancer PSAV Prostate cancer progression: alkaline phosphatase, CgA	612/700	Accrual completed: Analysis pending [21]

(continued)

Table 31.1 (continued)

Study design	Cohort	Agent	Endpoints	Sample size	Status
Phase II, placebo control	Watchful waiting	Se-yeast (200, 800 µg*) Average duration 45 months *800 arm dropped in 2000 due to toxicity	PSAV, prostate cancer progression: alkaline phosphatase, CgA Bcl-2, Ki-67, thioredoxin reductase, glutathione peroxidase	159/220	Accrual completed: Analysis pending [21]
Phase II, placebo control	Healthy men	Se-yeast (240, 350 µg) Se-met (200 µg) 9 months	Plasma & urine selenium concentration DHT, T, PSA	0/300	Ongoing [22]
Phase II, placebo control	Preprostatectomy or prebrachy-therapy	Se-met (400 µg) 8–9 weeks	Androgen receptor (AR) gene expression in prostate tissue Expression of AR related genes, e.g., PSA, KLK2, CDC6, DHCR24	0/70	Ongoing [23]
Phase II, placebo control	Preprostatectomy	Se-met (400 µg), Finasteride (5 mg) 8–9 weeks	PSA gene expression- TUNEL, caspase-3, ELISA	0/164	Ongoing [24]
Phase II, placebo control	Preprostatectomy	Se-met (200 µg) 14–31 days	Prostate selenium concentration Serum & seminal vesicle selenium levels; PSA levels	68/68	Study completed: 22% increase in prostate selenium concentra-tion [25]
Phase III, placebo control	HGPIN	Se-met (200 µg) 3 years	Prostate cancer incidence- TUNEL, Ki-67	440/465	Accrual completed: Analysis pending [23]
Phase II, 2×2 placebo control	Preprostatectomy	Se-met (200 g), vitamin E (400 mg) 3–6 weeks	FeasibilityKi-67, NFkB, COX-2, p53 Tissue selenium levels	48/48	Accrual competed: Analysis pending [26]
Phase III, 2×2×2×2, placebo control	US male physicians	Vitamin E (400 mg), vitamin C (500 mg), multivitamin (Centrum Silver) 10 years	Total cancer risk; vascular events Prostate, colon cancer risk; myocardial infarction, cerebrovascular accident; macular degeneration; cognitive function	14,641	Ongoing: Vitamin E and vitamin C arms closed; multivitamin arm ongoing [27]
Phase I, placebo control	Preprostatectomy	Green Tea Catechins (800 mg PPE) 3–6 weeks	Tissue catechin levles Clusterin, MMPs, IGFs, 8-0H-dG	18/50	Ongoing [21]
Phase II, placebo Control	HGPIN	Green Tea Catechins (400 mg PPE) 12 months	Compliance, toxicity, quality of life Prostate Cancer NFkB, Ki-67, TUNEL	1/240	Ongoing [17]
Phase Ib, placebo control	Preprostatectomy	DIM (100, 200 mg) 3–4 weeks	Tissue DIM levels T, PSA, IGFs, AR localization Ki-67, TUNEL, caspase-3	45/45	Accrual completed: Analysis pending [28]
Phase II, placebo control	Preprostatectomy	Hecterol (10 µg) 4–6 weeks	Nuclear morphology HGPIN TUNEL, VEGF, IGFs	31/60	Study completed: Preliminary results – decrease in HGPIN; decrease TGF-β; increase IGFBP3 [29]

(continued)

Table 31.1 (continued)

Study design	Cohort	Agent	Endpoints	Sample size	Status
Phase II, historical and concurrent controls	Preprostatectomy	Sulindac sulfone (375 mg QD) 4 weeks	Apoptosis markers: bcl-2, Bax, Par-4, M30, TUNEL, PTEN PSA, HGPIN, MIB-1, DNA ploidy	105/130	Study completed: Prelminiary results – no differences in markers of apoptosis [30]
Phase II placebo control	Preprostatectomy	Celecoxib (400 mg b.i.d.) 4–6 weeks	Tissue PG levels COX-2, mRNA expression, DNA oxidation, p27, p21, PCNA, and Ki-67, PSA	64/65	Study completed: Preliminary results – no observed effects on PG, COX-2, and oxidized DNA base levels [31]
Phase III, placebo control "PCPT" (Prostate Cancer Prevention Trial: primary prevention)	Age > 55 PSA < 3 Digital rectal exam – within normal limits	Finasteride (5 mg/day) 7 years	7-Year period prevalence of prostate cancer Gleason Score, other cancers, toxicity	18,882	Study completed: Results – 24.8% decrease in 7-year period prevalence of prostate cancer [32]
Phase II, placebo control	Preprostatectomy	Finasteride (5 mg/day) 4–6 weeks	Effect of finasteride on IHC markers associated with high-grade Gleason Score	95/200	Ongoing [26]
Phase II, placebo control	Positive family history with negative biopsy	DFMO (500 mg QD) 1 year	Prostate polyamines levels (putrescine, spermine and spermadine), PSA	81/100	Study Completed: Results – significant change only in putrescine levels [33]
Phase II, placebo control	Preprostatectomy	Toremifene (40 mg QD) 3–6 weeks	HGPIN Index bcl-2, Ki-67, cd31 DHT, T, PSA, E	52/78	Study completed: Preliminary results – no effect on either HGPIN or biomarkers [34]

HGPIN Cohort

In the late 1990s, several small studies supported the position that the presence of HGPIN in a prostate biopsy was associated with an increased risk of cancer (as much as 40–50%) and that patients with HGPIN required close surveillance (follow-up and repeat biopsies). For example, in a study from Johns Hopkins, repeat biopsies identified cancer in 32.2% of 245 men with a prior diagnosis of HGPIN. The number of cores with high-grade PIN proved to be the only independent predictor of a cancer diagnosis: 30.2% with 1 or 2 cores, 40% with 3 cores, and 75% with >3 cores [10]. The more intensive follow-up and biopsy regimen suggested for an HGPIN diagnosis made this group of patients the potential candidates for

chemoprevention studies. Indeed, a few NCI-sponsored chemoprevention studies using this cohort were started during this time period and some are still underway including a phase 3, placebo-controlled trial of selenomethionine and a phase 2 study of polyphenon E. In recent years, however, larger, better-controlled studies have provided data showing that the subsequent risk of prostate cancer is not as great as originally observed and the standard of care is changing [11]. In fact, recent studies have shown that the cumulative risk of the detection of carcinoma on serial follow-up biopsies did not differ significantly between those with an initial diagnosis of HGPIN on biopsy compared with a control group, prompting reconsideration of repeat biopsy strategies for HGPIN patients [12].

Positive Family History Cohort

Epidemiological studies indicate that dominantly inherited susceptibility genes with high penetrance may cause as much as 5–10% of all prostate cancer cases, and as much as 30–40% of early onset disease [13]. Having a brother with prostate cancer may confer a greater risk than a father [14], possibly because the gene for the androgen receptor is located on the X-chromosome. The NCI is not currently sponsoring any chemoprevention trials in men with a positive family history.

Elevated PSA, Negative Biopsy Cohort

Men with an elevated PSA and a negative biopsy represent another potentially useful cohort for chemoprevention agent development. Although the absolute risk of finding prostate cancer on a subsequent biopsy is dependent upon the number of biopsy cores that have previously been examined, most men in this category will undergo repeat biopsies making them good candidates for clinical trials addressing intermediate biomarker endpoints. The NCI is currently sponsoring trials of high selenium yeast and soy in this cohort.

Active Surveillance Cohort

Since men with prostate cancer being followed with active surveillance (previously referred to as "watchful waiting") are routinely recommended to follow-up biopsies to monitor their disease status, these men represent another informative cohort for chemoprevention agent development. This group also provides an important population in whom to evaluate the usefulness of genomics and proteomics to predict the natural history of this heterogeneous disease. The NCI is currently sponsoring trials of high-selenium yeast, as well as lycopene and omega-3 fatty acids in this cohort.

Preprostatectomy Cohort

Men with localized prostate cancer planning to undergo definitive surgery represent another highly informative cohort. Study agents are generally administered for 3–6 weeks in this model, the period of time between the diagnostic biopsy and prostatectomy. Despite the short duration of drug exposure, valuable information can be obtained regarding the effect of the study drug on intermediate endpoint biomarkers and distribution of the candidate agent in prostate tissue, since the entire gland will become available at the time of surgery. As shown in Table 31.1, most of the drugs currently in phase 2 testing in the NCI prostate cancer chemoprevention agent development program are being evaluated in this cohort.

Chemoprevention Clinical Trial Program

The Prostate and Urologic Cancers Research Group in the Division of Cancer Prevention, NCI has sponsored a number of Phase I, II, and III chemoprevention trials that are completed or currently underway. A complete list of these trials is included in Table 31.1.

Five NCI-sponsored phase II prostate chemoprevention trials that were initiated in 2001–2003 have been completed and their data have been analyzed. All five trials employed the presurgical study design where men with localized prostate cancer are enrolled and the study agent is administered for the 3–6 weeks between diagnostic biopsy and radical prostatectomy. The primary endpoint is generally the bioavailability of the study agent in prostate tissue removed at prostatectomy. In addition, the study agent's effect on a variety of other intermediate biomarker endpoints can be studied. These usually include general measures of cell proliferation and apoptosis as well as molecular pathway-specific targets in prostate tissue.

The five completed trials examined the prostate tissue bioavailability and biomarker modulation for celecoxib, toremifene, 1-α hydroxyvitamin D2, exisulind, and genistein. Three of the five trials employed a randomized design with a placebo control group. Of the two studies without a placebo group, one study, the 1-α-hydroxyvitamin D2 trial, used a control group randomized to observation only, while the other, the exisulind trial, attempted a unique design using concurrent and historical untreated controls as the comparison group. Only one of the five trials, the celecoxib study, reached its full accrual goal. Hence, findings from the other four are difficult to interpret because of their small sample size and consequent low statistical power to detect the differences.

The celecoxib trial was conducted at the Sidney Kimmel Comprehensive Cancer Center at Johns Hopkins. This was a randomized, placebo controlled trial of celecoxib in men prior to receiving prostatectomy for clinically localized prostate cancer [31]. Sixty-four men were randomized to either celecoxib 400 mg twice daily or placebo for 4–6 weeks prior to prostatectomy. The primary endpoint was the modulation of prostate tissue prostaglandin (PG) levels by celecoxib. The investigators also examined fresh frozen prostate tissue levels of COX1 and COX2 mRNA as well as the presence of oxidized DNA bases. Paraffin-based, formalin-fixed tissue slides were used to examine celecoxib effects on markers of proliferation, apoptosis, and angiogenesis. Age, baseline PSA, race, and Gleason score were comparable across intervention groups, and the treatment regimen was well tolerated with no serious adverse events. However, despite achieving measurable prostate tissue levels of celecoxib in the intervention group, no significant treatment effects on PG levels, COX mRNA levels, or oxidized DNA base levels were observed. The investigators concluded they could not recommend further studies of celecoxib at 400 mg twice daily as a prostate cancer chemopreventive agent.

The four remaining Prostate Phase II Chemoprevention trials enrolled 34–71% of their requisite sample sizes. As such, low statistical power may have contributed to the lack of significant treatment effects reported by these trials. However, some findings suggest that with a larger study sample and, perhaps, with longer exposure time, a few of these agents may have promise. For example, in a study conducted at the University of Wisconsin using a synthetic analog of vitamin D, 1-α hydroxyvitamin D2, investigators found a lower percentage of patients with HGPIN in the synthetic vitamin D group after 1 month of intervention (23 vs. 50%, $p=0.15$). They also noted that patients in the vitamin D group exhibited consistent treatment group differences in the circulating plasma levels of two proteins that have been implicated in prostate cancer growth: lower levels of the growth factor, TGF-β2 ($p=0.07$), and higher levels of a growth factor binding protein, IGFBP3 ($p=0.04$).

Investigators at the Mayo Clinic conducted a trial to evaluate the effect of exisulind (a sulfone derivative of sulindac that has been developed as a proapoptotic agent for use in oncology) on molecular markers of apoptosis including bcl-2, Bax, Par-4, caspase-3, and PTEN. The trial employed an unusual design in that the trial was not randomized or placebo controlled. Administration of exisulind was begun 4 weeks before prostatectomy in enrolled patients. Pre-prostatectomy (i.e. base line biopsy) and post-prostatectomy levels of tissue biomarkers of apoptosis in treated patients ($n=44$) were

then compared with untreated prospective ($n=33$) and historical ($n=24$) controls selected from the same clinic population. After 4 weeks of intervention, no differences in the apoptosis markers chosen were observed. This study illustrates the importance of the randomized design, especially in clinical trials of modest size. For example, large group differences in Gleason scores for both biopsies and radical prostatectomy tissue were observed, perhaps due to differences in the time periods when cases were enrolled and controls were selected,. Only 28% of the combined prospective and historical controls had a Gleason score of 7 or greater on diagnostic biopsy compared with 48% of those in the exisulind group. This difference persisted in the prostatectomy specimens with 43% of controls having a Gleason score of 7 or greater compared with 61% of the exisulind group. These group differences in prostate cancer pathology may have contributed to the null findings regarding apoptosis.

The great advantage of the preprostatectomy study design employed in the trials described above is that the entire prostate gland can be examined following its surgical removal. This is a critical step in assessing a potential chemopreventive agent's bioavailability in prostatic tissue and its ability to modify important drug or disease specific molecular pathways. Two major drawbacks of this design are the relatively short duration of exposure to the agent and that the intervention is given to a patient who already has prostate cancer. Nevertheless, the presurgical model will continue to be an important early step in the clinical evaluation and development of chemoprevention agents.

Phase III Prostate Cancer Chemoprevention Trials

The Prostate Cancer Prevention Trial

Overview

Dihydrotestosterone (DHT) is the principal androgen supporting both benign and malignant prostate tissue and is an important molecular target for the chemoprevention of prostate cancer [35, 36]. Testosterone (T) is reduced to DHT by the 5-alpha-reductase enzymes [37]. Rennie et al. postulated the existence of at least two isoforms of this enzyme over two decades ago, based on their observation that 5-alpha reductase isolated from the stromal and epithelial compartments differed with regard to activity level (V_{max}) and sensitivity (K_i) to 5-alpha reductase inhibitors [38]. It was subsequently determined that the stromal isoenzyme (type 2) is the predominant form in benign prostatic hyperplasia, whereas both the stromal and epithelial (type 1) isoforms are present in localized prostate cancer [35, 39]. The Prostate Cancer Prevention Trial (PCPT) was the first large-scale, PCPT completed in the US. This phase III, placebo-controlled clinical trial evaluated finasteride, a selective inhibitor of the type 2 isoform of 5-alpha reductase, for the prevention of prostate cancer in healthy men. Between 1993 and 1996, the PCPT recruited 18,882 men aged 55 and older with a PSA of ≤3 ng/mL and a normal digital rectal examination (DRE). Study participants were randomized to receive 5 mg of finasteride or a matching placebo daily for 7 years and were followed with yearly PSA tests and DREs. Prostate biopsies were recommended for a PSA greater than 4.0 ng/mL or an abnormal DRE. Given that finasteride reduces serum PSA levels by about 50%, adjusted PSA values were reported to participants and their physicians to preserve the blind and to equalize the number of biopsies performed on the two study arms. In addition, all cancer-free men were asked to undergo an "end-of-study" prostate biopsy after 7 years on-study to reduce biases in prostate cancer detection that could have been introduced by the effects of finasteride on PSA and gland size. The primary study endpoint was the 7-year period prevalence of prostate cancer, a composite of incident cancers diagnosed "for-cause," i.e., elevated PSAs or abnormal DRE and prevalent cancers found at "end-of-study" biopsies. The PCPT was not designed to assess the effect of finasteride on prostate cancer mortality; it was neither large enough nor of sufficiently long duration [32].

Results

In February 2003, 15 months ahead of schedule, an independent Data and Safety Monitoring Committee (DSMC) charged with oversight of this clinical trial determined that the primary study endpoint had been reached: finasteride significantly reduced the risk of prostate cancer from 24.4 to 18.4% ($p<0.001$). Significant reductions were seen for incident as well as prevalent cancers, and the magnitude of risk reduction was similar for all risk groups based on age, race/ethnicity, family history, and entry PSA. In accordance with the DSMC recommendations, the trial was terminated, participants were unblinded, and the results were submitted for publication [32].

Adverse Events

Finasteride was well tolerated despite increases in hormone-related side effects such as erectile dysfunction, reduced ejaculate volume, loss of libido, and gynecomastia. In addition, men on the finasteride arm were more likely to temporarily discontinue study drug. A quality of life analysis reported by Moinpore et al., using the Sexual Activity Scale found that the effects of finasteride on sexual function, while statistically significant, were clinically minimal (an increase of 3.21 points out of 100 or about half the intraindividual variation) and decreased with time [40]. As expected, men on finasteride had fewer urinary complaints. Significant reductions were reported in benign prostatic hyperplasia, prostatitis, urinary retention, and transurethral prostate resections (TURPs) [32].

Does Finasteride Make the Grade?

Despite a clear benefit with regard to the primary study endpoint, finasteride was associated with a statistically significant increase in high-grade (HG) cancer. Overall, 6.4% of men on finasteride vs. 5.1% of men on placebo were diagnosed with high-grade (Gleason score 7–10) prostate cancer ($p=0.005$). In total, 43 more high-grade tumors were diagnosed on the finasteride arm (280 vs. 237) [32]. Although this finding dampened enthusiasm for the use of finasteride as a preventive agent [41], the lack of a temporal relationship between exposure to finasteride and the incidence of HG cancer raised doubts as to the causal nature of this association. For example, the 2.5-fold increase in the incidence of HG cancer seen after 1 year among men on finasteride did not increase over the next 6 years on drug. In addition, the total number of HG cancers detected in men who had the longest exposure to finasteride (i.e., at end-of-study biopsy) was nearly identical in the two arms: 92 on finasteride vs. 89 on placebo [32].

Assessment of tumor grade in the PCPT was based on Gleason scores determined on biopsy specimens, as not all men diagnosed with prostate cancer underwent prostatectomy. Given the profound effect of finasteride on prostate gland size (ultrasound measurement documented a 24.1% median decrease in prostate volume in men on the finasteride arm), the investigators addressed the possibility that this drug may have introduced detection-bias both for the diagnosis of prostate cancer and of high-grade disease [32]. Indeed, a comparison of Gleason scores determined at prostatectomy in 495 men who underwent surgery (~25% of the total number of men diagnosed with prostate cancer during the PCPT) showed the association between finasteride and HG disease to be no longer statistically significant [42]. To further explore the grade issue, more than 500 prostate biopsies on the two study arms with Gleason score$\geq$7 were examined for pathologic evidence of disease extent, a surrogate for aggressive behavior. High-grade cancers on the finasteride arm were found to be less extensive than those on the placebo arm with regard to positive cores (34 vs. 38%, $p=0.02$), bilaterality (22.8 vs. 30.6%, $p=0.05$), and perineural invasion (14.2 vs. 20.3%, $p=0.07$), suggesting that finasteride led to earlier detection of high-grade disease [42].

The effects of finasteride on the sensitivity of PSA, DRE, and biopsy for prostate cancer detection provide a strong underlying mechanism for detection-bias. For example, at a PSA threshold providing 90.5% specificity, the sensitivity for the detection of GS>7 prostate cancer was 53% on the finasteride arm vs. only 39.2% on the placebo arm [43]. Finasteride also significantly improved the sensitivity of DRE for the overall biopsy detection of prostate cancer. Although the sensitivity of DRE for the detection of GS$\geq$7 disease was also increased by finasteride, this difference did not reach statistical significance [44]. Finally, patients found to have high-grade disease at prostatectomy were significantly more likely to have had HG disease accurately diagnosed at the time of their prostate biopsy if they were on the finasteride arm (70 vs. 51%, $p=0.01$) [42].

PCPT: Conclusions

The PCPT provided a definitive answer to the primary study question: finasteride significantly reduced the 7-year period prevalence of prostate cancer [32]. Although finasteride was associated with an increase in high-grade disease, this was a secondary finding based on Gleason scores determined at biopsy, rather than on

prostatectomy specimens and was therefore subject to detection-bias. Subsequent analyses showed that finasteride significantly improved the diagnostic accuracy of PSA, DRE, and needle biopsy, leading to an underestimate of the magnitude of risk reduction and to an overestimate of the high-grade disease attributable to this agent [42, 45]. Finasteride has not yet been brought to the FDA for consideration of a prevention label, however, 5-alpha reductase inhibitors may represent a particularly useful class of agents for this purpose given their beneficial effects on urinary function and amelioration of complications associated with BPH [46].

The Reduction by Dutasteride of Prostate Cancer Events Trial

Reduction by Dutasteride of Prostate Cancer Events Trial (REDUCE) is a double-blind, placebo-controlled trial of dutasteride, 0.5 mg/day, for prostate cancer prevention. Dutasteride, an inhibitor of both the type 1 and 2 isoforms of 5-alpha reductase, has a more profound inhibitory effect on both serum and intraprostatic DHT levels than finasteride (described earlier) [47]. Although both isoenzymes are increased in high-grade prostate cancer, dutasteride is 45 times more effective than finasteride in inhibiting the type1 isoenzyme and twice as effective against the type 2 enzyme [35]. These observations suggest that the dual inhibitor may confer even greater protection against prostate cancer than finasteride [39].

REDUCE accrued 8,108 men aged 50–75 with PSA levels between 2.6 and 10 ng/dL (3.0–10 for men over 60 years) and a negative biopsy within 6 months of randomization. All participants were requested to have a follow-up 10-core prostate biopsy at 24 and 48 months postrandomization. The primary endpoint was the time to biopsy-proven prostate cancer. The secondary endpoints included the number and percent of cores positive for prostate cancer and the effect on Gleason score. Study results were presented by Gerald Andriole in abstract form at the April 2009 meeting of the American Urological Association. In summary, significantly fewer men randomized to dutasteride were diagnosed with prostate cancer over the course of the 4 year study (relative risk reduction 23.5%, $p<0.0001$). Unlike the PCPT, there was no statistically significant increase in high-grade prostate cancer, whether defined as GS

7–10 or 8–10. However, an increase in GS 8–10 cancers was noted on the dutasteride arm (19 cases or 0.6% on placebo vs. 29 cases or 0.9% on dutasteride, $p = 0.15$).

The Selenium and Vitamin E Cancer Prevention Trial

Selenium and Vitamin E Cancer Prevention Trial (SELECT) is a phase III randomized, placebo-controlled trial of selenium (200 mg/day from l-selenomethionine) and/or vitamin E (400 IU/day of *all rac*-a-tocopheryl acetate) supplementation for prostate cancer prevention [48]. Interest in these two agents was driven primarily by secondary analyses of two earlier randomized, placebo-controlled prevention trials. The first trial (Nutritional Prevention of Cancer study) [49] suggested that selenium could reduce prostate cancer incidence by as much as two-thirds. The second (Alpha Tocopherol Beta-Carotene Study) [50] suggested that vitamin E could decrease the incidence of prostate cancer incidence and mortality by more than 30%. The hypothesis that selenium and/or vitamin E would be effective in reducing prostate cancer risk was generally supported by epidemiologic, preclinical, and other clinical data [51–63].

The major eligibility requirements for SELECT were age ≥55 years for non-African American men (≥ least 50 years for African American men), serum PSA ≤4 ng/mL, and a nonsuspicious DRE. SELECT accrued 35,533 participants between July 2001 and July 2004. At baseline, white blood cells, red blood cells, plasma, and other tissue samples (e.g., toenails) were banked for subsequent ancillary correlative studies. Annual PSA tests and DREs was not mandatory since the benefits of this screening were (and still are) under debate when the trial opened and community standards regarding prostate cancer screening were expected to evolve over the course of this planned 7–12-year trial. Participants were seen every 6 months throughout the trial for adherence and adverse events monitoring [48].

The primary endpoint of SELECT was the clinical incidence of prostate cancer. The large sample size provided 96% power to detect a 25% decrease in prostate cancer for either of the single agents vs. placebo and 89% power to detect a 25% decrease for selenium plus vitamin E vs. an active single agent. Secondary endpoints included lung, colon, and total cancer incidence, cardiovascular events, death from any cause and toxicity. In addition, four prospectively conducted substudies addressing the usefulness of selenium and vitamin E in the prevention of macular degeneration, chronic obstructive lung disease, Alzheimer's disease, and colon polyps were performed in men already accrued to the parent study.

On 15 September 2008, following the second of five planned interim analyses, the DSMC recommended that the study supplements, vitamin E and selenium, be discontinued due to lack of efficacy. In addition, vitamin E was associated with a nonsignificant 13% increase in prostate cancer incidence ($p = 0.06$). A nonsignificant 7% increase in type 2 diabetes mellitus ($p = 0.16$) was observed in men on the selenium arm. Neither of these trends was seen in the combined vitamin E + selenium arm, which has raised some doubts regarding the validity of these observations. No significant differences were observed in any of the prespecified secondary endpoints, including toxicity [64].

These primary study findings underscore the importance of large-scale, randomized, clinical trials to definitively determine the risks and benefits of putative cancer preventive agents, including over-the-counter nutritional supplements. It should be emphasized that despite discontinuation of the study supplements, SELECT is not over. Most study participants have agreed to remain on-study and be followed in a blinded manner, which should help clarify the relationship between vitamin E and prostate cancer risk and between selenium and the risk of type 2 diabetes. It will also permit a more robust assessment of the secondary endpoints and substudies that make up a very important component of this clinical trial. Beyond that, the extensive biorepository, including prediagnostic serum and DNA from all study participants, will allow the conduct of correlative studies to better understand the biology of prostate cancer.

Conclusions

A great deal of progress had been made in the field of prostate cancer prevention over the past decade. Finasteride was definitively shown to reduce a man's risk of this disease, whereas selenium and vitamin E, in the doses and formulations tested, were shown to be ineffective in this regard. The NCI phase I/II prostate cancer chemoprevention agent development program continues to expand our understanding of promising chemoprevention agents with regard to metabolism, bioavailability, and modulation of intermediate end-point biomarkers. Future agent development studies will focus on novel prevention strategies, including vaccines, combinations of agents with complementary mechanisms, surrogate endpoints, and biomarkers of risk and benefit.

References

1. Lippman SM, Hong WK. Cancer prevention science and practice. Cancer Res 2002;62:5119–25.
2. Kinzler KW, Vogelstein B. Lessons from hereditary colorectal cancer. Cell 1996;87:159–70.
3. Jones PA, Baylin SB. The fundamental role of epigenetic events in cancer. Nat Rev Genet 2002;3:415–28.
4. Renan MJ. How many mutations are required for tumorigenesis? Implications from human cancer data. Mol Carcinog 1993;7:139–46.
5. Sakr WA. Prostatic intraepithelial neoplasia: A marker for high-risk groups and a potential target for chemoprevention. Eur Urol 1999;35:474–8.
6. Sporn MB, Suh N. Chemoprevention: an essential approach to controlling cancer. Nat Rev Cancer 2002;2:537–43.
7. Parnes HL, House MG, Kagan J, Kausal DJ, Lieberman R. Prostate cancer chemoprevention agent development: The National Cancer Institute, Division of Cancer Prevention portfolio. J Urol 2004;171:S68–74; discussion S5.
8. Bostwick DG, Qian J. Effect of androgen deprivation therapy on prostatic intraepithelial neoplasia. Urology 2001;58:91–3.
9. De Marzo AM, Marchi VL, Epstein JI, Nelson WG. Proliferative inflammatory atrophy of the prostate: implications for prostatic carcinogenesis. Am J Pathol 1999;155:1985–92.
10. Kronz JD, Allan CH, Shaikh AA, Epstein JI. Predicting cancer following a diagnosis of high-grade prostatic intraepithelial neoplasia on needle biopsy: data on men with more than one follow-up biopsy. Am J Surg Pathol 2001;25:1079–85.
11. Epstein JI, Herawi M. Prostate needle biopsies containing prostatic intraepithelial neoplasia or atypical foci suspicious for carcinoma: implications for patient care. J Urol 2006;175:820–34.
12. Godken N, Roehl KA, Catalona WJ, Humphrey PA. High-grade prostatic intraepithelial neoplasia in needle biopsy as risk factor for detection of adenocarcinoma: current level of risk in screening population. Urology 2005;65:538–42
13. Langeberg WJ, Isaacs WB, Stanford JL. Genetic etiology of hereditary prostate cancer. Front Biosci 2007;12:4101–10.
14. Noe M, Schroy P, Demierre MF, Babayan R, Geller AC. Increased cancer risk for individuals with a family history of prostate cancer, colorectal cancer, and melanoma and their associated screening recommendations and practices. Cancer Causes Control 2008;19:1–12.
15. Eastham J. Personal communication; 2009.
16. Carroll P. personal communication; 2008.
17. Kumar NB. Personal communication; 2008.
18. Bosland MC. Personal communication; 2008.
19. Kucuk O. Personal communication; 2006.
20. Bergan R. Personal communication; 2006.
21. Ahmann FR. Personal communication; 2008.
22. El-Bayoumy K. Personal communication; 2008.
23. Marshall J. Personal communication; 2008.
24. Ip C. Personal communication; 2008.
25. Sabichi AL, Lee JJ, Taylor RJ, et al. Selenium accumulation in prostate tissue during a randomized, controlled short-term trial of l-selenomethionine: a Southwest Oncology Group Study. Clin Cancer Res 2006;12:2178–84.
26. Kim J. Personal communication; 2007.
27. Gaziano JM, Glynn RJ, Christen WG, et al. Vitamins E and C in the prevention of prostate and total cancer in men: the Physicians' Health Study II randomized controlled trial. JAMA 2009;301:52–62.
28. Gee J. Personal communication; 2008.
29. Wilding G. Personal communication; 2008.
30. Leibovich BC. Personal communication; 2007.
31. Carducci MA WJ, Heath E, et al. A randomized , placebo-controlled trial of celecoxib in men prior to receiving prostatectomy for clinically localized adenocarcinoma of the prostate: Evaluation of drug-specific biomarker modulation. J Clin Oncol (ASCO Annu Meet Proc) 2007;25:235s.
32. Thompson IM, Goodman PJ, Tangen CM, et al. The influence of finasteride on the development of prostate cancer. N Engl J Med 2003;349:215–24.
33. Simoneau AR, Gerner EW, Nagle R, et al. The effect of difluoromethylornithine on decreasing prostate size and polyamines in men: results of a year-long phase IIb randomized placebo-controlled chemoprevention trial. Cancer Epidemiol Biomarkers Prev 2008;17:292–9.
34. Nelson BJ. Personal communication; 2006.
35. Tindall DJ, Rittmaster RS. The rationale for inhibiting 5alpha-reductase isoenzymes in the prevention and treatment of prostate cancer. J Urol 2008;179:1235–42.
36. Parnes HL, Thompson IM, Ford LG. Prevention of hormone-related cancers: prostate cancer. J Clin Oncol 2005;23:368–77.
37. Bartsch G, Rittmaster RS, Klocker H. Dihydrotestosterone and the concept of 5alpha-reductase inhibition in human benign prostatic hyperplasia. Eur Urol 2000;37:367–80.
38. Rennie PS, Bruchovsky N, McLoughlin MG, Batzold FH, Dunstan-Adams EE. Kinetic analysis of 5 alpha-reductase isoenzymes in benign prostatic hyperplasia (BPH). J Steroid Biochem 1983;19:169–73.
39. Thomas LN, Douglas RC, Lazier CB, et al. Levels of 5alpha-reductase type 1 and type 2 are increased in localized high grade compared to low grade prostate cancer. J Urol 2008;179:147–51.
40. Moinpour CM, Darke AK, Donaldson GW, et al. Longitudinal analysis of sexual function reported by men in the Prostate Cancer Prevention Trial. J Natl Cancer Inst 2007;99:1025–35.
41. Scardino PT. The prevention of prostate cancer – the dilemma continues. N Engl J Med 2003;349:297–9.

42. Lucia MS, Epstein JI, Goodman PJ, et al. Finasteride and high-grade prostate cancer in the Prostate Cancer Prevention Trial. J Natl Cancer Inst 2007;99:1375–83.

43. Thompson IM, Chi C, Ankerst DP, et al. Effect of finasteride on the sensitivity of PSA for detecting prostate cancer. J Natl Cancer Inst 2006;98:1128–33.

44. Thompson IM, Tangen CM, Goodman PJ, et al. Finasteride improves the sensitivity of digital rectal examination for prostate cancer detection. J Urol 2007;177:1749–52.

45. Thompson IM, Ankerst DP, Chi C, et al. Assessing prostate cancer risk: results from the Prostate Cancer Prevention Trial. J Natl Cancer Inst 2006;98:529–34.

46. McConnell JD, Roehrborn CG, Bautista OM, et al. The long-term effect of doxazosin, finasteride, and combination therapy on the clinical progression of benign prostatic hyperplasia. N Engl J Med 2003;349:2387–98.

47. Clark RV, Hermann DJ, Cunningham GR, Wilson TH, Morrill BB, Hobbs S. Marked suppression of dihydrotestosterone in men with benign prostatic hyperplasia by dutasteride, a dual 5alpha-reductase inhibitor. J Clin Endocrinol Metab 2004;89:2179–84.

48. Lippman SM, Goodman PJ, Klein EA, et al. Designing the Selenium and Vitamin E Cancer Prevention Trial (SELECT). J Natl Cancer Inst 2005;97:94–102.

49. Clark LC, Combs GF Jr., Turnbull BW, et al. Effects of selenium supplementation for cancer prevention in patients with carcinoma of the skin. A randomized controlled trial. Nutritional Prevention of Cancer Study Group. JAMA 1996;276:1957–63.

50. Heinonen OP, Albanes D, Virtamo J, et al. Prostate cancer and supplementation with alpha-tocopherol and beta-carotene: incidence and mortality in a controlled trial. J Natl Cancer Inst 1998;90:440–6.

51. Blot WJ, Li JY, Taylor PR, et al. Nutrition intervention trials in Linxian, China: supplementation with specific vitamin/mineral combinations, cancer incidence, and disease-specific mortality in the general population. J Natl Cancer Inst 1993;85:1483–92.

52. Yoshizawa K, Willett WC, Morris SJ, et al. Study of prediagnostic selenium level in toenails and the risk of advanced prostate cancer. J Natl Cancer Inst 1998;90:1219–24.

53. Redman C, Scott JA, Baines AT, et al. Inhibitory effect of selenomethionine on the growth of three selected human tumor cell lines. Cancer Lett 1998;125:103–10.

54. Menter DG, Sabichi AL, Lippman SM. Selenium effects on prostate cell growth. Cancer Epidemiol Biomarkers Prev 2000;9:1171–82.

55. Li H, Stampfer MJ, Giovannucci EL, et al. A prospective study of plasma selenium levels and prostate cancer risk. J Natl Cancer Inst 2004;96:696–703.

56. Willett W. Lessons from dietary studies in Adventists and questions for the future. Am J Clin Nutr 2003;78:539S–43S.

57. Coates RJ, Weiss NS, Daling JR, Morris JS, Labbe RF. Serum levels of selenium and retinol and the subsequent risk of cancer. Am J Epidemiol 1988;128:515–23.

58. Knekt P, Aromaa A, Maatela J, et al. Serum vitamin E and risk of cancer among Finnish men during a 10-year follow-up. Am J Epidemiol 1988;127:28–41.

59. Criqui MH, Bangdiwala S, Goodman DS, et al. Selenium, retinol, retinol-binding protein, and uric acid. Associations with cancer mortality in a population-based prospective case-control study. Ann Epidemiol 1991;1:385–93.

60. Hsing AW, Comstock GW, Abbey H, Polk BF. Serologic precursors of cancer. Retinol, carotenoids, and tocopherol and risk of prostate cancer. J Natl Cancer Inst 1990;82:941–6.

61. Comstock GW, Helzlsouer KJ, Bush TL. Prediagnostic serum levels of carotenoids and vitamin E as related to subsequent cancer in Washington County, Maryland. Am J Clin Nutr 1991;53:260S–4S.

62. Eichholzer M, Stahelin HB, Gey KF, Ludin E, Bernasconi F. Prediction of male cancer mortality by plasma levels of interacting vitamins: 17-year follow-up of the prospective Basel study. Int J Cancer 1996;66:145–50.

63. Chan JM, Stampfer MJ, Ma J, Rimm EB, Willett WC, Giovannucci EL. Supplemental vitamin E intake and prostate cancer risk in a large cohort of men in the United States. Cancer Epidemiol Biomarkers Prev 1999;8:893–9.

64. Lippman SM, Klein EA, Goodman PJ, et al. Effect of selenium and vitamin E on risk of prostate cancer and other cancers: the Selenium and Vitamin E Cancer Prevention Trial (SELECT). JAMA 2009;301:39–51.

Chapter 32
Diet and Prostate Cancer Incidence, Recurrence, and Progression Risk

June M. Chan and Erin L. Richman

Abstract Dramatic differences in rates of prostate cancer around the world and within immigrant populations have led researchers to investigate diet and lifestyle practices for prostate cancer risk. Epidemiologic studies over the past several decades have identified several dietary risk factors for prostate cancer incidence, and emerging data suggest that diet may also play a role after diagnosis. This chapter will summarize and integrate the findings of recent meta-analyses and current literature. Overall, data indicate that specific vegetables (e.g., cruciferous, tomatoes, soy/legumes/pulses) and nutrients (vitamin E, selenium, and lycopene) may prove beneficial in reducing the risk of developing prostate cancer, whereas calcium/calcium-rich foods/dairy products and processed or red meats may increase the risk.

Keywords Diet • Nutrition • Prostate cancer

Background

In 2008, it is estimated that more than 186,000 new cases of prostate cancer will be diagnosed in the United States, and more than 28,000 deaths due to prostate cancer will occur. Prostate cancer is the most common cancer in men in the US and the second most common cause of cancer death in men. Older age, African-American race, and family history of prostate cancer are well-established risk factors for prostate cancer incidence. Diet or exercise practices may also affect risk and possibly progression of this common cancer.

In the United States, African-American men are at the greatest risk of developing prostate cancer and approximately 20% (or one in five) of African-American men are diagnosed in their lifetime (assuming a lifespan of 85 years; www.seer.cancer.gov). Similarly, one out of six non-Hispanic white men, one in seven Hispanic men, and one in nine Asian/Pacific Islander men develop prostate cancer. Globally, prostate cancer is more common in the Americas, Western and Northern Europe, South Africa, Australia, and New Zealand. Asian and North African countries have historically lower rates of prostate cancer incidence.

It is interesting to note, however, that prostate cancer is on the rise in some of these low-risk countries. For example, countries such as China and Japan have historically had very low rates of prostate cancer, sometimes 30-fold less than the US. However, in recent decades, prostate cancer has been increasing in these countries, too. While their rates are still lower than in the US, they have experienced dramatic 50–100% increases in prostate cancer diagnosis and death rates [1, 2]. Researchers have hypothesized that some of this increase may be due to the "Westernization" of the diet in these traditionally low-risk countries.

Another reason that has led researchers to study the effects of diet and lifestyle on prostate cancer risk stems from studying immigrant populations. These are studies where investigators examine the risk of prostate cancer in a low-risk country, such as China, and compare this with first-generation and second-generation immigrants who live in higher risk countries such as the United States. For example, using data from the Surveillance Epidemiology and End Results (SEER) database, Cook et al. [2] reported the following incidence rates (presented here as cases per 100,000, for 1973–1986, adjusted to the world standard population) of prostate cancer among Chinese men in Shanghai, Chinese men born in

J.M. Chan (✉)
Epidemiology and Biostatistics, Urology, University of California, San Francisco, CA, USA
e-mail: june.chan@ucsf.edu

W.D. Figg et al. (eds.), *Drug Management of Prostate Cancer*,
DOI 10.1007/978-1-60327-829-4_32, © Springer Science+Business Media, LLC 2010

China but now living in the United States, and Chinese men born and living in the United States: 1.8, 23, and 37, respectively. These rates demonstrate how, within a single racial group, there are dramatic differences based on country of origin, birthplace, and country of current residence (please note that rates cannot be directly compared with other population rates, unless standardized to the same world population standard). The same trend was observed for Japanese and Filipino men in this study as well. Together, such data indicate that lifestyle factors that vary by culture and country may influence prostate cancer risk, even within a person's lifetime.

Methods

In this chapter, we will review dietary risk factors for prostate cancer incidence and comment briefly on other modifiable risk factors for this disease. The literature on diet and prostate cancer was recently summarized in 2007 by the World Cancer Research Fund and the American Institute for Cancer Research in their updated report, "Food, Nutrition, Physical Activity, and the Prevention of Cancer: a Global Perspective" (hereafter referred to as the WCRF-AICR report) [3]. This report conducted rigorous systematic literature reviews for individual cancer sites, including the review of 558 papers on diet and exercise as risk for prostate cancer, published from 1966 through April 2004. Details on the methodology employed in the WCRF–AICR report can be found elsewhere [3]. This chapter will summarize our understanding of dietary risk factors for prostate cancer by citing and integrating the findings of the WCRF–AICR report with newer papers published since April 2004. Wherever possible, we will comment on the quality of the evidence for a specific dietary item as a probable or possible risk factor for prostate cancer incidence.

The majority of published studies report on total prostate cancer as the main outcome; however, more recent literature also often examined advanced or aggressive disease outcomes as secondary analyses when data allowed. This is particularly relevant for prostate cancer because of changes in the distribution of early and advanced cases with the widespread use of PSA screening. In particular, more early stage cases are now diagnosed in countries that utilize PSA screening routinely, and it is estimated that a large proportion of early stage disease may actually be latent tumors with a different etiology than more aggressive phenotypes. Thus, risk factors may have a different association with early vs. advanced stage disease at diagnosis; and it may be important to subdivide overall prostate cancer into two distinct outcomes: those with a more clinically significant phenotype (characterized by higher PSA, stage, or grade at diagnosis) vs. those that have lower prognostic risk at diagnosis. Lastly, we will summarize the much more limited data available on diet and the risk of prostate cancer progression, recurrence, or mortality.

In assembling this review, we focused on data from case–control and cohort studies and randomized clinical trials. Each of these has strengths and weaknesses that are important to consider when interpreting results. Prospective diet and lifestyle data collection (from cohort or nested case–control studies) helps to minimize recall bias; whereas retrospective case–control studies are more vulnerable to this bias. The WCRF–AICR report also placed more weight on case–control studies where the controls were drawn from the population as opposed to hospital-based controls. Given that people who eat well often follow other health-seeking behaviors, it is important that studies consider confounding by other lifestyle factors (e.g., smoking, exercise, body size, etc) using multivariate analyses. Randomized clinical trials are often unfeasible designs for examining long-term cumulative effects of diet on cancer, given the inability to randomly assign daily food consumption over long time periods. Such trials are effective for examining specific nutritional supplements although these are still restricted to examining specific doses over relatively short intervention periods, and data on such trials are limited to date given the scope and cost of such studies. When assessing the effects of diet on prostate cancer recurrence, it is important to remember that biochemical recurrence correlates imperfectly with prostate cancer mortality; and the definition of recurrence may be study-specific. Such studies may also not always be able to adjust for confounding due to disease aggressiveness, as patients may make specific lifestyle changes based on their clinical features at diagnosis, which also strongly correlate with prognosis.

Diet and Prostate Cancer

Specific vegetables, fruits, and micronutrients may decrease the risk of prostate cancer, while dairy foods or foods high in calcium content and meat may increase risk.

In particular, cruciferous vegetables, foods rich in the carotenoid lycopene (e.g., tomatoes), legumes, soy, vitamin E, and selenium may protect against development of prostate cancer. In contrast, higher intakes of milk and other dairy foods, calcium, and processed meat or red meat (e.g., bacon, sausage, hot dogs) have been linked to elevations in prostate cancer incidence risk. Each of these will be discussed further below.

Vegetables and Fruits

Specific vegetables and fruits (e.g., cruciferous vegetables, legumes/pulses (including soy), tomatoes/tomato products) are considered possible protective risk factors for prostate cancer. Data on overall vegetable or fruit intake and other subgroups are less conclusive [3].

Legumes and Soy

Via meta-analyses the WCRF–AICR report (based on one cohort study and five population-based case–control studies) estimated that there was a statistically significant 3–7% decrease in prostate cancer risk per one serving increase per week of legumes/pulses [3]. Since the publication of that report, an additional four case–control studies have been published, all of which observed an inverse trend for consumption of soy, tofu, or a traditional Taiwanese vegetarian soy- and wheat protein-based diet [4–7]. Two of these studies used population-based controls [6, 7]. These studies were conducted in China, Scotland, Taiwan, and Japan.

An additional study conducted among Japanese, Korean, and American men reported differences between prostate cancer cases and controls with regard to the ability to convert the soy isoflavone daidzein into equol. Asian cases were less likely to produce equol than Asian controls, and Asian men were roughly twice as likely to produce equol as the American men in the study, although numbers for this comparison were small. Of four cohort studies published since the Global Perspective [8–11], three reported overall null associations for total prostate cancer and soy or legume consumption [8–10]. Although, one of these, a large cohort study of Japanese men, observed a statistically significant inverse association for soy products and localized prostate cancer [9]. The large Multi-Ethnic Cohort Study (4,404 cases identified among 82,483

men) reported statistically significant, small to moderate reductions in risk for overall and aggressive prostate cancer and legume consumption (RR = 0.89, 95% CI 0.89–0.99 for total prostate cancer and RR = 0.74, 95% CI 0.61–0.91 for aggressive disease) [11]. Mechanisms for legumes/soy remain unclear, although it is hypothesized that soy isoflavones that have estrogenic effects may inhibit testosterone-induced growth of the prostate. As effects have been reported for nonsoy legumes as well, other legume constituents such as dietary fiber, omega-3 fatty acids, protease inhibitors, and saponins are being investigated as well [11].

Cruciferous Vegetables

Results from three cohort studies reporting on cruciferous vegetable intake and prostate cancer risk have been somewhat equivocal, while eight case–control studies have generally reported inverse associations [3]. Since the WCRF–AICR report, a small cohort of 1,985 men exposed to asbestos reported a borderline statistically significantly risk reduction for broccoli consumption [12]. Cruciferous vegetables include broccoli, cauliflower, kale, cabbage, and Brussels sprouts. These vegetables are rich in the isothiocyanate sulforaphane and indole-3-carbinol, which have been shown to have anticancer properties, including induction of phase 1 and 2 enzymes that help eliminate carcinogens; effects on cell signaling, epigenetic regulation, and cell cycle arrest [13, 14]. Further support for a role of cruciferous vegetables in decreasing prostate cancer risk comes from evidence of an interaction with the glutathione S-transferase (GST) gene variants. GSTs are phase 2 enzymes involved in xenobiotic metabolism and excretion. Joseph et al. observed a stronger effect of high cruciferous vegetable consumption and prostate cancer risk among those with the GSTM1 present variant vs. null deletions in this gene [15].

Tomatoes and Lycopene

The WCRF–AICR report summarized data from 17 prospective studies (cohort or nested case–control) and 18 case–control studies on tomato intake (four prospective and seven case–control), dietary lycopene (three prospective and nine case–control), or circulating lycopene levels (four prospective and two case–control) [3].

The majority of studies observed moderate to strong inverse associations with increasing consumption of tomatoes or lycopene or circulating lycopene level.

Papers published subsequent to the WCRF–AICR report (two large prospective studies and two case–control studies) [16–19] have also been consistent in indicating moderate to strong risk reductions for dietary intakes of tomatoes (in particular, cooked tomatoes or tomato sauce) or lycopene or circulating lycopene levels. One case–control study conducted in Japanese men since the publication of WCRF–AICR report observed null results for tomato consumption, although the estimate was in the inverse direction [4]. Overall, some of the strongest evidence come from the large cohorts, the Health Professionals Follow-up Study and the Physicians Health Study.

The Health Professionals Follow-up Study observed more than a 30% risk reduction in prostate cancer risk for the highest vs. lowest quintile of plasma lycopene, and results were stronger for older men and those without a family history of prostate cancer [20]. In the Physicians Health Study, the odds ratio was 0.56 (95% CI = 0.34–0.91) for comparing extreme quintiles of circulating lycopene and the risk of aggressive prostate cancer [21]. We also observed a 20% decrease in the risk of prostate cancer recurrence and progression associated with increasing tomato sauce consumption by two servings per week after diagnosis relative to before prostate cancer diagnosis, in further analyses of the Health Professionals Follow-up Study [22].

Tomatoes are rich in the carotenoid lycopene that has antioxidant, antiproliferative, and prodifferentiation properties. Furthermore, initial studies suggest that lycopene supplements can also reduce transcript level of proinflammatory cytokines and reduce LDL cholesterol [3], each of which is hypothesized to influence the prostate microenvironment to predispose to cancer. In summary, tomatoes or cooked tomatoes or the carotenoid lycopene are a probable protective risk factor for prostate cancer.

Vitamin E

The WCRF–AICR report reviewed the data from six cohort studies and 14 case–control studies on either dietary vitamin E or serum levels of vitamin E. Overall, they concluded that the majority of studies demonstrated a decreased risk with increasing intake or level of vitamin E. Two subsequent cohort studies published

after the WCRF–AICR report also observed inverse associations for circulating levels of vitamin E or dietary vitamin E [23, 24]; although, one large prospective study reported null associations between plasma tocopherols and prostate cancer risk [17]. Supplemental vitamin E was associated with up to a 40% decreased risk of prostate cancer mortality, in secondary data analyses of a randomized clinical trial.

In some studies, a potential interaction with smoking has been observed, whereby the benefit of vitamin E was limited to men with a current or past history of smoking [25]. While data are not entirely consistent with regard to vitamin E assessed in the diet vs. supplements vs. circulation, the literature suggests that vitamin E, in general, is a possible protective risk factor for prostate cancer.

Vitamin E refers to up to eight different compounds of similar structure and biological function that are divided into the tocopherols and tocotrienols. Gamma tocopherol is the major form of vitamin E consumed in the human diet, whereas alpha-tocopherol is the main form of vitamin E consumed in supplements and measured in tissues. Vitamin E has antioxidant, anti-inflammatory, antiproliferative, and proapoptotic functions that may protect against prostate cancer development or progression.

Selenium

Secondary analyses of a randomized clinical trial and several prospective studies have observed a 50–65% reduction in prostate cancer risk associated with greater selenium intake or physiologic measures of selenium, and in vitro and in vivo studies indicate that selenium may have multiple effects on prostate cancer including antiproliferative, proapoptotic, antiangiogenic, and antioxidant properties [26–37]. The WCRF–AICR report concluded that there was strong evidence from clinical trials and cohort studies that selenium probably protects against prostate cancer.

Subsequent to this review, a nested case–control study from the Physicians' Health Study reported a strong interaction between the valine(V)/alanine(A)-polymorphism (rs4880) in *SOD2* and plasma selenium levels and risk of total and aggressive prostate cancer [38]. Men who were in the highest quartile of selenium, and had the AA genotype, had a 53% lower risk of total prostate cancer (odds ratio (OR) = 0.47, 95% CI 0.26–0.85) and a 65% lower risk of aggressive prostate cancer (OR = 0.35, 95% CI 0.15–0.82), compared to men who were in the lowest quartile of selenium and had the VA or VV genotypes (*p*-values for interaction 0.05 and 0.01, respectively). At the time of this writing, vitamin E and selenium are the focus of the large, ongoing, national, randomized, blinded, placebo-controlled, Selenium and Vitamin E Cancer Prevention Trial (SELECT) (See Chapter 31: Prostate Cancer Chemoprevention Strategies for detailed information on the SELECT trial).

Recently, a large prospective cohort study reported an elevated risk of prostate cancer associated with more than daily usage of multivitamins, in particular, among men also taking individual supplements (e.g., selenium, folate, vitamin E, beta-carotene, zinc) or who had a family history of prostate cancer [39]. Such a potential adverse interaction for higher dosing of specific nutrients warrants further investigation.

Milk, Dairy, and Calcium

Milk, calcium, or dairy products have been associated with a greater risk of prostate cancer in most observational studies. The WCRF–AICR report reviewed ten cohort studies and 13 case–control studies investigating milk and dairy foods, as well as nine cohort studies and 12 case–control studies focused on dietary calcium intake. They concluded that there was suggestive evidence that milk and dairy products are possible risk factors for prostate cancer; and diets high in calcium are a probable cause of prostate cancer. One [40] out of three [4, 7] additional case–control studies and four [41–44] out of seven cohort studies [10, 45, 46] published after the WCRF–AICR report also observed positive associations between some measure of milk, dairy, or calcium and prostate cancer risk. The four prospective studies observing positive associations were large well-conducted cohorts in several different countries [41–44].

Subsequent secondary results from a randomized clinical trial on calcium supplements and colorectal adenomas reported a null to inverse association between prostate cancer and calcium supplements [47]. It has been hypothesized that this apparent discrepancy may be because calcium has different actions on prostate cancer development at different times in the disease course or depending on clinical phenotype. Most of the cases observed in the trial tended to be earlier stage cases than that reported in the observational studies. The leading hypothesized mechanism by which dairy or milk intake may affect prostate cancer risk involves the effects of calcium intake on circulating levels of $1,25(OH)_2D_3$, the most biologically active form of vitamin D, which has been shown to inhibit growth of prostate cancer cells.

Meat, Poultry, Fat, and Prostate Cancer

The WCRF–AICR report concluded that data were too limited or inconsistent to draw conclusions regarding relationships between meat, fats, fish, and prostate cancer; although, processed meat was considered a suggestive risk factor.

Results of ecologic and case–control studies have consistently suggested a positive association between total meat intake and prostate cancer [48, 49], yet most prospective cohort studies have reported null associations [44, 45, 50–53].

For example, 9 of 12 case–control studies conducted between 1966 and 1999 reported a positive association between total meat intake and prostate cancer, three out of which were statistically significant, while only two out of eleven prospective cohort studies conducted between 1979 and 2008 reported a positive association, eight reported no association, and one reported an inverse association [44, 45, 48, 50–54]. This discrepancy may be due to issues such as recall bias or inappropriate control selection, or may also partially be explained by a greater role of meat intake in the progression, rather than initiation of prostate cancer. If this was the case, an association may be found in a case–control study with hospital-based cases, but not in a cohort study where incident prostate cancer may include indolent disease identified by PSA screening. Another possible explanation for the null findings of most cohort studies is the variability in nutrient composition and cooking practices for different types of meat, which may have different associations with prostate cancer.

Red and Processed Meat

Several studies have looked at red or processed meat and prostate cancer risk. The results have been inconsistent for red meat, with five out of ten cohort studies reporting a positive association and five reporting no association [44, 48, 51, 52, 55, 56]. Fewer studies have looked at processed meat and prostate cancer, but three of five cohort studies reported a positive association between processed meat and total prostate cancer [44, 52, 53, 55, 56], and four out of six reported a positive association between processed meat and advanced/metastatic prostate cancer, albeit nonsignificant [44, 51–53, 55, 56]. Thus, the evidence suggests processed meat, and possibly red meat, may be positively associated with prostate cancer progression.

Poultry

Overall, total poultry intake has not been associated with prostate cancer incidence or mortality [44, 50–52]. However, a recent cohort study reported a nonsignificant 1.65-fold increase in the risk of advanced prostate cancer when comparing highest vs. lowest quintiles of chicken intake. Another cohort study reported a nonsignificant positive association between chicken or turkey with skin and metastatic prostate cancer but a nonsignificant inverse association between chicken or turkey without skin and metastatic prostate cancer [50, 51]. This suggests a possible increased risk of advanced prostate cancer associated with either a component of poultry skin or perhaps a diet or lifestyle factor correlated with choosing to eat the skin on poultry; although, none of the results have been significant and the evidence is currently sparse.

Biological Mechanisms for Meat and Poultry

The observed associations between processed meat, red meat, and potentially poultry with skin intake and prostate cancer may be mediated by high levels of dietary animal fat, heme, zinc, and/or carcinogens found on meat such as heterocyclic amines (HA) and *N*-nitroso compounds (NNC). Meat is a major source of animal fat in the diet, and ecologic studies have reported a positive correlation between per capita fat intake and prostate cancer incidence and mortality [49]. Animal and in vitro studies provide evidence to

support this hypothesis. For example, mice injected with DU145 prostate cancer cells and fed a high-fat, linoleic acid-rich diet developed twice the tumor mass compared to similarly injected mice fed a low-fat diet. Mice fed a low-fat diet exhibited significantly less proliferative behavior compared to mPIN epithelial cells of mice on a high-fat diet [57, 58]. Potential mechanisms to explain these findings include changes in hormone metabolism, cell membrane composition, cell signal transduction, and proinflammatory eicosanoid synthesis due to high animal fat intake, all of which may promote prostate cancer cell growth [48]. However, recent epidemiologic studies generally do not support an association between total, saturated, or animal fat intake and total prostate cancer incidence [45, 52, 54, 59], and the WCRF–AICR report deemed the data on fats and prostate cancer as too low quality, too inconsistent, or too sparse to allow conclusions to be reached [3].

Additionally, 8 out of 13 case–control, nested case–control, or cohort studies have reported a positive association between alpha-linolenic acid (ALA) intake and prostate cancer, particularly for advanced prostate cancer [60–62]. A recent cohort study reported a significant approximately two-fold increased risk of advanced prostate cancer comparing men in highest vs. lowest quintile of ALA intake, but no association between ALA intake and total prostate cancer was reported[62]. Conversely, animal studies have reported no change in prostate tumor growth in mice fed with ALA-rich diets compared with mice fed with linoleic acid-rich diets, and the mechanism by which ALA may increase the risk of advanced prostate cancer has yet to be elucidated [60].

Along with animal fats, meat is a major dietary source of heme compounds and zinc. Heme compounds, including oxymyoglobin, deoxymyoglobin, hemoglobin, and deoxyhemoglobin, are hydrolyzed to amino acids, peptides, and a heme group in the gastrointestinal tract. The heme group can then catalyze oxidative reactions, causing tissue damage throughout the body [63]. Zinc is found in high levels in the prostate and is necessary for testosterone synthesis and therefore may also contribute to prostate carcinogenesis [48].

HAs and NNCs are other agents that may potentially be involved in the observed association between processed meat, red meat, and poultry with skin and prostate carcinogenesis. Heterocyclic amines (HA) are potent mutagens formed when beef, pork, chicken, and fish are cooked to higher degrees of doneness with heat-intensive methods [64–66]. *2-amino-1-methyl-6-phenylimidazol[4,5-b]pyridine* (PhIP) is the predominant carcinogenic HA in the US diet [67–69] and is found predominantly in well-done chicken, beef, and pork [70–72]. PhIP intake in humans has been linked to increased risk of prostate, gastrointestinal, breast, and lung cancers [64]; it has been shown to covalently bind to and damage DNA [73–76], and it induces prostate, colon, intestinal, and mammary adenocarcinomas in rats [77–84].

In epidemiologic studies, consumption of cooked meats and associated HA have been linked to increased risk of prostate and other cancers [85–96], although a few studies report no such associations [97–99]. Differences in findings may be partly explained by differences in meat intake and doneness preference assessment methods [64].

NNCs are another category of mutagens that could explain the observed positive associations between meat and prostate cancer, particularly processed meats. Processed meats that have been smoked or cured using nitrites, such as bacon, are a major dietary source of NNCs [100]. NNCs are also formed endogenously through the reaction of secondary and tertiary amino compounds (found in meat) with nitrite or other nitrosating agents in the gastrointestinal tract. Hughes et al. reported that a high-meat diet (420 g/day) resulted in NNC exposures comparable to that of tobacco smoke and NNCs have been shown to induce tumors in multiple organs in rats [100, 101].

Fish and Marine Omega-3 Fatty Acids

The results for fish intake and prostate cancer risk have been inconsistent and, similar to meat from land animals, may depend on the type of fish and stage of prostate cancer studied. Three out of four case–control studies reported an inverse association between total fish intake and prostate cancer risk, one of which was significant [102]. In contrast, only two out of eight cohort studies reported a significant positive association between total fish intake and total prostate cancer, while six reported no association [44, 52–54, 102–104]. Fewer studies have looked at advanced prostate cancer and total fish intake, and the results were once again inconsistent.

One cohort study reported a significant inverse association between total fish intake and advanced prostate cancer among health professionals in the United States, but no association for total prostate cancer, and another cohort study reported a significant inverse association between total fish intake and prostate cancer mortality in Sweden, while two nested-case control studies, one in the Netherlands and the other in Los Angeles and Hawaii, reported no association between total fish intake and advanced prostate cancer [52, 53, 102, 103]. Additionally, one cohort study reported a nonsignificant 27% reduction in risk of prostate cancer progression comparing men in the fourth quartile of postdiagnostic fish intake to the lowest quartile [22].

Thus, the evidence suggests that total fish intake may be inversely associated with prostate cancer progression, but more research is needed to confirm these results. Furthermore, similar to the possible opposing associations between poultry with skin and poultry without skin and prostate cancer, a cohort study in Sweden reported a significant inverse association for dark meat fish consumption and total prostate cancer incidence, but a significant positive association for cod/saithe/fish finger and shellfish consumption and total prostate cancer [105].

The potential inverse association between fish consumption and prostate cancer development and/or progression is thought to be due to the high level of omega-3 polyunsaturated fatty acids in dark meat fish. The main marine omega-3 fatty acids, eicosapentaenoic acid (EPA) and docosahexaenoic acid (DHA), have consistently been shown to inhibit prostate cancer cell growth in vitro and in animal studies [106]. Marine omega-3 fatty acids inhibit the synthesis of proinflammatory eicosanoids from arachodonic acid (AA), by competing for the cycolooxygenase-2 enzyme and inhibiting lipoxygenase activity. AA-derived eicosanoids, such as prostaglandins, leukotrienes, and hydroxyeicosatetraenoic acids, have been shown to increase cellular proliferation, impede immune surveillance, induce angiogenesis, and inhibit apoptosis and have been linked to tumor development and progression in animal, in vitro, and human studies [106]. Hence, a high level of marine omega-3 fatty acids in the diet may decrease the risk of prostate cancer and/or slow prostate cancer progression by inhibiting the synthesis of these compounds.

Diet and Prostate Cancer Progression and Survival

There are limited data on diet after diagnosis and prostate cancer recurrence or survival risk, although several studies of diet and prostate cancer incidence observed stronger associations for risk of advanced or fatal prostate cancer. In a large prospective cohort study, we observed that higher tomato sauce and fish intake *after* diagnosis was associated with reduced risk of prostate cancer recurrence/progression, independent of tumor features, treatment, and prediagnostic diet [22]. Also, one case–control and two cohort studies have reported a significant positive association between saturated fat intake and prostate cancer survival or biochemical recurrence after radical prostatectomy, suggesting a possible role of saturated fat in the progression of prostate cancer [107–109]. Several small intervention studies conducted in different populations of prostate cancer survivors have examined effects of various plant-based, low-fat diets, or tomato-rich diets, soy supplements, and lycopene or other antioxidant supplements [110–113]. Most of these have reported possible beneficial effects on PSA levels or other intermediary biomarkers, providing additional preliminary provocative data for a role of diet after diagnosis.

Conclusions

In conclusion, evidence to date suggests that specific vegetables (e.g., cruciferous, tomatoes, soy/legumes/pulses) and nutrients (vitamin E, selenium, lycopene) may prove beneficial in reducing the risk of developing prostate cancer, whereas calcium/dairy and processed meats may increase risk. Emerging data also suggest that diet after diagnosis may help delay recurrence or progression of cancer in men with localized disease, and further research is warranted given the increasing numbers of men living with this disease.

References

1. Sim HG, Cheng CW. Changing demography of prostate cancer in Asia. Eur J Cancer 2005;41:834–45.
2. Cook LS, Goldoft M, Schwartz SM, Weiss NS. Incidence of adenocarcinoma of the prostate in Asian immigrants to the United States and their descendants. J Urol 1999; 161:152–5.
3. World Cancer Research Fund and American Institute for Cancer Research. Food, nutrition, physical activity, and the prevention of cancer: a global perspective. Washington D.C.: American Institute for Cancer Research; 2007.
4. Sonoda T, Nagata Y, Mori M, et al. A case-control study of diet and prostate cancer in Japan: possible protective effect of traditional Japanese diet. Cancer Sci 2004;95:238–42.
5. Chen YC, Chiang CI, Lin RS, Pu YS, Lai MK, Sung FC. Diet, vegetarian food and prostate carcinoma among men in Taiwan. Br J Cancer 2005;93:1057–61.
6. Heald CL, Ritchie MR, Bolton-Smith C, Morton MS, Alexander FE. Phyto-oestrogens and risk of prostate cancer in Scottish men. Br J Nutr 2007;98:388–96.
7. Li XM, Li J, Tsuji I, Nakaya N, Nishino Y, Zhao XJ. Mass screening-based case-control study of diet and prostate cancer in Changchun, China. Asian J Androl 2008;10:551–60.
8. Allen NE, Sauvaget C, Roddam AW, et al. A prospective study of diet and prostate cancer in Japanese men. Cancer Causes Control 2004;15:911–20.
9. Kurahashi N, Iwasaki M, Sasazuki S, Otani T, Inoue M, Tsugane S. Soy product and isoflavone consumption in relation to prostate cancer in Japanese men. Cancer Epidemiol Biomarkers Prev 2007;16:538–45.
10. Smit E, Garcia-Palmieri MR, Figueroa NR, et al. Protein and legume intake and prostate cancer mortality in Puerto Rican men. Nutr Cancer 2007;58:146–52.
11. Park SY, Murphy SP, Wilkens LR, Henderson BE, Kolonel LN. Legume and isoflavone intake and prostate cancer risk: the Multiethnic Cohort Study. Int J Cancer 2008;123:927–32.
12. Ambrosini GL, de Klerk NH, Fritschi L, Mackerras D, Musk B. Fruit, vegetable, vitamin A intakes, and prostate cancer risk. Prostate Cancer Prostatic Dis 2008;11:61–6.
13. Clarke JD, Dashwood RH, Ho E. Multi-targeted prevention of cancer by sulforaphane. Cancer Lett 2008;269:291–304.
14. Higdon JV, Delage B, Williams DE, Dashwood RH. Cruciferous vegetables and human cancer risk: epidemiologic evidence and mechanistic basis. Pharmacol Res 2007;55:224–36.
15. Joseph MA, Moysich KB, Freudenheim JL, et al. Cruciferous vegetables, genetic polymorphisms in glutathione S-fransferases M1 and T1, and prostate cancer risk. Nutr Cancer 2004;50(2):206–13.
16. Jian L, Lee AH, Binns CW. Tea and lycopene protect against prostate cancer. Asia Pac J Clin Nutr 2007;16 suppl 1:453–7.
17. Key TJ, Appleby PN, Allen NE, et al. Plasma carotenoids, retinol, and tocopherols and the risk of prostate cancer in the European Prospective Investigation into Cancer and Nutrition study. Am J Clin Nutr 2007;86:672–81.
18. Kirsh VA, Mayne ST, Peters U, et al. A prospective study of lycopene and tomato product intake and risk of prostate cancer. Cancer Epidemiol Biomarkers Prev 2006;15:92–8.
19. McCann SE, Ambrosone CB, Moysich KB, et al. Intakes of selected nutrients, foods, and phytochemicals and prostate cancer risk in western New York. Nutr Cancer 2005;53:33–41.
20. Wu K, Erdman JW, Jr., Schwartz SJ, et al. Plasma and dietary carotenoids, and the risk of prostate cancer: a Nested Case-Control Study. Cancer Epidemiol Biomarkers Prev 2004;13:260–9.

21. Gann PH, Ma J, Giovannucci E, et al. Lower prostate cancer risk in men with elevated plasma lycopene levels: results of a prospective analysis. Cancer Res 1999;59:1225–30.

22. Chan JM, Holick CN, Leitzmann MF, et al. Diet after diagnosis and the risk of prostate cancer progression, recurrence, and death (United States). Cancer Causes Control 2006;17:199–208.

23. Weinstein SJ, Wright ME, Lawson KA, et al. Serum and dietary vitamin E in relation to prostate cancer risk. Cancer Epidemiol Biomarkers Prev 2007;16:1253–9.

24. Wright ME, Weinstein SJ, Lawson KA, et al. Supplemental and dietary vitamin E intakes and risk of prostate cancer in a large prospective study. Cancer Epidemiol Biomarkers Prev 2007;16:1128–35.

25. Chan JM, Gann PH, Giovannucci EL. Role of diet in prostate cancer development and progression. J Clin Oncol 2005;23:8152–60.

26. Peters U, Foster CB, Chatterjee N, et al. Serum selenium and risk of prostate cancer-a nested case-control study. Am J Clin Nutr 2007;85:209–17.

27. Brinkman M, Reulen RC, Kellen E, Buntinx F, Zeegers MP. Are men with low selenium levels at increased risk of prostate cancer? Eur J Cancer 2006;42:2463–71.

28. Allen NE, Morris JS, Ngwenyama RA, Key TJ. A case–control study of selenium in nails and prostate cancer risk in British men. Br J Cancer 2004;90:1392–6.

29. Brooks JD, Metter EJ, Chan DW, et al. Plasma selenium level before diagnosis and the risk of prostate cancer development. J Urol 2001;166:2034–8.

30. Vogt TM, Ziegler RG, Graubard BI, et al. Serum selenium and risk of prostate cancer in U.S. blacks and whites. Int J Cancer 2003;103:664–70.

31. Nomura AM, Lee J, Stemmermann GN, Combs GF. Serum selenium and subsequent risk of prostate cancer. Cancer Epidemiol Biomarkers Prev 2000;9:883–7.

32. Yoshizawa K, Willett WC, Morris SJ, et al. Study of prediagnostic selenium level in toenails and the risk of advanced prostate cancer. J Natl Cancer Inst 1998;90:1219–24.

33. van den Brandt PA, Zeegers MP, Bode P, Goldbohm RA. Toenail selenium levels and the subsequent risk of prostate cancer: a prospective cohort study. Cancer Epidemiol Biomarkers Prev 2003;12:866–71.

34. Li H, Stampfer MJ, Giovannucci EL, et al. A prospective study of plasma selenium levels and prostate cancer risk. J Natl Cancer Inst 2004;96:696–703.

35. Helzlsouer KJ, Huang HY, Alberg AJ, et al. Association between alpha-tocopherol, gamma-tocopherol, selenium, and subsequent prostate cancer. J Natl Cancer Inst 2000;92:2018–23.

36. Clark LC, Combs GF, Jr., Turnbull BW, et al. Effects of selenium supplementation for cancer prevention in patients with carcinoma of the skin. A randomized controlled trial. Nutritional Prevention of Cancer Study Group. JAMA 1996;276:1957–63.

37. Duffield-Lillico AJ, Reid ME, Turnbull BW, et al. Baseline characteristics and the effect of selenium supplementation on cancer incidence in a randomized clinical trial: a summary report of the Nutritional Prevention of Cancer Trial. Cancer Epidemiol Biomarkers Prev 2002;11:630–9.

38. Li H, Kantoff PW, Giovannucci E, et al. Manganese superoxide dismutase polymorphism, prediagnostic antioxidant status, and risk of clinical significant prostate cancer. Cancer Res 2005;65:2498–504.

39. Lawson KA, Wright ME, Subar A, et al. Multivitamin use and risk of prostate cancer in the National Institutes of Health-AARP Diet and Health Study. J Natl Cancer Inst 2007;99:754–64.

40. Torniainen S, Hedelin M, Autio V, et al. Lactase persistence, dietary intake of milk, and the risk for prostate cancer in Sweden and Finland. Cancer Epidemiol Biomarkers Prev 2007;16:956–61.

41. Ahn J, Albanes D, Peters U, et al. Dairy products, calcium intake, and risk of prostate cancer in the prostate, lung, colorectal, and ovarian cancer screening trial. Cancer Epidemiol Biomarkers Prev 2007;16:2623–30.

42. Allen NE, Key TJ, Appleby PN, et al. Animal foods, protein, calcium and prostate cancer risk: the European Prospective Investigation into Cancer and Nutrition. Br J Cancer 2008;98:1574–81.

43. Kurahashi N, Inoue M, Iwasaki M, Sasazuki S, Tsugane AS. Dairy product, saturated fatty acid, and calcium intake and prostate cancer in a prospective cohort of Japanese men. Cancer Epidemiol Biomarkers Prev 2008;17:930–7.

44. Rohrmann S, Platz EA, Kavanaugh CJ, Thuita L, Hoffman SC, Helzlsouer KJ. Meat and dairy consumption and subsequent risk of prostate cancer in a US cohort study. Cancer Causes Control 2007;18:41–50.

45. Neuhouser ML, Barnett MJ, Kristal AR, et al. (n-6) PUFA increase and dairy foods decrease prostate cancer risk in heavy smokers. J Nutr 2007;137:1821–7.

46. Park Y, Mitrou PN, Kipnis V, Hollenbeck A, Schatzkin A, Leitzmann MF. Calcium, dairy foods, and risk of incident and fatal prostate cancer: the NIH-AARP Diet and Health Study. Am J Epidemiol 2007;166:1270–9.

47. Baron JA, Beach M, Wallace K, et al. Risk of prostate cancer in a randomized clinical trial of calcium supplementation. Cancer Epidemiol Biomarkers Prev 2005;14:586–9.

48. Kolonel LN. Fat, meat, and prostate cancer. Epidemiol Rev 2001;23:72–81.

49. Platz EA, Giovannucci E. Prostate cancer. In: Schottenfeld D, Fraumeni JF, eds. Cancer epidemiology and prevention. 3 ed. New York: Oxford University Press; 2006:1128–50.

50. Koutros S, Cross AJ, Sandler DP, et al. Meat and meat mutagens and risk of prostate cancer in the Agricultural Health Study. Cancer Epidemiol Biomarkers Prev 2008;17:80–7.

51. Michaud DS, Augustsson K, Rimm EB, Stampfer MJ, Willet WC, Giovannucci E. A prospective study on intake of animal products and risk of prostate cancer. Cancer Causes Control 2001;12:557–67.

52. Park SY, Murphy SP, Wilkens LR, Henderson BE, Kolonel LN. Fat and meat intake and prostate cancer risk: the multiethnic cohort study. Int J Cancer 2007;121:1339–45.

53. Schuurman AG, van den Brandt PA, Dorant E, Goldbohm RA. Animal products, calcium and protein and prostate cancer risk in The Netherlands Cohort Study. Br J Cancer 1999;80:1107–13.

54. Veierod MB, Laake P, Thelle DS. Dietary fat intake and risk of prostate cancer: a prospective study of 25,708 Norwegian men. Int J Cancer 1997;73:634–8.

55. Cross AJ, Peters U, Kirsh VA, et al. A prospective study of meat and meat mutagens and prostate cancer risk. Cancer Res 2005;65:11779–84.

56. Rodriguez C, McCullough ML, Mondul AM, et al. Meat consumption among Black and White men and risk of prostate cancer in the Cancer Prevention Study II Nutrition Cohort. Cancer Epidemiol Biomarkers Prev 2006;15:211–6.

57. Connolly JM, Coleman M, Rose DP. Effects of dietary fatty acids on DU145 human prostate cancer cell growth in athymic nude mice. Nutr Cancer 1997;29:114–9.

58. Kobayashi N, Barnard RJ, Said J, et al. Effect of low-fat diet on development of prostate cancer and Akt phosphorylation in the Hi-Myc transgenic mouse model. Cancer Res 2008;68:3066–73.

59. Crowe FL, Key TJ, Appleby PN, et al. Dietary fat intake and risk of prostate cancer in the European Prospective Investigation into Cancer and Nutrition. Am J Clin Nutr 2008;87:1405–13.

60. Astorg P. Dietary N-6 and N-3 polyunsaturated fatty acids and prostate cancer risk: a review of epidemiological and experimental evidence. Cancer Causes Control 2004; 15:367–86.

61. Koralek DO, Peters U, Andriole G, et al. A prospective study of dietary alpha-linolenic acid and the risk of prostate cancer (United States). Cancer Causes Control 2006;17:783–91.

62. Leitzmann MF, Stampfer MJ, Michaud DS, et al. Dietary intake of n-3 and n-6 fatty acids and the risk of prostate cancer. Am J Clin Nutr 2004;80:204–16.

63. Tappel A. Heme of consumed red meat can act as a catalyst of oxidative damage and could initiate colon, breast and prostate cancers, heart disease and other diseases. Med Hypotheses 2007;68:562–4.

64. Keating GA, Layton DW, Felton JS. Factors determining dietary intakes of heterocyclic amines in cooked foods. Mutat Res 1999;443:149–56.

65. Keating GA, Sinha R, Layton D, et al. Comparison of heterocyclic amine levels in home-cooked meats with exposure indicators (United States). Cancer Causes Control 2000;11:731–9.

66. Thompson LH, Tucker JD, Stewart SA, et al. Genotoxicity of compounds from cooked beef in repair-deficient CHO cells versus Salmonella mutagenicity. Mutagenesis 1987; 2:483–7.

67. Felton JS, Knize MG. New mutagens from cooked food. Prog Clin Biol Res 1990;347:19–38.

68. Felton JS, Knize MG, Shen NH, Andresen BD, Bjeldanes LF, Hatch FT. Identification of the mutagens in cooked beef. Environ Health Perspect 1986;67:17–24.

69. Felton JS, Knize MG, Wood C, et al. Isolation and characterization of new mutagens from fried ground beef. Carcinogenesis 1984;5:95–102.

70. Sinha R, Knize MG, Salmon CP, et al. Heterocyclic amine content of pork products cooked by different methods and to varying degrees of doneness. Food Chem Toxicol 1998;36:289–97.

71. Sinha R, Rothman N, Brown ED, et al. High concentrations of the carcinogen 2-amino-1-methyl-6-phenylimidazo-[4,5-b]pyridine (PhIP) occur in chicken but are dependent on the cooking method. Cancer Res 1995;55:4516–9.

72. Sinha R, Rothman N, Salmon CP, et al. Heterocyclic amine content in beef cooked by different methods to varying degrees of doneness and gravy made from meat drippings. Food Chem Toxicol 1998;36:279–87.

73. Lawson T, Kolar C. Human prostate epithelial cells metabolize chemicals of dietary origin to mutagens. Cancer Lett 2002;175:141–6.

74. Martin FL, Cole KJ, Muir GH, et al. Primary cultures of prostate cells and their ability to activate carcinogens. Prostate Cancer Prostatic Dis 2002;5:96–104.

75. Williams JA, Martin FL, Muir GH, Hewer A, Grover PL, Phillips DH. Metabolic activation of carcinogens and expression of various cytochromes P450 in human prostate tissue. Carcinogenesis 2000;21:1683–9.

76. Di Paolo OA, Teitel CH, Nowell S, Coles BF, Kadlubar FF. Expression of cytochromes P450 and glutathione S-transferases in human prostate, and the potential for activation of heterocyclic amine carcinogens via acetyl-coA-, PAPS- and ATP-dependent pathways. Int J Cancer 2005;117:8–13.

77. Ghoshal A, Preisegger KH, Takayama S, Thorgeirsson SS, Snyderwine EG. Induction of mammary tumors in female Sprague-Dawley rats by the food-derived carcinogen 2-amino-1-methyl-6-phenylimidazo[4,5-b]pyridine and effect of dietary fat. Carcinogenesis 1994;15:2429–33.

78. Ito N, Hasegawa R, Imaida K, et al. Carcinogenicity of 2-amino-1-methyl-6-phenylimidazo[4,5-b]pyridine (PhIP) in the rat. Mutat Res 1997;376:107–14.

79. Ito N, Hasegawa R, Sano M, et al. A new colon and mammary carcinogen in cooked food, 2-amino-1-methyl-6-phenylimidazo[4,5-b]pyridine (PhIP). Carcinogenesis 1991; 12:1503–6.

80. Ochiai M, Ogawa K, Wakabayashi K, et al. Induction of intestinal adenocarcinomas by 2-amino-1-methyl-6-phenylimidazo[4,5-b]pyridine in Nagase analbuminemic rats. Jpn J Cancer Res 1991;82:363–6.

81. Ohgaki H, Hasegawa H, Kato T, et al. Carcinogenicity in mice and rats of heterocyclic amines in cooked foods. Environ Health Perspect 1986;67:129–34.

82. Shirai T, Cui L, Takahashi S, et al. Carcinogenicity of 2-amino-1-methyl-6-phenylimidazo [4,5-b]pyridine (PhIP) in the rat prostate and induction of invasive carcinomas by subsequent treatment with testosterone propionate. Cancer Lett 1999;143:217–21.

83. Shirai T, Sano M, Tamano S, et al. The prostate: a target for carcinogenicity of 2-amino-1-methyl-6-phenylimidazo[4,5-b]pyridine (PhIP) derived from cooked foods. Cancer Res 1997;57:195–8.

84. Stuart GR, Holcroft J, de Boer JG, Glickman BW. Prostate mutations in rats induced by the suspected human carcinogen 2-amino-1-methyl-6-phenylimidazo[4,5-b]pyridine. Cancer Res 2000;60:266–8.

85. De Stefani E, Fierro L, Barrios E, Ronco A. Tobacco, alcohol, diet and risk of prostate cancer. Tumori 1995;81:315–20.

86. Ewings P, Bowie C. A case-control study of cancer of the prostate in Somerset and east Devon. Br J Cancer 1996; 74:661–6.

87. Kampman E, Slattery ML, Bigler J, et al. Meat consumption, genetic susceptibility, and colon cancer risk: a United States multicenter case-control study. Cancer Epidemiol Biomarkers Prev 1999;8:15–24.

88. Lang NP, Butler MA, Massengill J, et al. Rapid metabolic phenotypes for acetyltransferase and cytochrome P4501A2 and putative exposure to food-borne heterocyclic amines

increase the risk for colorectal cancer or polyps. Cancer Epidemiol Biomarkers Prev 1994;3:675–82.

89. Mills PK, Beeson WL, Phillips RL, Fraser GE. Cohort study of diet, lifestyle, and prostate cancer in Adventist men. Cancer 1989;64:598–604.

90. Murtaugh MA, Ma KN, Sweeney C, Caan BJ, Slattery ML. Meat consumption patterns and preparation, genetic variants of metabolic enzymes, and their association with rectal cancer in men and women. J Nutr 2004;134:776–84.

91. Norrish AE, Ferguson LR, Knize MG, Felton JS, Sharpe SJ, Jackson RT. Heterocyclic amine content of cooked meat and risk of prostate cancer. J Natl Cancer Inst 1999;91:2038–44.

92. Probst-Hensch NM, Sinha R, Longnecker MP, et al. Meat preparation and colorectal adenomas in a large sigmoidoscopy-based case-control study in California (United States). Cancer Causes Control 1997;8:175–83.

93. Sinha R, Kulldorff M, Curtin J, Brown CC, Alavanja MC, Swanson CA. Fried, well-done red meat and risk of lung cancer in women (United States). Cancer Causes Control 1998;9:621–30.

94. Sinha R, Rothman N. Role of well-done, grilled red meat, heterocyclic amines (HCAs) in the etiology of human cancer. Cancer Lett 1999;143:189–94.

95. Ward MH, Sinha R, Heineman EF, et al. Risk of adenocarcinoma of the stomach and esophagus with meat cooking method and doneness preference. Int J Cancer 1997;71:14–9.

96. Zheng W, Gustafson DR, Sinha R, et al. Well-done meat intake and the risk of breast cancer. J Natl Cancer Inst 1998;90:1724–9.

97. Augustsson K, Skog K, Jagerstad M, Dickman PW, Steineck G. Dietary heterocyclic amines and cancer of the colon, rectum, bladder, and kidney: a population-based study. Lancet 1999;353:703–7.

98. Lyon JL, Mahoney AW. Fried foods and the risk of colon cancer. Am J Epidemiol 1988;128:1000–6.

99. Muscat JE, Wynder EL. The consumption of well-done red meat and the risk of colorectal cancer. Am J Public Health 1994;84:856–8.

100. Lijinsky W. N-Nitroso compounds in the diet. Mutat Res 1999;443:129–38.

101. Hughes R, Cross AJ, Pollock JR, Bingham S. Dose-dependent effect of dietary meat on endogenous colonic N-nitrosation. Carcinogenesis 2001;22:199–202.

102. Terry PD, Rohan TE, Wolk A. Intakes of fish and marine fatty acids and the risks of cancers of the breast and prostate and of other hormone-related cancers: a review of the epidemiologic evidence. Am J Clin Nutr 2003;77:532–43.

103. Augustsson K, Michaud DS, Rimm EB, et al. A prospective study of intake of fish and marine fatty acids and prostate cancer. Cancer Epidemiol Biomarkers Prev 2003;12:64–7.

104. Terry P, Lichtenstein P, Feychting M, Ahlbom A, Wolk A. Fatty fish consumption and risk of prostate cancer. Lancet 2001;357:1764–6.

105. Hedelin M, Chang ET, Wiklund F, et al. Association of frequent consumption of fatty fish with prostate cancer risk is modified by COX-2 polymorphism. Int J Cancer 2007;120:398–405.

106. Terry PD, Terry JB, Rohan TE. Long-chain (n-3) fatty acid intake and risk of cancers of the breast and the prostate: recent epidemiological studies, biological mechanisms, and directions for future research. J Nutr 2004;134:3412S–20S.

107. Fradet Y, Meyer F, Bairati I, Shadmani R, Moore L. Dietary fat and prostate cancer progression and survival. Eur Urol 1999;35:388–91.

108. Strom SS, Yamamura Y, Forman MR, Pettaway CA, Barrera SL, DiGiovanni J. Saturated fat intake predicts biochemical failure after prostatectomy. Int J Cancer 2008;122:2581–5.

109. Bairati I, Meyer F, Fradet Y, Moore L. Dietary fat and advanced prostate cancer. J Urol 1998;159:1271–5.

110. Aronson WJ, Glaspy JA, Reddy ST, Reese D, Heber D, Bagga D. Modulation of omega-3/omega-6 polyunsaturated ratios with dietary fish oils in men with prostate cancer. Urology 2001;58:283–8.

111. Ornish D, Weidner G, Fair WR, et al. Intensive lifestyle changes may affect the progression of prostate cancer. J Urol 2005;174:1065-9; discussion 9–70.

112. Schroder FH, Roobol MJ, Boeve ER, et al. Randomized, double-blind, placebo-controlled crossover study in men with prostate cancer and rising PSA: effectiveness of a dietary supplement. Eur Urol 2005;48:922-30; discussion 30–1.

113. Chen L, Stacewicz-Sapuntzakis M, Duncan C, et al. Oxidative DNA damage in prostate cancer patients consuming tomato sauce-based entrees as a whole-food intervention. J Natl Cancer Inst 2001;93:1872–9.

Chapter 33
Inflammation as a Target in Prostate Cancer

Marshall Scott Lucia, James R. Lambert, Elizabeth A. Platz, and Angelo M. De Marzo

Abstract Epidemiological studies have implicated chronic infections and inflammation as major risk factors for a variety of human cancers. Emerging evidence suggests that chronic inflammation is important for the development of prostate cancer and foci of inflammation (i.e., lymphocytes and macrophages) and is extremely common in the prostate. Multiple mechanisms have been investigated in studies examining the role of inflammation in prostate cancer initiation and development. In this chapter, we review the current state of thinking on the causes of prostatic inflammation, inflammatory genes potentially involved in prostatic inflammation and carcinogenesis, and the role of inflammation in the development of prostate cancer. An understanding of the role of chronic inflammation in the development of prostate cancer will provide new therapeutic strategies to combat the disease.

Keywords Carcinogenesis • Chemoprevention • Chemotherapy • Cytokines • Inflammation • Oxidative stress • Prostate cancer

It is estimated that 20% of all human malignancies, including those of the colon, liver, stomach, bladder, cervix, and lung, result from chronic inflammation and/or chronic infections [1]. Although not yet proven, epidemiologic and histopathologic evidence is accumulating to incriminate chronic inflammation in the pathogenesis of prostate cancer. As the molecular pathways that orchestrate inflammatory processes become better defined, so do their potential

M.S. Lucia (✉)
Department of Pathology, University of Colorado, Denver, Aurora, CO, USA
e-mail: scott.lucia@ucdenver.edu

roles in carcinogenesis. Inflammation due to tissue injury by infectious agents or other stimuli serves in the eradication of pathogens, clearing of debris, epithelial regeneration, stromal remodeling, and vascularization to heal the wound and restore function of the tissue. Once the repair is completed, the inflammatory reaction typically subsides. However, when inflammation becomes prolonged or unrelenting, these same processes may provide the critical ingredients for the development and progression of cancer, particularly in situations where epithelial mutagenesis has occurred.

Chronic Inflammation of the Prostate

Areas of inflammation are extremely common in the prostate, with studies reporting a prevalence of >95% in resection specimens particularly involving the peripheral zone of the prostate where prostate cancer typically occurs [2–4]. Macrophages, T-cells and B-cells, characteristically present even in normal prostate [2], are increased in the aged and hyperplastic prostate [3–5]. The majority (70–80%) of lymphocytes are CD3+ T lymphocytes, >90% of which express $\alpha\beta$ T-cell receptor (TCR) [5–8]. A small percentage (<5%) express $\gamma\delta$ TCR that respond to nonconventional phosphoantigens and demonstrate antitumor cytotoxic activity, although these cells may be present in higher numbers in cancerous tissues [9]. Both type 1 (Th1) and type 2 (Th2) immune responses, defined by differential cytokine production, have been found in hyperplastic tissues [10].

Inflammation is often found to involve areas of focal prostatic atrophy [4, 11]. A spectrum of focal atrophic lesions that are associated with variable

W.D. Figg et al. (eds.), *Drug Management of Prostate Cancer*,
DOI 10.1007/978-1-60327-829-4_33, © Springer Science+Business Media, LLC 2010

degrees of chronic inflammation have been described on a histological basis and grouped under the term proliferative inflammatory atrophy (PIA), with the recognition that many of these lesions have demonstrated increased proliferation and therefore may be a form of repair [11, 12]. Like prostate cancer, PIA occurs predominantly in the peripheral zone of the prostate (as opposed to the more centrally-located transition zone where benign hyperplasia tends to occur) and increases in frequency with advancing age [4, 11, 12]. PIA lesions have also been suggested as representing early events in prostatic carcinogenesis [4, 11, 13].

Possible Causes of Prostatic Inflammation

Although chronic inflammation in the prostate is a common occurrence, the cause of prostatic inflammation is unknown. Infectious, hormonal, dietary, and/or physico-chemical factors have the potential to produce a chronic inflammatory process in the prostate. It is also possible that once one or more of these insults triggers an initial inflammatory response, it could lead to the development of an autoimmune reaction to prostatic antigens that continues well after the inciting agent is cleared.

Infectious Agents

A variety of bacteria (sexually and nonsexually transmitted) and viruses have been detected in the prostate (reviewed in [4]); some of these agents may reach the prostate and elicit an inflammatory response [14]. Although generally felt to be acute or self-limited in condition, the potential for infections to become chronic or unrelenting is not known. Certainly, asymptomatic infections can occur. Several small scale case–control epidemiologic studies have observed mildly increased risks for prostate cancer in men with histories of sexually-transmitted infections [15, 16]. Meta-analyses calculated odds ratio of 1.4–1.5 for men with a history of any sexually-transmitted infection, 1.4 for a history of gonor-

rhea, and 1.6–2.3 for a history of syphilis [15, 16], although in these studies recall bias cannot be excluded. A higher risk of prostate cancer was also identified in a prospective study in men who carried antibodies against the protozoan *Trichomonas vaginalis* [17]. A number of viruses including herpes viruses, cytomegalovirus, and human papilloma virus may also infect the prostate; however, little evidence exists to support a causal role in prostate cancer (reviewed in [18]). Whereas these studies have focused on classical pathogens, it is also possible that an as yet unidentified microbe or virus may be involved in the pathogenesis of prostate cancer. Recently, a new γ retrovirus, xenotropic murine leukemia-related virus (XMRV) was detected in prostate cancer specimens using a DNA microarray-based analysis [19]. The virus was detected primarily in men with a specific germline mutation of RNASEL (see below), the gene that encodes for the antiviral enzyme RNaseL, suggesting that prolonged infection in the prostate may be a result of genetic predisposition. While intriguing, it is yet unknown whether this virus might also be found in the prostates of men without a diagnosis of prostate cancer. Although all of these results suggest that an infectious cause may be potentially responsible for a certain proportion of prostate cancer, this may not be necessarily due to direct oncogenic actions of an infectious agent. Prolonged infection could trigger an inflammatory reaction that persists despite clearance of the organism by the unmasking of self antigens in an autoimmune manner. In support of this, T-cell responses against histone peptides and prostate-specific antigen (PSA) have been detected in the prostate [20, 21].

Hormones

It has long been recognized that androgens are involved in prostatic carcinogenesis [22], forming the basis for androgen ablation therapy for advanced prostate cancer. In rodent models, estrogens can potentiate prostatic carcinogenesis when combined with androgen [23]. Estrogens in the presence of androgen causes increased prostatic inflammation in animal models [24]. Although the mechanism by which this occurs is unclear, it may involve upregulation of nuclear factor kappa B (NF-κB) [24].

Dietary Factors

The potential for cell and DNA damage by reactive oxygen and/or nitrogen species elaborated during an immune response to infectious agents or other elicitors may be countered by antioxidants. In some studies, higher exposure to lycopene (a free-radical scavenger), selenium (an element required for activity of an anti-oxidant enzyme), and vitamin E, at least in smokers, have each been observed to be inversely associated with prostate cancer risk [25–27].

Epidemiological studies also suggest an association between consumption of animal fat and red and processed meat and prostate cancer incidence and mortality [28]. It is hypothesized that certain dietary compounds are selectively taken up in the prostate, thereby acting as either direct carcinogens (initiators and/or promoters) or indirectly by stimulating a localized inflammatory reaction. For example, the heterocyclic amine, 2-amino-1-methyl-6-phenylimidazo[4,5-b]pyridine (PhIP), is a carcinogen formed during the cooking of meats at high temperature [28]. Administration of PhIP to laboratory rats produces carcinomas of the ventral prostate [29]. Interestingly, despite observed increases in mutation frequency in all four lobes of the rat prostate upon PhIP administration (initiating activity), carcinomas only developed in the ventral prostate where there was also a ventral lobe-specific increase in inflammatory cells, particularly macrophages and mast cells associated with epithelial injury and atrophy analogous to PIA (promoting activity) [29].

Prostatic and Urinary Factors

The prostatic epithelium produces a variety of factors that can stimulate or inhibit inflammatory reactions. For example, PSA, a major serine protease produced by prostatic epithelial cells, has been shown to stimulate a T-cell immune reaction in patients with prostatitis/pelvic pain syndrome [21]. Inspissated prostatic secretions, or corpora amylacea, may erode into the stroma where they often produce a profound chronic inflammatory reaction [4]. Increased ejaculation frequency has been associated with a lower risk for prostate cancer [30]. Functional purging or "flushing" of the prostate may reduce epithelial contact with

carcinogens that are concentrated in urine or prostatic secretions, reduce the likelihood of corpora amylacea forming, reduce risk of infection, and stimulate healthy epithelial turnover. Obstruction or urine reflux may lead to increased prostatic inflammation through chemical irritation, increased exposure to infectious agents, or pressure-induced epithelial injury with subsequent production of inflammatory cytokines.

Functional mature prostatic epithelium also produces potential inhibitors of inflammation including transforming growth factor-beta (TGF-β) and prostate-derived factor (PDF) (aka macrophage inhibitory cytokine, MIC-1). It is therefore plausible that in normal prostate, there is a balance between pro-inflammatory and anti-inflammatory processes. When this balance is perturbed either by an increase in pro-inflammatory or a decrease in anti-inflammatory factors or both by one or more dietary, infectious, hormonal or physicochemical insults, a chronic inflammatory condition occurs. Progressive damage to the prostatic tissues may then "fuel the fire" to produce an autoimmune reaction forming the "primordial soup" of eventual carcinogenesis.

Inflammatory Genes in Prostate Cancer

Heredity plays an important role in prostatic carcinogenesis with an estimated one-quarter of all prostate cancer occurring in family clusters [31–33]. Several of the genes associated with prostate cancer risk encode products that play critical roles in inflammatory pathways. Pedigree analysis has identified three genes, RNASEL, PDF, and MSR1, which are linked to prostate cancer [34–36]. Variants in genes encoding other components of the immune response, including interleukins (IL-6, IL-8, IL-10) and toll-like receptors (TLRs) have also been evaluated for their associations with prostate cancer in case–control studies [37].

RNASEL

The hereditary prostate cancer 1 (HPC1) region on chromosome 1 was the first susceptibility region identified in familial prostate cancer [34]. Subsequent studies demonstrated that the HPC1 locus harbors the gene encoding ribonuclease L (RNASEL). RNaseL functions in the innate immune system by degrading single-stranded viral RNAs. Sustained activation of RNaseL leads to a mitochondrial-mediated pathway of apoptosis that eliminates virally infected cells [38]. Mutations in RNASEL lead to production of RNaseL with impaired ability to promote apoptosis of virally infected cells. Several studies examining the role of RNASEL as a prostate cancer susceptibility gene have been reported. While some studies demonstrate confirmatory evidence, others do not [39], suggesting either population differences or environmental factors may modulate the role of RNASEL in prostatic carcinogenesis.

A common genetic variant in RNASEL resulting in reduced enzymatic activity of RNaseL (R462Q) has been implicated in up to 13% of prostate cancers. The XMRV virus was primarily detected in individuals homozygous for this mutation [19]. Activation of RNaseL in DU145 human prostate cancer cells induced the putative pro-apoptotic suppressor of prostate cancer, PDF.

Prostate-Derived Factor

PDF is a secretory protein with homology to members of the TGF-β superfamily and has previously been identified as nonsteroidal anti-inflammatory drug (NSAID)-activated gene (NAG-1) and MIC-1 [40, 41]. PDF was first identified as a gene involved in macrophage activation, and its expression is induced by NSAIDs in human colorectal carcinoma cells [40, 41]. Together, these findings support a role for PDF in inflammatory processes and may provide insight into the proposed tumor-suppressive activities of PDF.

PDF mRNA is highly expressed in human prostate epithelium suggesting a role in prostate homeostasis, and several studies have shown that PDF inhibits prostate cancer cell growth and induces apoptosis [42–44]. PDF resides on chromosome 19 in a region identified as a susceptibility locus in genome-wide studies on prostate cancer incidence [35]. Additionally, a genetic polymorphism in PDF has been described that changes the basic amino acid histidine (H) to aspartic acid (D) at position 6 of the mature PDF protein [45]. This change has been associated with a lower risk of sporadic and familial prostate cancer [35]. However,

a similar study found the H6D polymorphism to be only marginally associated with a lower risk of prostate cancer development, but it was associated with increased risk of progression once the tumor had been established [46]. Thus, the role of PDF in prostate cancer initiation and progression is not clear.

Macrophage Scavenger Receptor (MSR1)

Macrophage scavenger receptor (MSR1) is a candidate prostate cancer susceptibility gene identified through linkage analysis of HPC [36]. The MSR1 gene encodes a homotrimeric class A receptor that is primarily expressed in macrophages. It is termed a "scavenger receptor" due to the diverse array of ligands it binds including gram-positive and gram-negative bacteria and lipoproteins. MSR1 action has been linked to a variety of normal and pathologic processes including inflammation and immunity. Mice defective for MSR1 function are more susceptible to bacterial infection suggesting an anti-inflammatory role for MSR1 [47, 48].

Although a number of studies have demonstrated an increased frequency of MSR1 mutations in men with prostate cancer, studies on the role of these variants and prostate cancer risk have yielded inconsistent results. Interestingly, MSR1 mutations have been identified to have a more reproducible effect on prostate cancer risk in African-American men [49]. Although studies to date have not defined MSR1 as a major prostate cancer gene per se, they do suggest that MSR1 may, in combination with environmental cues such as pathogen infection, modify prostate cancer risk.

Interleukins

Case–control studies have evaluated sequence variants in the genes encoding IL-8 and IL-10 among others and prostate cancer risk with mixed results. IL-8 is a pro-inflammatory cytokine often found at elevated levels in the semen of men with chronic prostatitis [50] and is also associated with prostatic angiogenesis [51]. IL-10 is considered an anti-inflammatory cytokine with immunoregulatory functions including downregulation of Th1. Further work is necessary to evaluate the hypothesis that sequence variants in IL-8 and/or IL-10 are involved in prostatic inflammation and development of prostate cancer.

Toll-Like Receptors

TLRs are transmembrane proteins expressed by cells of the innate immune system. TLRs recognize invading pathogens and activate signaling pathways leading to inflammatory immune responses that clear the infection. In humans, the TLR family includes eleven proteins (TLR1–TLR11). Different TLRs serve as receptors for a wide variety of ligands including bacterial cell-wall components, viral RNA or immunomodulatory compounds.

Several studies have explored the possible connection between TLR signaling and prostate cancer. Sequence variants in several TLR genes including TLR-4 and the TLR-1–6–10 cluster have been linked to prostate cancer risk [52, 53]. Further investigations are required to understand the biological consequences of TLR signaling and prostate cancer risk. However, because TLR signaling is so critically related to innate immunity, it is intriguing to speculate a central role for TLR-signaling in prostatic inflammation and prostate cancer development.

Chronic Inflammation in the Development of Prostate Cancer

The "immune surveillance" theory has long held that inflammation is a consequence of the host response against a cancer rather than a cause [54]. However, recent evidence suggests that the cytokine environment of tumor-associated inflammatory cells actually suppresses cell-mediated antitumor immune surveillance activities [55, 56]. Indeed, studies now suggest that longstanding inflammation through a number of interrelated mechanisms acting in a concerted fashion may serve to favor tumor growth and spread. These include the elaboration of cytokines and growth factors that favor tumor cell growth, generation of mutagenic reactive oxygen and nitrogen species (ROS and RNS), and induction of cyclooxygenase-2 and prostaglandin (PG) synthesis.

Cytokines and Growth Factors

Chronic inflammation produces an environment rich in cytokines and growth factors that govern cell-to-cell communication and may contribute to malignant progression [57]. Tumor necrosis factor-α (TNF-α), a pro-inflammatory cytokine produced predominantly by macrophages/monocytes upon exposure to a wide range of stimuli, has an important role in orchestrating inflammatory events, host responses to pathogens, and wound healing by inducing a cascade of other cytokines and growth factors such as COX-2, angiogenic factors, and matrix metalloproteins (MMPs) [58]. Production of TNF-α in cultured prostate cancer cells suppresses androgen receptor expression and may contribute to loss of androgen responsiveness [59]. TNF-α may also directly stimulate tumor cell proliferation through activation of NF-κB [60]. The NF-κB family of transcription factors includes key regulators of genes involved in cell growth and differentiation such as c-myc, cyclin-D1, and IL-6 and inhibitors of apoptosis such as Bcl-2 (Fig. 33.1) [61]. NF-κB may also regulate angiogenesis through modulation of vascular endothelial growth factor (VEGF) [61, 62].

VEGF stimulates endothelial proliferation, induces angiogenesis, regulates vascular permeability and is a key target for antiangiogenic chemotherapeutic agents [63, 64]. Although VEGF expression is limited to basal cells in the normal prostate, it is also expressed in prostate cancer and prostatic intraepithelial neoplasia (PIN) [65]. In addition to NF-κB, VEGF production is induced by prostaglandin E2 (PGE2) and TNF-α.

A variety of interleukins and chemokines produced by inflammatory cells during the inflammatory response may have the potential to stimulate tumor cell proliferation, survival, and metastasis. Interleukins such as IL-1 and IL-8 have been shown to stimulate growth of cancer cells in vitro [66, 67]. IL-1 modulates the expression of MMPs that facilitate cell migration [68]. IL-8 is a potent inducer of angiogenesis [69]. Finally, CXC group chemokines, such as gro-α and CXC-12, may contribute to carcinogenesis by direct stimulation of tumor cell growth, regulation of angiogenesis, or aid in tumor cell chemotaxis [68, 70, 71].

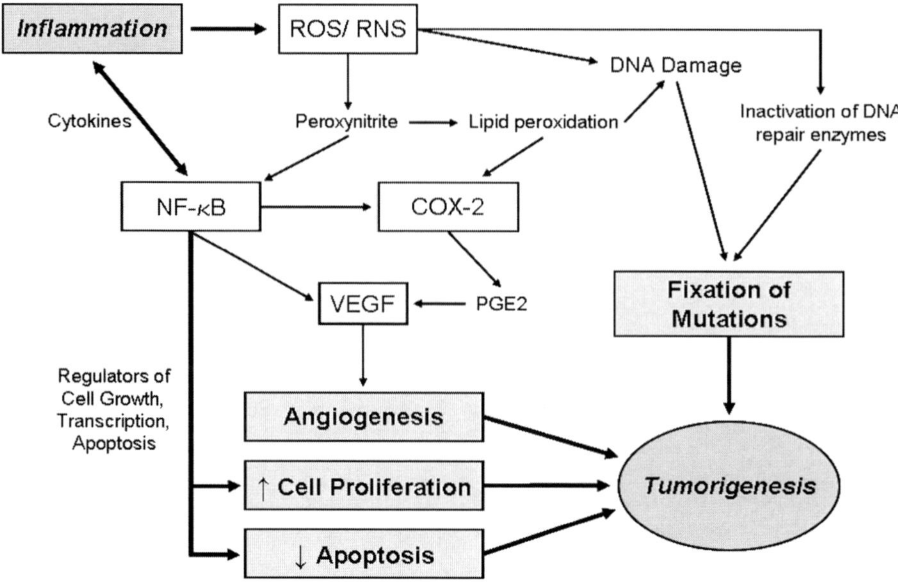

Fig. 33.1 Complex interaction between reactive oxygen species (ROS), reactive nitrogen species (RNS), nuclear factor kappa B (NF-κB), cyclooxygenase-2 (COX-2), vascular endothelial growth factor (VEGF), and cellular processes promoting tumorigenesis. *PGE2* prostaglandin E2

Oxidative Stress

Condemning evidence implicating inflammation in prostate carcinogenesis comes from molecular changes that occur in inflamed benign prostatic tissues such as PIA. Epithelial cells in PIA overexpress the glutathione S-transferases (GST) GSTP1 and GSTA1, suggesting that PIA lesions are under oxidative stress, possibly in part due to reactive species generated during the inflammatory response [11, 72]. Reactive oxygen species (ROS), such as superoxide and hydrogen peroxide, are highly reactive intermediate by-products of oxidative metabolism. ROS are produced in relatively high quantities by activated macrophages in response to a variety of stimuli as part of the "respiratory burst." ROS may also be produced in many cell types in response to inflammatory cytokines and during the metabolism of many known carcinogens [73]. Reactive nitrogen species (RNS) include nitric oxide (NO) and its reactive intermediates. NO is a gas with free-radical properties that has a number of diverse actions including neurotransmission, vasodilatation, induction of apoptosis, p53 regulation, and modulation of epithelial proliferation [74]. RNS are produced in relatively high quantities by inflammatory cells and most other cell types by the inducible form of the

enzyme NO synthase (iNOS, NOS2) in response to stimulation with inflammatory cytokines, such as TNF-α and IL-1 [75].

ROS and RNS may contribute to carcinogenesis by damaging cellular lipids, proteins, and DNA (see Fig. 33.1). For instance, ROS and RNS together form peroxynitrite that directly damages cellular lipids and proteins [74]. ROS are also directly mutagenic to DNA causing the formation of 8-hydroxyguanine (8-OHG) [76]. As a defense against such insults, ROS can be neutralized by intracellular antioxidants (e.g., vitamin E, carotenoids) and cellular enzymes (e.g., glutathione peroxidase, which requires selenium for activity and glutathione-S-transferases) [77]. Oxidative and nitrosative stress refers to an imbalance between the production of reactive intermediates and these antioxidant defenses. GSTP1 is the primary GST present in prostatic epithelial cells. It is responsible for inactivating oxidant carcinogens via conjugation to reduced glutathione [77]. Inactivation of the GSTP1 gene by CpG island methylation occurs in a very high proportion of prostate cancer and PIN specimens [78]. Other major antioxidant enzymes including copper-zinc superoxide dismutase, manganese superoxide dismutase, and catalase were also shown to have lower expression in PIN and prostate cancer compared to benign epithelium

[79]. The transition of PIA lesions to prostate cancer may be supported by the observation that in tissues taken from men with prostate cancer, the proportion of methylated GSTP1 promoter region CpG sites is 0% in normal epithelium and BPH, approximately 6% in PIA, 70% in HGPIN, and over 90% in adenocarcinoma [13].

Measures of oxidative stress can be increased by androgens in human prostate cancer cell lines [80]. In situations of increased oxidative and/or nitrosative stress, progressive damage to epithelial cells leads to cell death triggering replacement by proliferation of resident progenitor cells. DNA synthesis in the presence of mutagenic reactive intermediates is thus at increased risk of mutagenesis. Damage to DNA repair enzymes via hydroxylation (ROS) or nitrosylation (RNS) may alter their activity, thereby exacerbating mutagenesis [81]. The cumulative result is an imbalance between the rate of mutagenesis and the ability to repair mutations (without error), allowing for their progressive accumulation [82].

Cyclooxygenase-2

Cyclooxygenase (COX) is a key enzyme in the synthesis of PGs and other eicosanoids from arachidonic acid (AA) and exists in two isoforms. COX-1 is constitutively expressed in many tissues, whereas COX-2 is not usually expressed or expressed at very low levels in epithelial tissues but is predominantly expressed by inflammatory cells such as macrophages. Oxidative stress can rapidly induce COX-2 in epithelial cells, either directly through lipid peroxidation [83] or indirectly through induction of NF-κB (see Fig. 33.1) [84]. COX-2 may also be induced by TNF-α and interleukin-1 produced by inflammatory cells [85]. Overexpression of COX-2 is associated with increased tumorigenesis in animal models and alterations in cellular adhesion and apoptosis in epithelial cells [86]. COX-2 stimulates angiogenesis in tumors by induction of PGE2 and VEGF [87]. Conversely, suppression of COX-2 inhibits angiogenesis and tumor growth [87]. While studies have shown that COX-2 may or may not be elevated in prostate cancers per se, benign tissues that are inflamed such as PIA show elevated COX-2 expression [88]. In vitro studies showed that COX-2 inhibitors decreased growth and increased apoptosis in prostate cancer cell lines [89]. Apoptosis due to inhibition of COX-2 is a result of shunting of AA metabolism to stimulate the production of ceramide, a mediator of apoptosis [90]. Thus, nonsteroidal anti-inflammatory agents (NSAIDs) or specific COX-2 inhibitors to inhibit COX-2 and PG synthesis may have therapeutic or chemopreventive potential (Fig. 33.2). Studies using animal models of prostate carcinogenesis and metastasis demonstrated suppression of tumor growth and metastasis with nonsteroidal anti-inflammatory agents (NSAIDs) or selective COX-2 inhibitors [91, 92].

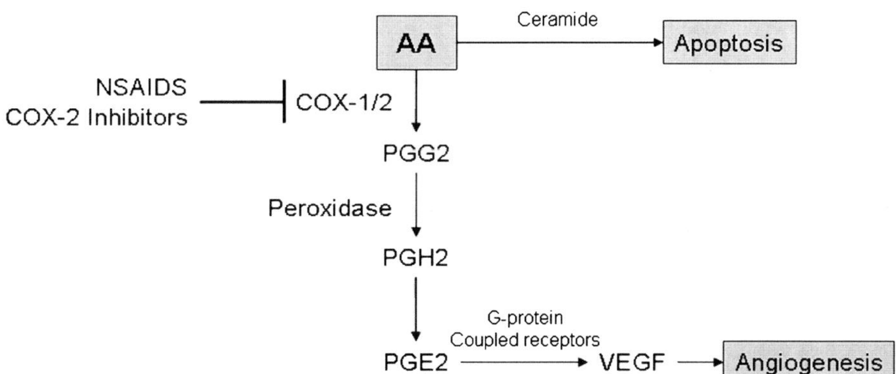

Fig. 33.2 Schematic diagram highlighting prostaglandin E2 (PGE2) synthesis from arachidonic acid (AA). PGE2, interacting with G-protein coupled receptors, leads to increased angiogenesis through upregulation of VEGF. Inhibition of cyclooxygenase-2 (COX-2) by nonsteroidal anti-inflammatory drugs (NSAIDS) and/or selective COX-2 inhibitors inhibits angiogenesis and promotes apoptosis through channeling of AA through ceramide. *PGG2* prostaglandin G2; *PGH2* prostaglandin H2

Inflammation in Metastasis

The role of inflammation in metastasis is not very well defined. The observation that matrix metalloprotiens (MMPs) are produced by leukocytes present within tumors suggests that matrix remodeling in areas of chronic inflammation may promote cell motility and intravasation of tumor cells [93]. Induction of angiogenesis in regions of chronic inflammation may also promote tumor metastasis. Perhaps most damning in the implication of chronic inflammation and metastatic dissemination of cancer cells comes from a study on the regulation of the metastasis suppressor Maspin by IκB kinaseα (IKKα). IKKα is activated by receptor activator of NF-κB ligand (RANKL), a cytokine produced by inflammatory cells. An inverse correlation was observed, both in a mouse model and human tissue, between IKKα activation and Maspin production, suggesting that RANKL produced by inflammatory cells associated with prostate tumors activates IKKα leading to downregulation of Maspin and enhancement of metastasis [62].

Targeting Inflammation in the Management of Prostate Cancer

When designing clinical trials targeting inflammation in prostate cancer, both the protumorigenic and antitumorigenic roles of inflammatory cells and processes must be considered. Strategies aimed at interfering with the above protumorigenic processes while bolstering antitumorigenic cell-mediated immunity would be ideal. For the latter, emerging evidence suggests that stimulating antitumor T-cell responses using aminobisphosphonates (activation of $\gamma\delta$ T cells) or stimulating hsp70 activity holds promise for treatment of advanced prostate cancer [94, 95].

Coupling increased cell proliferation with mutagenesis forms the key recipe for carcinogenesis. Formation of new vasculature (angiogenesis) and stimulation of cell motility then sets the stage for tumor progression. As reviewed herein, factors produced by inflammatory cells may participate during all stages of carcinogenesis including early events of tumor initiation and promotion (Fig. 33.3). Thus, key

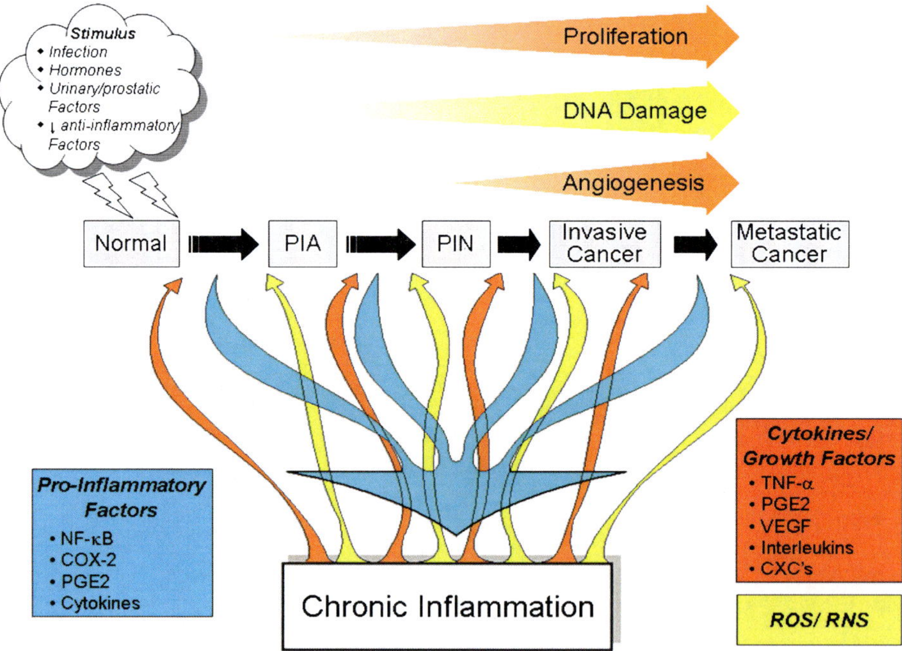

Fig. 33.3 The interplay between pro-inflammatory factors produced by prostatic epithelium during progression of prostatic carcinogenesis and reciprocal products of chronic inflammation. Following stimulation by one or more stimuli (*white cloud*), pro-inflammatory factors (*blue box* and *arrow*) stimulate production of protumorigenic cytokines and growth factors (*orange box* and *arrows*) and reactive oxygen/nitrogen species (ROS/RNS, *yellow box* and *arrows*) promoting progression of tumorigenesis through increased cell proliferation coupled with progressive DNA damage and angiogenesis. *PIA* proliferative inflammatory atrophy; *PIN* prostatic intraepithelial neoplasia

regulatory elements in the inflammatory response, such as NF-κB and COX-2, represent legitimate targets for chemoprevention and therapeutic strategies. In support of this, a case–control study reported a 55% risk reduction for prostate cancer with selective COX-2 inhibitors after adjusting for age and potential confounders [96]. A meta-analysis of 91 epidemiologic studies showed significant risk reductions for a number of human malignancies, including a 39% risk reduction for prostate cancer in patients daily taking NSAIDS [97]. There was an inverse association between NSAID intake and prostate cancer risk. COX-2 inhibitors have also been used in clinical trials in men with rising PSA after radical prostatectomy and/or radiation therapy for prostate cancer. Although outcomes data have not been reported, use of COX-2 inhibitors slowed PSA doubling times, suggesting an effect on tumor progression [98, 99]. Non-COX-2-dependent mechanisms may be responsible for some of the anticancer effects of these drugs [100]. To date, use of COX-2 inhibitors for chemoprevention is limited due to the potential for adverse cardiovascular effects; future refinement of these agents to minimize cardiovascular toxicity is warranted.

Combating oxidative stress through the use of antioxidants is particularly attractive for chemoprevention since these agents are usually well tolerated, and intake can be increased through the diet by taking supplements. Antioxidants such as lycopene (tomato products), resveratrol (grape products, peanuts), selenium, and vitamin E are being evaluated clinically. The effect of these agents may involve other anticancer actions (e.g., cell cycle inhibition) in addition to antioxidant properties.

Conclusion

As more is learned about the multiple pathways involved in carcinogenesis, newer targets for intervention will emerge. Eventually, we could envision combination strategies targeting many pathways simultaneously using pharmacological and dietary approaches. While rationale for control of inflammation is sound for chemoprevention, it may also be strong for adjuvant therapy. Since more conservative approaches toward the management of prostate cancer, including expectant management and targeted focal

therapies, are being introduced, the role of anti-inflammatory/antioxidant agents for prostate cancer therapy must also be pursued.

References

1. Kuper H, Adami HO, Trichopoulos D. Infections as a major preventable cause of human cancer. J Intern Med 2000; 248(3):171–183.
2. Bostwick DG, de la RG, Dundore P, Corica FA, Iczkowski KA. Intraepithelial and stromal lymphocytes in the normal human prostate. Prostate 2003; 55(3):187–193.
3. Theyer G, Kramer G, Assmann I et al. Phenotypic characterization of infiltrating leukocytes in benign prostatic hyperplasia. Lab Invest 1992; 66(1):96–107.
4. De Marzo AM, Platz EA, Sutcliffe S et al. Inflammation in prostate carcinogenesis. Nat Rev Cancer 2007; 7(4): 256–269.
5. Steiner G, Gessl A, Kramer G, Schollhammer A, Forster O, Marberger M. Phenotype and function of peripheral and prostatic lymphocytes in patients with benign prostatic hyperplasia. J Urol 1994; 151(2):480–484.
6. Steiner GE, Stix U, Handisurya A et al. Cytokine expression pattern in benign prostatic hyperplasia infiltrating T cells and impact of lymphocytic infiltration on cytokine mRNA profile in prostatic tissue. Lab Invest 2003; 83(8): 1131–1146.
7. Steiner GE, Djavan B, Kramer G et al. The picture of the prostatic lymphokine network is becoming increasingly complex. Rev Urol 2002; 4(4):171–177.
8. Steiner GE, Newman ME, Paikl D et al. Expression and function of pro-inflammatory interleukin IL-17 and IL-17 receptor in normal, benign hyperplastic, and malignant prostate. Prostate 2003; 56(3):171–182.
9. Groh V, Rhinehart R, Secrist H, Bauer S, Grabstein KH, Spies T. Broad tumor-associated expression and recognition by tumor-derived gamma delta T cells of MICA and MICB. Proc Natl Acad Sci U S A 1999; 96(12): 6879–6884.
10. Kramer G, Mitteregger D, Marberger M. Is benign prostatic hyperplasia (BPH) an immune inflammatory disease? Eur Urol 2007; 51(5):1202–1216.
11. De Marzo AM, Marchi VL, Epstein JI, Nelson WG. Proliferative inflammatory atrophy of the prostate: implications for prostatic carcinogenesis. Am J Pathol 1999; 155(6):1985–1992.
12. De Marzo AM, Platz EA, Epstein JI et al. A working group classification of focal prostate atrophy lesions. Am J Surg Pathol 2006; 30(10):1281–1291.
13. Nakayama M, Bennett CJ, Hicks JL et al. Hypermethylation of the human glutathione S-transferase-pi gene (GSTP1) CpG island is present in a subset of proliferative inflammatory atrophy lesions but not in normal or hyperplastic epithelium of the prostate: a detailed study using laser-capture microdissection. Am J Pathol 2003; 163(3):923–933.
14. Sutcliffe S, Zenilman JM, Ghanem KG et al. Sexually transmitted infections and prostatic inflammation/cell

damage as measured by serum prostate specific antigen concentration. J Urol 2006; 175(5):1937–1942.

15. Dennis LK, Dawson DV. Meta-analysis of measures of sexual activity and prostate cancer. Epidemiology 2002; 13(1):72–79.

16. Taylor ML, Mainous AG, III, Wells BJ. Prostate cancer and sexually transmitted diseases: a meta-analysis. Fam Med 2005; 37(7):506–512.

17. Sutcliffe S, Giovannucci E, Alderete JF et al. Plasma antibodies against Trichomonas vaginalis and subsequent risk of prostate cancer. Cancer Epidemiol Biomarkers Prev 2006; 15(5):939–945.

18. Strickler HD, Goedert JJ. Sexual behavior and evidence for an infectious cause of prostate cancer. Epidemiol Rev 2001; 23(1):144–151.

19. Urisman A, Molinaro RJ, Fischer N et al. Identification of a novel Gammaretrovirus in prostate tumors of patients homozygous for R462Q RNASEL variant. PLoS Pathog 2006; 2(3):e25.

20. Savage PA, Vosseller K, Kang C et al. Recognition of a ubiquitous self antigen by prostate cancer-infiltrating CD8+ T lymphocytes. Science 2008; 319(5860):215–220.

21. Ponniah S, Arah I, Alexander RB. PSA is a candidate self-antigen in autoimmune chronic prostatitis/chronic pelvic pain syndrome. Prostate 2000; 44(1):49–54.

22. Dehm SM, Tindall DJ. Molecular regulation of androgen action in prostate cancer. J Cell Biochem 2006; 99(2):333–344.

23. Harkonen PL, Makela SI. Role of estrogens in development of prostate cancer. J Steroid Biochem Mol Biol 2004; 92(4):297–305.

24. Ho E, Boileau TW, Bray TM. Dietary influences on endocrine-inflammatory interactions in prostate cancer development. Arch Biochem Biophys 2004; 428(1):109–117.

25. Giovannucci E. Tomato products, lycopene, and prostate cancer: a review of the epidemiological literature. J Nutr 2005; 135(8):2030S–2031S.

26. Heinonen OP, Albanes D, Virtamo J et al. Prostate cancer and supplementation with alpha-tocopherol and beta-carotene: incidence and mortality in a controlled trial. J Natl Cancer Inst 1998; 90(6):440–446.

27. Duffield-Lillico AJ, Dalkin BL, Reid ME et al. Selenium supplementation, baseline plasma selenium status and incidence of prostate cancer: an analysis of the complete treatment period of the Nutritional Prevention of Cancer Trial. BJU Int 2003; 91(7):608–612.

28. Knize MG, Felton JS. Formation and human risk of carcinogenic heterocyclic amines formed from natural precursors in meat. Nutr Rev 2005; 63(5):158–165.

29. Nakai Y, Nelson WG, De Marzo AM. The dietary charred meat carcinogen 2-amino-1-methyl-6-phenylimidazo[4,5-b]pyridine acts as both a tumor initiator and promoter in the rat ventral prostate. Cancer Res 2007; 67(3):1378–1384.

30. Leitzmann MF, Platz EA, Stampfer MJ, Willett WC, Giovannucci E. Ejaculation frequency and subsequent risk of prostate cancer. JAMA 2004; 291(13):1578–1586.

31. Lichtenstein P, Holm NV, Verkasalo PK et al. Environmental and heritable factors in the causation of cancer – analyses of cohorts of twins from Sweden, Denmark, and Finland. N Engl J Med 2000; 343(2):78–85.

32. Page WF, Braun MM, Partin AW, Caporaso N, Walsh P. Heredity and prostate cancer: a study of World War II veteran twins. Prostate 1997; 33(4):240–245.

33. Gronberg H, Damber L, Damber JE. Studies of genetic factors in prostate cancer in a twin population. J Urol 1994; 152(5 Pt 1):1484–1487.

34. Smith JR, Freije D, Carpten JD et al. Major susceptibility locus for prostate cancer on chromosome 1 suggested by a genome-wide search. Science 1996; 274(5291): 1371–1374.

35. Lindmark F, Zheng SL, Wiklund F et al. H6D polymorphism in macrophage-inhibitory cytokine-1 gene associated with prostate cancer. J Natl Cancer Inst 2004; 96(16):1248–1254.

36. Xu J, Zheng SL, Komiya A et al. Germline mutations and sequence variants of the macrophage scavenger receptor 1 gene are associated with prostate cancer risk. Nat Genet 2002; 32(2):321–325.

37. Sun J, Turner A, Xu J, Gronberg H, Isaacs W. Genetic variability in inflammation pathways and prostate cancer risk. Urol Oncol 2007; 25(3):250–259.

38. Castelli JC, Hassel BA, Wood KA et al. A study of the interferon antiviral mechanism: apoptosis activation by the 2-5A system. J Exp Med 1997; 186(6):967–972.

39. Schaid DJ. The complex genetic epidemiology of prostate cancer. Hum Mol Genet 2004; 13 Spec No 1:R103–R121.

40. Bootcov MR, Bauskin AR, Valenzuela SM et al. MIC-1, a novel macrophage inhibitory cytokine, is a divergent member of the TGF-beta superfamily. Proc Natl Acad Sci U S A 1997; 94(21):11514–11519.

41. Baek SJ, Kim KS, Nixon JB, Wilson LC, Eling TE. Cyclooxygenase inhibitors regulate the expression of a TGF-beta superfamily member that has proapoptotic and antitumorigenic activities. Mol Pharmacol 2001; 59(4):901–908.

42. Tan M, Wang Y, Guan K, Sun Y. PTGF-beta, a type beta transforming growth factor (TGF-beta) superfamily member, is a p53 target gene that inhibits tumor cell growth via TGF-beta signaling pathway. Proc Natl Acad Sci U S A 2000; 97(1):109–114.

43. Paralkar VM, Vail AL, Grasser WA et al. Cloning and characterization of a novel member of the transforming growth factor-beta/bone morphogenetic protein family. J Biol Chem 1998; 273(22):13760–13767.

44. Shim M, Eling TE. Protein kinase C-dependent regulation of NAG-1/placental bone morphogenic protein/MIC-1 expression in LNCaP prostate carcinoma cells. J Biol Chem 2005; 280(19):18636–18642.

45. Fairlie WD, Moore AG, Bauskin AR, Russell PK, Zhang HP, Breit SN. MIC-1 is a novel TGF-beta superfamily cytokine associated with macrophage activation. J Leukoc Biol 1999; 65(1):2–5.

46. Hayes VM, Severi G, Southey MC et al. Macrophage inhibitory cytokine-1 H6D polymorphism, prostate cancer risk, and survival. Cancer Epidemiol Biomarkers Prev 2006; 15(6):1223–1225.

47. Gough PJ, Greaves DR, Gordon S. A naturally occurring isoform of the human macrophage scavenger receptor (SR-A) gene generated by alternative splicing blocks modified LDL uptake. J Lipid Res 1998; 39(3):531–543.

48. Peiser L, De Winther MP, Makepeace K et al. The class A macrophage scavenger receptor is a major pattern recognition receptor for Neisseria meningitidis which is independent of lipopolysaccharide and not required for secretory responses. Infect Immun 2002; 70(10):5346–5354.

49. Sun J, Hsu FC, Turner AR et al. Meta-analysis of association of rare mutations and common sequence variants in the MSR1 gene and prostate cancer risk. Prostate 2006; 66(7):728–737.

50. Alexander RB, Ponniah S, Hasday J, Hebel JR. Elevated levels of proinflammatory cytokines in the semen of patients with chronic prostatitis/chronic pelvic pain syndrome. Urology 1998; 52(5):744–749.

51. Kim SJ, Uehara H, Karashima T, Mccarty M, Shih N, Fidler IJ. Expression of interleukin-8 correlates with angiogenesis, tumorigenicity, and metastasis of human prostate cancer cells implanted orthotopically in nude mice. Neoplasia 2001; 3(1):33–42.

52. Zheng SL, ugustsson-Balter K, Chang B et al. Sequence variants of toll-like receptor 4 are associated with prostate cancer risk: results from the Cancer Prostate in Sweden Study. Cancer Res 2004; 64(8):2918–2922.

53. Sun J, Wiklund F, Zheng SL et al. Sequence variants in Toll-like receptor gene cluster (TLR6-TLR1-TLR10) and prostate cancer risk. J Natl Cancer Inst 2005; 97(7):525–532.

54. Burnet FM. Immunological surveillance in neoplasia. Transplant Rev 1971; 7:3–25.

55. Langowski JL, Zhang X, Wu L et al. IL-23 promotes tumour incidence and growth. Nature 2006; 442(7101):461–465.

56. O'Byrne KJ, Dalgleish AG. Chronic immune activation and inflammation as the cause of malignancy. Br J Cancer 2001; 85(4):473–483.

57. Balkwill F, Mantovani A. Inflammation and cancer: back to Virchow? Lancet 2001; 357(9255):539–545.

58. Beutler BA. The role of tumor necrosis factor in health and disease. J Rheumatol Suppl 1999; 57:16–21.

59. Mizokami A, Gotoh A, Yamada H, Keller ET, Matsumoto T. Tumor necrosis factor-alpha represses androgen sensitivity in the LNCaP prostate cancer cell line. J Urol 2000; 164(3 Pt 1):800–805.

60. Li Q, Verma IM. NF-kappaB regulation in the immune system. Nat Rev Immunol 2002; 2(10):725–734.

61. Naugler WE, Karin M. NF-kappaB and cancer-identifying targets and mechanisms. Curr Opin Genet Dev 2008; 18(1): 19–26.

62. Luo JL, Tan W, Ricono JM et al. Nuclear cytokine-activated IKKalpha controls prostate cancer metastasis by repressing Maspin. Nature 2007; 446(7136):690–694.

63. Breen EC. VEGF in biological control. J Cell Biochem 2007; 102(6):1358–1367.

64. Aita M, Fasola G, Defferrari C et al. Targeting the VEGF pathway: Antiangiogenic strategies in the treatment of non-small cell lung cancer. Crit Rev Oncol Hematol 2008; 68(3):183–196.

65. Kollermann J, Helpap B. Expression of vascular endothelial growth factor (VEGF) and VEGF receptor Flk-1 in benign, premalignant, and malignant prostate tissue. Am J Clin Pathol 2001; 116(1):115–121.

66. Ito R, Kitadai Y, Kyo E et al. Interleukin 1 alpha acts as an autocrine growth stimulator for human gastric carcinoma cells. Cancer Res 1993; 53(17):4102–4106.

67. Bar-Eli M. Role of interleukin-8 in tumor growth and metastasis of human melanoma. Pathobiology 1999; 67(1):12–18.

68. Brigati C, Noonan DM, Albini A, Benelli R. Tumors and inflammatory infiltrates: friends or foes? Clin Exp Metastasis 2002; 19(3):247–258.

69. Xie K. Interleukin-8 and human cancer biology. Cytokine Growth Factor Rev 2001; 12(4):375–391.

70. Coussens LM, Werb Z. Inflammation and cancer. Nature 2002; 420(6917):860–867.

71. Moore BB, Arenberg DA, Stoy K et al. Distinct CXC chemokines mediate tumorigenicity of prostate cancer cells. Am J Pathol 1999; 154(5):1503–1512.

72. Parsons JK, Nelson CP, Gage WR, Nelson WG, Kensler TW, De Marzo AM. GSTA1 expression in normal, preneoplastic, and neoplastic human prostate tissue. Prostate 2001; 49(1):30–37.

73. Kovacic P, Jacintho JD. Mechanisms of carcinogenesis: focus on oxidative stress and electron transfer. Curr Med Chem 2001; 8(7):773–796.

74. Sawa T, Ohshima H. Nitrative DNA damage in inflammation and its possible role in carcinogenesis. Nitric Oxide 2006; 14(2):91–100.

75. Zidek Z. Role of cytokines in the modulation of nitric oxide production by cyclic AMP. Eur Cytokine Netw 2001; 12(1):22–32.

76. Shen Z, Wu W, Hazen SL. Activated leukocytes oxidatively damage DNA, RNA, and the nucleotide pool through halide-dependent formation of hydroxyl radical. Biochemistry 2000; 39(18):5474–5482.

77. Hayes JD, Pulford DJ. The glutathione S-transferase supergene family: regulation of GST and the contribution of the isoenzymes to cancer chemoprotection and drug resistance. Crit Rev Biochem Mol Biol 1995; 30(6):445–600.

78. Nelson WG, De Marzo AM, Deweese TL. The molecular pathogenesis of prostate cancer: implications for prostate cancer prevention. Urology 2001; 57(4 Suppl 1):39–45.

79. Bostwick DG, Alexander EE, Singh R et al. Antioxidant enzyme expression and reactive oxygen species damage in prostatic intraepithelial neoplasia and cancer. Cancer 2000; 89(1):123–134.

80. Ripple MO, Henry WF, Rago RP, Wilding G. Prooxidant-antioxidant shift induced by androgen treatment of human prostate carcinoma cells. J Natl Cancer Inst 1997; 89(1): 40–48.

81. Hirst DG, Robson T. Nitrosative stress in cancer therapy. Front Biosci 2007; 12:3406–3418.

82. Jackson AL, Loeb LA. The contribution of endogenous sources of DNA damage to the multiple mutations in cancer. Mutat Res 2001; 477(1–2):7–21.

83. Uchida K. A lipid-derived endogenous inducer of COX-2: a bridge between inflammation and oxidative stress. Mol Cells 2008; 25(3):347–351.

84. Lu Y, Wahl LM. Oxidative stress augments the production of matrix metalloproteinase-1, cyclooxygenase-2, and prostaglandin E2 through enhancement of NF-kappa B activity in lipopolysaccharide-activated human primary monocytes. J Immunol 2005; 175(8):5423–5429.

85. Fosslien E. Molecular pathology of cyclooxygenase-2 in neoplasia. Ann Clin Lab Sci 2000; 30(1):3–21.

86. Cao Y, Prescott SM. Many actions of cyclooxygenase-2 in cellular dynamics and in cancer. J Cell Physiol 2002; 190(3):279–286.

87. Gately S, Li WW. Multiple roles of COX-2 in tumor angiogenesis: a target for antiangiogenic therapy. Semin Oncol 2004; 31(2 Suppl 7):2–11.

88. Zha S, Gage WR, Sauvageot J et al. Cyclooxygenase-2 is up-regulated in proliferative inflammatory atrophy of the prostate, but not in prostate carcinoma. Cancer Res 2001; 61(24):8617–8623.

89. Kirschenbaum A, Liu X, Yao S, Levine AC. The role of cyclooxygenase-2 in prostate cancer. Urology 2001; 58(2 Suppl 1):127–131.

90. Sheng H, Shao J, Morrow JD, Beauchamp RD, DuBois RN. Modulation of apoptosis and Bcl-2 expression by prostaglandin E2 in human colon cancer cells. Cancer Res 1998; 58(2):362–366.

91. Narayanan BA, Narayanan NK, Pittman B, Reddy BS. Regression of mouse prostatic intraepithelial neoplasia by nonsteroidal anti-inflammatory drugs in the transgenic adenocarcinoma mouse prostate model. Clin Cancer Res 2004; 10(22):7727–7737.

92. Narayanan BA, Narayanan NK, Pttman B, Reddy BS. Adenocarcina of the mouse prostate growth inhibition by celecoxib: downregulation of transcription factors involved in COX-2 inhibition. Prostate 2006; 66(3):257–265.

93. Le NT, Xue M, Castelnoble LA, Jackson CJ. The dual personalities of matrix metalloproteinases in inflammation. Front Biosci 2007; 12:1475–1487.

94. Dieli F, Vermijlen D, Fulfaro F et al. Targeting human {gamma}{delta} T cells with zoledronate and interleukin-2 for immunotherapy of hormone-refractory prostate cancer. Cancer Res 2007; 67(15):7450–7457.

95. Kottke T, Sanchez-Perez L, Diaz RM et al. Induction of hsp70-mediated Th17 autoimmunity can be exploited as immunotherapy for metastatic prostate cancer. Cancer Res 2007; 67(24):11970–11979.

96. Harris RE, Beebe-Donk J, Alshafie GA. Cancer chemoprevention by cyclooxygenase 2 (COX-2) blockade: results of case control studies. Subcell Biochem 2007; 42:193–212.

97. Harris RE, Beebe-Donk J, Doss H, Burr DD. Aspirin, ibuprofen, and other non-steroidal anti-inflammatory drugs in cancer prevention: a critical review of non-selective COX-2 blockade (review). Oncol Rep 2005; 13(4):559–583.

98. Smith MR, Manola J, Kaufman DS, Oh WK, Bubley GJ, Kantoff PW. Celecoxib versus placebo for men with prostate cancer and a rising serum prostate-specific antigen after radical prostatectomy and/or radiation therapy. J Clin Oncol 2006; 24(18):2723–2728.

99. Pruthi RS, Derksen JE, Moore D et al. Phase II trial of celecoxib in prostate-specific antigen recurrent prostate cancer after definitive radiation therapy or radical prostatectomy. Clin Cancer Res 2006; 12(7 Pt 1):2172–2177.

100. Sooriakumaran P, Langley SE, Laing RW, Coley HM. COX-2 inhibition: a possible role in the management of prostate cancer? J Chemother 2007; 19(1):21–32.

Part VII
Drug Development

Chapter 34
Challenges for the Development of New Agents in Prostate Cancer

Ajjai S. Alva, Deborah A. Bradley, and Maha Hussain

Abstract Development of novel therapeutic agents in advanced prostate cancer presents particular challenges due to multiple factors including advanced age at diagnosis with competing causes of death and difficulties in assessing responses in bone (the predominant site of metastatic disease). Over the last 2 decades, few non hormonal drugs have met the regulatory requirements for approval in advanced prostate cancer. These include mitoxantrone (1996), zoledronic acid (2002) and docetaxel (2004). Sipuleucel-T, an autologous cell based vaccine and cabazitaxel were approved in 2010. Despite these breakthroughs, the general landscape for new and effective treatments in prostate cancer remains challenging. The aim of this review is to discuss the specific obstacles in the development of novel agents in prostate cancer and potential strategies to overcome them.

Keywords Prostate cancer • Novel targeted agents • Challenges • End-points • Drug development

Introduction

Prostate cancer is a major public health problem. Despite the reported reduction in prostate cancer mortality, in 2008, over 28,000 men are destined to die from their disease [1]. The primary cause of mortality is metastatic castration-resistant prostate cancer (CRPC). Historically, few treatment options were available to this group of patients. However, a paradigm shift occurred when palliation was demonstrated with mitoxantrone therapy in the mid 1990s [1, 2] followed by a modest but unequivocal survival benefit with docetaxel-based chemotherapy in two pivotal phase III trials in 2004 [3, 4], a major advance in a disease once thought to be chemoresistant.

Over the last several years, a great deal of progress has been made in understanding prostate cancer biology leading to a plethora of new agents being investigated in first, second, and even third-line settings. Trial designs and modestly active agents in the context of a complex disease make approval of new agents difficult.

The difficulties in conducting clinical trials in prostate cancer are not new. Historically, several attempts were made to address the issue of screening for antitumor activity by enrolling only patients with measurable disease or looking at alternative endpoints [2–4]. However, based on disappointing trial results, several reviews, decades ago, concluded that chemotherapy had no real role in treatment of prostate cancer [5–7]. Several features of the disease and the patient population continue to present challenges in the development of new agents for this disease. Prostate cancer is a complex disease with marked inter and intrapatient heterogeneity, both at a clinical and molecular level [8]. Prostate cancer patients are generally older, with confounding comorbidities, and the disease manifests mostly in bone which is a difficult organ to assess. Second- and third-line hormone therapies are widely prevalent and their ease of use coupled with the desire to minimize toxicities owing to older age and patient comorbidities may play a role in delaying enrollment

M. Hussain (✉)
Comprehensive Cancer Center, University of Michigan, Ann Arbor, MI, USA
e-mail: mahahuss@umich.edu

W.D. Figg et al. (eds.), *Drug Management of Prostate Cancer*,
DOI 10.1007/978-1-60327-829-4_34, © Springer Science+Business Media, LLC 2010

in clinical trials. Despite all these issues, the results of several recent trials clearly indicate that when an active agent is combined with adequate trial design, it is possible to obtain positive clinically meaningful results as reflected by phase III trials that led to FDA approval of mitoxantrone, zoledronic acid, and docetaxel [9–14].

Defining Appropriate Clinical Endpoints Based on Stage of Development

Screening for Antitumor Effect: "The Phase II Setting"

Objective Response: How Defined?

For agents to make it to a phase III trial, it must be established with reasonable certainty that an agent has antitumor activity. With few exceptions, the latter, historically, has been based on measurable disease response in the vast majority of solid tumors. This poses a problem in prostate cancer in that even in the contemporary era, only 30–40% of patients have measurable soft tissue disease [9, 10]. Therefore, limiting accrual to patients with measurable disease is neither practical nor reflective of the disease population at large. It is instructive, however, to note that with the taxanes, particularly docetaxel, evidence of significant objective antitumor activity was evident early in its development as reflected by measurable disease response in 28–55% of patients with an impressive median survival of up to 23 months [15–18]. This data was compelling and led to phase III testing [9, 10]. Similarly, more recently measurable disease responses were also noted with ixabepilone [19, 20].

Objective measurable disease response is clearly useful if present, however, for the vast majority of patients with metastatic prostate cancer; alternatives including better assessment of response in bone are needed. With better assessments lacking, one useful measure for screening for antitumor activity in CRPC, at least with use of cytotoxic therapy, has been PSA response. The role of PSA as an indicator of response was first reported in 1989 [21]. Following that report, several phase II trials utilized PSA as a marker of response [22–24]. Retrospective analyses of phase II trials suggested a correlation between a 50% or greater

decline in PSA and survival [23, 25, 26] leading to a consensus recommendation by the Prostate-Specific Antigen Working Group [27] for use of PSA as an outcome measure in clinical trials. However, controversy remains regarding the optimum posttreatment PSA percentage decline, time for PSA evaluation in relationship to initiation of treatment, duration of posttreatment PSA decline, and definition of PSA progression. Retrospective analysis of several large clinical trials with known primary outcomes and PSA data available have helped to provide information related to PSA changes and prognosis (discussed below).

Time-to-Event End Points

One key objective of therapy is better control of the disease activity (to delay disease progression) with the aim of reducing disease-related morbidities and maximizing quality of life. Clinically, this is meaningful to patients. Recognizing that response is one element of the control process and driven by the development of agents that may not exert an overt cytotoxic effect or have mechanisms of action that are cytostatic, efforts have focused on using time to progression (TTP) or progression-free survival (PFS) as the primary endpoints to capture antitumor effect. These endpoints have been successfully utilized in a variety of cancers where it also led to FDA approvals. An example in the genitourinary arena is sorafenib's FDA approval based on improvement in PFS in renal cell carcinoma [28, 29]. Of note is that if response rate was the driving factor, this drug would not have made it this far as it is associated with an objective response rate of less than 5% [28, 29].

Challenges in Using Time-to-Event Endpoints in CRPC

TTP does not incorporate death, while PFS includes progression and death from any cause. Both are appealing, but challenging. The challenges in evaluating PFS and TTP are similar. Ideally, trials should be controlled and blinded, progression must be prospectively defined, and plans to handle missing data must be prospectively determined. Timing of tumor assessments must be symmetrical in all study arms. If progression is to be determined radiographically, independent radiology review may be ideal for the analysis and interpretation of trial results, though may not be practical and is costly for phase II settings.

Because bone is the predominant site of disease and often the only site of disease in patients with metastatic prostate cancer, ability to assess response in bone plays a major role in time-to-event endpoints. Response of bone lesions in clinical trials has been based on radionuclide bone scans. Although considered to be the standard screening technique for assessing the entire skeleton for metastases, it is well recognized that bone scanning lacks the specificity needed to accurately assess response vs. flare. These limitations stem from the fact that bone scans measure only osteoblastic metabolic activity and do not evaluate structural integrity of bone nor actual growth nor apoptosis of the cancer cells themselves.

The problem of assessing response in bone has been well illustrated in development of atrasentan, an endothelin antagonist, hypothesized to interfere with the development and progression of osteoblastic bone metastases [30–33] in prostate cancer. Results of a double-blind, randomized, placebo-controlled, multinational phase II trial [34] investigating two dose levels of atrasentan showed a nonsignificant trend towards an increase in TTP with a significant increase in time to PSA progression in patients treated with atrasentan. In this trial, bone scans were only done at baseline and at progression. Interim bone scan assessments were not mandated per protocol. Based on the phase II trial results, a phase III trial compared TTP between atrasentan and placebo. Bone scans were performed as part of the efficacy analysis every 12 weeks. The study was closed early by an Independent Data Safety Monitoring Committee after reviewing an unexpectedly high number of early progressions. Of note, >50% of patients reached the progression endpoint within 100 days of trial entry, mostly due to bone scan progressions. Intention to treat analysis of the 809 patients accrued prior to trial closure showed a nonsignificant trend towards an increase in TTP favoring the atrasentan arm [35, 36]. When the analysis was limited to patients with bone metastases, a significant increase in TTP was observed [35, 36]. In review, the study that mandated bone scans showed early radiologic progression in the absence of clinical symptoms in most patients raising concern whether response was appropriately assessed given the limitations of bone scans.

As a result of this trial and others, a recent update to consensus recommendations for clinical trial conduct in advanced prostate cancer (Prostate Cancer Working Group 2) was published [37]. The key change in these recommendations is to focus on time-to-event measures rather than response and to ensure adequate drug exposure before declaring futility.

The Phase III Setting

The gold standard in assessing clinical benefit of anticancer therapies in prostate cancer as well as other malignancies has been survival outcomes assessed in prospective randomized phase III trials. Although necessary, these trials are costly, requiring large numbers of patients often followed over many years. Survival has proven to be an achievable endpoint in metastatic CRPC [9, 10]. However, whenever survival is the measure in a trial where a large number of trial participants have a disease with a relatively long natural history, the observed results maybe confounded by competing causes of mortality, and subsequent treatment. This has not been a critical issue in this stage of the disease, though it is very relevant in earlier stages of prostate cancer.

Patient-Reported Outcomes

Patient-reported outcomes such as symptom benefit are clinically important and have served as an endpoint for drug approval. Several problems confound the assessment of symptoms of advanced prostate cancer, including the fact that the symptoms of this disease often overlap with intercurrent conditions and older age and side effects of therapy. Therefore, any efficacy with respect to patient reported outcome can only be established by conducting randomized, controlled, double-blinded trials with a prospectively defined primary endpoint using validated measuring instruments, analysis methodology, and a clinically meaningful effect size.

Patient-reported outcomes led to approval of mitoxantrone, in combination with prednisone for the treatment of metastatic CRPC patients with pain related to disease. Its efficacy was demonstrated in an open-label phase III trial of 161 symptomatic patients that used prospectively defined endpoint of palliative response. Twenty-nine percent of the patients in the mitoxantrone + prednisone arm, compared to 12% in the prednisone alone arm, demonstrated a two-point improvement on a six-point pain intensity scale that was at least 6 weeks in duration, and was accompanied by a stable analgesic score [11].

Although this endpoint provides direct evidence of clinical benefit to patients, it has not been correlated with improvement in survival; optimal tools have not yet been defined, and many methodological problems remain unresolved, therefore is rarely used as a primary endpoint for assessing drug efficacy today. Patient-related outcomes have also become of more limited value because patients with metastatic CRPC enrolling in clinical trials today are often asymptomatic or have few symptoms attributable to disease. This is in stark contrast to the 80s and 90s when most patients presented with advanced clinically morbid disease.

Composite Endpoints

No single ideal endpoint has been described yet in this disease that is suitable for all disease stages and drugs. A composite endpoint can be appropriate when the benefit of a drug is multifaceted. In metastatic prostate cancer, zoledronic acid was approved for treatment of patients with progressive bone metastases using a composite endpoint [13, 14]. In this phase III trial, 643 men with asymptomatic or minimally symptomatic CRPC and evidence of bone metastases were randomized to zoledronic acid or placebo. The endpoint was occurrence of any skeletal-related event at 15 months as defined by pathological fracture, spinal cord compression, surgery, or radiation therapy to bone or change in antineoplastic treatment for bone pain. At 15 months, patients treated with zoledronic acid experienced fewer skeletal-related events as compared to patients treated with placebo (33 vs. 44%, $P=0.02$). Results of this study led to FDA approval of zoledronic acid in patients with CRPC with bone metastases.

More recently, a composite endpoint was utilized to investigate satraplatin, a novel orally bioavailable platinum compound, in the second line setting for men with CRPC. In a large multinational randomized phase III trial comparing satraplatin plus prednisone to placebo plus prednisone, the Satraplatin and Prednisone Against Refractory Cancer (SPARC) trial, a coprimary endpoint of overall survival and PFS (defined as a composite endpoint based on first occurrence of tumor progression, skeletal event, symptomatic progression, or death) was utilized. Secondary and exploratory endpoints included time to pain progression, pain response, tumor response, and PSA response. Final results of this 950 patient trial have been presented [38, 39]. A 33% improvement in PFS in favor of satraplatin was reported (11.1 vs. 9.7 weeks and HR 0.67 95% CI 0.57–0.77; $P<0.0001$), but no benefit in overall survival was demonstrated (61.3 vs. 61.4 week andHR=0.97; 95% CI 0.83–1.13). All other prespecified endpoints were statistically significant in favor of satraplatin. Of interest, a significant number of patients went on to receive third-line chemotherapy. It is doubtful that further treatment can explain the lack of a survival benefit considering there is no effective third-line therapy.

Use of Alternative Clinical Endpoints

Development of surrogate endpoints that can be objectively measured and lead to a quicker determination of whether an agent is of benefit or not to patients is an area of active investigation and significant interest in prostate cancer research.

Biomarkers

A biomarker is a characteristic that is objectively measured and evaluated as an indicator of normal biologic processes, pathogenic processes, or pharmacologic responses to a therapeutic intervention [40]. There has been significant interest in use of biomarkers as surrogates in clinical trials. In order for a biomarker to qualify as a valid surrogate endpoint, (1) the biomarker must be a prognostic marker of the true clinical endpoint, (2) treatment-mediated changes in the potential surrogate must be prognostic, and (3) effects of treatments on the marker must be associated with effects of treatments on the true clinical endpoint [41].

PSA

PSA has served as a biomarker for diagnosis, prognosis and monitoring for disease activity, and response to therapy in different settings of prostate cancer. The observation that systemic and local therapies impact the PSA level has led to the use of PSA in the daily clinical practice to guide therapeutic decisions. This clearly impacts on the integrity of clinical trials that have harder clinical endpoints, not to mention, causing difficulties when reconciling PSA changes with objective disease measures when they are in opposite directions. To date, there are no data from prospective randomized clinical trials that have validated these practices to produce level one supporting evidence. Despite this, given the limitations of studies with overt clinical endpoints, with the reproducible and quantitative nature of PSA, enormous interest has been focused on developing and evaluating PSA-based endpoints.

PSA Response

The role of PSA decline as an indicator of response in CRPC was first reported in 1989 [21]. Following this report, several phase II trials utilized PSA as a marker of antitumor response with retrospective analyses suggesting a correlation between a 50% or greater decline in PSA and survival [23, 25, 26]. In 1999, recommendations by the Prostate-Specific Antigen Working Group [27] were published. These aimed at streamlining design and outcome reporting for phase II clinical trials in prostate cancer. PSA decline was suggested as one outcome measure. However, controversy remains regarding the optimum posttreatment PSA percentage decline in relation to baseline PSA, time for PSA evaluation in relation to initiation of treatment, duration of posttreatment PSA decline, and definition of PSA progression. Retrospective analysis of several large clinical trials with known primary outcomes and PSA data available have helped to provide information related to PSA changes and prognosis such that specific PSA endpoints can be validated in prospective trials.

In newly metastatic disease treated with androgen deprivation therapy (ADT), the PSA level after 7 months of ADT strongly correlated with risk of death in a secondary analysis of the first 1.345 patients registered to SWOG 9346 (INT-0162) [42]. In this phase III trial, hormone naïve patients with metastatic disease were treated 7 months of induction ADT. Patients who achieved a PSA of 4.0 ng/mL or less on months 6 and 7 were randomized to continuous vs. intermittent ADT. After controlling for prognostic factors, patients with a PSA of 4 or less to more than 0.2 ng/mL had less than

one-third the risk of death as those with a PSA of more than 4 ng/mL ($P<0.001$). Patients with PSA of 0.2 ng/mL or less had less than one-fifth the risk of death as patients with a PSA of more than 4 ng/mL ($P<0.001$) and had significantly better survival than those with PSA of more than 0.2–4 ng/mL or less ($P<0.001$). Median survival was 13 months for patients with a PSA of more than 4 ng/mL at the end of induction (95% CI, 11–16 months), 44 months for patients with PSA of more than 0.2–4 ng/mL or less (95% CI 39–55 months), and 75 months for patients with PSA of 0.2 ng/mL or less (95% CI 62–91 months) suggesting that PSA level at 7 months may be a useful endpoint in this patient population.

Secondary analysis of SWOG 9916, a randomized phase III trial comparing docetaxel and estramustine to mitoxantrone and prednisone in patients with metastatic CRPC evaluated PSA changes as potential surrogate markers for survival [43]. Three-month PSA level declines of 20–40%, a 2-month PSA decline of 30%, and PSA velocity at 2 and 3 months met the Prentice's surrogacy criteria. The optimal biochemical surrogate was a 30% PSA decline 3 months after treatment initiation. A PSA decline of ≥30% within 3 months of chemotherapy initiation also had the highest degree of surrogacy in analysis of data from the TAX327 trial, a multinational phase III trial comparing different schedules of docetaxel and prednisone to mitoxantrone and prednisone in the same patient population, although surrogacy was more modest in this trial [44]. If validated, PSA decline as a surrogate endpoint in future trials has the potential to substantially alter the design and duration of future phase III studies. These findings are being prospectively confirmed in two randomized cooperative group trials (SWOG-0421 and CALGB 90401).

PSA Progression

In hormone-sensitive and CRPC, PSA progression heralds clinical progression [45] and has been an accepted indicator of worsening disease, though no data exist regarding what constitutes an appropriate definition for PSA progression. So far criteria have been consensus-based [27, 37]. Several definitions including definitions proposed by the Prostate-Specific Antigen Working Group [27] and the Prostate Cancer

Working Group [37] were recently explored using PSA data from two SWOG trials with hormone sensitive (S9346) and CRPC (S9916) [46]. The Prostate-Specific Antigen Working Group 1999 and the Prostate Cancer Working Group 2008 were both strongly predictive of overall survival indicating that both consensus definitions are useful. However, whether PSA progression or PSA response is a more useful endpoint to consider remains unanswered.

Limitations of PSA Based End-Points

Although PSA endpoints have been are attractive to overcome some of the difficulties encountered in assessing outcome by means of other endpoints, e.g., bone scans or pain relief, it is not established how well the posttherapy PSA changes capture the biologic effect of therapy on the tumor. As described above, different PSA-based endpoints may correlate with disease prognosis, can thus support their use for patient selection and stratification in clinical trials, and may also provide evidence of activity of a drug in a Phase 2 trial. The data described above suggest a potential PSA role, however, routine application await prospective validation of PSA as a surrogate for clinical benefit. Because PSA changes can be drug class-specific and disease state-specific, its validation as a surrogate or intermediate marker needs to be established for each drug class and disease state combination. Pending prospective validation, however, several strong leads in different disease settings, discussed above, suggest that PSA may be a useful intermediate biomarker in some settings.

Biochemical Markers of Bone Turnover

Biochemical markers of bone turnover can be classified as markers of bone resorption and bone formation reflecting osteoclastic and osteoblastic activity respectively. Originally used to evaluate treatment of metabolic bone disease, over the last several years, the potential utility of bone turnover to measure efficacy of bone targeted therapy in cancer has been realized [13, 47, 48]. Given that bone is the predominant site and often only site of disease in 85–90% of men with metastatic prostate cancer [9, 10], the use of bone turnover markers to monitor therapy has been of particular interest in this disease. Although in prostate cancer, bone metastases are mostly osteoblastic in nature, it is well recognized that prostate cancer metastases result from a heterogeneous mixture of osetoblastic and osteolytic lesions [49–52]. It has been shown that osteoblastic metastases form on trabecular bone at sites of previous osteoclast resorption and that such resorption is required for subsequent osteoblastic bone formation [53, 54]. These findings suggest that prostate cancer induces bone production through an overall increase in bone remodeling [55–57]; thus, investigation of markers of osteoblastic and osteoclastic activity are relevant in evaluating baseline disease activity and monitoring therapeutic response.

In prostate cancer, investigation of bone turnover markers has largely been limited to studies of bisphosphonate use. In this setting, elevated markers of osteolytic activity (N-telopeptide) and osteoblastic activity (bone-specific alkaline phosphatase) have been associated with adverse clinical outcomes including shorter time to skeletal events, disease progression, and death [13, 47, 48]. Additionally, a correlation between baseline values of N-telopeptide, bone-specific alkaline phosphatase, PSA, and number of bone lesions have also been shown [48, 58], suggesting baseline markers of osteolytic and osteoblastic activity correlate with tumor burden. There is little data published on the effect of chemotherapy on bone makers. This is in large part secondary to the ability of PSA to serve as a surrogate of response in traditional cytoxic therapies. However, as the potential treatment armamentarium available has increased to include targeted therapeutics that may not be cytotoxic, standard clinical endpoints of efficacy such as tumor response rates may not be as applicable as they are. Therefore, the role of bone turnover markers is again being investigated to aid in assessing treatment response, especially in bone targeted therapy [34, 59–61]. Results from phase II and III studies of atrasentan, an investigational agent that inhibits the endothelin-A receptor resulting in decreased osteoblast activity, has shown no significant responses as assessed by classical measures, yet it appeared to result in an increase in TTP in patients with bone metastatses [5, 6, 40]. Investigation of bone markers in these studies has also demonstrated suppression of biochemical markers of bone turnover supporting the potential role of bone turnover markers in investigating efficacy of novel agents. Clearly for bone turnover markers to be of use as a response measure, their role must be first validated. To do so, changes in bone turnover marker have been included as a secondary endpoint in S0241, a phase III trial investigating the addition of atrasentan to docetaxcl + prednisone.

Circulating Tumor Cells

Other biomarkers being evaluated include circulating tumor cells (CTC). CTCs have been demonstrated in multiple solid tumors and have been of clinical interest for several decades. Recent technology advances with improved sensitivity and specificity have made it feasible to measure and characterize CTCs leading to resurgence into their investigation. The largest body of knowledge utilizing CTCs to monitor treatment response comes from the breast cancer literature. Cristofanelli et al. have shown that number of CTCs before treatment is an independent predictor of PFS and overall survival in patients with metastatic breast cancer [62] and that detection of elevated CTCs during therapy is an accurate indication of rapid disease progression and mortality [63]. Recent studies in CRPC are evaluating the ability of CTCs to be used as a surrogate of overall survival. Moreno et al. investigated CTCs in peripheral blood of CRPC patients pre and posttherapy [64]. At every time point, including baseline, patients with less than 5 CTCs/7.5 mL had a significantly improved overall survival compared to those with more than 5 CTCs. Patients who had a reduction in CTCs to less than 5 CTCs/7.5 mL at 2–5 weeks after treatment had significantly improved survival compared to those who had persistently high CTCs. Multivariate analyses of the 240 evaluable patients in this study revealed CTC number as the strongest independent predictor of outcome. The Cellsearch ™ system used in the above study has been granted an expanded clearance by the FDA for monitoring therapy in CRPC patients and is now commercially available. If validated in larger prospective trials, CTCs could serve as convenient and early indicators of treatment efficacy in trials of new agents or combination therapy in CRPC.

Conclusions

The gold standard in assessing clinical benefit of anticancer therapies in prostate cancer, as well as other malignancies, has been survival outcomes assessed in prospective randomized phase III trials. Significant progress has been made over the last decade in understanding the biology of prostate cancer development and progression. As a result, most drugs chosen for study today are based on sound rationale, aimed at targeting specific biological changes thought to be crucial mediators in disease progression. However, with a plethora of targets identified and multiple promising agents available for investigation, the challenge now is how to prioritize to swiftly eliminate inactive or marginal agents and to enable promising therapies to be taken to definitive phase III clinical trials. To do this efficiently, alternative endpoints and tools that are applicable to the complex nature of this disease are necessary, particularly in the phase II setting so that a "go/no-go" decision can be made regarding an agent as to its worthiness of more definitive testing.

References

1. Jemal A, Siegel R, Ward E, et al. Cancer statistics, 2008. CA Cancer J Clin 2008;58:71–96.
2. Schmidt JD, Gibbons RP, Johnson DE, Prout GR, Scott WW, Murphy GP. Chemotherapy of advanced prostatic cancer. Evaluation of response parameters. Urology 1976;7:602–10.
3. Slack NH, Murphy GP. Criteria for evaluating patient responses to treatment modalities for prostatic cancer. Urol Clin North Am 1984;11:337–42.
4. Slack NH, Brady MF, Murphy GP. Stable versus partial response in advanced prostate cancer. Prostate 1984;5:401–15.
5. Eisenberger MA. Chemotherapy for prostate carcinoma. NCI Monogr 1988;(7):151–63.
6. Yagoda A, Petrylak D. Cytotoxic chemotherapy for advanced hormone-resistant prostate cancer. Cancer 1993;71: 1098–109.
7. Tannock IF. Is there evidence that chemotherapy is of benefit to patients with carcinoma of the prostate? J Clin Oncol 1985;3:1013–21.
8. Shah RB, Mehra R, Chinnaiyan AM, et al. Androgen-independent prostate cancer is a heterogeneous group of diseases: lessons from a rapid autopsy program. Cancer Res 2004;64:9209–16.
9. Petrylak DP, Tangen CM, Hussain MH, et al. Docetaxel and estramustine compared with mitoxantrone and prednisone for advanced refractory prostate cancer. N Engl J Med 2004;351:1513–20.

10. Tannock IF, de Wit R, Berry WR, et al. Docetaxel plus prednisone or mitoxantrone plus prednisone for advanced prostate cancer. N Engl J Med 2004;351:1502–12.

11. Tannock IF, Osoba D, Stockler MR, et al. Chemotherapy with mitoxantrone plus prednisone or prednisone alone for symptomatic hormone-resistant prostate cancer: a Canadian randomized trial with palliative end points. J Clin Oncol 1996;14:1756–64.

12. Kantoff PW, Halabi S, Conaway M, et al. Hydrocortisone with or without mitoxantrone in men with hormone-refractory prostate cancer: results of the cancer and leukemia group B 9182 study. J Clin Oncol 1999;17:2506–13.

13. Saad F, Gleason DM, Murray R, et al. A randomized, placebo-controlled trial of zoledronic acid in patients with hormone-refractory metastatic prostate carcinoma. J Natl Cancer Inst 2002;94:1458–68.

14. Saad F, Gleason DM, Murray R, et al. Long-term efficacy of zoledronic acid for the prevention of skeletal complications in patients with metastatic hormone-refractory prostate cancer. J Natl Cancer Inst 2004;96:879–82.

15. Petrylak DP, Macarthur R, O'Connor J, et al. Phase I/II studies of docetaxel (Taxotere) combined with estramustine in men with hormone-refractory prostate cancer. Semin Oncol 1999;26:28–33.

16. Savarese DM, Halabi S, Hars V, et al. Phase II study of docetaxel, estramustine, and low-dose hydrocortisone in men with hormone-refractory prostate cancer: a final report of CALGB 9780. Cancer and Leukemia Group B. J Clin Oncol 2001;19:2509–16.

17. Kreis W, Budman D. Daily oral estramustine and intermittent intravenous docetaxel (Taxotere) as chemotherapeutic treatment for metastatic, hormone-refractory prostate cancer. Semin Oncol 1999;26:34–8.

18. Petrylak DP, Macarthur RB, O'Connor J, et al. Phase I trial of docetaxel with estramustine in androgen-independent prostate cancer. J Clin Oncol 1999;17:958–67.

19. Galsky MD, Small EJ, Oh WK, et al. Multi-institutional randomized phase II trial of the epothilone B analog ixabepilone (BMS-247550) with or without estramustine phosphate in patients with progressive castrate metastatic prostate cancer. J Clin Oncol 2005;23:1439–46.

20. Hussain M, Tangen CM, Lara PN, Jr., et al. Ixabepilone (epothilone B analogue BMS-247550) is active in chemotherapy-naive patients with hormone-refractory prostate cancer: a Southwest Oncology Group trial S0111. J Clin Oncol 2005;23:8724–9.

21. Ferro MA, Gillatt D, Symes MO, Smith PJ. High-dose intravenous estrogen therapy in advanced prostatic carcinoma. Use of serum prostate-specific antigen to monitor response. Urology 1989;34:134–8.

22. Seidman AD, Scher HI, Petrylak D, Dershaw DD, Curley T. Estramustine and vinblastine: use of prostate specific antigen as a clinical trial end point for hormone refractory prostatic cancer. J Urol 1992;147:931–4.

23. Smith DC, Dunn RL, Strawderman MS, Pienta KJ. Change in serum prostate-specific antigen as a marker of response to cytotoxic therapy for hormone-refractory prostate cancer. J Clin Oncol 1998;16:1835–43.

24. Vollmer RT, Dawson NA, Vogelzang NJ. The dynamics of prostate specific antigen in hormone refractory prostate carcinoma: an analysis of cancer and leukemia group B study 9181 of megestrol acetate. Cancer 1998;83:1989–94.

25. Kelly WK, Scher HI, Mazumdar M, Vlamis V, Schwartz M, Fossa SD. Prostate-specific antigen as a measure of disease outcome in metastatic hormone-refractory prostate cancer. J Clin Oncol 1993;11:607–15.

26. Scher HI, Kelly WM, Zhang ZF, et al. Post-therapy serum prostate-specific antigen level and survival in patients with androgen-independent prostate cancer. J Natl Cancer Inst 1999;91:244–51.

27. Bubley GJ, Carducci M, Dahut W, et al. Eligibility and response guidelines for phase II clinical trials in androgen-independent prostate cancer: recommendations from the Prostate-Specific Antigen Working Group. J Clin Oncol 1999;17:3461–7.

28. Ratain MJ, Eisen T, Stadler WM, et al. Phase II placebo-controlled randomized discontinuation trial of sorafenib in patients with metastatic renal cell carcinoma. J Clin Oncol 2006;24:2505–12.

29. Escudier B, Eisen T, Stadler WM, et al. Sorafenib in advanced clear-cell renal-cell carcinoma. N Engl J Med 2007;356:125–34.

30. Nelson JB, Hedican SP, George DJ, et al. Identification of endothelin-1 in the pathophysiology of metastatic adenocarcinoma of the prostate. Nat Med 1995;1:944–9.

31. Yin JJ, Mohammad KS, Kakonen SM, et al. A causal role for endothelin-1 in the pathogenesis of osteoblastic bone metastases. Proc Natl Acad Sci U S A 2003;100:10954–9.

32. Pirtskhalaishvili G, Nelson JB. Endothelium-derived factors as paracrine mediators of prostate cancer progression. Prostate 2000;44:77–87.

33. Thakkar SG, Choueiri TK, Garcia JA. Endothelin receptor antagonists: rationale, clinical development, and role in prostate cancer therapeutics. Curr Oncol Rep 2006;8:108–13.

34. Carducci MA, Padley RJ, Breul J, et al. Effect of endothelin-A receptor blockade with atrasentan on tumor progression in men with hormone-refractory prostate cancer: a randomized, phase II, placebo-controlled trial. J Clin Oncol 2003;21:679–89.

35. Lipton A, Sleep DJ, Hulting SM, Isaacson JD, Allen AR. Benefit of atrasentan in men with hormone refractory prostate cancer metastatic to bone. J Clin Oncol 2004;22:4687.

36. Sleep DJ, Nelson JB, Petrylak DP, Isaacson JD, Carducci MA. Clinical benefit of atrasentan for men with metastatic hormone-refractory prostate cancer metastatic to bone. J Clin Oncol 2006;24:4630.

37. Scher HI, Halabi S, Tannock I, et al. Design and end points of clinical trials for patients with progressive prostate cancer and castrate levels of testosterone: recommendations of the Prostate Cancer Clinical Trials Working Group. J Clin Oncol 2008;26:1148–59.

38. Sternberg CN, Petrylak D, Witjes F, et al. Satraplatin (S) demonstrates significant clinical benefits for the treatment of patients with HRPC: results of a randomized phase III trial. J Clin Oncol 2007;25:abstract 5019.

39. Sartor A, Petrylak D, Witjes J, et al. Satraplatin in patients with advanced hormone-refractory prostate cancer (HRPC): overall survival (OS) results from the phase III satraplatin and prednisone against refractory cancer (SPARC) trial. J Clin Oncol 2008;20 Suppl:abstract 5003.

40. Biomarkers and surrogate endpoints: preferred definitions and conceptual framework. Clin Pharmacol Ther 2001;69:89–95.

41. Prentice RL. Surrogate endpoints in clinical trials: definition and operational criteria. Stat Med 1989;8:431–40.

42. Hussain M, Tangen CM, Higano C, et al. Absolute prostate-specific antigen value after androgen deprivation is a strong independent predictor of survival in new metastatic prostate cancer: data from Southwest Oncology Group Trial 9346 (INT-0162). J Clin Oncol 2006;24:3984–90.

43. Petrylak DP, Ankerst DP, Jiang CS, et al. Evaluation of prostate-specific antigen declines for surrogacy in patients treated on SWOG 99-16. J Natl Cancer Inst 2006;98:516–21.

44. Armstrong AJ, Garrett-Mayer E, Ou Yang YC, et al. Prostate-specific antigen and pain surrogacy analysis in metastatic hormone-refractory prostate cancer. J Clin Oncol 2007;25:3965–70.

45. Eisenberger M, Crawford E, McLeod D, Hussain M, Loehrer P, Blumenstein B. The prognostic significance of prostate specific antigen (PSA) in stage D2 prostate cancer (PC) interim evaluation of intergroup study 0105 (Meeting abstract). Proceedings of the 1995 ASCO Annual Meeting 1995;14:abstract 613.

46. Hussain M, Goldman B, Tangen C, Higano C, Petrylak D, Crawford E. Use of prostate-specific antigen progression (PSA-P) to predict overall survival (OS) in patients (pts) with metastatic prostate cancer (PC): data from S9346 and S9916. J Clin Oncol 2008;20 Suppl:abstract 5015.

47. Brown JE, Cook RJ, Major P, et al. Bone turnover markers as predictors of skeletal complications in prostate cancer, lung cancer, and other solid tumors. J Natl Cancer Inst 2005;97:59–69.

48. Coleman RE, Major P, Lipton A, et al. Predictive value of bone resorption and formation markers in cancer patients with bone metastases receiving the bisphosphonate zoledronic acid. J Clin Oncol 2005;23:4925–35.

49. Keller ET, Brown J. Prostate cancer bone metastases promote both osteolytic and osteoblastic activity. J Cell Biochem 2004;91:718–29.

50. Berruti A, Piovesan A, Torta M, et al. Biochemical evaluation of bone turnover in cancer patients with bone metastases: relationship with radiograph appearances and disease extension. Br J Cancer 1996;73:1581–7.

51. Vinholes J, Coleman R, Eastell R. Effects of bone metastases on bone metabolism: implications for diagnosis, imaging and assessment of response to cancer treatment. Cancer Treat Rev 1996;22:289–331.

52. Percival RC, Urwin GH, Harris S, et al. Biochemical and histological evidence that carcinoma of the prostate is associated with increased bone resorption. Eur J Surg Oncol 1987;13:41–9.

53. Zhang J, Dai J, Qi Y, et al. Osteoprotegerin inhibits prostate cancer-induced osteoclastogenesis and prevents prostate tumor growth in the bone. J Clin Invest 2001;107:1235–44.

54. Carlin BI, Andriole GL. The natural history, skeletal complications, and management of bone metastases in patients with prostate carcinoma. Cancer 2000;88:2989–94.

55. Karsenty G. Bone formation and factors affecting this process. Matrix Biol 2000;19:85–9.

56. Parfitt AM. The mechanism of coupling: a role for the vasculature. Bone 2000;26:319–23.

57. Boyce BF, Hughes DE, Wright KR, Xing L, Dai A. Recent advances in bone biology provide insight into the pathogenesis of bone diseases. Lab Invest 1999;79:83–94.

58. Pectasides D, Nikolaou M, Farmakis D, et al. Clinical value of bone remodelling markers in patients with bone metastases treated with zoledronic acid. Anticancer Res 2005;25:1457–63.

59. Vogelzang N, Nelson J, Schulman C, et al. Meta-analysis of clinical trials of atrasentan 10 mg in metastatic hormone-refractory prostate cancer. J Clin Oncol 2005;23:4563.

60. Carducci M, Nelson JB, Saad F, et al. Effects of atrasentan on disease progression and biological markers in men with metastatic hormone-refractory prostate cancer: phase 3 study. J Clin Oncol 2004;22:4508.

61. Lara PN, Jr., Stadler WM, Longmate J, et al. A randomized phase II trial of the matrix metalloproteinase inhibitor BMS-275291 in hormone-refractory prostate cancer patients with bone metastases. Clin Cancer Res 2006;12:1556–63.

62. Cristofanilli M, Budd GT, Ellis MJ, et al. Circulating tumor cells, disease progression, and survival in metastatic breast cancer. N Engl J Med 2004;351:781–91.

63. Hayes DF, Cristofanilli M, Budd GT, et al. Circulating tumor cells at each follow-up time point during therapy of metastatic breast cancer patients predict progression-free and overall survival. Clin Cancer Res 2006;12:4218–24.

64. Moreno JSD, Shaffer D, Montgomery B, et al. Multi-center study evaluating circulating tumor cells (CTCs) as a surrogate for survival in men treated for castration refractory prostate cancer (CRPC). J Clin Oncol. 2007 ASCO Annual Meeting Proceedings Part I. 2007;25(20 Suppl):5016.

Chapter 35
FDA Approval of Prostate Cancer Treatments

Yang-Min Ning, Ramzi N. Dagher, and Richard Pazdur

Abstract The United States Food and Drug Administration has approved more than ten drugs for the treatment of prostate cancer, which include hormonal, supportive, and cytotoxic agents. Although these drugs have remarkably improved the management of patients with the disease, new treatments are greatly needed for achieving better clinical outcomes. Regulatory evaluation of newer agents under development is highly challenging, especially for agents intended for patients with advanced metastatic disease resistant to castration and/or docetaxel. Substantial evidence of efficacy and safety must be demonstrated for an agent to receive marketing approval. The evidence must be based on adequate, well-designed, and well-conducted clinical trials that provide quantitative assessments of measured clinical benefits and risks of the agent. Although improvements in survival and/or patient-reported outcomes continue to be valid endpoints for approving new claims or agents, effective surrogates that can reliably measure and predict clinical benefit remain to be established for accelerating drug development for the disease. Furthermore, appropriate utilization of trial results is very important. Subgroup analysis and/or post-hoc analysis results are not acceptable for regulatory action in general. Productive collaboration between all stakeholders and the agency is one of the keys for successful development of prostate cancer treatments.

Keywords Drug approval • Drug development • Endpoints • FDA • Post-hoc analysis • Prostate cancer • Subgroup analysis • Surrogate endpoints • Survival

Introduction

Medical treatment of prostate cancer dates back to the well-known landmark findings in the 1940s that androgen deprivation, achieved through either orchiectomy or estrogen administration, can retard advanced prostate cancer and alleviate disease-related symptoms. From a regulatory perspective, effective modern drug management of prostate cancer began with the approval of leuprolide for palliative treatment of prostate cancer in 1985 [1]. Since then, more than ten drugs have been approved by the United States Food and Drug Administration (FDA) for the treatment of the disease. These drugs can be classified into three groups: hormonal agents, cytotoxic agents, and supportive agents. Currently, many agents are under development for the disease, especially for metastatic castration-resistant prostate cancer (CRPC).[1]

In this chapter, we will review the general FDA approval process for anticancer drugs, summarize the approved drugs for the treatment of prostate cancer with an emphasis on the drugs approved in the last decade, and discuss the current challenges in evaluating new drugs being developed.

---

[1]CRPC denotes the progressive recurrent disease setting of prostate cancer despite the low plasma levels of testosterone (<50 ng/dL) achieved by medical or surgical castration, a clinical phenomenon that is historically defined as androgen-independent or hormone-refractory prostate cancer. CRPC becomes well accepted now in that it is more conceptually appropriate than the other terms in reflecting the nature of the disease setting. Therefore, CRPC will be used in the review wherever a description of the disease setting is needed.

Y.-M. Ning (✉)
Office of Oncology Drug Products, The U.S. Food and Drug Administration, Silver Spring, MD, USA
e-mail: ningy@mail.nih.gov

W.D. Figg et al. (eds.), *Drug Management of Prostate Cancer*,
DOI 10.1007/978-1-60327-829-4_35, © Springer Science+Business Media, LLC 2010

General FDA Approval Process for Anticancer Drugs

In the United States, FDA regulates all commercial marketing claims of therapeutic products. Since the passage of the Federal Food and Drugs Act in 1906, the requirements for approval of a product have evolved with the enactment of several legislative initiatives. Substantial evidence of safety and efficacy must be demonstrated prior to drug approval [2, 3].

Anticancer drugs are reviewed by the Office of Oncology Drug Products (OODP) in the Center for Drug Evaluation and Research (http://www.fda.gov/cder/Offices/OODP). The OODP-regulated products include traditionally termed "drugs" and biologic anticancer products (antibodies and oligonucleotides). OODP is engaged in all stages of clinical development, from evaluating and advising on pre-submissions of an investigational new drug (IND) application, INDs, the design and conduct of trials oriented for a new drug application (NDA), and NDA submissions, to approval of anticancer drugs, following up on postmarketing commitments, assisting further postmarketing development, and monitoring safety of marketed drugs.

Experimental drugs must be developed under an IND application prior to marketing approval. Regulatory evaluation objectives vary with the stages of development. In early stages, mainly involving Phase 1 IND studies, evaluations focus on the completeness of preclinical evidence supporting the use of anticancer drugs in humans and the safety of the drugs for initiation of clinical studies. Clinical protocols are evaluated for their appropriateness based on preclinical information, study eligibility criteria, treatment plans and modifications, and proposed monitoring plans for the safety of study subjects. Major safety endpoints of a study include assessment of the study agent's tolerability and acute toxicity, dose-limiting toxicity, maximum tolerated dose, and determination of dosing schedules for further development.

Phase 2 studies are intended to evaluate antitumor activity of an agent in addition to gathering more safety information about the agent. In later stages of development, evaluations generally concentrate on the design and conduct of trials intended to support an NDA application. FDA evaluation will be provided to sponsors if they request end-of-phase 2 discussions of their development plans and/or special protocol assessments for protocols before the conduct of Phase 3 trials.

Substantial evidence of efficacy and safety must be demonstrated for an anticancer drug to receive FDA approval for an intended indication. The evidence must be based on adequate and well-controlled clinical trials that reliably provide quantitative assessments of measured clinical benefits and risks of study drugs [4]. To evaluate such evidence, the design of a trial will be considered in FDA review, which generally relates to the proposed study population, randomization and/or blinding, comparators, efficacy endpoints, and pre-specified and/or interim analysis plans. Selection of appropriate endpoints and prespecification of analysis plan should be discussed with the Agency prior to initiating the trial.

The accepted regulatory anticancer endpoints can be classified into three types: prolongation of life (overall survival, OS), symptom relief or quality of life improvement (i.e., pain reduction or other patient-reported outcomes), and established surrogate(s) for a longer life or a better life [5–9]. Historically, anticancer drugs were approved based on the response rate alone until the mid-1980s, when the Oncologic Drugs Advisory Committee (ODAC), a group of oncology experts that provide independent scientific advice based on reasoned application of oncologic science [10], recommended the use of an improvement in patient's survival and symptoms for determining clinical benefit. In 1992, use of a surrogate endpoint that can reasonably likely predict clinical benefit was introduced under Subpart H for accelerated approval (AA) [4] of new drugs for life-threatening diseases such as cancer [11, 12]. The drugs approved under AA require further studies to demonstrate clinical benefit. Moreover, established surrogates can also be used for regular approval of new anticancer drugs when they are considered to consistently predict clinical benefit in selected clinical settings [7].

To accelerate anticancer drug development, endpoints for different cancers have been discussed in the OODP-sponsored workshops held in collaboration with other stakeholders over the last 5 years. Some of the discussions have been subsequently presented to the ODAC meetings for cancer-specific regulatory advice. Acceptance of different surrogate endpoints varies with the types of cancer and/or the types of regulatory approval being considered. In prostate cancer, surrogates have not been established for their use in regulatory action (ODAC meeting in 2005 [http://www.fda.gov/oc/advisory]). Persuasive treatment effects of study drugs in evaluation for marketing approval must be based on prespecified statistical plans [13]. Post-hoc analyses and/or subgroup analyses do not scientifically support a claim, but rather justify initiating trials to verify the results of these analyses.

Approved Prostate Cancer Treatments

Hormonal Agents

The approved hormonal agents can be classified by their mechanisms of action into three groups: gonadotropin-releasing hormone (GnRH) agonists, GnRH antagonists, and androgen receptor (AR) antagonists. Leuprolide, a GnRH agonist, is the first hormonal agent that received FDA approval in 1985 for palliative treatment of advanced prostate cancer, presenting an effective alternative for orchiectomy or use of estrogens [1]. Since then, different GnRH agonists and different formulations or delivery systems for longer drug action (up to 12 months) have also been approved. Use of these agonists has generally replaced orchiectomy or estrogen to achieve castration. However, GnRH agonists are associated with an initial testosterone surge before suppression. Contemplated by generating total androgen blockage, AR antagonists were developed and approved in the late 1980s and 1990s. Unlike a GnRH agonist, a GnRH antagonist does not cause the early testosterone flare, but can suppress testosterone as effectively as a GnRH agonist. The first GnRH antagonist, abarelix, was approved in 2003.

Efficacy endpoints for hormonal products are different for GnRH agents and AR antagonists. For the approval of GnRH products, either agonists or antagonists, serum testosterone was used as an established surrogate for castration. Survival was also used for the initial approval of goserelin in the metastatic disease setting. Avoidance of orchiectomy within 4–12 weeks of treatment was used for the approval of abarelix. AR antagonists were approved for use in conjunction with medical or surgical castration. None were approved as monotherapy [1]. The approved hormonal products are summarized in Table 35.1. Details about the basis for their approvals can be found at drugs@FDA.

Table 35.1 FDA-approved hormonal agents for treatment of prostate cancer

Class	Product	Year of approval
GnRH agonist[a]	Leuprolide	1985
	Goserelin	1987
	Triptorelin	2001
	Histrelin	2004
GnRH antagonist	Abarelix	2003
AR antagonist	Flutamide	1989
	Bicalutamide	1995
	Nilutamide	1996

[a] Generic products and products with different formulations not included

Supportive Agents

Zoledronic acid, a bisphosphonate agent that was initially approved in 2001 for tumor-related hypercalcemia, received regular approval in 2002 for use in patients with cancer bone metastasis to reduce skeletal-related events (SRE) [14]. Patients with progressive prostate cancer who have received at least one hormonal therapy were included in the drug's approval evaluation. In addition, the drug was also studied in patients with other malignancies, including multiple myeloma and breast cancer. The efficacy endpoint in the trials was SREs, consisting of pathological fracture, radiation therapy to bone, surgery to bone, cord compression, and change in chemotherapy for bone pain (prostate cancer only). The efficacy endpoint was analyzed either as the proportion of patients with SRE or time to first SRE. In the prostate cancer study, efficacy analyses showed statistically significant reductions in skeletal morbidity in patients treated with the drug administered at 4 mg every 3–4 weeks for 12 months when compared with placebo-treated patients.

Cytotoxic Agents

Cytotoxic drugs that have been approved for treatment of advanced prostate cancer are estramustine, mitoxantrone, and docetaxel. Approval information is summarized in Table 35.2. Although other cytotoxic agents, including carboplatin, cyclophosphamide, and etoposide, are used by practicing oncologists to treat prostate cancer, these drugs are not approved for this indication.

Table 35.2 FDA-approved nonhormonal agents for treatment of prostate cancer

Drug	Year of approval	Approval type	Trial design	End point
Zoledronic acid	2001	Regular	RCT[a]	SRE[b]
Estramustine	1981	Regular	RCT	Response rate including stable disease
Mitoxantrone	1996	Regular	RCT	Response rate in pain reduction
Docetaxel	2004	Regular	RCT	Survival

[a]RCT denotes randomized clinical trial

[b]Skeletal-related events, including pathological fracture, radiation therapy or surgery to bone, cord compression, and change in chemotherapy for bone pain

Estramustine

Estramustine is a chemically conjugated antineoplastic agent that combines estradiol with nornitrogen mustard. FDA approved this drug for metastatic and/or progressive carcinoma of the prostate in 1981 [15]. Prior to estramustine, diethylstilbestrol (DES) was the primary drug for the treatment of advanced prostate cancer. The approval of estramustine was based on the results of randomized studies comparing estramustine with DES in small-sized populations that included both orchiectomized and nonorchiectomized patients. The key efficacy evaluation relied on the differences in the rate of disease progression or in the rate of no disease progression between the estramustine and DES arms. These efficacy endpoints considered stable disease as a component of the calculation of response rate. Stable disease is not acceptable now as an adequate assessment of a treatment effect. Because of the historical differences and the evolution of clinical trial practices and regulatory standards in the last 20 years, discussing the studies and results that led to the approval of estramustine is less meaningful for today's evaluation of prostate cancer drugs. The use of estramustine for prostate cancer appears to have been replaced by other agents.

Mitoxantrone

Mitoxantrone was approved in 1996 for palliative treatment of metastatic CRPC. This approval was based on the results of a randomized trial comparing mitoxantrone plus prednisone to prednisone alone in patients with symptomatic metastatic CRPC [16]. A total of 161 patients with tumor-related pain were randomized equally to each arm.

The primary endpoint was palliative response, defined as a two-point decrease in pain as assessed by a six-point pain scale completed by patients (or complete loss of pain if initially 1+) without an increase in analgesic medication and maintained for two consecutive evaluations at least 3 weeks apart, which was assessed based on McGill Pain Questionnaire (MPQ). Palliative response rate was 29% in patients who received the combination compared with 12% in patients receiving prednisone alone *(P* = 0.01). The duration of palliation was longer in patients receiving mitoxantrone (median 43 and 18 weeks; $P < 0.0001$, log-rank). Patients who were initially randomized to prednisone alone but had no response were allowed to receive mitoxantrone, and their response rate was 22%. Regarding the secondary endpoints, the key finding was that most responding patients had an improvement in quality-of-life scales and a decrease in serum prostate-specific antigen level. No difference in overall survival was found between the two arms. Nevertheless, the trial was not designed for detecting a survival difference. In addition, the drug safety profile was acceptable.

The endpoint for the mitoxantrone approval relied on the clinical benefit observed, although there was only a group (about 1/3) of patients who benefited from the combination treatment. More importantly, the approval helped change the previous views that prostate cancer was chemotherapy resistant. Furthermore, the pain control benefit was corroborated by the results of another similar but larger randomized trial of mitoxantrone in the same disease setting [17]. Despite the clinical benefit, the use of mitoxantrone in the patient population has diminished after the approval of docetaxel.

Docetaxel

In 2004, docetaxel was approved for use in combination with prednisone for the treatment of metastatic CRPC. This was based on the results of TAX327, a randomized, international trial designed to evaluate docetaxel for the treatment of metastatic CRPC [18, 19]. A total of 1,006 patients were randomized to one of three treatment arms: mitoxantrone + prednisone, weekly docetaxel + prednisone, or docetaxel once every 3 weeks (q3w) + prednisone.

The prespecified primary endpoint was overall survival. The treatment with docetaxel q3w + prednisone demonstrated a statistically significant survival advantage over the mitoxantrone control arm, with median survival times of 18.9 vs. 16.5 months, respectively, $P=0.0094$. In contrast, the weekly docetaxel arm did not show a statistically significant survival advantage over the control arm. Similarly, another randomized Phase 3 trial that compared docetaxel plus estramustine with mitoxantrone plus prednisone (SWOG 9916) also demonstrated a survival advantage of docetaxel over mitoxantrone, according to the published literature [20].

A recent reanalysis of survival benefit in TAX327, preformed 3.5 years after the initial analysis, showed that the survival advantage has persisted, with median survival times of 19.2 months in the docetaxel q3w arm when compared with 16.3 months in the control arm, $P=0.004$, further substantiating the drug's efficacy [21].

The secondary endpoints, including pain response rate and duration, PSA response rate and duration, tumor response, time to-pain progression, time-to-PSA progression, and time-to tumor progression, were not used in the approval decision-making [19]. They were considered as exploratory and not supportive of the indication as pursued, since their analysis plans were not prespecified for adjustment for multiplicity or their ordering. In addition, the data for their analyses were partially available at the time of evaluation.

Challenges in Approval of Prostate Cancer Treatments

Numerous agents for prostate cancer are currently under development. Some of them appear to be promising based on the evidence reported in recent oncology meetings. Like all other drugs, for a prostate cancer drug to receive regulatory approval, the results of adequate and well-conducted trials of the drug have to provide substantial evidence of efficacy and safety to assure effective clinical use in an intended population. In general, study drugs that have passed through the early phases of clinical development undergo intensive investigations for establishing their efficacy or clinical benefits. Nevertheless, their safety should always be a top concern during all phases of development. This could be exemplified by the recent termination of a Phase 3 trial of a study drug in combination with docetaxel in patients with CRPC because of a higher rate of sudden deaths in patients receiving the combination treatment [22].

Therefore, the following discussions will focus on both endpoints acceptable for demonstrating efficacy for prostate cancer treatments and appropriate utilization of exploratory analyses in support of a new claim for the disease.

As discussed earlier, the three types of endpoints, including prolongation of life, improvement in health-related quality of life, and established surrogate(s) likely for predicting either of them, are also applicable for evaluating efficacy of drugs/agents for prostate cancer. Clearly, overall survival and reliable patient-reported outcomes have been used for approving prostate cancer treatments. Several surrogate endpoints that are commonly used in early phase studies in prostate cancer, such as PSA response rate, prolongation of PSA doubling time, and time-to-tumor progression, have not been validated or accepted as evidence of efficacy for approving prostate cancer treatments.

The OODP held a public workshop in June 2004 to discuss various trial endpoints for the disease [23]. The relative advantages and disadvantages of various surrogate endpoints such as PSA response, bone scan-based progression, time to disease progression, and progression-free-survival were discussed in the different disease settings. No consensus was reached about these surrogates because of insufficient evidence about their prediction of clinical benefit. This was further discussed and confirmed in the ODAC meeting in March 2005. Overall survival remains the standard endpoint in the Phase 3 metastatic setting to confirm clinical benefit. Recently, the Prostate Cancer Clinical Trials Working Group has published its recommendations toward standardizing outcome measures, especially the surrogates, in evaluation of systemic treatment trials in patients with progressive CRPC, and encouraged incorporation of these recommendations into Phase 3 trials that assess overall survival to validate or refine the surrogates [24].

Recent retrospective analyses of the PSA data from studies TAX327 and SWOG9916 showed a good survival correlation of PSA declines of 30% or more at the first 3 months, with a hazard ratio of 0.50 ($P<0.001$) in TAX327 and a hazard ratio of 0.43 ($P<0.001$) in SWOG9916, respectively, when compared with those without the PSA declines [25, 26]. These analyses suggest that a 30% PSA decline 3 months after treatment initiation may serve as a useful surrogate for predicting clinical benefit for cytotoxic agents. The validation of this surrogate in prospective studies is required before it can be used for future trial design and regulatory action. Prospective validation of this surrogate has been considered in two randomized trials that use overall survival as the primary endpoint for evaluating two different targeted agents in combination with docetaxel in patients with metastatic CRPC [26]. If positive, the results of these studies may help establish the first surrogate in this disease setting.

Use of nonvalidated surrogate endpoints for trials intended to support an NDA should be avoided. Combining various nonvalidated surrogates with validated endpoints in a composite endpoint (e.g., progression-free survival that includes the assessment of disease progression by PSA, bone scan, soft tissue, symptoms, or death) complicates the interpretation of the composite endpoint [24, 27].

One common challenge is whether statistically underpowered analyses of secondary endpoints or results of post-hoc or subgroup analyses are acceptable as a basis for marketing approval when the primary endpoint of a trial is not satisfied as prespecified. These analyses should be viewed as exploratory or hypothesis-generating. These analyses cannot be viewed as definitive evidence of efficacy to support marketing approval of an intended indication. Statistically, no prespecified alpha level is generally reserved for conducting a formal analysis of the endpoints not prespecified in analysis plans. Thus, the "significant results" of such analyses may be produced by chance alone and do not necessarily signify true treatment differences [28].

Selection of appropriate endpoints that measure the clinical benefit of a treatment effect is a cornerstone for efficacy evaluation of prostate cancer treatments. Selected trial endpoints and general trial designs should be discussed with the FDA prior to conduct of trials to accelerate drug development. Clinical benefits suggested by exploratory analyses such as subgroup or post-hoc analyses do not necessarily represent substantial evidence of efficacy to support marketing approval, but rather to justify initiating prospective controlled trials to verify the exploratory findings.

Summary

For the last two decades, the FDA has approved more than ten drugs for treatment of prostate cancer, which include hormonal, supportive, and cytotoxic agents. Although these drugs have remarkably improved the management of patients with the disease, evaluation of newer agents under development is highly challenging, especially for agents intended for patients with advanced metastatic disease resistant to castration and/or docetaxel. Although improvements in survival and/or patient-reported outcomes continue to be valid endpoints for approving new claims or agents, effective surrogates that can reliably predict clinical benefit remain to be established for the disease. In addition to adequate conduct of well-designed clinical trials, appropriate utilization of trial results is also very important. Subgroup analysis and/or post-hoc analysis results are not acceptable for regulatory action in general. Productive collaboration between all stakeholders and the agency is one of the keys for accelerating the development of prostate cancer treatments.

Footnotes

The views expressed herein are the results of independent work and do not necessarily represent the views or findings of the US FDA or the US government.

The authors have no financial interests or relationships with the commercial sponsors of any products discussed or mentioned in the review.

References

1. Fourcroy J. Regulatory history of hormone therapy for prostate cancer. Mol Urol 1998; 2:215–220
2. Dagher RN, Pazdur R. The role of FDA in the regulation of anticancer drugs. Curr Cancer Ther Rev 2006; 2: 327–329

3. Roberts Jr. TG. Food and Drug administration role in oncology product development. In Cancer Chemotherapy and Biotherapy: Principles and Practice 4th edition, ed by Chabner BA and Longo DL. Philadelphia, PA, Lippincott Williams & Wilkins, 2006

4. 21 Code of Federal Regulations, Part 314

5. FDA Guidance for Industry: clinical trial endpoints for the approval of cancer drugs and biologics. May 2007; http://www.fda.gov/downloads/Drugs/GuidanceCompliance RegulatoryInformation/Guidances/ucm071590.pdf

6. Pazdur R. Endpoints for assessing drug activity in clinical trials. Oncologist 2008; 13: 19–21

7. Johnson JR, Willimas G, Pazdur R. End points and United States FDA approval of oncology drugs. J Clin Oncol 2003; 21: 1404–1411

8. Rock EP, Kenedy DL, Furness MH, et al. Patient-reported outcomes supporting anticancer product approvals. J Clin Oncol 2007; 25(32): 5094–5099

9. Williams G, Pazdur R, Temple R. Assessing tumor-related signs and symptpoms to support cancer drug approval. J Biopharm Stat 2004; 14: 5–21

10. Farrell AT, Papadouli I, Hori A, et al. The advisory process for anticancer drug regulation: a global perspective. Ann Oncol 2006; 17: 889–896

11. Dagher R, Johnson J, Willimas G, et al. Accelerated approval of oncology products: a decade of experience. JNCI 2004; 96: 1500–1509

12. Flemming TR. Surrogate endpoints and FDA's accelerated approval process. Health Aff 2005; 24: 67–78

13. International Conference on Harmonization of techiniqual requirements for registration of pharmaceuticals for human use. Part E9, Statistical principles for clinical trials. 1998

14. Ibrahim A, Scher N, Willimas G, et al. Approval summary for zoledronic acid for treatment of multiple myelopma and cancer bone metastases. Clin Cancer Res 2003; 9: 2392–2399

15. Benson Jr. RC, Murphy GP. Drug therapy of prostate cancer. Urology 1982; 19: 621–622

16. Tannock IF, Osaba D, Stockler MR, et al. Chemotherapy with mitoxantrone plus prednisone or prednisone alone for symptomatic hormone-resistant prostate cancer: a Canadian randomized trial with palliative end points. J Clin Oncol 1996; 14: 1756–1764

17. Kantoff PW, Halabi S, Conaway M, et al. Hydrocortisone with or without mitoxantrone in men with hormone-refractory prostate cancer: results of the CALGB 9182 study. J Clin Oncol 1999; 17: 2506–2513

18. Tannock IF, de Wit R, Berry WR, et al. Docetaxel plus prednisone or mitoxantrone plus prednisone for advanced prostate cancer. NEJM 2004; 351: 1502–1512

19. Dagher R, Li N, Abraham S, et al. Approval summary: docetaxel in combination with prednisone for the treatment of androgen-independent hormone-refractory prostate cancer. Clin Cancer Res 2004; 10: 8147–8151

20. Petrylak DP, Tangen CM, Hussain MH, et al. Docetaxel and estramustine compared with mitoxantrone and prednisone for advanced refractory prostate cancer. NEJM 2004; 351: 1513–1520

21. Berthold DR, Pond GR, Soban F, et al. Docetaxel plus prednisone or mitoxantrone plus prednisone for advanced prostate cancer: updated survival in the TAX 327 study. J Clin Oncol 2008; 26: 242–245

22. Vaishampayan U, Hussain M. Update in systemic therapy of prostate cance: improvement in quality and duration of life. Expert Rev 2008; 8: 269–281

23. FDA project on cancer drug approval endpoints: http://www. fda.gov/Drugs/DevelopmentApprovalProcess/Development Resources/CancerDrugs/ucm094586.htm

24. Scher HI, Halabi S, Tannock I, et al. Design and end points of clinical trials for patients with progressive prostate cancer and castrate levels of testosterone: recommendations of the prostate cancer clinical trials working group. J Clin Oncol 2008; 26: 1148–1159

25. Armstrong AJ, Garrett-Mayer E, Ou Yang YC, et al. Prostate-specific antigen and pain surrogacy analysis in metastatic hormone-refractory prostate cancer. J Clin Oncol 2007; 25: 3956–3970

26. Petrylak DP, Ankerst DP, Jiang CS et al. Evaluation of prostate-specific antigen declines for surrogacy in patients treated on SWOG 99-16. JNCI 2006; 98: 516–521

27. Panageas KS, Ben-Porat L, Dickler MN, et al. When you look matters: the effect of assessment schedule on progression-free survival. JNCI 2007; 99: 428–432

28. Wang R, Lagakos SW, Ware JH, et al. Statistics in medicine-reporting of subgroup analyses in clinical trials. NEJM 2007; 357(21): 2189–2194

Chapter 36
Applications of Proteomics in Prostate Cancer

Mitchell Gross, Edward Macrohon Nepomuceno, and David B. Agus

Abstract Prostate-specific antigen (PSA) is the most commonly used circulating protein biomarker, which guides the diagnosis and treatment of prostate cancer. However, limitations in sensitivity and specificity limit utility of PSA when used as a diagnostic marker in screening population or as a prognostic, theragnostic, or surrogate biomarker in patients with recurrent or advanced prostate cancer. Accordingly, there is a need to discover new biomarkers to improve diagnosis, risk stratification, and therapeutic monitoring in prostate cancer. Proteomics, as an emerging technology, offers great promise in providing the cancer research community with biomarkers to guide therapeutic decision-making. However, caution must be used as new biomarkers are discovered and subject to appropriate validation before they can be applied to mainstream clinical settings.

Keywords Proteomic · Mass spectrometry · Biomarker (diagnostic, prognostic, predictive, pharmacogenomic) · Theragnostic · Prostate-specific antigen · Immunohisto-chemistry

Introduction

Prostate cancer (CaP) results from alterations and deregulations in control of growth, motility, and survival. It is generally believed that a more complete and fundamental understanding of the processes, which are altered in cancer, can be uncovered at a molecular level and that this insight will lead to new, improved, and personalized treatment approaches.

Proteomics denotes the large scale identification and monitoring of proteins in biologic systems. A fundamental goal of proteomic research is to uncover the basic mechanisms and pathways that contribute to the process of transformation. Over the last few decades, proteomic technologies have been applied in an attempt to understand complex biologic processes including prostate cancer. In general, these approaches have not yet been successful at contributing fundamental insights into clinical disease. Most recently, technological advances have provided new and improved tools to allow unprecedented sensitivity, quantification, and completeness for proteomic analysis of complex biologic tissues. Moreover, the integration of proteomic with genomic and transcription profiling technologies provides an unprecedented complete and complex data set to understand the fundamental processes, which underlie the development and progression of prostate cancer and therapeutic response. We focus on the application of these technologies, which may fundamentally change the care of prostate cancer.

Cancer Biomarkers Overview

Biomarkers are quantifiable measurements, which can be used as indicators of an underlying biologic process [1]. For cancer biomarkers, in particular, there is a developing framework, which separates biomarkers according to potential utilities in terms of diagnostic, prognostic, predictive, and therapeutic monitoring (Table 36.1) [2, 3]. The promise of individualized therapy hinges on the use of predictive biomarkers to direct therapies in

D.B. Agus (✉)
USC Westside Prostate Cancer Center, Keck School of Medicine of USC, Beverly Hills, CA, USA
e-mail: agus@usc.edu

W.D. Figg et al. (eds.), *Drug Management of Prostate Cancer*,
DOI 10.1007/978-1-60327-829-4_36, © Springer Science+Business Media, LLC 2010

Table 36.1 Classification of cancer biomarkers

Diagnostic	Definitively establish the presence of cancer
Prognostic	Predict the probably outcome of cancer regardless of therapy; may be used to stratify patients for more aggressive therapy
Prediction/ theragnostic	Predict response to a specific therapy
Pharmacodynamic/ therapeutic monitoring	Determine whether a therapy is having the intended effect on the disease based on changes over time; "pharmacodynamic marker that therapy is affecting its intended target to produce the desired result"

Adapted from Table 1.1 [2]

specific patients. Predictive biomarkers represent a relatively new and increasingly important paradigm in oncology as molecular biomarkers are directly linked to cancer biology and molecular therapeutics. However, there are only a few examples of predictive biomarkers in oncology. Well-studied examples include amplification of the human epidermal growth factor-2 (HER2) oncogene and the utility of a HER2-directed antibody (trastuzumab), expression of the estrogen receptor protein with estrogen-inhibiting therapies in breast cancer, and the presence of the BCR-ABL oncogenic translocation and the activity of ABL-tyrosine kinase inhibitors in chronic myelogenous leukemia [4, 5]. More recently, some molecular characteristics have been identified, which function as predictive biomarkers in other cancers including the presence of epidermal growth factor receptor (EGFR) mutations with EGFR tyrosine kinase inhibitors in lung cancer and *KRAS* mutations with resistance to EGFR antibody in colon cancer [6, 7]. Multi-gene signatures have also been developed as predictive markers for patients with breast cancer [8]. Development of predictive biomarkers represents an important unmet need for prostate cancer.

For prostate and other cancers, currently used prognostic biomarkers are relatively coarsely defined clinico-pathologic variables such as clinical stage, histologic subtype, and performance status. The focus of much of the previous research efforts has been to develop tissue or blood-based prognostic biomarkers for prostate cancer. In some studies, there is a suggestion that these markers may add to standard prognostic biomarkers such as prostate-specific antigen (PSA), Gleason grade,

and tumor stage. However, most of these reports are limited to single cohorts and have not been validated in multi-institution studies. Further, many of these tissue or blood-based markers do not have direct relevance in treatment decision making (i.e., they are not predictive). Taken together, these considerations have prevented the routine application of protein-based biomarkers, other than PSA, from entering routine clinical practice.

Current Status of Tissue-Based Protein Biomarkers

Tissue-Based Diagnostic Markers

Classical histology (tissue morphology based hematoxylin and eosin staining) is the "gold standard" diagnostic biomarker used to differentiate cancer from normal tissue. Ultimately, histology depends on patterns and differential staining of proteins with eosin and nucleic acid with hematoxylin. Techniques to examine protein expression patterns in tissue based on immunohistochemistry (IHC) are well-established in anatomic pathology. A common use of IHC in prostate cancer is to confirm a diagnosis of CaP in small areas of atypical glands submitted in limited tissue samples obtained from routine prostate biopsy. Loss of a basal cell marker (p63 or high molecular weight cytokeratin) along with increased expression of a marker for dysplastic or cancerous epithelium (alpha-methylacyl-CoA racemase) is helpful to distinguish cancerous from normal acini [9]. Occasionally, IHC is used to confirm the tissue of origin in locally advanced or metastatic CaP [10]. Generally, metastatic prostate cancer expresses androgen receptor (AR), prostate acid phosphotase (PAP), and PSA.

Tissue-Based Prognostic Markers

The Gleason grading system provides important prognostic information in patients with prostate cancer and is commonly used (along with clinical stage and serum PSA) to guide initial therapeutic decisions for patients with prostate cancer [11–15]. Prognostic nomograms incorporating these and other clinical factors have been widely reported and used to predict progression-free interval following primary therapy with surgery or radiation [16].

There are a few reports describing the utility of gene expression studies as a prognostic biomarker in prostate cancer. Approaches based on gene expression analysis in fresh frozen tissue have shown preliminary evidence of producing prognostic information for patients with CaP [17–19]. These studies share a similar experimental approach in that microarrays are used to compare gene expression with pathologic variables in primary prostate cancer specimens. Perhaps due to small methodological variations and other technical limitations, no gene or protein prognostic marker was shared by these (and subsequent) studies. However, individual studies did contribute specific information about tissue-based prognostic markers. Lapointe et al. showed that expression of MUC1 and AZGP1 (zinc-α-2-glycoporotein) was associated with an increased and decreased risk of recurrence, respectively [17]. Similarly, True et al. identified increased protein expression of monoamine oxidase A (*MAOA*), and defender against death (DAD1) in higher grade prostate cancers [18]. Perhaps attributed to limitations in the immune reagents, quantization, and sample variability, none of these IHC-based markers are used in clinical practice to guide the care of patients with prostate cancer.

Other studies have explored potential utility for tissue-based prognostic markers with IHC based on putative roles and function derived from the preclinical and related studies (summarized in Table 36.2) [20]. Individually, these studies produce interesting insights into processes that contribute to the development and progression of prostate cancer. However, many studies are based on IHC-techniques, which are difficult to standardize or have not been validated in subsequent studies or with larger cohorts of unselected patients. More importantly, these prognostic markers have not been directly linked to treatment decision making (i.e., they are not predictive biomarkers). Therefore, most of these prognostic markers have not entered routine clinical practice.

Table 36.2 Examples of tissue-based prognostic protein biomarkers

Biomarker	Source	Technique	Comment	References
p27	Tissue	IHC	Cyclin-dependent kinase inhibitor involved with cell cycle arrest and apoptosis	[21, 22]
			Low levels of p27 expression associated with adverse prognosis in patients undergoing prostatectomy	
			In patients with positive margins, a low p27 is associated with a higher risk of recurrence	
			Levels at the time of prostate biopsy are associated with time to PSA failure	
Caveolin-1	Tissue, Serum	IHC Sandwich immunoassay	Structural protein involved in regulation of membrane trafficking, cell adhesion, and signaling	[23]
			High expression correlates with Gleason score, positive surgical margins, and lymph node involvement	
Androgen receptor (AR)	Tissue	IHC	High levels of AR expression in prostatectomy samples correlate with clinical stage, lymph node status, extracapsular extension, seminal vesicle invasion, and Gleason score	[24–26]
			High AR expression was predictive of higher probability of recurrence	
Estrogen receptor-β (ERβ)	Tissue	IHC	Expression may be lower in some high grade prostate cancer	[27, 28]
			High expression may be related to shorter progression free survival	
Ki-67	Tissue	IHC	Marker for cellular proliferation	[29–31]
			High expression correlates with decreased progression free survival in postradiation setting	

Current Status of Blood-Based Protein Biomarkers

Blood is a particularly attractive tissue to develop clinically important biomarkers, especially for patients with prostate cancer. The utility of tissue-based markers may be limited by the heterogeneity of prostate epithelial cells often mixed with normal glands and stroma. Especially for IHC-based techniques, heterogeneous expression patterns and difficulties in standardization present significant challenges to validating important biomarkers using these techniques. Further, direct access to cancer tissue is particularly limited in patients with prostate cancer as often the only tissue available for subsequent analysis are core biopsies obtained many years before development of more aggressive, metastatic disease. The promise of blood-based biomarkers addresses many of these limitations. Blood may be repeatedly sampled in many stages of the disease, and large collections of blood exist to perform biomarker discovery and validation experiments for diagnostic and prognostic studies. Relatively standardized collection and processing techniques applying to blood and blood-based markers may not be as liable and may be more robust than tissue-based studies.

Aside from PSA, other blood borne protein markers have been studied as diagnostic, prognostic, and predictive biomarkers in prostate cancer [32]. Some studies report that levels of human glandular kallikrein (hK2, a serine-protease related to PSA) or levels of antigen derived from prostate cancer nuclear matrix (early prostate cancer antigen-2, EPCA-2) may add to the diagnostic accuracy of serum PSA [29–31, 33, 34]. Other studies have focused on blood borne prognostic and predictive markers. Chromogranin A (CGA) and neuron-specific enolase (NSE) represent neuroendocrine proteins, which are expressed, at variable levels, in primary and metastatic prostate cancer deposits. Both markers are commonly elevated in the blood in recurrent prostate cancer and have shown to add independent prognostic information to models, which also incorporate PSA [35–38]. As metastatic involvement of bone is one of the most common clinical scenarios in patients with advanced prostate cancer, bone markers have been studied as markers that predict the development of metastatic disease. In a study that compared the accuracy of ten bone metabolism markers as diagnostic and predictive marker, osteoprotegerin (OPG) had high diagnostic and prognostic validity of all markers tested, and remained significant in multivariate models [39]. Total or bone-specific alkaline phosphatases are prognostic in advanced prostate cancer [40–42]. Other prognostic models for advanced CaP have shown that elevations in relatively nonspecific immune markers (such as lactate dehydrogenase C-reactive protein, or interleukin-6) are associated with poor outcomes [40–45].

PSA as an Example of a Widely Used Blood-Based Biomarker

PSA is an androgen-regulated secreted protein, which is expressed by both normal and malignant prostate epithelial cells and is widely used as a serum marker for prostate cancer [46]. As a diagnostic marker, PSA elevation ($\geq$4 ng/mL) is a relatively sensitive (~80–90%) biomarker [47–49]. However, as PSA is also produced by noncancerous prostate epithelium and levels can be elevated by benign prostate hypertrophy, prostate inflammation, and other factors, PSA as a diagnostic biomarker lacks specificity [46]. Depending on population age and other risk factors, occult prostate cancers may be found in approximately 25% of patients with normal PSA levels ($\leq$4 ng/mL) [50]. Insights into the normal biology of PSA have led to studies that try to improve on the sensitivity and specificity of PSA as a diagnostic biomarker. In prostate cancer cells, disruption of the basement membrane allows the PSA molecule and its modified forms to be more readily released directly into the blood stream. With less exposure to the seminal proteases present in the lumen, fewer cleaved PSA products are available in the serum. Thus, the ratio of free PSA to total PSA (fPSA/tPSA) or "PSA index" is lower in patients with prostate cancer and can be used to distinguish cases with intermediate PSA levels (i.e., 4–10 ng/mL) [46]. Various truncated forms of the proPSA have also been suggested as potential biomarkers for patients with prostate cancer, which could increase the specificity of PSA testing [51].

PSA is also widely used as a prognostic biomarker for many stages and forms of prostate cancer. At the time of diagnosis, many risk prediction models routinely identify pretherapy PSA level as an independent factor, which predicts progression free survival [11, 13–15]. Most, but not all, patients with recurrent CaP demonstrate elevated levels of PSA. For recurrent prostate cancer, PSA levels contribute to multivariable models to predict survival for castration-resistant prostate cancer (CRPC) [41, 42]. The most important use of PSA in recurrent prostate cancer is to monitor therapy response. As PSA is an androgen-regulated secreted protein, decreases in PSA levels are expected following androgen-deprivation therapy. Further, PSA kinetics and the extent of the PSA nadir are useful ways to monitor therapy response [52–54]. For most patients, a PSA elevation despite androgen-deprivation therapy is a harbinger of androgen-independent progression. For CRPC, changes in PSA levels, such as a confirmed PSA decline of 50% compared with baseline, are commonly incorporated into reports from HRPC therapeutic trials, based on standardized reporting guidelines [55]. Most recently, a 30% decrease in PSA in response to docetaxel-based first-line chemotherapy for CRPC has been shown to function as a surrogate for overall survival in this population [40].

Although PSA is a widely used diagnostic, prognostic, and activity marker for prostate cancer, a significant limitation remains such that changes in PSA levels cannot be used to predict therapy. Further, decreases of PSA in response to therapy remain as a yet not validated surrogate for overall survival in response to taxane-based chemotherapy.

Overview of Proteomic Technologies

Proteomics refers to the study of the total set of proteins present in a complex biologic tissue at a particular point in time. Depending on the experimental question, subproteomes can be defined to include the sets of all proteins expressed in an organism, tissue (blood or prostate), or isolated cells. Subproteomes can also be defined based on protein location (cytoplasmic, nuclear, secreted), function (tyrosine kinases), and modifications (phosphorylation, glycosylation). Advancements in the technology of mass spectrometry are providing a method of high-throughput protein identification and quantification to present a complete representation of protein expression from many types of samples. As with other emerging technologies, attention must be paid to method development as small differences in technique may produce large differences in results. In general, the proteomic methods can be divided

into four main steps: sample preparation, protein separation, protein identification, and quantification.

Sample Preparation

Sample preparation is one of the most important, and often most overlooked, part of any proteomic experiment. The choice of tissue to be analyzed is the first critical decision point in any such study. Analysis may focus on an individual cell type, tumor tissue, or the whole organism. Focus on a pure cell population may be important for experimental purposes, but complex isolation techniques may limit the applicability of the results to clinical laboratories. Studies that begin with minimally processed tissues, such as tumor samples, may have to overcome noninformative levels of normal proteins to detect small changes in important proteins in a subset of critical cells. Blood may be a particularly useful protein-rich tissue to be analyzed as it continuously samples all tissues in the body.

Protein stability is also an important consideration. Some proteins are inherently stable and may remain unchanged at ambient temperatures for long periods of time, while other proteins, and in particular posttranslational modifications, are particularly labile [56]. The action of proteases and other enzymes present in biologic tissue may also obscure important biologic variations in protein content. Sample preparation protocols most balance a need to maintain and preserve protein complexity with an understanding of practical considerations and potential clinical utility. For example, the semi-standardized collection and processing of blood into plasma may preserve protein content because EDTA-mediated inhibition of proteases [57]. However, more detailed proteomic investigations are starting to show that relatively minor variations in variables such as "clot time," "storage temperature," and number of "freeze thaw cycles" may produce important differences in protein content [58, 59].

Protein/Peptide Separation

One of the primary challenges in analyzing any proteomic experiment is the vast range of protein concentrations found in biologic systems. Proteins comprise both the relatively invariant structural elements in cells and tissues as well as highly variable and liable elements, which direct major cellular processes. The problem presented by the range of protein concentrations found in biologic tissue is best demonstrated in blood (plasma). Concentrations for blood-resident proteins range from ~50 g/L for albumin down to ~10^{-8}–10^{-9} g/L for many cytokines and peptide hormones; a concentration range that spans about ten orders of magnitude [60]. Unfortunately, the resolving power of most mass spectrometers only spans about 4–5 orders of magnitude. Therefore, in the absence of any fractionation, the ability to detect and quantify proteins of mid to lower levels of abundance is severely limited by high-abundant and relatively noninformative proteins.

A variety of approaches have been developed to address the problem of sample fractionation for proteomic analysis. For many years, two-dimensional gel chromatography, which separates proteins based on electrical charge and size, has commonly been used in front of proteomic analysis [61]. More recently, liquid chromatography (LC) has become a standard method for proteomic separation. LC-based separation protocols are appealing as they effectively subfractionate a complex sample into a series of much simpler samples, which are sequentially presented to the mass spectrometer. LC is also convenient as it can be used in line with many mass spectrometers. A somewhat standardized approach includes a proteolysis step, with trypsin, to produce protein fragments (peptides) within a relatively narrow size range (typically ~10 amino acids or about 1,000–2,000 Da). Depending on the goals of the experiment, LC-MS protocols may be optimized to focus proteomic analysis on the sub-proteomes of specific biologic interest. For unbiased proteomics-based biomarker discovery (short gun proteomics), the LC-MS setup has commonly been used as it can produce the most complete representation of clinical tissues to date [62, 63].

Another approach to address the problem of dynamic range and sensitivity is to use affinity methods to enrich, or deplete, samples (prior to trypsinization) to focus proteomic techniques on the most informative proteins. Immuno-affinity columns have been developed to deplete high-abundance protein from blood including albumin, immunoglobin, and transferring [64–66]. Conversely, affinity methods may be used to enrich samples for proteins of interest. For example, phosphorylated species can be isolated

based on their differential affinity to immobilized metal species and phosphotyrosine-specific antibodies [67, 68]. Similar work was recently developed for isolating and analyzing glycosylated species in blood [69]. Protein glycosylation, and in particular N-linked glycosylation, is prevalent in proteins destined for extra cellular environments. These include proteins on the extracellular side of the plasma membrane, secreted proteins, and proteins contained in body fluids (e.g., blood serum). Therefore, many commonly used cancer biomarkers (including PSA, CA-125, and alphafetoprotein) are glycosylated.

Protein Identification and Protein Quantification

Mass spectrometry (MS) characterizes the composition of a sample mixture based on the mass to charge ratio (m/z ratio). MS instruments require an ionizing source to produce gas-phase ions. The two common forms of ionization are as follows: electrospray ionization (ESI), in which peptides in a liquid sample are converted to gas-phase ions through high voltage, heat, and drying gases; and matrix-assisted laser desorption ionization (MALDI), in which ions are produced when peptides are mixed with a photoreactive matrix followed by laser irradiation [70, 71]. An advantage of ESI is that the input may include direct infection of the efflux from a liquid chromatographic prefractionation step (such as LC) and is amenable to high-throughput configurations. Disadvantages of MALDI are that neither it generally may not be used "in-line" with other fractionation techniques nor can the process be easily automated for high-throughput applications. Following ionization, peptide/proteins are analyzed to determine their m/z ratio. Common detection techniques are time-of-flight (TOF), which measures the time it takes for the ion to travel from the ion source to the detector plate, (more massive objects take more time) and Fourier transform-ion cyclotron resonance (FT-ICR), which analyzes the electrical field produced by ions orbiting in a strong magnetic field (more massive ions circulate more slowly) [72]. MS-based technologic advances are such that the most accurate instruments commonly used in proteomic experiments (FT-ICR) can determine the mass of a typical peptide (~1,000 Da) to within 0.001 Da (~10 parts per million) [71]. Many mass spectrometers are capable of "tandem operation" (MS/MS). In this configuration, parent ions can be selected and concentrated by a magnetic quadropole and then fragmented to produce daughter ions; the pattern and weights of these ions can be used to deduce the precise amino acid sequence of the parent peptide [73]. Together, the accuracy and resolution provided by modern MS instruments allows for an increasingly complete identification of all proteins present in biologic samples [74].

Protein quantification presents another important challenge for MS-based techniques. In most configurations, the size of the m/z peak is qualitatively related to the abundance of the underlying peptide. However, experimental variability including that produced by prefractionation methods, the abundance of other ion species, among others precludes a precise measurement of quantization from standard MS data. In many experimental situations, one is most interested in comparing protein levels between samples, rather than deriving an absolute quantity. Isotope and dye-based labeling protocols have been developed to allow pairwise comparison of biologic samples [75, 76].

Selective reaction monitoring and multiple reaction monitoring (SRM/MRM) is a technique for "targeted proteomics," which combines protein identification and quantization into a single high-throughput experimental configuration. A fundamental principle of MS instruments is that precision improves with the square root of the number of ions measured [77]. Triple-quadrapole MS instruments allow for selective retention of ions within a precise mass/charge window for subsequent analysis. In this way, the accuracy of measurement is greatly enhanced. In all analytical chemistry, simultaneous detection and quantization of an internal standard along with the analyte of interest is desirable as a way to standardize for systematic measurement errors. The mass accuracy of triple-quadrapole MS instruments allows for the addition of known amounts of chemically similar peptides with different mass/charge ration via the incorporation of unnatural isotope abundances. These isotopically labeled peptides can be used as internal standards to provide accurate quantization of samples and to account for nonstochastic differentiation in sample preparation and ionization efficiencies. Lastly, SRM can unambiguously identify target peptides based on fragmentation signatures. Therefore, SRM utilizes the capability of triple-quadrapole mass spectrometers to select for ions of interest (to improve precision) with the addition of isotope-substituted monitor peptides (for quantization) and CID (for identification). In this way, SRM assays can be designed to monitor analyte peptides with high precision (CV<10%). SRM assays (ion selection and monitor peptides) are often combined to produce multiple reaction monitoring and provide accurate measurements of abundances of multiple proteins. Recently, several groups have reported the limit of detection for proteins (including PSA) spiked into human serum in the 1–10 ng/mL range by combining prefractionation with MRM [78, 79].

Examples of Proteomic Applications for Prostate Cancer

A number of groups have reported preliminary results, which seek to apply serum proteomic analysis to develop an improved screening test for prostate and other cancers [80–82]. These studies applied a low-resolution form of whole protein serum profiling based on surface-enhanced laser desorption ionization time-of-flight (SELDI-TOF) spectrometry. SELDI is a modification of MALDI, which seeks to streamline protein separation with analysis in a high-throughput system. Analytes are placed directly onto metal plates (chips) coated with substances to mimic the separation properties of substances such as ion-exchange resins, hydrophobic separation (C4, C18), immobilized metal surfaces, among others. The chips are then washed (to remove unbound material), matrix is added, and bound proteins are analyzed by TOF MS. There have been some reported successes with this technology in proteomic analysis of blood, including a use in prostate cancer diagnostics [82]. Significant efforts have been undertaken in an attempt to standardize and validate SELDI-TOF for early cancer diagnosis [83]. However, the SELDI-TOF techniques utilized are limited by the small dynamic range, poor mass range (proteins only approximately 5–30 kDa), and poor ability to perform protein identification and validation. In addition, reanalysis of some of the original SELDI-TOF data revealed the presence of significant nonbiologic experimental bias between subjects with cancer and controls, which may have been the result of differences in specimen handling before MS data was collected [84]. Overall, these and other issues have significantly decreased the enthusiasm for utilizing SELDI-TOF to develop prostate cancer biomarkers.

A very active area for the application of proteomics for the study of prostate cancer involves target identification toward discovering prognostic and predictive biomarkers. Proteins secreted or shed by prostate cancer cells grown in tissue culture may reflect circulating markers, which directly reflect the status of prostate cancer cells in patients [85]. Proteomic techniques can be used to identify and quantify these proteins in the hopes discovering clinically useful biomarkers for patient care. In a study utilizing quantitative proteomics based on an isotope-coded affinity tag (ICAT) technique, Martin et al. identified over 600 proteins present in the conditioned media from the LNCaP human prostate cancer cell line [86]. Interestingly, most of the proteins identified in the media were predicted to be present inside the cells (cytoplasmic or nuclear), based on annotated databases, while only about a quarter of proteins were predicted to be expressed in compartments directly exposed to the extracellular space (as cell-bound or secreted proteins). The study also identified about 50 novel proteins regulated by androgen-stimulation. Recently, we reported the results utilizing SELDI-TOF to study androgen-regulated proteins utilizing a similar experimental design. In this study, we identified beta-2-microglobulin (β2M) as an androgen-regulated secreted protein, which is highly expressed in prostate cancer cells and tissues, and is elevated in the serum of prostate cancer patients [87]. Discovery efforts have applied proteomic technologies to study important therapeutic targets include the androgen receptor and microtubules [88, 89]. More generally, proteomic techniques are well suited to study specific cancer phenotypes such as therapy resistance. A particularly promising approach is to combine proteomic and genomic analyses to understand entire biologic networks, which may underlie a disease-specific phenotype [90, 91].

Summary

Technologic development and maturation of proteomic technologies is poised to give clinical sciences important analytical tools to study human disease. There is a high likelihood that a combination of protein identification and quantization tools, including IHC and MS-based technologies to provide individualized information, reflect the molecular characterization of cancer. As these assays are developed, attention must be focused on issues such as reproducibility and validation to ensure the results of these studies will have maximal applicability to patient care. The success of these approaches may lead to better diagnostic, prognostic, and predictive markers to direct therapy for prostate cancer.

References

1. Biomarkers Definitions Working Group. Biomarkers and surrogate endpoints: preferred definitions and conceptual framework. Clin Pharmacol Ther 2001;69(3):89–95.
2. Patlak M, Nass SJ, National Cancer Policy Forum (U.S.), United States. Department of Health and Human Services. Developing biomarker-based tools for cancer screening, diagnosis, and treatment: the state of the science, evaluation, implementation, and economics: workshop summary. Washington, D.C.: National Academies Press; 2006.
3. Sawyers CL. The cancer biomarker problem. Nature 2008;452(7187):548–52.
4. Yeon CH, Pegram MD. Anti-erbB-2 antibody trastuzumab in the treatment of HER2-amplified breast cancer. Invest New Drugs 2005;23(5):391–409.
5. Sawyers CL. Rational therapeutic intervention in cancer: kinases as drug targets. Curr Opin Genet Dev 2002;12(1):111–5.
6. Amado RG, Wolf M, Peeters M, et al. Wild-type KRAS is required for panitumumab efficacy in patients with metastatic colorectal cancer. J Clin Oncol 2008;26(10):1626–34.
7. Sequist LV, Bell DW, Lynch TJ, Haber DA. Molecular predictors of response to epidermal growth factor receptor antagonists in non-small-cell lung cancer. J Clin Oncol 2007;25(5):587–95.
8. Morris SR, Carey LA. Gene expression profiling in breast cancer. Curr Opin Oncol 2007;19(6):547–51.
9. Epstein JI. Diagnosis and reporting of limited adenocarcinoma of the prostate on needle biopsy. Mod Pathol 2004;17(3):307–15.
10. Varadhachary GR, Abbruzzese JL, Lenzi R. Diagnostic strategies for unknown primary cancer. Cancer 2004;100(9):1776–85.
11. Bianco FJ Jr, Wood DP Jr, Cher ML, Powell IJ, Souza JW, Pontes JE. Ten-year survival after radical prostatectomy: specimen Gleason score is the predictor in organ-confined prostate cancer. Clin Prostate Cancer 2003;1(4):242–7.
12. Epstein JI, Allsbrook WC Jr, Amin MB, Egevad LL. Update on the Gleason grading system for prostate cancer: results of an international consensus conference of urologic pathologists. Adv Anat Pathol 2006;13(1):57–9.
13. Graefen M, Karakiewicz PI, Cagiannos I, et al. Validation study of the accuracy of a postoperative nomogram for recurrence after radical prostatectomy for localized prostate cancer. J Clin Oncol 2002;20(4):951–6.

14. Kattan MW, Zelefsky MJ, Kupelian PA, Scardino PT, Fuks Z, Leibel SA. Pretreatment nomogram for predicting the outcome of three-dimensional conformal radiotherapy in prostate cancer. J Clin Oncol 2000;18(19):3352–9.

15. Stephenson AJ, Scardino PT, Eastham JA, et al. Preoperative nomogram predicting the 10-year probability of prostate cancer recurrence after radical prostatectomy. J Natl Cancer Inst 2006;98(10):715–7.

16. Karakiewicz PI, Hutterer GC. Predictive models and prostate cancer. Nat Clin Pract 2008;5(2):82–92.

17. Lapointe J, Li C, Higgins JP, et al. Gene expression profiling identifies clinically relevant subtypes of prostate cancer. Proc Natl Acad Sci U S A 2004;101(3):811–6.

18. True L, Coleman I, Hawley S, et al. A molecular correlate to the Gleason grading system for prostate adenocarcinoma. Proc Natl Acad Sci U S A 2006;103(29):10991–6.

19. Singh D, Febbo PG, Ross K, et al. Gene expression correlates of clinical prostate cancer behavior. Cancer Cell 2002;1(2):203–9.

20. Chin JL, Reiter RE. Molecular markers and prostate cancer prognosis. Clin Prostate Cancer 2004;3(3):157–64.

21. Freedland SJ, deGregorio F, Sacoolidge JC, et al. Preoperative p27 status is an independent predictor of prostate specific antigen failure following radical prostatectomy. J Urol 2003;169(4):1325–30.

22. Yang RM, Naitoh J, Murphy M, et al. Low p27 expression predicts poor disease-free survival in patients with prostate cancer. J Urol 1998;159(3):941–5.

23. Mouraviev V, Li L, Tahir SA, et al. The role of caveolin-1 in androgen insensitive prostate cancer. J Urol 2002;168 (4 Pt 1):1589–96.

24. Cordon-Cardo C, Kotsianti A, Verbel DA, et al. Improved prediction of prostate cancer recurrence through systems pathology. J Clin Invest 2007;117(7):1876–83.

25. Li R, Wheeler T, Dai H, Frolov A, Thompson T, Ayala G. High level of androgen receptor is associated with aggressive clinicopathologic features and decreased biochemical recurrence-free survival in prostate: cancer patients treated with radical prostatectomy. Am J Surg Pathol 2004;28(7): 928–34.

26. Wako K, Kawasaki T, Yamana K, et al. Expression of androgen receptor through androgen-converting enzymes is associated with biological aggressiveness in prostate cancer. J Clin Pathol 2008;4:448–54.

27. Torlakovic E, Lilleby W, Berner A, et al. Differential expression of steroid receptors in prostate tissues before and after radiation therapy for prostatic adenocarcinoma. Int J Cancer 2005;117(3):381–6.

28. Torlakovic E, Lilleby W, Torlakovic G, Fossa SD, Chibbar R. Prostate carcinoma expression of estrogen receptor-beta as detected by PPG5/10 antibody has positive association with primary Gleason grade and Gleason score. Hum Pathol 2002;33(6):646–51.

29. Bettencourt MC, Bauer JJ, Sesterhenn IA, Mostofi FK, McLeod DG, Moul JW. Ki-67 expression is a prognostic marker of prostate cancer recurrence after radical prostatectomy. J Urol 1996;156(3):1064–8.

30. Cowen D, Troncoso P, Khoo VS, et al. Ki-67 staining is an independent correlate of biochemical failure in prostate cancer treated with radiotherapy. Clin Cancer Res 2002; 8(5):1148–54.

31. Halvorsen OJ, Haukaas S, Hoisaeter PA, Akslen LA. Maximum Ki-67 staining in prostate cancer provides independent prognostic information after radical prostatectomy. Anticancer Res 2001;21(6A):4071–6.

32. Bok RA, Small EJ. Bloodborne biomolecular markers in prostate cancer development and progression. Nat Rev Cancer 2002;2(12):918–26.

33. Leman ES, Cannon GW, Trock BJ, et al. EPCA-2: a highly specific serum marker for prostate cancer. Urology 2007;69(4):714–20.

34. Nam R, Diamandis E, Toi A, et al. Serum human glandular Kallikrein-2 protease levels predict the presence of prostate cancer among men with elevated prostate-specific antigen. J Clin Oncol 2000;18(5):1036.

35. Berruti A, Dogliotti L, Mosca A, et al. Circulating neuroendocrine markers in patients with prostate carcinoma. Cancer 2000;88(11):2590–7.

36. Berruti A, Mosca A, Tucci M, et al. Independent prognostic role of circulating chromogranin A in prostate cancer patients with hormone-refractory disease. Endocrine Relat Cancer 2005;12(1):109–17

37. Culine S, El Demery M, Lamy PJ, Iborra F, Avances C, Pinguet F. Docetaxel and cisplatin in patients with metastatic androgen independent prostate cancer and circulating neuroendocrine markers. J Urol 2007;178(3 Pt 1):844–8; discussion 848.

38. Taplin ME, Bubley GJ, Ko YJ, et al. Selection for androgen receptor mutations in prostate cancers treated with androgen antagonist. Cancer Res 1999;59(11):2511–5.

39. Jung K, Lein M, Stephan C, et al. Comparison of 10 serum bone turnover markers in prostate carcinoma patients with bone metastatic spread: diagnostic and prognostic implications. Int J Cancer 2004;111(5):783–91

40. Armstrong AJ, Garrett-Mayer E, Ou Yang YC, et al. Prostate-specific antigen and pain surrogacy analysis in metastatic hormone-refractory prostate cancer. J Clin Oncol 2007;25(25):3965–70.

41. Armstrong AJ, Garrett-Mayer ES, Yang YC, de Wit R, Tannock IF, Eisenberger M. A Contemporary Prognostic Nomogram for Men with Hormone-Refractory Metastatic Prostate Cancer: a TAX327 Study Analysis. Clin Cancer Res 2007;13(21):6396–403.

42. Halabi S, Small EJ, Kantoff PW, et al. Prognostic model for predicting survival in men with hormone-refractory metastatic prostate cancer. J Clin Oncol 2003;21(7):1232–7.

43. George DJ, Halabi S, Shepard TF, et al. Prognostic significance of plasma vascular endothelial growth factor levels in patients with hormone-refractory prostate cancer treated on Cancer and Leukemia Group B 9480. Clin Cancer Res 2001;7(7):1932–6.

44. Graff J, Lalani AS, Lee S, et al. C-reactive protein as a prognostic marker for men with androgen-independent prostate cancer (AIPC): results from the ASCENT trial. Proc Am Soc Clin Oncol 2007;25(18 S):abstract 5074.

45. Humphrey PA, Halabi S, Picus J, et al. Prognostic significance of plasma scatter factor/hepatocyte growth factor levels in patients with metastatic hormone-refractory prostate cancer: results from cancer and leukemia group B 150005/9480. Clin Genitourin Cancer 2006;4(4):269–74

46. Balk SP, Ko YJ, Bubley GJ. Biology of prostate-specific antigen. J Clin Oncol 2003;21(2):383–91.

47. Catalona WJ, Smith DS, Ratliff TL, et al. Measurement of prostate-specific antigen in serum as a screening test for prostate cancer. N Engl J Med 1991;324(17):1156–61.

48. Labrie F, Dupont A, Suburu R, et al. Serum prostate specific antigen as pre-screening test for prostate cancer. J Urol 1992;147(3 Pt 2):846–51; discussion 851–2.

49. Brawer MK, Chetner MP, Beatie J, Buchner DM, Vessella RL, Lange PH. Screening for prostatic carcinoma with prostate specific antigen. J Urol 1992;147(3 Pt 2):841–5.

50. Thompson IM, Pauler DK, Goodman PJ, et al. Prevalence of prostate cancer among men with a prostate-specific antigen level < or =4.0 ng per milliliter. N Engl J Med 2004;350(22): 2239–46.

51. Mikolajczyk SD, Marker KM, Millar LS, et al. A truncated precursor form of prostate-specific antigen is a more specific serum marker of prostate cancer. Cancer Res 2001;61(18):6958–63.

52. D'Amico AV, Moul JW, Carroll PR, et al. Intermediate end point for prostate cancer-specific mortality following salvage hormonal therapy for prostate-specific antigen failure. J Natl Cancer Inst 2004;96(7):509–15.

53. Kwak C, Jeong SJ, Park MS, Lee E, Lee SE. Prognostic significance of the nadir prostate specific antigen level after hormone therapy for prostate cancer. J Urol 2002;168(3): 995–1000.

54. Slovin SF, Wilton AS, Heller G, Scher HI. Time to detectable metastatic disease in patients with rising prostate-specific antigen values following surgery or radiation therapy. Clin Cancer Res 2005;11(24 Pt 1):8669–73.

55. Bubley GJ, Carducci M, Dahut W, et al. Eligibility and response guidelines for phase II clinical trials in androgen-independent prostate cancer: recommendations from the Prostate-Specific Antigen Working Group. J Clin Oncol 1999;17(11):3461–7.

56. Boyanton BL Jr, Blick KE. Stability studies of twenty-four analytes in human plasma and serum. Clin Chem 2002;48(12): 2242–7.

57. Evans MJ, Livesey JH, Ellis MJ, Yandle TG. Effect of anti-coagulants and storage temperatures on stability of plasma and serum hormones. Clin Biochem 2001;34(2):107–12.

58. Banks RE, Stanley AJ, Cairns DA, et al. Influences of blood sample processing on low-molecular-weight proteome identified by surface-enhanced laser desorption/ionization mass spectrometry. Clin Chem 2005;51(9):1637–49.

59. Hsieh SY, Chen RK, Pan YH, Lee HL. Systematical evaluation of the effects of sample collection procedures on low-molecular-weight serum/plasma proteome profiling. Proteomics 2006;6(10):3189–98.

60. Anderson NL, Anderson NG. The human plasma proteome: history, character, and diagnostic prospects. Mol Cell Proteomics 2002;1(11):845–67.

61. Rabilloud T. Two-dimensional gel electrophoresis in proteomics: old, old fashioned, but it still climbs up the mountains. Proteomics 2002;2(1):3–10.

62. McDonald WH, Yates JR III. Shotgun proteomics: integrating technologies to answer biological questions. Curr Opin Mol Ther 2003;5(3):302–9.

63. Wu L, Han DK. Overcoming the dynamic range problem in mass spectrometry-based shotgun proteomics. Expert Rev Proteomics 2006;3(6):611–9.

64. Gong Y, Li X, Yang B, et al. Different immunoaffinity fractionation strategies to characterize the human plasma proteome. J Proteome Res 2006;5(6):1379–87.

65. Liu T, Qian WJ, Mottaz HM, et al. Evaluation of multiprotein immunoaffinity subtraction for plasma proteomics and candidate biomarker discovery using mass spectrometry. Mol Cell Proteomics 2006;5(11):2167–74.

66. Pieper R, Su Q, Gatlin CL, Huang ST, Anderson NL, Steiner S. Multi-component immunoaffinity subtraction chromatography: an innovative step towards a comprehensive survey of the human plasma proteome. Proteomics 2003;3(4):422–32.

67. Kalume DE, Molina H, Pandey A. Tackling the phosphoproteome: tools and strategies. Curr Opin Chem Biol 2003;7(1): 64–9.

68. Mann M, Jensen ON. Proteomic analysis of post-translational modifications. Nat Biotechnol 2003;21(3):255–61.

69. Zhang H, Yi EC, Li XJ, et al. High throughput quantitative analysis of serum proteins using glycopeptide capture and liquid chromatography mass spectrometry. Mol Cell Proteomics 2004;4(2):144–55.

70. Fenn JB, Mann M, Meng CK, Wong SF, Whitehouse CM. Electrospray ionization for mass spectrometry of large biomolecules. Science 1989;246(4926):64–71.

71. Karas M, Hillenkamp F. Laser desorption ionization of proteins with molecular masses exceeding 10,000 daltons. Anal Chem 1988;60(20):2299–301.

72. Katz JE, Mallick P, Agus DB. A perspective on protein profiling of blood. BJU Int 2005;96(4):477–82.

73. Aebersold R, Mann M. Mass spectrometry-based proteomics. Nature 2003;422(6928):198–207.

74. Luethy R, Kessner DE, Katz JE, et al. Precursor-ion mass re-estimation improves peptide identification on hybrid instruments. J Proteome Res 2008;7(9):4031–9

75. Tao WA, Aebersold R. Advances in quantitative proteomics via stable isotope tagging and mass spectrometry. Current Opin Biotechnol 2003;14(1):110–8.

76. Unlu M, Morgan ME, Minden JS. Difference gel electrophoresis: a single gel method for detecting changes in protein extracts. Electrophoresis 1997;18(11):2071–7.

77. MacCoss MJ, Toth MJ, Matthews DE. Evaluation and optimization of ion-current ratio measurements by selected-ion-monitoring mass spectrometry. Anal Chem 2001; 73(13):2976–84.

78. Keshishian H, Addona T, Burgess M, Kuhn E, Carr SA. Quantitative, multiplexed assays for low abundance proteins in plasma by targeted mass spectrometry and stable isotope dilution. Mol Cell Proteomics 2007;6(12):2212–29

79. Stahl-Zeng J, Lange V, Ossola R, et al. High sensitivity detection of plasma proteins by multiple reaction monitoring of N-glycosites. Mol Cell Proteomics 2007;6(10):1809–17.

80. Adam BL, Qu Y, Davis JW, et al. Serum protein fingerprinting coupled with a pattern-matching algorithm distinguishes prostate cancer from benign prostate hyperplasia and healthy men. Cancer Res 2002;62(13):3609–14.

81. Petricoin EF, Ardekani AM, Hitt BA, et al. Use of proteomic patterns in serum to identify ovarian cancer. Lancet 2002;359(9306):572–7.

82. Petricoin EF III, Ornstein DK, Paweletz CP, et al. Serum proteomic patterns for detection of prostate cancer. J Natl Cancer Inst 2002;94(20):1576–8.

83. Semmes OJ, Feng Z, Adam BL, et al. Evaluation of serum protein profiling by surface-enhanced laser desorption/ionization time-of-flight mass spectrometry for the detection of prostate cancer: I. Assessment of platform reproducibility. Clin Chem 2005;51(1):102–12.

84. Sorace JM, Zhan M. A data review and re-assessment of ovarian cancer serum proteomic profiling. BMC Bioinformatics 2003;4(1):24.

85. Sardana G, Marshall J, Diamandis EP. Discovery of candidate tumor markers for prostate cancer via proteomic analysis of cell culture-conditioned medium. Clin Chem 2007;53(3):429–37.

86. Martin DB, Gifford DR, Wright ME, et al. Quantitative proteomic analysis of proteins released by neoplastic prostate epithelium. Cancer Res 2004;64(1):347–55.

87. Gross M, Top I, Laux I, et al. Beta-2-microglobulin is an androgen-regulated secreted protein elevated in serum of patients with advanced prostate cancer. Clin Cancer Res 2007;13(7):1979–86.

88. Bhat KM, Setaluri V. Microtubule-associated proteins as targets in cancer chemotherapy. Clin Cancer Res 2007;13(10):2849–54.

89. Jasavala R, Martinez H, Thumar J, et al. Identification of putative androgen receptor interaction protein modules: cytoskeleton and endosomes modulate androgen receptor signaling in prostate cancer cells. Mol Cell Proteomics 2007;6(2):252–71.

90. Lin B, White JT, Lu W, et al. Evidence for the presence of disease-perturbed networks in prostate cancer cells by genomic and proteomic analyses: a systems approach to disease. Cancer Res 2005;65(8):3081–91.

91. Tu LC, Yan X, Hood L, Lin B. Proteomics analysis of the interactome of N-myc downstream regulated gene 1 and its interactions with the androgen response program in prostate cancer cells. Mol Cell Proteomics 2007;6(4):575–88.

Index

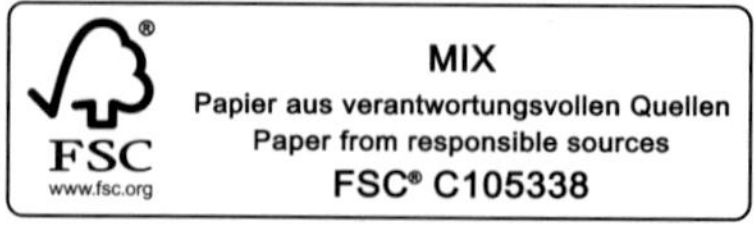

Printed by Books on Demand, Germany